Writing DNP Clinical Case Narratives

Demonstrating and Evaluating Competency in Comprehensive Care

Janice Smolowitz, EdD, DNP, ANP-BC, DCC, is Senior Associate Dean and Professor of Clinical Nursing and Co-Director of the Doctor of Nursing Practice (DNP) program at Columbia University School of Nursing (CUSN). She has been a member of the faculty since 1998. Dr. Smolowitz oversees the universal faculty practice plan at CUSN. In addition to her administrative responsibilities, Dr. Smolowitz teaches in the DNP program and chairs the DNP Portfolio and Comprehensive Examination Committees. She has been an invited member in several national committees, including the National Organization of Nurse Practitioner Faculty (NONPF) Practice Doctorate Nurse Practitioner Entry-Level Competencies (2006). She is a member of the American Board of Comprehensive Care, the Clinical Scholars Review, and the Parkinson's Study Group.

Dr. Smolowitz is a diplomate in comprehensive care and has practiced as an adult nurse practitioner for 18 years in primary adult health. For the past nine years she has practiced in the Movement Disorders Center of the Neurological Institute at Columbia University Medical Center. She participates in clinical research as both co-investigator and principal investigator.

Judy Honig, EdD, DNP, CPNP, is Associate Dean of Student Affairs, Associate Professor of Clinical Nursing, and Director of the DNP program at CUSN. She has been a faculty member since 1988. In addition to her administrative and practice responsibilities, Dr. Honig conducts research related to the health status of minority children, participates in curriculum development and clinical and classroom teaching, and is a member of the CUSN DNP Portfolio Committee.

Dr. Honig has served on several national committees pertaining to the DNP degree, including the American Association of Colleges of Nursing (AACN) Task Forces for the Practice Doctorate and DNP Essentials, NONPF's Clinical Leadership Committee, and National Association of Pediatric Nurse Practitioners' (NAPNAP) DNP Position Statement Committee.

Dr. Honig has practiced as a pediatric nurse practitioner for 25 years and has been an attending faculty nurse practitioner at Children's Hospital of New York since 1994. She has a faculty practice in an urban pediatric primary care facility and maintains a practice in behavioral pediatrics.

Courtney Reinisch, DNP, FNP-BC, DCC, is an Assistant Professor of Clinical Nursing at CUSN. She has been a member of the faculty since 2007. Dr. Reinisch teaches in the DNP and master's degree programs. She is a member of the CUSN DNP Portfolio Committee and Comprehensive Examination Committee, as well as the CUSN Curriculum Committee. Most recently, she has participated in the Emergency Nurses Association working group for validation methods for nurse practitioners in the emergency department setting. She presented her portfolio as the Terminal Scholarly Project at NONPF in 2008.

Dr. Reinisch is a diplomate in comprehensive care. She has practiced as a bilingual family nurse practitioner for 10 years, providing care to underserved populations in urban and suburban settings in both family practice and emergency medicine. She has implemented institutional practice changes through quality improvement initiatives, creating a model for an expanded advanced practice nursing role in the emergency department. This model is being replicated in emergency departments nationally.

Writing DNP Clinical Case Narratives

Demonstrating and Evaluating Competency in Comprehensive Care

Janice Smolowitz, EdD, DNP
Judy Honig, EdD, DNP
Courtney Reinisch, DNP

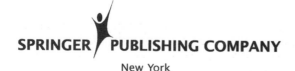

SPRINGER PUBLISHING COMPANY

New York

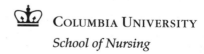

COLUMBIA UNIVERSITY
School of Nursing

Springer Publishing Company, LLC
11 West 42nd Street
New York, NY 10036
www.springerpub.com

Acquisitions Editor: Margaret Zuccarini
Production Editor: Gayle Lee
Project Manager: Becca Mosher, Publication Services, Inc.
Cover Design: Steve Pisano
Composition: Publication Services, Inc.

ISBN: 978-0-8261-0530-1
E-book ISBN: 978-0-8261-0531-8
10 11 12/ 5 4 3 2 1

The author and the publisher of this Work have made every effort to use sources believed to be reliable to provide information that is accurate and compatible with the standards generally accepted at the time of publication. Because medical science is continually advancing, our knowledge base continues to expand. Therefore, as new information becomes available, changes in procedures become necessary. We recommend that the reader always consult current research and specific institutional policies before performing any clinical procedure. The author and publisher shall not be liable for any special, consequential, or exemplary damages resulting, in whole or in part, from the readers' use of, or reliance on, the information contained in this book. The publisher has no responsibility for the persistence or accuracy of URLs for external or third-party Internet Web sites referred to in this publication and does not guarantee that any content on such Web sites is, or will remain, accurate or appropriate.

Library of Congress Cataloging-in-Publication Data

Writing DNP clinical case narratives : demonstrating and evaluating competency in comprehensive care / [edited by] Janice Smolowitz, Judy Honig, and Courtney Reinisch.
   p. ; cm.
 Includes bibliographical references and index.
 ISBN 978-0-8261-0530-1 (alk. paper)
 1. Nurse practitioners. 2. Nursing—Study and teaching (Graduate) 3. Nursing—Case studies. I. Smolowitz, Janice. II. Honig, Judy. III. Reinisch, Courtney.
 [DNLM: 1. Education, Nursing, Graduate. 2. Nurse Clinicians—education. 3. Nurse Practitioners—education. 4. Nursing Care—methods. WY 18.5 W956 2010]
 RT82.8.W75 2010
 610.73092—dc22

                                                                    2010010321

Printed in the United States of America by Hamilton Printing Company.

Contents

Section I: The DNP, Comprehensive Patient Care, Clinical Competencies, and Clinical Case Narrative Writing

Section II: DNP Approach and Clinical Case Narratives in the Pediatric and Adolescent Population

Section III: DNP Approach and Clinical Case Narratives in Chronic Care

Section IV: DNP Approach and Clinical Case Narratives in Mental Health Care

Section V: DNP Approach and Clinical Case Narratives in Adult Care

Section VI: DNP Approach and Clinical Case Management in Anesthesia Care

Appendices

Contributors

Laura Ardizzone, DNP, CRNA
Assistant Professor of Clinical Nursing
Columbia University School of Nursing
New York, NY

Kimberly Attwood, PhD, DNP, FNP, GNP
Columbia University School of Nursing
New York, NY

Patricia Auer, DNP, ANP, GNP, DCC
Primary Care Provider/Manager
Hudson Headwaters Health Network Program
Saratoga Springs, NY

Dawn Bucher, DNP, FNP, DCC
Assistant Professor of Clinical Nursing
Columbia University School of Nursing
New York, NY

David F. Cann, DNP, CRNA
Columbia University School of Nursing
New York, NY

Sara Sheets Cook, DNP, RN
Vice Dean; Dorothy M. Rogers Professor of Clinical Nursing
Columbia University School of Nursing
New York, NY

Leanne M. Currie, DNSc, RN
Assistant Professor of Nursing
Columbia University School of Nursing
New York, NY

Susan Doyle-Lindrud, DNP, ANP, DCC
Associate Director, Clinical Research Services
The Cancer Institute of New Jersey
New Brunswick, NJ

Marybeth Duffy, DNP, FNP
New York Presbyterian Hospital
New York, NY

Cindy B. Freeman, DNP, P/MHNP
Track Director, Psychiatric Mental Health Nurse Practitioner Program
The University of Texas-Houston-Health Science Center
Houston, TX

Norma Hannigan, DNP, FNP, DCC
Assistant Professor of Clinical Nursing
Columbia University School of Nursing
New York, NY

Mary Huang, DNP, PNP
Assistant Clinical Professor of Nursing
Columbia University School of Nursing
New York, NY

Rita Marie John, DNP, EdD, PNP, DCC
Assistant Professor of Clinical Nursing
Columbia University School of Nursing
New York, NY

Kevin Johnson, DNP, CRNA
Assistant Chief, Anesthesia Services
Mailand Medical Center
Dallas, TX

Mary P. Johnson, DNP, ACNP
Assistant Professor of Clinical Nursing
Columbia University School of Nursing
New York, NY

Mellen Lovrin, DNP, P/MHNP
Instructor in Clinical Nursing
Columbia University School of Nursing
New York, NY

Rachel Lyons, DNP, PNP
Assistant Clinical Professor of Nursing
Columbia University School of Nursing
New York, NY

Sabrina Opiola McCauley, DNP, NNP, PNP
Instructor of Clinical Nursing
Columbia University School of Nursing
New York, NY

Mary O'Neil Mundinger, DrPH
Dean; Centennial Professor of Health Policy
Columbia University School of Nursing
New York, NY

Lora E. Peppard, DNP, P/MHNP
Columbia University School of Nursing
New York, NY

Dallas D. Regan, DNP, ACNP, DCC
Columbia University School of Nursing
New York, NY

Rebekah L. Ruppe, DNP, CNM
Assistant Professor of Clinical Nursing
Columbia University School of Nursing
New York, NY

Carrie Lyn Sammarco, DNP, FNP
Staff Associate/Nurse Practitioner
Weill Cornell Medical College
New York, NY

Marisa Wallace, DNP, FNP
Assistant Clinical Professor of Nursing
Columbia University School of Nursing
New York, NY

Lynne Beth Weissman, DNP, PNP
Dominican College
Assistant Professor of Nursing
Coordinator of the Graduate FNP Program
Orangeburg, NY

Preface

The Doctor of Nursing Practice (DNP) program at the Columbia University School of Nursing (CUSN) is designed to prepare advanced practice nurses to be comprehensive care providers, with the knowledge and skills necessary to provide fully accountable health care for patients across clinical sites and over time. A competency-based approach is used to educate and evaluate DNP student performance in comprehensive care.

The American Association of Colleges of Nursing (AACN) publication *Essentials of Doctoral Education for Advanced Nursing Practice* (AACN, 2006) outlines eight competencies that form the basis for DNP curricula and course objectives. All DNP students are expected to demonstrate achievement of the AACN essentials. The AACN also recommends that all DNP programs include an integrative practicum and terminal scholarly project that represent the culmination and synthesis of the DNP curriculum. DNP students enrolled in tracks that are clinically focused must demonstrate mastery of a variety of clinical competencies that focus on direct patient care, including full accountability and coordination of care across settings and time, translation and evaluation of research for practice, and interdisciplinary collaboration (NONPF, 2006). Schools of nursing are developing mechanisms to measure doctoral-level clinical competencies. At CUSN students demonstrate mastery of comprehensive care competencies through clinical case narrative writing.

CUSN faculty members have been developing and refining the clinical case narrative format for the past seven years. Case narrative writing is an academic exercise that promotes a systematic reflective process for DNP students to apply to all patient care encounters. This format is grounded in clinical and doctoral competency, which is incorporated into students' approach to patient care.

The clinical case narrative provides a framework wherein students can systematically document clinical encounters with patients, and faculty members can assess DNP students' performance. The descriptive nature of the narrative provides a basis for understanding the complex cognitive processes employed during the provision of care. The case narrative requires in-depth reflection, high-level analysis and synthesis, and critical appraisal and application of clinical evidence. This iterative process of case narrative thinking and writing is a consistent thread throughout the DNP curriculum and is transformative for students. The process is internalized by DNP students and becomes an enduring method of reflective, evidence-based clinical care.

The purpose of this book is to provide DNP faculty and students with a reliable and detailed guide to use when implementing a format to document the care provided. Case narratives differ from the traditional case study format.

When writing case narratives, students make public the decision-making process, identify the evidence that supports the decision, discuss the robustness of the evidence, analyze the effectiveness of the clinical decision, and critically reflect on the overall case.

Text Organization

This book is divided into six sections. The first section discusses comprehensive patient care, introduces the complexities of clinical competencies and their integration into clinical practice, and discusses case narratives as a template for demonstrating clinical competency. The subsequent sections of the book discuss the DNP approach to specific patient populations. Each section includes DNP case narratives written by CUSN DNP students who have provided direct patient care in ambulatory and inpatient settings. These narratives serve as exemplars of the format and can be critically examined in the classroom setting to promote discussion of the provision of evidence-based comprehensive care. General guidelines for writing specific types of notes in different clinical settings are provided in the appendices.

Case Narrative Organization

Each case narrative is based on an actual patient encounter. Some case narratives depict a single encounter that illustrates several competencies. The majority of case narratives depict complex management over time to demonstrate application of the competencies at the DNP level. All narratives include the reason for selecting the case, assessment, care provided, and outcomes. Evidence is cited throughout the narrative to support each decision-making nexus. With each citation, the evidence is briefly summarized in italics and "leveled" according to the Oxford Centre for Evidence-Based Medicine (Centre for Reviews and Dissemination, 2009). After appropriate sections in the narrative, when a component of the competency is demonstrated, it is indicated in bold font. Readers may then make their own determination whether it has been sufficiently met. DNP students have the opportunity to document their critical thinking process at difficult decision points in critical appraisal sections, which are identified by a box format. The narrative concludes with the competency defense, in which DNP students explain how each competency in the narrative was satisfied. Readers are able to reflect and comment on students' justification and determine if the competency was successfully fulfilled.

Case Narratives as Clinical Tool

Clinical case narratives are important tools that support the education of doctoral nurse clinicians. Their in-depth description and reflection provide a model through which students can demonstrate their ability to employ the complex cognitive processes needed to discern the appropriate provision of care. Narratives provide faculty with a student-generated product that they can use to analyze and evaluate the level of reflection, analysis, synthesis, critical appraisal, and application of the clinical evidence required of students at this level of practice.

Case Narratives as Clinical Scholarship

Clinical case narratives are an example of innovative clinical scholarship. Scholarship in the traditional model of nursing has been defined in terms of scientific inquiry through research. With the paradigm shift in nursing education and the emphasis on evidence-based practice, new forms of scholarship are emerging. Clinical case narratives are an example of scholarship in nursing that "can be defined as those activities that systematically advance the teaching, research, and practice of nursing through rigorous inquiry that 1) is significant to the profession, 2) is creative, 3) can be documented, 4) can be replicated or elaborated, and 5) can be peer-reviewed through various methods" (AACN, 1999).

The book is meant to provide DNP faculty and students with a methodical guide for writing case narratives that can be used as a process evaluation format during the development of clinical expertise and as an outcome assessment to measure the synthesis of knowledge and the attainment of clinical competencies. Writing and presenting case narratives create opportunities for doctoral students to think systematically, critically appraise and individualize the evidence, and engage in clinical sholarship.

Janice Smolowitz, EdD, DNP, ANP-BC, DCC
Judy Honig, EdD, DNP, CPNP
Courtney Reinisch, DNP, FNP-BC, DCC

References

American Association of Colleges of Nursing (AACN). (1999). *AACN position statement on defining scholarship in the discipline of nursing.* Washington, DC: Author.
American Association of Colleges of Nursing. (2006). *The essentials of doctoral education for advanced nursing practice.* Retrieved July 6, 2009, from http://www.aacn.nche.edu/DNP/pdf/Essentials.pdf
Centre for Reviews and Dissemination. (2009). *Systematic reviews: CRD's guidance for undertaking reviews in health.* Retrieved January 19, 2010, from http://www.york.ac.uk/inst/crd/pdf/Systematic_Reviews.pdf.
National Organization of Nurse Practitioner Faculties (NONPF). (2006). *Practice doctorate nurse practitioner entry-level competencies.* Retrieved January 19, 2010, from http://www.nonpf.com/nonpf2005/PracticeDoctorateResourceCenter/CompetencyDraftFinalApril2006.pdf

Acknowledgments

We are indebted to those who pioneered comprehensive care in advanced practice nursing. We wish to thank Dr. Mary Mundinger of Columbia University School of Nursing for her vision and perseverance. She created the ideal academic environment and universal faculty practice in which this new level of practice was implemented, tested, and validated, and became the foundation for the doctoral clinician. Under Dr. Mundinger's leadership, engagement in comprehensive, evidenced-based practice at the highest level is embedded in the culture of doctoral-level practitioners. We also recognize physician colleagues, Dr. Michael Weisfeld, formerly of Columbia University Medical Center, now at Johns Hopkins, and Dr. William Speck, both of whom showed vision and courage in their support of this expanded nursing role. As a result of their commitment to improving patient outcomes, they facilitated the breakdown of systematic barriers so patients could have access to care by advanced practice nurses at Columbia University Medical Center.

We wish to express our gratitude to the members of the Council for Comprehensive Care, who provided clarity and focus about comprehensive care competencies and the doctor of nursing practice role in the provision of comprehensive care. Given the changing landscape of health care and health care financing today, the council has kept us cognizant of the context in which the DNP role is evolving, and has encouraged us to proactively define ourselves.

Finally, we acknowledge the work of the faculty and students in the Columbia University Doctor of Nursing Practice program, whose personal insights expanded and transformed the case-narrative format in the DNP residency in order to advance the doctoral role in comprehensive care.

The editors express their appreciation to Margaret Zuccarini of Springer Publishing for her gracious invitation to prepare a book on DNP clinical case narrative writing and Gayle Lee for her support in facilitating the completion of this text.

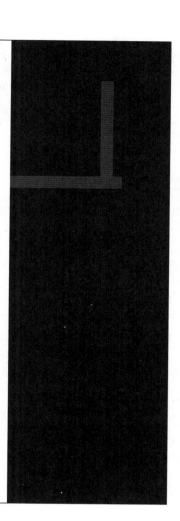

The DNP, Comprehensive Patient Care, Clinical Competencies, and Clinical Case Narrative Writing

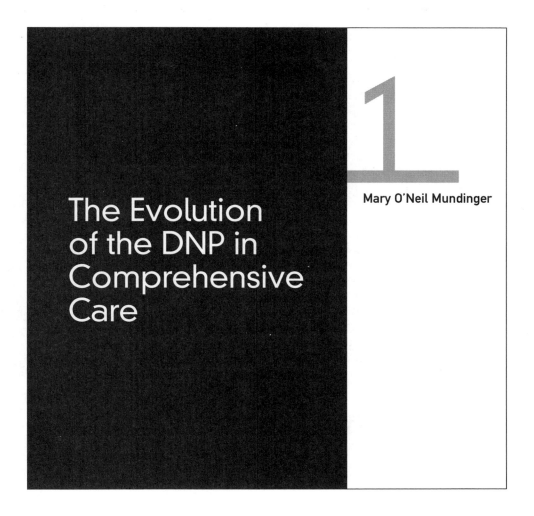

The Evolution of the DNP in Comprehensive Care

1

Mary O'Neil Mundinger

Over the past 40 years, two convergent and interdependent themes have emerged in the health professions; the cascade of new medical knowledge and the corresponding demand from patients for more targeted care have led to the unprecedented development of specialty and subspecialty roles in medicine. As physicians have been increasingly drawn to new, challenging frontiers of practice and well-paid careers, the generalist underpinning for our health care system has eroded. During the same years that new science was flowering in medicine, the seeds of independent comprehensive care were taking root in nursing.

THE EMERGENCE OF THE NURSE PRACTITIONER MODEL

In the early 1960s, community health nurses were the most independent of nurses. Visiting patients in their homes or community centers, they were faced with diagnostic and treatment challenges for which they knew they needed additional knowledge. Their patients—particularly those with chronic illnesses—had health care needs that required new and expanded skills. Lee

Ford, RN, and Henry Silver, MD, at the University of Colorado answered this challenge in 1965 with a unique, new training program that produced the first "nurse practitioners" (NPs) in community health nursing. These NPs were taught to conduct more comprehensive physical and medical assessments and to act on their findings. At the same point in time, national health policy underwent a dramatic change that would prove to be one of the most serendipitous events in the field of advanced practice nursing.

That year (1965), federal law was passed establishing Medicare and Medicaid. These new laws—federal Medicare for the elderly and disabled, and Medicaid, a federal-state partnership for care of the poor—opened access for care to millions who had never had it before. The resources for primary care—the first access point for detection and treatment of illness—were profoundly underdeveloped for the overwhelming new demand. The nurse practitioner model, originally developed for community health nurses, soon became associated with primary care delivery and moved, with the speed of all ideas spawned in a time of need, to rural and inner-city areas, where these newly educated NPs became primary care providers. In only seven years, by 1972, those who completed this nascent training program were authorized to receive direct reimbursement (discounted from MD fees) from Medicare and Medicaid for clinic visits in rural and underserved areas.

NURSES MOVED INTO PRIMARY CARE AS PHYSICIANS MOVED OUT

During the 1970s and 1980s, there was resurgent interest in physician careers in primary care, particularly the new family practice role—a combination of obstetrics, pediatrics, and general medicine. This mission harkened back to the revered and by then mythical family doctor who handled most of an individual's health care needs. By 1970, however, physicians also had many new career choices, all better paying with fewer demands on their time than primary or family practice often required. There was more prestige in specialty practice, and patients were becoming accustomed to seeing specialists, especially because the major users of specialty care had Medicare and did not need referrals from their generalist physician. Concurrently, nursing was developing formal degree programs for primary care NPs, who were making inroads, state by state, in acquiring prescriptive privileges and independence to see patients without MD supervision.

This progression—nurses moving into primary care as physicians moved out—did not generate significant MD concern other than the desire to control and supervise nurses in their expanded roles. In the late 1980s, however, things began to change. Nursing was in decline as a profession, and schools were struggling to maintain enrollments. During the years when the NP model of care was becoming established, nursing schools, especially in universities and on medical center campuses, were focused on developing research programs. Schools aspired to have research faculty with PhDs who engaged in sponsored research, but these scientists were also expected to educate nurses who required significant clinical mentoring. Research, when done successfully, is all-encompassing. It is difficult indeed to be a fully engaged and funded researcher, actively publishing and developing new science, and also to be an active up-to-date clinician mentoring novice clinicians. Many schools wanted to have an all-doctoral faculty, in line with other health profession schools, but found that researchers were not best suited (or most willing) to be clinical supervisors, and students could tell if their mentors were not fully engaged or current in the clinical endeavor.

COLUMBIA UNIVERSITY SCHOOL OF NURSING'S MODEL OF CLINICAL EDUCATION

Columbia University School of Nursing (CUSN), not immune to national trends, concluded that a new model of education was needed to remedy this disconnect. Recruiting distinguished researchers was a crucial element of building the configuration needed, but a new academic clinical component was added. Those who taught clinical courses would themselves be immersed in clinical practice at the highest level of their own education. As part of their academic assignment, Columbia nursing faculty with practices in primary care or specialty practices would take students and introduce them to current practice at its very best. The model thrived. Clinicians devoted to caring for patients became faculty members without leaving the patient care roles they valued. Students had enviable clinical experts as their teachers, and researchers were free to pursue their science and share their scholarship with students. Amazingly, nursing had adopted the academic-medical model.

In the early 1990s, nursing faculty practice—expert clinicians and teachers—had taken off at Columbia Presbyterian Medical Center, which was developing a major primary care presence for families in the hospital's broad neighborhood and was applying for New York State funding to do so. The academic health center physicians had already established a premier clinical presence in every aspect of medicine except primary care, and there were inadequate physician resources in the center to meet the primary care goals of the hospital. William Speck, MD, then president of the hospital, asked the nursing school to provide that resource. With a new and vibrant faculty cohort in the school, the resource that both the hospital and medical center needed was in place. The opportunity to become a recognized primary care entity in a major academic health center, combined with a patient population with a great unmet need for general care, presented a unique opportunity to conduct a rigorous evaluation of primary care delivered by nurses. If NPs were to become a recognized and high-quality resource for patients in a sphere of practice where MDs had set the standard, a randomized clinical trial comparing NPs with primary care MDs would be the most useful and strongest evaluation.

The year 1993—similar to 1965—was an auspicious year for a great leap forward for Columbia nursing; many challenges and opportunities were aligned in a way to foster this advancement. Primary care resources remained deeply inadequate in the community; the hospital needed state funding to construct its new building; medical center physicians were increasingly devoted to specialty—not generalist—practices and were willing to cede primary care to reliably competent nurses; and the School of Nursing had developed a new but thriving faculty practice model. Even with all of these building blocks in place and with benefits clear to all the players, such a radical change in an academic health center practice environment required visionary, magnanimous physicians and courageous, smart nurses who all agreed to be measured by existing standards. This was the environment that created the opportunity for the randomized controlled trial (RCT) from which the new clinical doctorate could emerge.

PARTICIPATION OF FACULTY NPS IN A RANDOMIZED CONTROLLED TRIAL

It was a transformative time. The chair of Medicine, Myron Weisfeldt, MD, along with Bill Speck, MD, and their joint leadership on the hospital medical board, approved medical participation in the clinical trial and authorized hospital admitting privileges for the faculty NPs in the trial. This authorization was necessary to reduce variables between the trial participants (MDs and NPs) so that the evaluation of outcomes and competencies could be fairly compared. The third extraordinary physician to endorse the trial and NP authority was Herbert Pardes, then dean of the Columbia College of Physicians and Surgeons and vice president of Columbia Presbyterian Medical Center. Without his support and that of Drs. Weisfeldt and Speck, none of the major nursing clinical advancements at Columbia for the last decade could have occurred. These three physicians didn't just concur; they planned, advocated, informed, and educated and took a lot of political heat.

CUSN faculty NPs signed up for the clinical trial without missing a beat. Of course, they were aware of the potential for failure, of not meeting the bar. But they understood the opportunity to be the first vetted pioneers in the full scope and authority of primary care. They were setting a new standard for the profession, and their courage and confidence were palpable. The school established a group practice for the trial as the Center for Advanced Practice, or CAP.

The RCT evaluated broad aspects of care for over 1,300 (primarily Medicaid) patients for more than a year (Mundinger et al., 2000). No differences were found between MD care and NP care in any category. Although the results have been broadly interpreted as showing that NPs can do what MDs can in primary care, it is critical to understand that the NPs in the trial were educated and experienced beyond traditional NP education. They learned to admit and co-manage critically ill patients; to take a call in a group practice in which the call could be from a patient they had never seen; to perform emergency department evaluations and make judgments about who should treat a patient; to choose a specialist referral and to utilize referral recommendations; to read and interpret x-rays and more complicated lab tests; and to master sophisticated differential diagnostic skills. They learned all of this from their medical colleagues at Columbia, who prepared them for the randomized trial; thus the CAP faculty added crucial medical skills to the strong nursing competencies they had already mastered.

ESTABLISHMENT OF FACULTY PRACTICE: CAPNA

In 1997, with the trial completed and analysis begun, CAP faculty established a new primary care practice, Columbia Advanced Practice Nurse Associates (CAPNA). Admitting privileges at the medical center hospital had become permanent (and also awarded to all faculty NPs who met the same standard). New York State was a welcoming environment for independent nursing practice; full prescriptive privileges were authorized, and only a "collaborative" (consultative) MD relationship was required in order for NPs to establish their own practice. With its seven-year history of successful primary care faculty practice, Columbia nursing succeeded in obtaining agreements from commercial insurers to reimburse CAPNA practitioners directly and at MD rates. With hospital privileges, insurance contracts, and collaborative MD relationships in place, CAPNA opened in midtown Manhattan and began seeing commercially insured patients.

Organized medicine, unmoved by NPs caring for poor or rural underserved patients, was mobilized by the CAPNA practice, which might pose a competitive threat to physicians caring for affluent, insured individuals. The American Medical Association (AMA), the Medical Society of the State of New York (MSSNY), and other inflamed medical groups opposed the NPs. Robert Graham, executive vice president of the American Academy of Family Physicians, stated that what the nurses are doing "comes very close to practicing medicine, which, of course, requires a medical degree and a license" (Lardner, 1998), and the MSSNY executive vice president pledged to work full-time to shut down the CAPNA practice. Unannounced visits by New York State medical officials with accompanying letters and threats to take legal action were common occurrences. There were some amused responses in the media about the differential medical response to NP care for the well insured as compared to the poor and Medicare-insured elderly for whom NPs had provided primary care for over three decades without a whisper of concern from organized medicine. A pharmaceutical firm gave $1 million for a sophisticated ad campaign in support of CAPNA, and *60 Minutes* aired a celebratory piece on CAPNA, narrated by Morley Safer. More commercial insurers came on board, and patients signed up for care. The public good had won out, at least for a few years.

THE COLUMBIA DNP MODEL, COLLABORATION ON THE CREATION OF CACC, AND THE AACN ESSENTIALS

In 1999, Columbia nursing set forth the plans for a new degree in nursing—the first clinical doctorate—designed to teach nurses the skills that the CAP nurses first learned informally six years before as preparation for the trial comparing MD and NP practice, and that the CAPNA practice had formalized in 1997. The degree, the doctor of nursing practice (DNP), was approved by the Trustees of Columbia University in 2004. In hopes and confidence that the year's long university review would be positive, CUSN offered the course of study during the university review to clinical faculty who became the students who would pioneer the new academic degree. To provide a clear firewall between students and faculty, several MD colleagues from the medical school and PhD faculty from CUSN served as course directors and teachers. The pioneer faculty students formalized and increased their learning as they earned the first DNP degrees in history.

From 1999, when the DNP degree plan began at CUSN, until the university approved and granted the first degrees in February 2005, several supporting activities were completed. Knowing that a clinical doctorate in nursing would be highly desirable to nurses and that schools would quickly act to develop such a degree, Columbia invited 20 health policy and nursing leaders to join a new group, the Council for the Advancement of Primary Care, to develop and promulgate standards for this new program of study. Deans from academic health center nursing schools and physicians involved with broad national health policy issues joined the council and have met annually since 2000 to further the standardization mission. In 2003 representatives from eight of the council nursing schools published the competencies that a DNP graduate should achieve (CUSN, 2003). In 2005 the council changed its name to the Council for the Advancement of Comprehensive Care (CACC) to reflect the understanding that DNP clinical education encompassed a broader set of skills and knowledge than primary care alone.

During this same innovative period at Columbia, nursing nationally awoke to the idea of moving advanced practice to the doctoral level; the Columbia model, forged over 20 years of evolution and evaluation, took hold across the country. The American Association of Colleges of Nursing (AACN) voted to phase out MS degree programs in advanced practice nursing by 2015 in favor of the clinical doctorate (AACN, 2005). AACN committees were formed to determine the "essentials" of the new degree, and the resulting document was similar to the 2003 CACC competencies document except in one respect. Whereas CACC focuses on direct patient care as "practice," the AACN DNP essentials apply to DNP programs developed in other areas of "practice" than the clinical realm. Practice could also be administration, or health policy as conducted by a nurse. Although an inclusive stance by an organization representing all collegiate nursing schools—the great majority of which have no faculty prepared to develop an advanced clinical practice degree program—is understandable, this lack of distinction of DNP direct care competency (practice) has blurred and potentially weakened the public's understanding of who a DNP is and what this professional can do.

Indeed, as DNP programs proliferate, very few have developed clinical doctoral education at a demonstrably different level than their preceding MS degree programs. Other "essentials" for the new degree are more likely to be clearly doctoral level (informatics, use of evidence, for example), but the "practice" essential is variable. Some DNP programs appear to be clinical research or have a clinical project as the capstone achievement. Some DNP programs clearly have no advanced patient care outcomes (administration or informatics as the "practice" essential) or are offered as online programs.

COMPREHENSIVE CARE CERTIFICATION EXAM FOR DNP GRADUATES

The confusion and disparate focus of the DNP degree required action for clarification and standardization. CACC, established to standardize the degree, changed its mission to standardize the clinical competencies for graduates of DNP programs that focus on comprehensive care. The decision was reached that a national certification examination could become the clarifying competency standard where the degree had failed to do so. The council sought proposals from existing certifying agencies, and in 2007 it selected the National Board of Medical Examiners (NBME).

In 2007 CACC entered into a contract with the NBME to develop an exam utilizing the test pool of questions from the previous Step 3 of the United States Medical Licensing Exams. NBME and CACC representatives developed an exam that was comparable in content and similar in format and that would measure the same set of competencies and apply similar performance standards as Step 3 of the United States Medical Licensing Examination, which is administered to physicians as one component of qualifying for licensure. CACC established a subsidiary group, the American Board of Comprehensive Care (ABCC), which would function as an independent, certifying body for DNP candidates who successfully completed the certification process.

During 2007 and 2008, as over 200 schools of nursing prepared to develop and offer DNP degrees, several conservative medical groups—including the American Academy of Family Practice Physicians, the American College of Physicians, and the American Medical Association—continued to formulate policy and make statements antagonistic to the degree and the certification. They lobbied NBME to withdraw from the partnership with CACC and sought state regulatory change to prohibit DNPs from using their newly earned title of "Doctor."

To date, these efforts have failed. As the new degrees are established and strengthened and as certification of DNPs expands, the nurses with this new degree, new title, and new competencies are thriving. As in 1935 and 1965, the political context and public need are aligned for radical social advancement. DNPs are qualified and welcomed, by most of the medical profession and increasingly by an informed public, as an answer to critical gaps in the health care system.

Comprehensive care—primary access and broad scope of care—is already in great demand and in great shortage. With health care reform imminent, DNPs are a wise solution to universal coverage with goals of cost-effective, evidence-based care at the core of reform. Medicare and Medicaid fostered the rise of NPs, and universal coverage will open a wide door of access for DNPs.

Primary care has outgrown its early 1970s definition of coordinated, first-contact care. The needs of patients already require more than the most recent definition from a 1996 Institute of Medicine study: "Primary care is the provision of integrated, accessible health care services by clinicians who are accountable for addressing a large majority of personal health care needs, developing a sustained partnership with patients, and practicing in the context of family and community" (Institute of Medicine, 1996). Primary care, as an encompassing form for generalist care, is outdated. It has never been more necessary to have a wise clinician overseeing the spectrum of generalist and specialist care needed: someone who has authority across sites and over time for patients; someone who can select specialists and communicate a shared strategy for patients; someone whose diagnostic skills are honed to a sharp edge of differential acumen; and someone who understands the distinction between strong and not-so-strong evidence and knows how to apply it appropriately for patients.

Comprehensive care *is* a specialty, but it is one that every individual needs and deserves. DNP education is formulated to develop comprehensive care competencies. Patients, physicians, policymakers, and the broader public are embracing this new role. The doctor of nursing practice with its accompanying clinical certification has arrived and faces a promising and rewarding future.

References

American Association of Colleges of Nursing (AACN). (2005). *2005 annual report: Annual state of the schools.* Washington, DC: American Association of Colleges of Nursing, 2005.

Columbia University School of Nursing (CUSN). (2003). *Competencies of a clinical doctorate.* New York: Columbia University School of Nursing.

Institute of Medicine. (1996). *Primary care: America's health in a new era.* M.S. Donaldson, K.D. Yordy, K.N. Lohr, & N.A. Vanselow (Eds.). Washington, DC: National Academy Press.

Lardner, James. (1998, July 27). For nurses, a barrier broken. *U.S. News & World Report, 125*(4), 58.

Mundinger, M.O., Kane, R.L., Lenz, E.R., Totten, A.M., Tsai, W.Y., Cleary, P.D., Friedewald, W.T., Siu, A.L., & Shelanski, M.L. (2000). Primary care outcomes in patients treated by nurse practitioners or physicians. *Journal of the American Medical Association, 283*(1), 59–68.

2

Development of DNP Competencies in Comprehensive Care

Judy Honig
Janice Smolowitz

The evolution of clinical competencies at Columbia University School of Nursing's doctor of nursing practice (CUSN DNP) has been and remains a dynamic, iterative, reflective process. This process has benefited from the critical review and insights of health policy experts, leaders of nursing organizations, deans of schools of nursing, and DNP student residents over the past 10 years. The prevailing guidance has been the vision and understanding that doctorally prepared advanced practice nurses, equipped with expanded knowledge and skills, can improve the access, efficiency, and quality of health care for diverse populations across clinical settings over time.

The CUSN DNP competencies are inexorably linked to the CUSN DNP program, which is based on empirical evidence from outcome studies that utilized the medical model to demonstrate parity between care provided by physicians and nurse practitioners (NPs) (Brown & Grimes, 1995; Carroll & Fay, 1997; Jones & Clark, 1997; Kleinpell-Nowell & Weiner, 1999; Safriet, 1992; Spitzer, Sackett, & Sibley, 1974; U.S. Congress, Office of Technology Assessment, 1986), culminating in a randomized controlled trial (RCT) that demonstrated that primary care faculty physicians and faculty NPs provide the same quality of care, achieve the same patient satisfaction, and utilize resources at the same cost (Mundinger et al., 2000). The faculty NPs in the RCT were indistinguishable from the physician group in terms of accountability to patients. Both groups had admitting privileges and followed patients across settings and over time. The faculty NP role with expanded responsibility and accountability provided the model upon which the comprehensive care competencies and CUSN DNP program were built (Smolowitz & Honig, 2008).

FIRST PHASE OF COMPETENCY DEVELOPMENT

Prior to the RCT, the scope of practice as provided by the CUSN faculty NPs had not been explored in the literature. This was a new concept for NPs. Following publication of the RCT, CUSN faculty NPs examined their clinical practices to delineate the broadened role and added skills required to provide comprehensive primary care. A detailed examination of the skill sets of these NPs was conducted. Interviews and focus groups were held to identify, clarify, and validate the expanded scope of knowledge and practice competencies required. Expanded knowledge enabled the faculty NPs to provide diagnostically complex care across settings and over time, utilize sophisticated informatics and decision-making technology, and assimilate in-depth knowledge of biophysical, psychosocial, and behavioral sciences. This in-depth study established the need to formalize the educational process and provided the first draft of the CUSN DNP competencies.

SECOND PHASE OF COMPETENCY DEVELOPMENT

During the second phase of competency development, CUSN faculty reviewed the newly developed competencies and compared them with established competencies, including the National Organization of Nurse Practitioner Faculties (NONPF) domains and core competencies (NONPF, 2000), *Graduate Education in Internal Medicine: A Resource Guide to Curriculum Development* (1997), and the primary care competencies outlined in *Primary Care: America's Health in a New Era* (IOM, 1996) to determine consistency and the need for incorporation into CUSN doctoral-level competencies.

This first version of the CUSN competencies utilized the structure and format of the NONPF domains and competencies of nurse practitioner practice (2000) as a foundation. Individual NONPF competencies were expanded or enhanced, and new domains were developed to reflect clinical practice at the doctoral level. Specific competencies developed by physician boards to reflect this level of clinical practice were integrated into the CUSN competencies. The first draft of the clinical doctorate competencies was approved by CUSN faculty in 2001.

THIRD PHASE OF COMPETENCY DEVELOPMENT

This draft was brought to the Council for the Advancement of Comprehensive Care (CACC) for review. CACC, spearheaded by Dr. Mary Mundinger, is a consortium of school of nursing deans, health policy experts, and nursing leaders who are committed to ensuring high standards of comprehensive care and doctoral nursing practice.

CACC members who had been discussing the provision of comprehensive care utilized the Institute of Medicine (IOM) (1996, p. 1) definition: "provision of integrated, accessible health care services by clinicians who are accountable for addressing a large majority of personal health care needs, developing a sustained partnership with patients, and practicing in the context of family and community." This definition emphasizes prevention, risk assessment, cultural competence, and coordination of services for a diverse population of patients. Advances in science and technology, including genomics, had created new preventive, diagnostic, and treatment options for patients. In addition, the site of care delivery had shifted away from the hospital to multiple alternative settings.

CACC members conceptualized the doctor of nursing practice (DNP) as a clinician with the necessary skills, education, and competencies, as identified in the IOM definition of primary care, to provide comprehensive care to maintain and improve the health status of patients over time and across sites. They envisioned the DNP as an expert clinician, educated to address the health care challenges created by an increasing number of complex and chronic health care conditions, the growth of information and biomedical technology, the aging and increasingly diverse population, and identified disparities in care.

CACC involvement in the competencies began the third phase of competency development. Deans of nursing schools who were members of CACC and leaders in the national movement to launch the clinical doctorate, who were committed to standardization without prescription, nominated one of their faculty members to serve on the Consensus Committee for DNP Competencies. This committee, chaired by Dr. J. Honig, was charged with the task of discussing and revising the competencies drafted by CUSN faculty. The seven members of the committee included program directors and experienced and practicing advanced practice nurses (APNs) with research doctorates. As a result of the review process, the Consensus Committee agreed that the competencies represented core competencies for doctoral-level advanced nursing practice. This committee of experts, with multiple-specialty APN perspectives, agreed that the core competencies for doctoral-level advanced nursing transcended differences and explicated the commonalities across populations and specialties.

FOURTH PHASE OF COMPETENCY DEVELOPMENT

During the fourth phase, the Consensus Committee report on the competencies was presented at a national meeting of CACC. The competencies were examined, critiqued, revised, and published (CACC, 2003). The 2003 competencies provided the foundation for the educational and content standards for the clinical doctorate at CUSN.

FIFTH PHASE OF COMPETENCY DEVELOPMENT

The first CUSN DNP class graduated in 2005. The experience of these graduates was presented at a national meeting of CACC, initiating the fifth phase of competency development. A new CACC subcommittee, chaired by Dr. J. Smolowitz, was charged with reexamining the 2003 competencies in light of the experiences of CUSN DNP graduates and examples of health care professionals' competencies, including the Outcome Project of the Accreditation Council Graduate Medical Education (ACGME, 2007), the Royal College of General Practitioners guide (RCGP, 2009), and the draft of the American Association of Colleges of Nursing *Essentials* (AACN, 2006). The subcommittee revised the 2003 competencies. A draft was presented to CACC and was approved by CACC members. These competencies were published in the *Competencies of a Clinical Nursing Doctorate* (CACC, 2006).

SIXTH PHASE OF COMPETENCY DEVELOPMENT

The competencies underwent further revisions as a result of DNP faculty and student input. As part of routine outcome evaluations, the competencies were reexamined, and it was determined that further refinement was warranted. The competencies were reconceptualized into complex sets of behaviors. They were collapsed into eleven behavioral competencies, which were essentially the same as the multiple competencies within the nine domains initially used. This iteration of the competencies was published in *Case Studies: The Doctor of Nursing Practice, Setting the Standard in Health Care* (CUSN, 2005). This change occurred during the period when the NONPF competency structure was being reviewed and revised and stand-alone DNP competencies were being developed for NP faculty (NONPF, 2006). These competencies were subsequently benchmarked against the NONPF doctoral competencies (2006) and found to be consistent in content with a detailed focus on provision of direct, comprehensive patient care.

SEVENTH PHASE OF COMPETENCY DEVELOPMENT

In 2006 the American Association of Colleges of Nursing (AACN) published the *Essentials of Doctoral Education for Advanced Nursing Practice*. The CUSN DNP Competency Committee benchmarked the CUSN DNP competencies against the AACN essentials and found them to be consistent and in some cases to exceed the competencies outlined in the AACN document. In particular, the CUSN DNP competencies provided much more depth and breadth for Essential VIII that emphasized comprehensive care. See Table 2.1.

EIGHTH PHASE OF COMPETENCY DEVELOPMENT

A natural continuous process of reevaluation of the competencies occurred as CUSN DNP residents and faculty utilized the competencies to discuss case narratives and assess and evaluate direct patient care provided in multispecialty settings. These discussions resulted in the most current version of the DNP competencies, which were developed and piloted at CUSN in 2009 and adopted by CACC in 2010.

Comparison of Columbia University School of Nursing DNP Competencies in Comprehensive Care, AACN Essentials, and NONPF Practice Doctorate Nurse Practitioner Entry-Level Competencies.

CUSN (2010)	AACN (2006)	NONPF (2006)
DNP graduates will demonstrate expertise in the provision, coordination, and direction of comprehensive care to patients, including those who present in healthy states and those who present with complex, chronic, and/or co-morbid conditions, across clinical sites and over time.	The following *DNP Essentials* outline the curricular elements and competencies that must be present in programs conferring the Doctor of Nursing Practice degree [. . .] The *DNP Essentials* delineated here address the foundational competencies that are core to all advanced nursing practice roles.	At completion of the program, the NP graduate of the nursing practice doctorate will possess the existing NONPF NP core competencies and the following competencies.
DOMAIN 1. COMPREHENSIVE CLINICALCARE Competency 1. Evaluate patient needs based on age, developmental stage, family history, ethnicity, individual risk, including genetic profile to formulate plans for health promotion, anticipatory guidance, counseling, and disease prevention services for healthy or sick patients and their families in any clinical setting.	Essential I: Scientific Underpinnings for Practice Essential VII: Clinical Prevention and Population Health for Improving the Nation's Health Essential VIII: Advanced Nursing Practice	Independent Practice (1) Practices independently by assessing, diagnosing, treating, and managing undifferentiated patients. (2) Assumes full accountability for actions as a licensed independent practitioner. Scientific Foundation (1) Critically analyzes data for practice by integrating knowledge from arts and sciences within the context of nursing's philosophical framework and scientific foundation.

(continued)

DNP Comprehensive Care Competencies *(Continued)*

CUSN (2010)	AACN (2006)	NONPF (2006)
DOMAIN 1. COMPREHENSIVE CLINICAL CARE Competency 2. Evaluate population or geographically-based health risk utilizing principles of epidemiology, clinical prevention, environmental health, and biostatistics.	Essential II: Organizational and Systems Leadership for Quality Improvement and Systems Thinking Essential VII: Clinical Prevention and Population Health for Improving the Nation's Health Essential VIII: Advanced Nursing Practice	Practice Inquiry (1) Applies clinical investigative skills for evaluation of health outcomes at the patient, family, population, clinical unit, systems, and/or community levels. Health Delivery System (3) Manages risks to individuals, families, populations, and health care systems.
DOMAIN 1. COMPREHENSIVE CLINICALCARE Competency 3. Formulate differential diagnoses, and diagnostic strategies and therapeutic interventions with attention to scientific evidence, safety, cost, invasiveness, simplicity, acceptability, adherence, and efficacy for patients who present with new conditions and those with ambiguous or incomplete data, complex illnesses, comorbid conditions, and multiple diagnoses in all clinical settings.	Essential III: Clinical Scholarship and Analytical Methods for Evidence-Based Practice Essential VIII: Advanced Nursing Practice	Independent Practice (1) Practices independently by assessing, diagnosing, treating, and managing undifferentiated patients. (2) Assumes full accountability for actions as a licensed independent practitioner. Scientific Foundation (1) Critically analyzes data for practice by integrating knowledge from arts and sciences within the context of nursing's philosophical framework and scientific foundation. (2) Translates research and data to anticipate, predict, and explain variations in practice. Quality (1) Uses best available evidence to enhance quality in clinical practice.

DOMAIN 1. COMPREHENSIVE CLINICAL CARE
Competency 4. Appraise acuity of patient condition, determine need to transfer patient to higher acuity setting, coordinate, and manage transfer to optimize patient outcomes.

Essential VI: Interprofessional Collaboration for Improving Patient and Population Health Outcomes

Essential VIII: Advanced Nursing Practice

Independent practice
(1) Practices independently by assessing, diagnosing, treating, and managing undifferentiated patients.
(2) Assumes full accountability for actions as a licensed independent practitioner.

Scientific foundation
(1) Critically analyzes data for practice by integrating knowledge from arts and sciences within the context of nursing's philosophical framework and scientific foundation.

Leadership
(1) Assumes increasingly complex leadership roles.
(2) Provides leadership to foster interprofessional collaboration.
(3) Demonstrates a leadership style that uses critical and reflective thinking.

Quality
(1) Uses best available evidence to enhance quality in clinical practice.

Health Delivery System
(1) Applies knowledge of organizational behavior and systems.
(2) Demonstrates skills in negotiating, consensus building, and partnering.

(continued)

2.1 DNP Comprehensive Care Competencies *(Continued)*

CUSN (2010)	AACN (2006)	NONPF (2006)
DOMAIN 1. COMPREHENSIVE CLINICAL CARE **Competency 5.** Evaluate and direct care during hospitalization, and design a comprehensive discharge plan for patients from an acute care setting.	Essential VI: Interprofessional Collaboration for Improving Patient and Population Health Outcomes Essential VIII: Advanced Nursing Practice	**Independent practice** (1) Practices independently by assessing, diagnosing, treating, and managing undifferentiated patients. (2) Assumes full accountability for actions as a licensed independent practitioner. **Leadership** (1) Assumes increasingly complex leadership roles. (2) Provides leadership to foster interprofessional collaboration. (3) Demonstrates a leadership style that uses critical and reflective thinking. **Quality** (1) Uses best available evidence to enhance quality in clinical practice. **Health Delivery System** (1) Applies knowledge of organizational behavior and systems. (2) Demonstrates skills in negotiating, consensus building, and partnering. **Practice Inquiry** (1) Applies clinical investigative skills for evaluation of health outcomes at the patient, family, population, clinical unit systems, and/or community health.

DOMAIN 1. COMPREHENSIVE CLINICAL CARE
Competency 6. Direct comprehensive care for patient in a subacute setting to maximize quality of life and functional status.

Essential VI: Interprofessional Collaboration for Improving Patient and Population Health Outcomes
Essential VIII: Advanced Nursing Practice

Health Delivery System
(2) Demonstrates skills in negotiating, consensus building, and partnering.
(3) Manages risks to individuals, families, populations, and healthcare systems.

DOMAIN 1. COMPREHENSIVE CLINICAL CARE
Competency 7. Facilitate and guide the process of palliative care and/or planning end of life care by discussing diagnoses and prognosis, clarifying and validating patient desires and priorities, and promoting informed choices and shared decision making by patient, family, and members of the health care team.

Essential I: Scientific Underpinnings for Practice
Essential III: Clinical Scholarship and Analytical Methods for Evidence-Based Practice
Essential VIII: Advanced Nursing Practice

Independent Practice
(2) Assumes full accountability for actions as a licensed independent practitioner.

Ethics
(1) Applies ethically sound solutions to complex issues.

Policy
(1) Analyzes ethical, legal, and social factors in policy development.

DOMAIN 2. INTERDISCIPLINARY AND PATIENT-CENTERED COMMUNICATION
Competency 1. Assemble a collaborative interdisciplinary network, refer and consult appropriately while maintaining primary responsibility for comprehensive patient care.

Essential II: Organizational and Systems Leadership for Quality Improvement and Systems Thinking
Essential VI: Interprofessional Collaboration for Improving Patient and Population Health Outcomes
Essential VIII: Advanced Nursing Practice

Quality
(2) Evaluates how organizational, structural, financial, marketing, and policy decisions impact cost, quality, and accessibility of health care.
(3) Demonstrates skills in peer review that promote a culture of excellence.

Health Delivery System
(1) Applies knowledge of organizational behavior and systems.
(2) Demonstrates skills in negotiating, consensus building, and partnering.

(continued)

CUSN (2010)	AACN (2006)	NONPF (2006)
DOMAIN 2. INTERDISCIPLINARY AND PATIENT-CENTERED COMMUNICATION Competency 2. Coordinate and manage the care of patients with chronic illness utilizing specialists, other disciplines, community resources, and family, while maintaining primary responsibility for direction of patient care and ensuring the seamless flow of information among providers as the focus of care transitions across ambulatory to acute, sub acute settings, and community settings.	Essential II: Organizational and Systems Leadership for Quality Improvement and Systems Thinking Essential VI: Interprofessional Collaboration for Improving Patient and Population Health Outcomes Essential VIII: Advanced Nursing Practice	Quality (1) Uses best available evidence to enhance quality in clinical practice. (2) Evaluates how organizational, structural, financial, marketing, and policy decisions impact cost, quality, and accessibility of health care. Leadership (1) Assumes increasingly complex leadership roles. (2) Provides leadership to foster interprofessional collaboration. (3) Demonstrates a leadership style that uses critical and reflective thinking. Health Delivery System (1) Applies knowledge of organizational behavior and systems. (2) Demonstrates skills in negotiating, consensus building, and partnering. Health Delivery System (4) Facilitates development of culturally relevant health care systems. Independent Practice (1) Practices independently by assessing, diagnosing, treating, and managing undifferentiated patients.
DOMAIN 3. SYTEMS AND CONTEXT OF CARE Competency 1. Construct and evaluate outcomes of a culturally sensitive, individualized intervention that incorporates shared decision-making and addresses the specific needs of a patient in context of family and community.	Essential II: Organizational and Systems Leadership for Quality Improvement and Systems Thinking Essential III: Clinical Scholarship and Analytical Methods for Evidence-Based Practice Essential VIII: Advanced Nursing Practice	

(2) Assumes full accountability for actions as a licensed independent practitioner.

Leadership
(1) Assumes increasingly complex leadership roles.
(3) Demonstrates a leadership style that uses critical and reflective thinking.

Quality
(1) Uses best available evidence to enhance quality in clinical practice.

Practice Inquiry
(1) Applies clinical investigative skills for evaluation of health outcomes at the patient, family, population, clinical unit, systems, and/or community levels.

Health Delivery System
(1) Applies knowledge of organizational behavior and systems.
(2) Demonstrates skills in negotiating, consensus building, and partnering.
(3) Manages risks to individuals, families, populations, and health care systems.

Quality
(1) Uses best available evidence to enhance quality in clinical practice.
(2) Evaluates how organizational, structural, financial, marketing, and policy decisions impact cost, quality, and accessibility of health care.

Essential II: Organizational and Systems Leadership for Quality Improvement and Systems Thinking
Essential V: Health Care Policy for Advocacy in Health Care
Essential VIII: Advanced Nursing Practice

DOMAIN 3. SYSTEMS AND CONTEXT OF CARE
Competency 2. Evaluate gaps in health care access that compromise optimal patient outcomes, and apply current knowledge of the organization and financing of health care systems to advocate for the patient and to ameliorate negative impact.

(continued)

CUSN (2010)	AACN (2006)	NONPF (2006)
DOMAIN 3. SYSTEMS AND CONTEXT OF CARE Competency 3. Synthesize the principles of legal and ethical decision-making and analyze dilemmas that arise in patient care, interprofessional relationships, research, or practice management to improve outcomes.	Essential I: Scientific Underpinnings for Practice Essential VIII: Advanced Nursing Practice	**Practice Inquiry** (1) Applies clinical investigative skills for evaluation of health outcomes at the patient, family, population, clinical unit, systems, and/or community levels. (2) Provides leadership in the translation of new knowledge into practice. **Quality** (1) Uses best available evidence to enhance quality in clinical practice. (3) Demonstrates skills in peer review that promote a culture of excellence.
DOMAIN 3. SYSTEMS AND CONTEXT OF CARE Competency 4. Integrate principles of business, finance, economics, and/or health policy to design an initiative that benefits a group of patients, practice, community, and/ or population.	Essential II: Organizational and Systems Leadership for Quality Improvement and Systems Thinking Essential V: Health Care Policy for Advocacy in Health Care	**Quality** (1) Uses best available evidence to enhance quality in clinical practice. (2) Evaluates how organizational, structural, financial, marketing, and policy decisions impact cost, quality and accessibility of health care. (3) Demonstrates skills in peer review that promote a culture of excellence. **Policy** (1) Analyzes ethical, legal, and social factors in policy development. (2) Influences health policy.

DOMAIN 4. BUILIDNG AND USING EVIDENCE FOR BEST CLINICAL PRACTICES AND SCHOLARSHIP

Competency 1. Synthesize and analyze evidence from practice, clinical information systems, and patient databases using informatics tools to identify deficits and improve delivery of care.

Essential III: Clinical Scholarship and Analytical Methods for Evidence-Based Practice

Essential IV: Information Systems/Technology and Patient Care Technology for the Improvement and Transformation of Health Care

Essential VIII: Advanced Nursing Practice

Practice Inquiry
(1) Applies clinical investigative skills for evaluation of health outcomes at the patient, family, population, clinical unit, systems, and/or community levels.
(2) Provides leadership in the translation of new knowledge into practice.
(4) Disseminates evidence from inquiry to diverse audiences using multiple methods.

Quality
(1) Uses best available evidence to enhance quality in clinical practice.
(2) Evaluates how organizational, structural, financial, marketing, and policy decisions impact cost, quality, and accessibility of health care.
(3) Demonstrates skills in peer review that promote a culture of excellence.

Health Delivery System
(1) Applies knowledge of organizational behavior and systems.
(2) Demonstrates skills in negotiating, consensus building, and partnering.
(3) Manages risks to individuals, families, populations, and health care systems.
(4) Facilitates development of culturally relevant health care systems.

2.1 DNP Comprehensive Care Competencies (Continued)

CUSN (2010)	AACN (2006)	NONPF (2006)
		Practice Inquiry
		(1) Applies clinical investigative skills for evaluation of health outcomes at the patient, family, population, clinical unit, systems, and/or community levels.
		(2) Provides leadership in the translation of new knowledge into practice.
		(4) Disseminates evidence from inquiry to diverse audiences using multiple methods.
		Technology and Information Literacy
		(1) Demonstrates information literacy in complex decision making.
		(2) Translates technical and scientific health information appropriate for user need.
		(3) Participates in the development of clinical information system.
DOMAIN 4. BUILIDNG AND USING EVIDENCE FOR BEST CLINICAL PRACTICES AND SCHOLARSHIP	Essential III: Clinical Scholarship and Analytical Methods for Evidence-Based Practice	**Policy**
Competency 2. Evaluate quality of care against standards using reliable and valid methods and measures and propose innovative, interdisciplinary models that enhance outcomes.	Essential V: Health Care Policy for Advocacy in Health Care	(1) Analyzes ethical, legal, and social factors in policy development.
		(2) Influences health policy.
		(3) Evaluates the impact of globalization on health care policy development.

(continued)

DOMAIN 4. BUILIDNG AND USING EVIDENCE FOR BEST CLINICAL PRACTICES AND SCHOLARSHIP

Competency 3. Critically appraise and synthesize research findings and other evidence using a systematic methodology and interdisciplinary models to inform practice and policy for optimal patient outcomes.

Essential I: Scientific Underpinnings for Practice

Essential III: Clinical Scholarship and Analytical Methods for Evidence-Based Practice

Essential V: Health Care Policy for Advocacy in Health Care

Essential VIII: Advanced Nursing Practice

Quality
(1) Uses best available evidence to enhance quality in clinical practice.
(2) Evaluates how organizational, structural, financial, marketing, and policy decisions impact cost, quality, and accessibility of health care.
(3) Demonstrates skills in peer review that promote a culture of excellence.

Practice Inquiry
(1) Applies clinical investigative skills for evaluation of health outcomes at the patient, family, population, clinical unit systems, and/or community health.
(2) Provides leadership in the translation of new knowledge into practice.
(4) Disseminates evidence from inquiry to diverse audiences using multiple methods.

DOMAIN 4. BUILIDNG AND USING EVIDENCE FOR BEST CLINICAL PRACTICES AND SCHOLARSHIP

Competency 4. Assess and critically appraise clinical scholarship through participation in the peer review process for the purpose of disseminating knowledge to the professional community.

Essential III: Clinical Scholarship and Analytical Methods for Evidence-Based Practice

Essential VI: Interprofessional Collaboration for Improving Patient and Population Health Outcomes

Quality
(3) Demonstrates skills in peer review that promote a culture of excellence.

Practice Inquiry
(1) Applies clinical investigative skills for evaluation of health outcomes at the patient, family, population, clinical unit systems, and/or community health.
(2) Provides leadership in the translation of new knowledge into practice.

2.1 DNP Comprehensive Care Competencies (Continued)

CUSN (2010)	AACN (2006)	NONPF (2006)
		(4) Disseminates evidence from inquiry to diverse audiences using multiple methods.
		Technology and Information Literacy
		(1) Demonstrates information literacy in complex decision making.
		(2) Translates technical and scientific health information appropriate for user need.
		(3) Participates in the development of clinical information system.

Competencies will continue to be reviewed and revised. The dynamic state of health care technology and scientific discovery requires constant surveillance of the relevance and adequacy of the outcome competencies. The CUSN DNP competencies provide a blueprint for educational content and graduate certification of a clinical nursing doctorate. The establishment of this doctoral level of education, with well-defined and distinctive competencies, will contribute to quality and access to comprehensive care.

The developmen t of the competencies of a clinical nursing doctorate was made possible by funding from the Teagle Foundation, the W.K. Kellogg Foundation, the Robert Wood Johnson Foundation, and Pfizer Inc.

Acknowledgments 2003
Columbia University School of Nursing
University of Illinois at Chicago College of Nursing
University of Iowa College of Nursing
Rush University College of Nursing
University of Texas Health Sciences Center at Houston School of Nursing
Yale University School of Nursing
University of Washington School of Nursing

Acknowledgments 2006
Columbia University School of Nursing
University of California School of Nursing
University of Tennessee School of Nursing
Vanderbilt University School of Nursing
Rand Corporation

References

Accreditation Council Graduate Medical Education (ACGME). (2007). *ACGME Outcome Project.* Retrieved August 17, 2009, from http://www.acgme.org/outcome/comp/GeneralCompetenciesStandards21307.pdf

American Association of Colleges of Nursing (AACN). (2006). *The essentials of doctoral education for advanced nursing practice.* Retrieved July 6, 2009, from http://www.aacn.nche.edu/DNP/pdf/Essentials.pdf

Brown, S.A., & Grimes, D.E. (1995). A meta-analysis of nurse practitioners and nurse midwives in primary care. *Nursing Research, 44*(6), 332–339.

Carroll, T.L., & Fay, V.P. (1997). Measuring the impact of advanced practice nursing on achieving cost-quality outcomes: Issues and challenges. *Nursing Administration Quarterly, 21*(4), 32–40.

Columbia University School of Nursing (CUSN). (2005). *Case studies: The doctor of nursing practice, setting the standard in health care.* New York: Columbia University School of Nursing.

Council for the Advancement of Comprehensive Care (CACC). (2003). *Competencies of a clinical nursing doctorate.* New York: Columbia University School of Nursing.

Council for the Advancement of Comprehensive Care (CACC). (2006). *Competencies of a clinical nursing doctorate.* New York: Columbia University School of Nursing.

Ende, J., Kelley, M.A., Ramsey, P.G., Sox, H.C. (1997). *Graduate Education in Internal Medicine: A Resource Guide to Curriculum Development.* The Report of the Federated Council for

Internal Medicine Task Force on Internal Medicine Residency Curriculum. FCIM, Inc. Philadelphia, PA.

Institute of Medicine (IOM). (1996). *Primary care: America's health in a new era.* Washington, DC: National Academies Press.

Jones, M.E., & Clark, D. (1997). Increasing access to health care: A study of pediatric nurse practitioner outcomes in a school-based clinic. *Journal of Nursing Care Quality, 11*(4), 53–59.

Kleinpell-Nowell, R., & Weiner, T.M. (1999). Measuring advanced practice nursing outcomes. *AACN Clinical Reviews, 10* (3), 356–368.

Mundinger, M.O., Kane, R.L., Lenz, E.R., Totten, A.M., Tsai, W.Y., Cleary, P.D., Friedewald, W.T., Siu, A.L., & Shelanski, M.L. (2000). Primary outcomes in patients treated by nurse practitioners or physicians: A randomized trial. *Journal of the American Medical Association, 283,* 59–68.

National Organization of Nurse Practitioner Faculties (NONPF). (2000). *Domains and competencies of nurse practitioner practice.* Washington, DC: National Organization of Nurse Practitioner Faculties.

National Organization of Nurse Practitioner Faculties (NONPF). (2006). *Practice doctorate nurse practitioner entry-level competencies.* Retrieved January 20, 2010, from http://www.nonpf. com/nonpf2005/PracticeDoctorateResourceCenter/CompetencyDraftFinalApril2006.pdf

Royal College of General Practitioners (RCGP). (2009). *RCGP guide to revalidation for general practitioners.* Retrieved August 17, 2009, from http://www.rcgp.org.uk/PDF/PDS _Guide_to_Revalidation_for_GPs.pdf

Safriet, B.J. (1992). Health care dollars and regulatory sense: The role of the nurse practitioner. *Yale Journal on Regulation, 9,* 417–488.

Smolowitz, J. and Honig, J. (2008). DNP portfolio: Scholarly project for doctor of nursing practice. *Clinical Scholars Review, 1*(1), 19–23.

Spitzer, W.O., Sackett, D.L., Sibley, J.C., et al. (1974). The Burlington randomized trial of the nurse practitioner. *New England Journal of Medicine, 290*(5), 151–156.

U.S. Congress, Office of Technology Assessment. (1986). *Nurse practitioners, physician assistants, and certified nurse-midwives: A policy analysis* (Health Technology Case Study 37). OTA-HCA-37. Washington, DC: U.S. Government Printing Office.

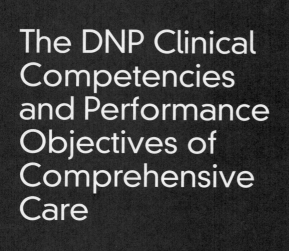

The DNP Clinical Competencies and Performance Objectives of Comprehensive Care

3

Judy Honig
Courtney Reinisch
Janice Smolowitz

The Columbia University School of Nursing doctor of nursing practice (CUSN DNP) curriculum is designed to prepare advanced practice nurses as comprehensive care providers and applies a competency-based approach to educate and to evaluate DNP students. The CUSN competencies of a doctor of nursing practice in comprehensive care (see Table 2.1) form the framework for the curriculum and are integrated throughout the coursework and practica. The direct care competencies are linked to performance objectives that students are expected to achieve and to substantiate in written clinical case narratives.

DOCTOR OF NURSING PRACTICE COMPETENCIES FOR COMPREHENSIVE CARE

Competencies for graduates of the practice doctorate in nursing have been on the national agenda for the nursing profession since 2000, when the notion of a clinical doctorate in nursing was conceived. CUSN began the process of describing doctoral-level competencies in 2000, and published versions appeared in 2003 (CACC), 2005 (CUSN), and 2006 (CACC). The American Association of Colleges of Nursing (AACN) published *The Essentials of Doctoral Education for Advanced Nursing Practice* (2006), and the National Organization of Nurse Practitioner Faculties (NONPF) published the *Practice Doctorate Nurse Practitioner Entry-Level Competencies* (2006). The current CUSN competencies overlap with, and in some domains extend beyond, the AACN and NONPF competencies.

As part of the ongoing evaluation of the CUSN DNP program, it was important to assert that the fundamental structure for the CUSN DNP is consistent with foundational competencies that emerged from the AACN and NONPF. When the competencies for these organizations became available in 2006, the 2006 CUSN DNP competencies were benchmarked against them and again in 2010 when the CUSN DNP competencies were revised (see Table 2.1). In addition, the curricular content of the DNP program was mapped against the CUSN competencies to ensure that all competencies were addressed sufficiently.

Students have academic and clinical experiences that are directed at one or more of the competencies. The competencies also provide the structure for student assessment. Students are expected to meet each of the competencies and to demonstrate their attainment through written case narratives, presentations, publications, and other professional activities.

THE DOCTOR OF NURSING PRACTICE AS A COMPREHENSIVE HEALTH CARE PROVIDER

With the changing demography and diversity of the population and major advances in clinical science and health care delivery systems, the conventional definition of primary care—first-contact, coordinated, and comprehensive care—is expanded and needs to be transitioned into a well-organized personalized health care system that is qualitatively different than it has been in the past. As clinical and medical information becomes more available to patients and patients assume a more active role in directing their own care, the comprehensive care provider's role is expanded to include the expert clinician who views the patient in multiple contexts, interprets and analyzes health care choices, and engages the patient in a collaborative relationship. This redefined primary care is emerging from within the advanced practice nurse (APN) community and is driven by the clinical doctorate. APN/DNP clinicians have the educational background and practice perspective to adopt this new paradigm of primary care—comprehensive care. The crucial educational component of the DNP program is to provide the student with an academic, mentored, integrative clinical experience (residency) in which the student can assimilate and synthesize knowledge in the provision of comprehensive patient care. The outcome measures of this assimilation are in-depth, reflective, evidence-based clinical case narratives.

DIRECT CARE COMPETENCIES AND PERFORMANCE OBJECTIVES

With the increased knowledge and skills necessary for the provision of comprehensive care across settings and over time, CUSN DNP faculty developed a series of detailed, cognitively complex competencies that address the role of the advanced practice nurse in comprehensive care. These competencies form a subset of the CUSN DNP competencies and correspond to Essential 8 in the AACN framework. These specialized competencies, referred to as the Direct Care Competencies, provide direction for the curriculum in direct care and for the assessment of the student as a clinical expert in comprehensive care. Each direct care competency is composed of several performance objectives, which are behaviors that are demonstrated in the provision of direct patient care. The performance objectives describe each competency using measurable behaviors. Students use the performance objectives to determine how to meet and to document attainment of the competency. Table 3.1 presents the direct care competencies and performance objectives. These competencies provide a framework for DNP residents and faculty to assess students' ability to provide clinically complex, culturally sensitive, comprehensive care across settings and over time for patients in the context of family and community. Students demonstrate attainment of the direct care competencies through case presentations in class and by writing competency-based clinical case narratives. CUSN DNP graduates report that clinical case narrative writing is a transformational professional experience.

3.1	Doctor of the Nursing Practice Comprehensive Care Competencies and Performance Objectives for Direct Patient Care
Domain (D) 1. Comprehensive Clinical Care	
Competency (C) 1	**Performance Objective (PO)**
Evaluate patient needs based on age, developmental stage, family history, ethnicity, individual risk, including genetic profile, to formulate plans for health promotion, anticipatory guidance, counseling, and disease prevention services for healthy or sick patients and their families in any clinical setting.	A. Identify a potential genetic risk. B. Diagnose a genetic condition. C. Evaluate individual patient needs based on age, developmental stage, family history, ethnicity, and individual risk. D. Formulate a plan that addresses health promotion, anticipatory guidance, and/or disease prevention for the individual. E. Develop a plan that addresses health promotion, anticipatory guidance, and/or disease prevention for the family.

(continued)

3.1 Doctor of the Nursing Practice Comprehensive Care Competencies and Performance Objectives for Direct Patient Care *(Continued)*

Domain (D) 1. Comprehensive Clinical Care	
Competency (C) 2	**Performance Objective (PO)**
Evaluate population or geographically-based health risk utilizing principles of epidemiology, clinical prevention, environmental health, and biostatistics.	A. Assess the patient/family *at risk* for a condition incorporating epidemiological principles and/or environmental factors that contribute to risk/incidence of disease. B. Assess the patient/family *with* a condition incorporating epidemiological principles and/or environmental factors that contribute to risk/incidence of disease.
Competency (C) 3	**Performance Objective (PO)**
Formulate differential diagnoses, and diagnostic strategies and therapeutic interventions with attention to scientific evidence, safety, cost, invasiveness, simplicity, acceptability, adherence, and efficacy for patients who present with new conditions and those with ambiguous or incomplete data, complex illnesses, comorbid conditions, and multiple diagnoses in all clinical settings.	A. Formulate a differential diagnosis for a patient who presents with new undifferentiated signs and symptoms. B. Formulate a differential diagnosis for a patient who presents with ambiguous or incomplete data, complex illnesses, comorbid conditions, and potential multiple diagnoses. C. Discuss the rationale for the differential diagnosis. D. Discuss the rationale for the diagnostic evaluation with attention to scientific evidence, safety, cost, invasiveness, simplicity, acceptability, adherence, and efficacy. E. Discuss the rationale for the therapeutic intervention with attention to scientific evidence, safety, cost, invasiveness, simplicity, acceptability, adherence, and efficacy.
Competency (C) 4	**Performance Objective (PO)**
Appraise acuity of patient condition, determine need to transfer patient to higher acuity setting, coordinate, and manage transfer to optimize patient outcomes.	A. Assess the acuity of patient status. B. Determine the most appropriate treatment setting based on level of acuity. C. Formulate a transfer plan. D. Implement plan to transfer the patient to a higher level of care utilizing written and oral communication. E. Coordinate care during transition to the higher acuity setting.

(continued)

3.1 *(Continued)*

Domain (D) 1. Comprehensive Clinical Care	
Competency (C) 4	**Performance Objective**
	F. Co-manage care in person, or G. Co-manage care though written and verbal instructions. H. Recommendations for patient disposition from the higher acuity location. I. Coordination of post-discharge care.
Competency (C) 5	**Performance Objective (PO)**
Evaluate and direct care during hospitalization, and design a comprehensive discharge plan for patients from an acute care setting.	A. Assess the acuity of patient's condition and determine the most appropriate inpatient treatment setting based on level of acuity. B. Actively participate in the admission process to the appropriate inpatient treatment setting. C. Actively co-manage patient care during hospitalization. D. Formulate plan for ongoing care to be provided in a subacute setting, such as a long-term care facility, rehabilitation facility, or home or community setting. E. Coordinate ongoing comprehensive care to be provided in a subacute setting, such as a long-term care facility, rehabilitation facility, or home or community setting.
Competency (C) 6	**Performance Objective (PO)**
Direct comprehensive care for patient in a subacute setting to maximize quality of life and functional status.	A. Assess the acuity of the patient's condition to determine the need for subacute, long-term care. B. Determine the most appropriate subacute or chronic care treatment setting based on level of acuity, functional status, and availability of formal and informal caregiver resources. C. Coordinate ongoing comprehensive care provided in a subacute setting. D. Initiate referral to other health care professionals while maintaining primary responsibility for patient care in a subacute setting.

(continued)

3.1 Doctor of the Nursing Practice Comprehensive Care Competencies and Performance Objectives for Direct Patient Care *(Continued)*

Domain (D) 1. Comprehensive Clinical Care	
Competency (C) 6	**Performance Objective (PO)**
	E. Utilize consultant recommendations for decision-making while maintaining primary responsibility for care in a subacute setting.
Competency (C) 7	**Performance Objective (PO)**
Facilitate and guide the process of palliative care and/or planning end-of-life care by discussing diagnoses and prognosis, clarifying and validating patient desires and priorities, and promoting informed choices and shared decision-making by patient, family and members of the health care team.	**A.** Facilitate and guide the palliative care process by discussing diagnoses and prognosis, clarifying and validating patient desires and priorities, and promoting informed choices and shared decision-making by the patient, family, and members of the health care team. **B.** Facilitate and guide planning of end-of-life care by discussing diagnoses and prognosis, clarifying and validating patient desires and priorities, and promoting informed choices and shared decision-making by the patient, family, and members of the health care team.
Domain (D) 2. Interdisciplinary and Patient-Centered Communication	
Competency (C) 1	**Performance Objective (PO)**
Assemble a collaborative interdisciplinary network; refer and consult appropriately while maintaining primary responsibility for comprehensive patient care.	**A.** Initiate referral to other health care professionals while maintaining primary responsibility for patient care. **B.** Accept referrals from other health care professions and communicate consultation findings and recommendations to the referring provider and collaborative network. **C.** Utilize consultation recommendations for decision-making while maintaining primary responsibility for care. **D.** Evaluate outcomes of interventions.

(continued)

3.1 *(Continued)*

Domain (D) 2. Interdisciplinary and Patient-Centered Communication

Competency (C) 1	Performance Objective (PO)
	E. Provide ongoing patient follow-up and monitor outcomes of collaborative network interventions.

Competency (C) 2	Performance Objective (PO)
Coordinate and manage the care of patients with chronic illness utilizing specialists, other disciplines, community resources, and family, while maintaining primary responsibility for direction of patient care and ensuring the seamless flow of information among providers as the focus of care transitions across ambulatory to acute, subacute settings, and community settings.	A. Coordinate care for a patient with chronic illness as the focus of care transitions across ambulatory, acute, subacute, and/or community settings. B. Co-manage care for a patient with chronic illness as the focus of care transitions across ambulatory, acute, subacute, and/or community settings. C. Coordinate care for a patient with chronic illness utilizing specialists, other disciplines, community resources, and family. D. Direct care for patient with chronic illness and ensure the seamless flow of information among providers as the focus of care transitions across settings. E. Co-manage care for a patient with chronic illness utilizing shared decision-making and teaching. F. Co-manage care for a patient with chronic pain as the focus of care transitions across ambulatory, acute, subacute, and/or community settings.

Domain (D) 3. Systems and Context of Care

Competency (C) 1	Performance Objective (PO)
Construct and evaluate outcomes of a culturally sensitive, individualized intervention that incorporates shared decision-making and addresses the specific needs of a patient in context of family and community.	A. Assess culturally specific needs of patient in the context of family and community. B. Construct a culturally sensitive intervention to address the needs of the patient in the context of family and community. C. Evaluate outcomes of the intervention.

(continued)

3.1 Doctor of the Nursing Practice Comprehensive Care Competencies and Performance Objectives for Direct Patient Care *(Continued)*

Domain (D) 3. Systems and Context of Care	
Competency (C) 2	**Performance Objective (PO)**
Evaluate gaps in health care access that compromise optimal patient outcomes, and apply current knowledge of the organization and financing of health care systems to advocate for the patient and to ameliorate negative impact.	A. Identify gaps in access that compromise patient's optimum care. B. Identify gaps in reimbursement that compromise patient's optimum care. C. Demonstrate patient advocacy in the provision of continuous and comprehensive care. D. Apply current knowledge of the organization to ameliorate negative impact. E. Apply current knowledge of health care systems to ameliorate negative impact.
Competency (C) 3	**Performance Objective (PO)**
Synthesize the principles of legal and ethical decision-making and analyze dilemmas that arise in patient care, interprofessional relationships, research, or practice management to improve outcomes.	A. Synthesize ethical principles to address a complex practice dilemma. B. Apply ethical principles to resolve the dilemma. C. Synthesize legal principles to address a complex practice dilemma. D. Apply legal principles to resolve the dilemma.

References

American Association of Colleges of Nursing (AACN). (2006). *The essentials of doctoral education for advanced nursing practice*. Retrieved July 6, 2009, from http://www.aacn.nche.edu/DNP/pdf/Essentials.pdf

Council for the Advancement of Comprehensive Care (CACC). (2003). *Competencies of a clinical nursing doctorate*. New York: Columbia University School of Nursing.

Council for the Advancement of Comprehensive Care (CACC). (2006) *Competencies of a clinical nursing doctorate*. New York: Columbia University School of Nursing.

National Organization of Nurse Practitioner Faculties (NONPF). (2006). *Practice doctorate nurse practitioner entry-level competencies*. Retrieved from http://www.nonpf.com/nonpf2005/PracticeDoctorateResourceCenter/CompetencyDraftFinalApril2006.pdf

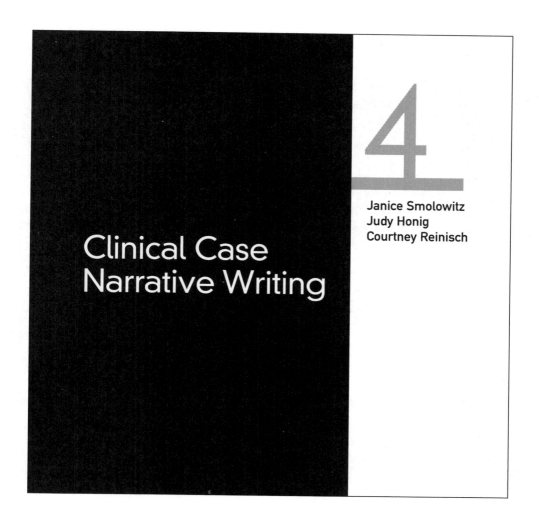

4

Clinical Case Narrative Writing

Janice Smolowitz
Judy Honig
Courtney Reinisch

The Columbia University School of Nursing doctor of nursing practice (CUSN DNP) program is designed to provide advanced practice nurses (APNs) with the knowledge and skills necessary to provide fully accountable, evidence-based care for patients across clinical sites and over time. The purpose of this degree is consistent with the Institute of Medicine's (IOM) definition of primary care as the "provision of integrated, accessible health care services by clinicians who are accountable for addressing a large majority of personal health care needs, developing a sustained partnership with patients, and practicing in the context of family and community" (IOM, 1996, p. 31). The DNP graduate is an expert clinician who views the patient in multiple contexts, interprets and analyzes health care choices, and engages the patient in a collaborative relationship.

The IOM report entitled *Health Professions Education* proposed reforming health professional education to enhance patient care, quality, and safety. This included "competency-based education for clinicians prepared to deliver patient-centered care as members of an interdisciplinary team, emphasizing evidence-based practice, quality improvement approaches, and informatics" (IOM, 2003, p. 3). The IOM called for well-defined clinical doctorates in direct care with standardized graduate competencies.

The publication *Essentials of Doctoral Education for Advanced Nursing Practice* (AACN, 2006) recognized the direct care role for APNs. The DNP APN is described as a clinician with expanded responsibility and accountability in the care and management of individuals and families and is also educated to identify and improve provision of care for a particular population at the aggregate and systems level. The National Organization of Nurse Practitioner Faculties (NONPF) also recognized the direct care role for the APN DNP graduate and defined doctoral competencies with emphasis on independent and interprofessional practice that requires advanced knowledge, skills, and abilities (NONPF, 2006).

AACN and NONPF, leaders in nursing education, have echoed the IOM's recommendations and published guidelines and strong position papers in support of doctoral education that prepares APNs with the necessary skills and competencies to provide comprehensive care. Schools of nursing must educate APN DNPs to address this need.

PORTFOLIO: THE TERMINAL SCHOLARLY PROJECT

The CUSN DNP portfolio is the terminal scholarly project (TSP) submitted in partial fulfillment of the requirements for the degree. The TSP is an intrinsic component of doctoral education that gives the student the opportunity to integrate knowledge amassed during the course of study and provides a foundation for future erudition. The portfolio is a compilation of accomplishments accrued by the student during learning activities and experiences and represents evidence of clinical competence. Portfolios have been used as an appraisal mechanism for professional performance, including the performance of health professionals (Carraccio & Englander, 2004; Cook, Kase, Middelton, & Monsen, 2003; Dannefer & Henson, 2007; Gadbury-Amyot et al., 2003; Lim, Chan, & Cheong, 1998; Kear & Bear, 2007; Melville, Rees, Brookfield, & Anderson, 2004).

The CUSN DNP competencies provide the framework for and are inherently linked to the DNP portfolio (see Table 2.1). All CUSN competencies are met in the portfolio.

CUSN students compile the portfolio during the DNP residency, which is the final integrative clinical experience. Students are assigned to faculty members who have earned the clinical doctorate and have clinical expertise in their specialty. The interaction between these advisors and students is continuous. The advisors encourage students to achieve scholarly products. During the residency, portfolio seminars are conducted in which students present their work for peer and faculty critique using an iterative process. When a student's work achieves the consensus standard determined by a series of inter-rater reviews, it is submitted to the DNP Portfolio Committee for final approval (Smolowitz & Honig, 2008).

CLINICAL CASE NARRATIVES

Clinical case narratives are a prominent and essential component of the DNP portfolio, enabling the student to demonstrate mastery of clinical competencies, translation of research into practice, and interdisciplinary collaboration; they also facilitate evaluation of the student's expertise in the provision, coordination, and direction of care to patients, including those who present in healthy states and those who present with complex, chronic, and/or comorbid conditions, across clinical sites and over time. Each clinical case narrative consists of actual patient encounters that occur during the residency. Each student's portfolio requires a minimum number of complex case narratives to provide sufficient evidence of achievement of this level of comprehensive practice.

CUSN faculty developed the clinical case narrative format to provide a framework wherein students are able to systematically document clinical encounters and faculty members are able to assess performance. The descriptive nature of the narrative provides a basis for understanding the complex cognitive processes employed in the provision of care. The case narrative requires in-depth reflection, high-level analysis and synthesis, and critical appraisal and application of clinical evidence. The clinical case narrative format ensures that all doctoral competencies are made explicit. Some clinical case narratives depict a single encounter that illustrates several competencies, but the majority depict complex management over time and across settings to demonstrate application of the competencies at the DNP level.

Writing the clinical case narratives requires reflection, synthesis of knowledge, and self-appraisal. This experience is transformational and provides the foundation for the pursuit of enduring clinical scholarship for those DNP APNs who choose to provide direct comprehensive care to patients across settings and over time in the context of family, community, and culture; it also provides a measurable outcome of competency-based, doctoral-level behaviors that can be evaluated by an academic committee (Smolowitz & Honig, 2008).

The following section of this chapter presents the format and components of the clinical case narrative. The CUSN faculty standardized this format to facilitate the process of writing and evaluating a clinical case narrative.

GENERAL CLINICAL CASE NARRATIVE FORMAT

The DNP resident demonstrates competence in the provision, coordination, and direction of care to patients, including those who present in healthy states and those who present with complex, chronic, and/or comorbid conditions, across clinical sites and over time. The ability to provide this care is documented in clinical case narratives that demonstrate the resident's ability to meet each of the CUSN doctoral competencies for comprehensive direct patient care. Each competency is composed of several performance objectives.

The following paragraphs describe the recommended format for clinical case narrative writing. Guidelines to assist the student in documenting specific aspects of care for different populations and settings are included in other chapters. It is expected that the DNP resident will utilize institutional guidelines and expert panel guidelines, as a basis for documentation, and adapt the format for specific cases to best illustrate his or her ability to meet the performance objectives and ultimately each CUSN doctoral competency for comprehensive direct patient care.

Privacy

Because the case narrative is written as part of the DNP educational process, it is imperative that patient privacy be protected. CUSN students are required to successfully complete Health Insurance Portability and Accountability Act

(HIPAA) training for researchers and clinicians. They observe HIPAA guidelines and de-identify all patient data in the written case narrative.

Introduction to the Clinical Case Narrative

Each case narrative begins with a paragraph that discusses the reason for selecting the case, the total number of encounters in the narrative, the type of site (ambulatory, home, acute, specialty practice, primary practice, etc.), the type of insurance (commercial, Medicaid, Medicare, self-pay), and the competency or competencies addressed in the case study. The introduction is the only section in which the care provided is described in the past tense.

Example of a Clinical Case Narrative Introduction

The case describes the care I provided for a 60-year-old female with Medicare insurance who presented for evaluation of emotional lability, abnormal gait, and changes in cognition. The case narrative focuses on three encounters that occurred over a period of two months in the ambulatory setting. This case narrative demonstrates my ability to meet the following CUSN doctoral competencies for direct patient care.

DOMAIN 1, COMPETENCY 1

Evaluate patient needs based on age, developmental stage, family history, ethnicity, and individual risk, including genetic profile, to formulate plans for health promotion, anticipatory guidance, counseling, and disease prevention services for healthy or sick patients and their families in any clinical setting.

PO 1A. Identify a potential genetic risk.
PO 1B. Diagnose a genetic condition.
PO 1C. Evaluate individual patient needs based on age, developmental stage, family history, ethnicity, and individual risk.
PO 1D. Formulate a plan that addresses health promotion, anticipatory guidance, and/or disease prevention for the individual.

In this example the DNP resident has listed the competency and only those performance objectives met in the case narrative. The patient's family was not available when care was provided; therefore, the DNP resident did not include PO 1E: Develop a plan that addresses health promotion, anticipatory guidance, and/or disease prevention for the family.

Summary of Care (provided prior to case narrative)

This note is written when the DNP resident assumes care for a patient known to a practice or addresses care prior to the time period that is the focus of the case narrative. For each identified active problem, a brief summary describes the patient care to date and the response to treatment. The following points should be included: initial diagnosis (time of diagnosis), relevant clinical findings, diagnostic tests, interventions, patient response to most recent therapeutic intervention, and proposed plan. The summary of care note precedes the encounter context.

Example: The patient is a 24-year-old white female who has been seen in the Multiple Sclerosis Center for approximately 20 months. She was referred by an ophthalmologist for evaluation of optic neuritis (ON). After a complete diagnostic evaluation that included MRI of the brain, cerebrospinal fluid examination, serum review, and neurological exam, she was diagnosed with multiple sclerosis (MS) and initiated on long-term injectable treatment, interferon beta-1a (Avonex).

While on treatment she continued to have relapses, including sensory, motor, and visual disturbances. She was treated with intravenous steroids for these relapses with benefit to her symptoms. She had reported mild depression and anxiety, especially regarding her diagnosis and "dealing with symptoms," as well as increased fatigue. She was started on fluoxetine (Prozac) 10 mg daily and was referred to a social worker at her last appointment. She was scheduled for today's appointment as a routine follow-up.

Encounter Context

The case narrative begins with the encounter context. This includes information to orient the reader to the initial encounter with regard to setting, time, context, patient demographics, and DNP role.

Example

Encounter Context

Encounter One (initial evaluation)

DNP role: I am an adult nurse practitioner and DNP resident seeing this patient for an initial consult visit.

Identifying Information

Site: Urban academic medical center.

Setting: Movement disorder specialty private office practice.

Reason for encounter: Initial evaluation, referral note on prescription pad from community physician.

Informant: Patient and home attendant. The home attendant has worked with this patient for three days. The home attendant has a referral note from a community physician that states "evaluate and treat patient for memory loss, mood changes, and leg movements." No other medical records are available.

Example

Encounter Context

Encounter One (postoperative day 0)

DNP role: I am an acute care nurse practitioner and DNP resident assuming responsibility of care for this patient.

Identifying information

Site: Urban academic medical center.

Setting: Adult surgical intensive care unit (SICU).

Reason for encounter: Patient admission to the SICU.

Informant: Chart review and surgical team report, as patient is mechanically ventilated and sedated following mitral valve replacement.

Patient Encounter or Encounters

This section forms the body of the narrative. The parts of each encounter vary depending on when the narrative begins. Some narratives begin with an initial comprehensive patient encounter. Other narratives begin with a focused or interval note that builds from the Summary of the Care provided prior to the case narrative, described previously.

Distinct templates are provided in subsequent documents to assist in identifying salient aspects of care that are *usually* addressed in the different types of encounters, populations, and settings.

All encounters are written in the present tense. Most encounters include *some or all* of the following information:

- Chief complaint (in patient's own words or from other source if patient is nonresponsive)
- History of present illness, which includes a relevant review of systems with pertinent positive and negative associated symptoms and risk factors for the presenting complaint
- Current health status, which includes active medical problems being treated that are not related to the presenting complaint
- Past health history
- Social history
- Family history, which may include a genogram
- Review of systems (not related to chief complaint)
- Physical examination

- Laboratory data review
- Impression
  - New or undifferentiated problems
    - For each new or undifferentiated problem or symptom, create a comprehensive list of possible diagnoses *in paragraph form* from most to least likely diagnosis based on the patient's history, which includes the presence and absence of pertinent findings, physical examination, diagnostic tests, and risk factors. Determine the probability of each diagnosis. State the most likely diagnosis and provide a rationale for the determination. This diagnosis and rationale will form the basis of the plan.
  - Ongoing health care needs
    - The status of each ongoing identified health care need is discussed. This assessment will form the basis for the ongoing plan of care.
    - When a previously identified acute or self-limiting health care need resolves, the problem is declared inactive and removed from the active problem list.
    - Health maintenance and immunizations should be addressed according to established guidelines. The patient's health maintenance needs are addressed at appropriate intervals and included in the plan of care under health maintenance.
- Plan: The plan of care may be written in varying formats as dictated by the clinical setting. Each plan should always include the following components.
  - Diagnostic tests
  - Referrals
  - Medications
  - Counseling and education
  - Health care maintenance
  - Follow-up
- An ICD9 code for each diagnosis identified in the impression

Citing and Leveling the Evidence

After appropriate sections of the case narrative, the scientific underpinnings for the clinical decision-making are given in italics. This evidence has usually been published within the past five years.

Sources should include primary sources, meta-analyses, or expert guidelines. The level of evidence for each source is cited using the Centre for Evidence-Based Medicine (CEBM) guideline: http://www.cebm.net/index.aspx?o=1025.

Example

Recurrent chest pain in the absence of coronary artery disease is a common problem that can lead to the excessive use of medical care. This review suggests a small to moderate benefit from psychological interventions, particularly those using a cognitive-behavioral framework. Patients with atypical chest pain who had negative coronary angiography were more likely to report more severe and prolonged symptoms than those who had not had the procedure (Kisely, Campbell, & Skerritt, 2005).

Oxford Centre for Evidence-Based Medicine (CEBM), level 1a.

Documentation of Performance Objectives

The performance objectives of a competency are met by behaviors that direct the outcome of the case narrative. After appropriate sections in the case narrative, the performance objective that was demonstrated by the DNP resident's actions is stated in *bold font*. Documentation explicates the DNP resident's actions, which may be illustrated by education, counseling, treatment interventions, referrals, consultations, or clinical decision-making.

Example: The patient has a congenital cardiac malformation, which is determined almost exclusively by genetics. I discuss this information with him and his wife. They state they understand that blood-related family members may wish to discuss this information with their health care providers. **(D1, C1, PO A, B).**

Critical Appraisal

When appropriate to a section of the case narrative, a detailed discussion of the DNP resident's thought processes is included as a critical appraisal section in a *box*. The critical appraisal may be particularly important to an ethical discussion or when there is conflicted or ambiguous evidence.

Situations such as this can leave health care providers with a delicate ethical dilemma: one between the fundamental ethical principles of autonomy and nonmaleficence. Autonomy is the patient's right to self-determination, whereas nonmaleficence is our responsibility as health care providers to do no harm.

The patient has made his wishes about his care explicitly clear, both in writing and during detailed conversations with his family. Furthermore, although not related to autonomy, his family is in full support of carrying out his wishes given his suffering with previous medical conditions.

Alternatively, health care providers have an ethical responsibility to do no harm to patients. In Western culture, withdrawal of care is considered by many to be giving up or somehow harming the patient. In this situation, the assessments of the neurologist, neurosurgeon, and attending surgeon were unified. There is little hope for recovery that would result in a meaningful life for this patient. The health care team honored the patient's wishes based on his right to autonomy.

Interim Summary Note

The interim summary note is utilized when the DNP resident does not need to provide detailed information about the care provided at specific visits over a period of time. This usually occurs when the patient's condition is stable and the issues addressed at the specific visits are not relevant to the performance objectives and competency that direct the case narrative. For each identified active problem, a brief summary describes the patient care during this intervening period.

Example: I saw the patient in my office every two months for the following six months. She lost 10 pounds by following a nutritious, low-sodium diet and increasing her activity by walking to work. Blood pressure control was achieved with enalapril (Vasotec) 5 mg daily. Her blood pressure at the last appointment, one month prior to today's appointment, was 120/70, and her pulse was 80. She denied any adverse effects from her medications and cardiac symptoms.

Case Summation

This brings the case narrative to its conclusion. This section discusses the outcome of the intervention and the plan for ongoing care, if not discussed in the final encounter.

Example: Stepmother reports that since the last visit three months ago, her child has not had another syncopal episode. He has consciously avoided the neck-stretching movement that preceded the episodes and feels that this has prevented the episodes from reccurring.

Competency Defense

In this final section of the narrative, the DNP resident discusses how each competency was attained. The DNP restates the competency and then critically appraises the care provided and utilizes evidence to demonstrate his or her ability to meet the competency. The defense of each competency is approximately one to two paragraphs in length.

Example

Domain 1, Competency 3. Formulate differential diagnoses and diagnostic strategies and therapeutic interventions with attention to scientific evidence, safety, cost, invasiveness, simplicity, acceptability, adherence, and efficacy for patients who present with new conditions and those with ambiguous or incomplete data, complex illnesses, comorbid conditions, and multiple diagnoses in all clinical settings.

    Defense. The patient's diagnoses were formulated using the DSM-IV criteria for bipolar I disorder, most recent episode mixed, and polysubstance abuse. Given his presenting symptoms, I identified that a polypharmacologic regimen would be essential to control his symptoms. The available evidence supports the efficacy of mood stabilization with antipsychotic therapy. Specifically, valproate (Depakote) was identified as an appropriate agent for use in the patient with mixed mania and comorbid substance abuse. Similarly, aripiprazole (Abilify) is indicated in the treatment of acute and chronic mixed and manic episodes in patients with bipolar I disorder. Because this patient presents with a history of depressive symptoms, antidepressant therapy must be considered. However, the addition of an antidepressant must be done with caution due to the risk of causing a switch in mood polarity. Bupropion (Welbutrin) has been associated with a lower risk for mood polarity switch, making it an ideal option for this patient. Although the literature does not consistently support the efficacy of cognitive behavioral therapy, it was identified as an important component of the treatment regimen.

Additional Documentation

At the end of the case, additional documentation may be provided that is relevant to the case but too detailed to include in the body of the narrative because it would distract from the competency focus. Primary among these documents are monograph-style drug lists that include all the medications discussed in the case narrative and that briefly identify salient indications, pharmacokinetics, and contraindications for the patient. Additional documentation can include pain scales, DSM criteria, validated assessment tools, and institution-specific policies and protocols.

Reference Style

Style should follow the *Publication Manual of the American Psychological Association* (APA), 5th edition.

References

American Association of Colleges of Nursing (AACN). (2005).*The essentials of doctoral education for advanced nursing practice.* Retrieved December 30, 2007, from http://www.aacn.nche.edu/DNP/pdf/Essentials.pdf

Carraccio, C., & Englander, R. (2004). Evaluating competence using a portfolio: A literature review and web-based application to the ACGME competencies. *Teach Learn Med, 16*(4), 381–387.

Cook, S.S., Kase, R., Middelton, L., & Monsen, R.B. (2003). Portfolio evaluation for professional competence: Credentialing in genetics for nurses. *Journal of Professional Nursing, 19*(2), 85–90.

Dannefer, E.F., & Henson, L.C. (2007). The portfolio approach to competency-based assessment at the Cleveland Clinic Lerner College of Medicine. *Academic Medicine, 82*(5), 493–502.

Gadbury-Amyot, C.C., Kim, J., Palm, R.L., Mills, G.E., Noble, E., & Overman, P.R. (2003). Validity and reliability of portfolio assessment of competency in a baccalaureate dental hygiene program. *Journal of Dental Education, 67*(9), 991–1002.

Institute of Medicine (IOM). (1996). *Primary care: America's health in a new era.* Washington, DC: National Academies Press.

Institute of Medicine (IOM). (2003). *Health professions education: A bridge to quality.* Washington, DC: National Academies Press.

Kear, M., & Bear, M. (2007). Using portfolio evaluation for program outcome assessment. *Journal of Nursing Education, 46*(3), 109–114. Retrieved January 14, 2008, from Research Library database.

Lim, J.L., Chan, N.F., & Cheong, P.Y. (1998). Experience with portfolio-based learning in family medicine for master of medicine degree. *Singapore Medical Journal, 39*(12), 543–546.

Melville, C., Rees, M., Brookfield, D., & Anderson, J. (2004). Portfolios for assessment of paediatric specialist registrars. *Medical Education, 38*(10), 1117–1125.

Mundinger, M.O., Kane, R.L., Lenz, E.R., Totten, A.M., Tsai, W.Y., Cleary, P.D., Friedewald, W.T., Siu, A.L., & Shelanski, M.L. (2000). Primary outcomes in patients treated by nurse practitioners or physicians: A randomized trial. *Journal of the American Medical Association, 283,* 59–68.

National Organization of Nurse Practitioner Faculties (NONPF) National Panel for NP Practice Doctorate Competencies. (2006). *Practice doctorate nurse practitioner entry-level competencies.* Retrieved December 30, 2007, from http://www.nonpf.com/NONPF2005/PracticeDoctorateResourceCenter/CompetencyDraftFinalApril2006.pdf

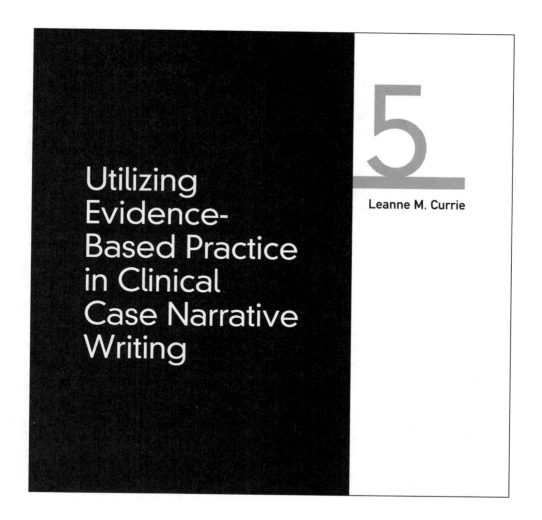

Utilizing Evidence-Based Practice in Clinical Case Narrative Writing

5

Leanne M. Currie

Evidence-based practice (EBP) is the process of identifying the best available evidence to guide patient-centered clinical decisions (Sackett, Straus, Richardson, Rosenberg, & Haynes, 2000). The American Nurses Association (ANA) 2004 Social Policy Statement expressly indicates that one of the six components of contemporary nursing practice is the "application of scientific knowledge to the process of diagnosis and treatment through the use of judgment and critical thinking" (American Nurses Association, 2004, 6). However, it has become increasingly difficult for individual clinicians to manage the vast amounts of information that are published on an annual basis. Indeed, it is not physically possible to keep current with all new information in one's domain. For example, Alper and colleagues (2004) estimated that an internal medicine provider would need to read approximately 240 relevant journals, including more than 7,000 journal articles, per month, which could take on average 627.5 hours in that month. Since there are only 720 hours in a month, there is not enough time to examine all possibly relevant information.

According to Cabana et al. (2000), several barriers to guideline use and EBP exist, including lack of awareness, lack of familiarity, lack of agreement, lack of self-efficacy (the perceived inability to implement new practice or to understand the research literature), lack of outcome expectancy (the perception that new practice won't work), and the inertia of previous practice (it's too hard to learn a new practice). These barriers likely lead to regional practice variation, whereby some guidelines are implemented but other guidelines are not implemented, often with underserved communities being the ones that have slower guideline adoption rates (Fisher, Bynum, & Skinner, 2009). One of the goals of EBP is to ensure that nationally recommended guidelines are adopted across all settings. This chapter provides an overview of the skills and knowledge required to apply evidence to practice in a patient-centered manner.

EVIDENCE-BASED PRACTICE

Evidence-based practice involves applying a set of skills to evaluate, translate, and integrate published research findings into clinical practice using a patient-centered approach (Sackett et al., 2000; Straus, Richardson, Glasziou, & Haynes, 2005). The Scottish epidemiologist Archie Cochrane is typically accredited with founding the evidence-based practice movement when he published a book entitled *Effectiveness and Efficiency: Random Reflections on Health Services* in 1972. He discussed the need for periodic critical summary of relevant randomized controlled trials. In 1981 Cochrane co-founded the Oxford Database of Perinatal Trials (ODPT), affectionately known as "Odd Pot," and this was followed by the Cochrane Pregnancy and Childbirth Database (CCPC) in 1992. Finally, in 1993, the Cochrane Collaboration was established as a not-for-profit entity that publishes systematic reviews on a wide range of topics. Around this time, Gordon Guyatt and David Sackett, both physicians at McMaster University in Canada, founded the Evidence-Based Medicine Working Group (Evidence-Based Medicine Working Group et al., 1992; Montori & Guyatt, 2008), and the term *evidence-based medicine* was coined.

These efforts were concurrent with the nursing movement toward increased utilization of research in practice (Closs & Cheater, 1994), and the past 10 years have seen a gradual transition from "research utilization" to "evidence-based practice" in nursing. Indeed, a growing number of evidence-based nursing texts and resources have been published, and several groups have developed models for evidence-based nursing, including Dicenso and colleagues (Dicenso, Guyatt, & Ciliska, 2005) and the Iowa Model of Evidence-Based Practice to Promote Quality of Care (Titler, 2006).

As EBP efforts move forward, several centers for EBP (or evidence-based medicine) have been founded. These centers, such as the Agency for Healthcare Research and Quality (AHRQ) in the United States and the Oxford Centre for Evidence-Based Medicine (CEBM) in the United Kingdom, have been valuable in providing online resources to support dissemination of evidence and evidence-based practice skills. In addition, the AHRQ has established Evidence-Based Practice Centers, of which 14 are currently funded and whose charge is to identify best practice recommendations via synthesis of research evidence (Agency for Healthcare Research and Quality, 2008).

In order to provide EBP skills, the Columbia University School of Nursing (CUSN) curriculum utilizes Sackett et al.'s (2000) *Evidence-Based Medicine* text, with additional resources integrated to support all steps of the EBP process.

According to Sackett, the EBP process has five steps: (1) formulate an answerable question, (2) identify the best available evidence, (3) critically appraise the evidence, (4) apply the evidence, and (5) evaluate the effectiveness of the evidence-based action. Each of these steps requires a set of specific skills, which are outlined in the following text.

Step 1: The PICO Question

The first step in the EBP process is formulating an answerable question. The structure used to formulate the clinical question is called PICO: the question should contain information about research related to a specific group of **P**atients, a specific **I**ntervention (or exposure) was studied as **C**ompared to another intervention (or exposure), and the research targeted a specific **O**utcome of interest. There are several formats to PICO questions, and these are contingent on the type of primary research required to answer the clinical question. Table 5.1 provides examples of PICO questions for different types of research studies, including questions that have resulted in reports published by CUSN DNP students.

Formulating the PICO question is relatively easy for most clinicians who identify clinical practice questions multiple times a day. However, some clinicians identify clinical questions that would require primary research, which are not relevant for a formal systematic review. Thus, formulation of the PICO question is an iterative process that is often clarified during step 2, identification of the evidence.

Step 2: Identify the Evidence

Identifying the evidence involves effectively using bibliographic resources from health science literature, which requires a relatively high level of information literacy. Information literacy is defined as the ability "to recognize when information is needed and . . . to locate, evaluate, and use effectively the needed information" (American Library Association, 1989, 2). The framework set forth by Haynes (2007), "The 5S evolution of information services for evidence-based healthcare decisions," is used to characterize the types of literature available. The 5S hierarchy categorizes research evidence from the least to the most easy to apply to practice: studies (least useful), syntheses, synopses, summaries, and systems (most useful).

Studies are published primary research studies that typically have gone through peer review but no other synthesis. As stated earlier, clinicians would need to read prolifically to capture all studies in their domain; therefore, studies are considered the least useful to busy clinicians. *Syntheses* are systematic reviews such as those conducted by the Cochrane collaboration; other evidence-based groups, such as the Joanna Briggs Institute (2009), that provide evidence-based resources for health care professionals in nursing, midwifery, medicine, and allied health; and other author groups. Syntheses are considered more useful than studies but still require effort to apply to practice. *Synopses* are brief, succinct descriptions of an individual study or a systematic review. Because they are typically one page long and are designed for easy reading, they are more useful to clinicians than studies or syntheses. Synopses are

5.1 Examples of PICO Questions for Specific Question Types

Type of Research	Patient	Intervention/ Exposure	Comparison	Outcome
Therapy[a]	Children with Type 1 diabetes	Continuous subcutaneous insulin infusion pump	Multiple daily injections	• HbA1c levels • Hypoglycemia
Therapy[b]	Adults with bipolar disorder	Omega-3 fatty acid supplementation	No supplement	Bipolar symptoms
Harm[c]	Women with previous c-section	Single-layer uterine suture	Double-layer uterine suture	Uterine rupture during subsequent trial of labor
Diagnosis[d]	European males	Prostate-specific antigen (PSA)	Prostate biopsy	Diagnostic accuracy of PSA
Prognosis[c]	Adults with lymphoma or leukemia	Donor lymphocyte infusion-induced graft versus lymphoma/ leukemia	Traditional hematopoietic stem cell transplantation (HCST)	Cancer remission and survival
Economic[e]	Patients with nonulcer dyspepsia infected with H. pylori	Drug treatment for H. pylori eradication	Placebo	• Dyspepsia • Health service costs

[a]Student project by Churchill & Ruppe (Churchill, Ruppe, & Smaldone, 2009).
[b]Student project by Turnbull & Cullen-Drill (Turnbull, Cullen-Drill, & Smaldone, 2008).
[c]Unpublished student projects.
[d]Diagnosis example (Harvey et al., 2009).
[e]Economic example (Moayyedi et al., 2000).

accessed via evidence-based journals, such as *Evidence-Based Nursing* (EBN), the *American College of Physicians (ACP) Journal Club,* or the *Database of Abstracts of Reviews of Effects* (DARE). *Summaries* are brief reports, two or three pages at most, on a given topic that summarize information from multiple sources (i.e., not only data from randomized controlled trials). Providers of summaries include the *British Medical Journal*'s (BMJ) "Clinical Evidence" and the ACP Physician's Information and Education Resource (PIER). Summaries are typically very useful but may become out of date quickly; therefore, they must have a method for frequent updates if new research comes to light. Finally, *systems* are computer-based clinical decision support systems that can provide current, patient-specific evidence to clinicians at the point of care (Bates et al., 2003).

According to Haynes (2007), systems are the least overwhelming, the quickest to use, and the easiest to apply of all types of resources. Furthermore, well-designed decision support systems have been shown to facilitate guideline adoption and prevent medical errors (Garg et al., 2005). However, decision support systems have been adopted slowly because developing such systems requires a large investment by health care organizations in time, expertise, and money; thus these systems are not likely to be ubiquitous for some time yet (Jha et al., 2009).

Several of the Web-based preappraised resources (syntheses, synopses, and summaries) have methods to characterize the quality of the study. For example, the BMJ's Clinical Evidence, a summary, uses a series of icons to denote the clinical applicability of summarized research findings, including two arrows pointing up to indicate "beneficial" and two question marks to indicate "unknown effectiveness." Use of such icons can facilitate easy scanning of these resources by busy clinicians. Web-based resources often have hyperlinks that can take the clinician directly to the individual research study on which a clinical recommendation is based. These tools can facilitate access to information for clinicians.

When preappraised resources fail to answer a clinical question and a systematic review must be conducted, clinicians must be skilled at finding individual articles. Students use subject headings (such as Medical Subject Headings—MeSH) and other search terms, in both *Medline* (PubMed) and in the *Cumulative Index of Nursing and Allied Health* (CINAHL). Students also use three important *Boolean search operators*: AND, OR, and NOT (Hersch, Stavri, & Detmer, 2006).

Step 3: Critically Appraise the Evidence

Once the unfiltered studies have been identified, they are critically appraised. To make this appraisal, the clinician must be able to comprehensively understand unfiltered published research reports. Students use the Oxford CEBM levels of evidence framework with critical appraisal questions from Straus et al. (2005) and systematic review guidelines from the Centre for Reviews and Dissemination (CRD) at York University in the United Kingdom (Centre for Reviews and Dissemination, 2009). Table 5.2 lists the levels of evidence based on the Oxford CEBM. Several other groups have developed tools for grading the evidence, and most systems have similar goals (Atkins et al., 2004). DNP students use the CEBM tool because it provides adequate information to justify each level of evidence in a summarized manner.

An understanding of basic epidemiological, biostatistical, and research principles is also required for critical appraisal of evidence. Gehlbach's *Interpreting the Medical Literature* (2006) is a valuable resource to help students understand research designs and applications of basic statistics. Types of study designs include randomized controlled trials (RCTs) and other experimental and quasi-experimental designs; epidemiological studies, including cohort, case-control, and descriptive designs; systematic reviews and meta-analyses; economic evaluations; and qualitative designs, including phenomenology,

5.2   CEBM Levels of Evidence

Level 1—Strongest Evidence (the BEST evidence)

1a—Systematic review/meta-analysis
1b—Individual well-designed studies (e.g., rigorous randomized controlled trials [RCTs]
   or cohort studies)

Level 2—Strong Evidence

2a—Systematic review of less rigorous studies
2b—Individual RCTs with design flaws or other less rigorous studies
2c—"Outcomes" research

Level 3—Moderate Strength Evidence

3a—Systematic review of yet less rigorous studies (case-control, nonconsecutive cohort)
3b—Individual case-control or nonconsecutive cohort study

Level 4—Weak Evidence

4—Case series or poor case-control study

Level 5—Weakest Evidence

5—Expert opinion without explicit critical appraisal

Source: *Oxford Centre for Evidence-Based Medicine Levels of Evidence* (Philips et al., 2009).

grounded theory, ethnography, and historical research. Although qualitative methods are typically not discussed in typical EBP texts, the topic is important because qualitative research often identifies new concepts and clarifies confusing research findings, and thus can be valuable for clinicians.

Study quality assessment involves establishing the internal and external validity of a given study. Validity is the extent to which a variable or intervention actually measures what it is supposed to measure or accomplishes what it is supposed to accomplish. Internal validity is the integrity of the study design and procedures, whereas external validity is whether or not the results can be applied to a larger population.

EBP skills include understanding basic epidemiological principles, such as estimating the treatment effects of therapeutic studies. Calculations such as relative risk (RR), relative risk reduction (RRR), absolute risk reduction (ARR), and numbers needed to treat (NNT) provide the necessary information to determine clinical relevance. Many research reports provide these data; however, if these data are not present in a research report, the DNP can perform these relatively simple calculations and thereby can identify the clinical applicability of study findings. Of these calculations, the most important estimate is the NNT, which is the number of patients needed to treat to see one beneficial outcome or to prevent one adverse outcome (Straus et al., 2005).

For studies that examine the accuracy of diagnostic and screening instruments, one must understand sensitivity and specificity, positive predictive value (PPV), and negative predictive value (NPV). For studies that report on prognosis, the key components of survival analysis are provided, including hazard ratios and survival curves. Finally, key processes of economic studies are presented with skills to perform critical appraisals of such studies.

In order to understand and interpret the findings reported in a research study, one must thoroughly understand the concept of statistical significance. Number lines visually model the relationship between *p*-values and alpha levels and between anchor points and confidence intervals. Figure 5.1 shows the use of number lines to characterize confidence intervals for continuous results and for ratio results. Although understanding statistical significance is a key part of the curriculum, it is clearly reinforced that statistical significance does not imply clinical significance, thus preserving the patient-centeredness of EBP.

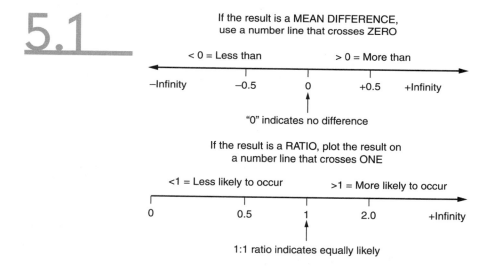

Step 4: Apply the Evidence

Once the evidence is critically appraised, the DNP student can apply it to practice. Using critical appraisal tools (CATs), students grade the evidence that is available for the clinical problem identified during the clinical experience (Straus et al., 2005). The case narrative exemplars provided in this text demonstrate students' critical appraisal of each resource and assignment of a level of evidence based on the CEBM levels of evidence. Evidence is summarized throughout each case to support each clinical decision, thus demonstrating the thoughtful application of evidence to practice. Each case narrative also clearly delineates patient preferences and patient-specific tailoring, taking into consideration details such as genetic risk factors, patient lab values, and cost. Advanced clinical skills and critical judgment of the DNP demonstrate the skillful application of evidence to practice.

Step 5: Evaluate the Practice Change

The final phase of the EBP process is evaluating practice change. Originally, this meant reflecting on one's practice behaviors, but evaluation of practice currently has a broader meaning, that of practice-based evidence (PBE). The vision for DNP practice and health care in general is to move toward PBE so that characteristics and outcomes of clinical practice can be evaluated over time. Furthermore, PBE can mean identifying new knowledge from practice, with systems designed to capture data as a byproduct of care (Lang, 2008). Proponents of PBE propose that data from routine clinical practice can be used to evaluate patient outcomes (Horn & Gassaway, 2007). Thus, rather than costly and complicated randomized controlled trials, clinical outcomes can be measured based on observational and retrospective studies.

Throughout the CUSN DNP program, clinicians develop plans to evaluate clinical practice change. They are provided with tools to evaluate their practice, such as benchmarking and evaluating guideline integration via informatics methods to ensure that data are captured as a byproduct of care. EBP skills provide a method for the DNP to critically appraise evidence and to use his or her clinical judgment to apply the evidence in a patient-centered manner.

References

Agency for Healthcare Research and Quality. (2008). *Evidence-based practice centers overview*. Retrieved September 8, 2009, from http://www.ahrq.gov/clinic/epc/

Alper, B.S., Hand, J.A., Elliot, S.G., Kinkade, S., Hauan, M.J., Onion, D.K., et al. (2004). How much effort is needed to keep up with the literature relevant for primary care? *Journal of the Medical Library Association, 92*(4), 429–437.

American Library Association. (1989). *Presidential Committee on Information Literacy: Final report*. Washington, DC: American Library Association. Retrieved January 20, 2010: http://www.ala.org/ala/mgrps/divs/acrl/publications/whitepapers/presidential.cfm

American Nurses Association. (2004). *Nursing: Scope and standards of practice*. Washington, DC: American Nurses Association. (A.N. Publishing). Retrieved January 20, 2010: www.nursingworld.org

Atkins, D., Eccles, M., Flottorp, S., Guyatt, G., Henry, D., Hill, S., et al. (2004). Systems for grading the quality of evidence and the strength of recommendations I: Critical appraisal of existing approaches. The GRADE Working Group. *BMC Health Services Research, 4*(1), 38.

Bates, D.W., Kuperman, G.J., Wang, S., Gandhi, T., Kittler, A., Volk, L., et al. (2003). Ten commandments for effective clinical decision support: Making the practice of evidence-based medicine a reality. *Journal of the American Medical Information Association, 10*(6), 523–530.

Cabana, M.D., Ebel, B.E., Cooper-Patrick, L., Powe, N.R., Rubin, H.R., & Rand, C.S. (2000). Barriers pediatricians face when using asthma practice guidelines. *Archives of Pediatric Adolescent Medicine, 154*(7), 685–693.

Centre for Reviews and Dissemination. (2009). *Systematic reviews: CRD's guidance for undertaking reviews in health*. Retrieved January 20, 2010 from http://www.york.ac.uk/inst/crd/pdf/Systematic_Reviews.pdf

Churchill, J.N., Ruppe, R.L., & Smaldone, A. (2009). Use of continuous insulin infusion pumps in young children with Type 1 diabetes: A systematic review. *Journal of Pediatric Health Care, 23*(3), 173–179.

Closs, S.J., & Cheater, F. (1994). Utilization of nursing research: Culture, interest and support. *Journal of Advanced Nursing, 19*(4), 762–773.

Cochrane, A.L. *Effectiveness and Efficiency: Random Reflections on Health Services.* London: Nuffield Provincial Hospitals Trust, 1972. (Reprinted in 1989 in association with BMJ. Reprinted in 1999 for Nuffield Trust by the Royal Society of Medicine Press, London.)

Dicenso, A., Guyatt, G., & Ciliska, D. (2005). *Evidence-based nursing: A guide to clinical practice.* Philadelphia: Mosby.

Evidence-Based Medicine Working Group, Guyatt, G., Cairns, J., Churchill, D., Cook, D., Haynes, B., et al. (1992). Evidence-based medicine: A new approach to teaching the practice of medicine. *Journal of the American Medical Association, 268*(17), 2420–2425.

Fisher, E.S., Bynum, J.P., & Skinner, J.S. (2009). Slowing the growth of health care costs—Lessons from regional variation. *New England Journal of Medicine, 360*(9), 849–852.

Garg, A.X., Adhikari, N.K.J., McDonald, H., Rosas-Arellano, M.P., Devereaux, P.J., Beyene, J., et al. (2005). Effects of computerized clinical decision support systems on practitioner performance and patient outcomes: A systematic review. *Journal of the American Medical Association, 293*(10), 1223–1238.

Gehlbach, S.H. (2006). *Interpreting the medical literature: Practical epidemiology for clinicians* (5th ed.). New York: McGraw-Hill Medical.

Harvey, P., Basuita, A., Endersby, D., Curtis, B., Iacovidou, A., & Walker, M. (2009). A systematic review of the diagnostic accuracy of prostate specific antigen. *BMC Urology, 9*(1), 14.

Haynes, B. (2007). Of studies, syntheses, synopses, summaries, and systems: The "5S" evolution of information services for evidence-based healthcare decisions. *Evidence-Based Nursing, 10*(1), 6–7.

Hersch, W., Stavri, P.Z., & Detmer, W.M. (2006). Information retrieval and digital libraries. In E.C. Shortliffe, J.J. Cimino (Eds.), *Biomedical informatics: Computer applications in health care and biomedicine.* New York: Springer.

Horn, S.D., & Gassaway, J. (2007). Practice-based evidence study design for comparative effectiveness research. *Medical Care Comparative Effectiveness and Safety: Emerging Methods, 45*(10), S50–S57.

Jha, A.K., DesRoches, C.M., Campbell, E.G., Donelan, K., Rao, S.R., Ferris, T.G., et al. (2009). Use of electronic health records in U.S. hospitals. *New England Journal of Medicine, 360*(16), 1628–1638.

Joanna Briggs Institute. (2009). *Joanna Briggs Institute model of evidence-based health care.* Retrieved January 20, 2010, from http://www.joannabriggs.edu.au/about/jbi_model.php

Lang, N.M. (2008). The promise of simultaneous transformation of practice and research with the use of clinical information systems. *Nursing Outlook, 56*(5), 232–236.

Moayyedi, P., Soo, S., Deeks, J., Forman, D., Mason, J., Innes, M., et al. (2000). Systematic review and economic evaluation of *Helicobacter pylori* eradication treatment for non-ulcer dyspepsia. *British Medical Journal, 321*(7262), 659–664.

Montori, V.M., & Guyatt, G. (2008). Progress in evidence-based medicine. *Journal of the American Medical Association, 300*(15), 1814–1816.

Philips, R., Ball, C., Sackett, D.L., Badenoch, D., Straus, S.E., Haynes, B., et al. (2009, March). *Oxford Centre for Evidence-Based Medicine levels of evidence.* Retrieved January 20, 2010, from http://www.cebm.net/index.aspx?o=1025

Sackett, D.L., Straus, S.E., Richardson, W.S., Rosenberg, W., & Haynes, R.B. (2000). *Evidence-based medicine: How to practice and teach EBM* (2nd ed.). Edinburgh & New York: Churchill Livingstone.

Straus, S.E., Richardson, W.S., Glasziou, P., & Haynes, R.B. (2005). *Evidence-based medicine: How to practice and teach EBM* (3rd ed.). Edinburgh: Churchill Livingstone.

Titler, M.G. (2006). Developing an evidence-based practice. In G. Lobiondo-Wood & J. Haber (Eds.), *Nursing research: Methods and critical appraisal for evidence-based practice* (6th ed.). St. Louis: Mosby.

Turnbull, T., Cullen-Drill, M., & Smaldone, A. (2008). Efficacy of omega-3 fatty acid supplementation on improvement of bipolar symptoms: A systematic review. *Archives of Psychiatric Nursing, 22*(5), 305–311.

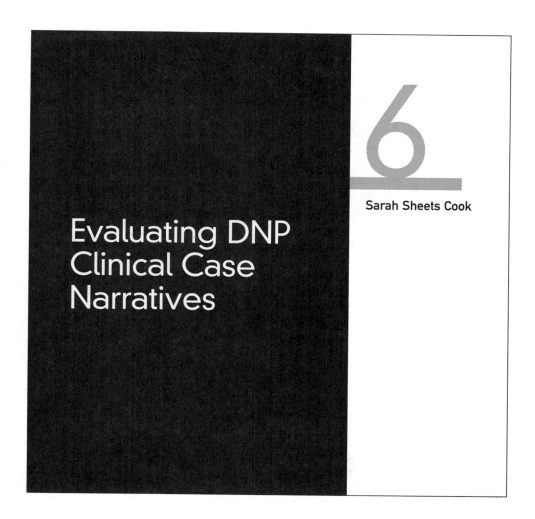

Sarah Sheets Cook

Evaluating DNP Clinical Case Narratives

The evaluation of competency achievement for the direct, cross-site clinical care doctorate in nursing practice (DNP) uses the DNP portfolio as evidence of scholarly practice at a level beyond the master's or single-site comprehensive care. Among the most compelling components of the DNP portfolio are the case narratives, which offer the candidate the opportunity to illuminate his or her aptitude at providing high-quality comprehensive care that embodies the essential competencies of the degree. The creation and format of these narratives are explicated in previous chapters in this section of the book. This chapter discusses methods for evaluating the narrative case studies.

At Columbia University School of Nursing (CUSN), the developmental evaluation of case narratives is a multistep process. During the year that candidates are taking didactic courses, they are required to present cases in class. The format used for this presentation is the same as the format required for the portfolio narrative cases. Before a case is presented, the candidate reviews the content with his or her clinical mentor (who often is a physician) to be sure the content is accurate. The student then posts the case to the shared files of the course with links to the relevant peer-reviewed articles used to support critical decisions in the case. All students read the narrative and articles prior to class and prepare for discussion based on their individual expertise. When the case is presented in class, it is critiqued by the candidate's peers for coherence, completeness, and utilization of the most current and relevant evidence to support clinical decisions. Candidates are required to present several cases, in different didactic courses, for example, in the DNP seminar courses, genetics/genomics course, and environmental/epidemiology course.

At the beginning of the residency, candidates are assigned a portfolio advisor. The DNP advisor is chosen from DNP faculty with an area of expertise or specialization congruent with that of the candidate. The advisor engages in a continuous dialogue with the candidate, throughout the residency, as case narratives are developed. Initially, the advisor provides process feedback, demonstrating to the candidate where the presented case varies from the required format and content. It is not uncommon for the first few narratives to require several revisions. Most candidates improve their narrative format and process consistency by the third or fourth case. The advisor also discusses the evidence chosen for justification of interventions, making sure that all the criteria the candidate proposes are addressed. It is especially important for the advisor to encourage a balance between current medical practice evidence and comprehensive nursing practice.

The residency mentor is an expert clinician who agrees to precept and directly supervise the DNP student during the residency to facilitate clinical experiences in multiple settings. Importantly, in partnership with the course director and portfolio advisor, the mentor participates in the case narrative writing and serves as the content expert.

Most of this process happens electronically using a Word program that allows electronic tracking for document review. Face-to-face discussion of narratives can happen as frequently as the candidate and advisor are able and wish to schedule such a meeting. However, if the candidate lives at a distance, online "discussion" using Skype or similar programs can facilitate a real-time discussion. After the narrative is in a form that satisfies the candidate, mentor, and advisor it is circulated among DNP residents, who provide input as peers with different perspectives. This review can occur during one of the monthly resident seminars or as an online discussion. Finally, the narrative is submitted to the Narrative Review Committee, which makes a final determination. Following that, the narrative becomes part of the portfolio for final, formal presentation to the Portfolio Committee. The Portfolio Committee may request further revisions until the case narrative is approved for inclusion in the DNP Portfolio.

Thus, there are several evaluation touch points over the two years of doctoral study in regard to case narratives. The first point is content validation with clinical colleagues and faculty during the didactic year. The second point is peer evaluation during class presentation of the case during the didactic and residency year. The third point is evaluation with the residency mentor, case narrative advisor, classmates, and ultimately the Narrative Case Review Committee and the Portfolio Committee.

Case narratives demonstrate candidate competency at achieving the CUSN direct care competencies (CACC, 2003), the American Association of Colleges of Nursing (ACCN) Essential VIII Advanced Nursing Practice (AACN, 2006), and the National Organization of Nurse Practitioner Faculties (NONPF) competencies for independent practice as a nurse practitioner (NONPF, Practice Doctorate Practitioner Entry-level Competencies, 2006). Evaluation of such presentations needs to assess not only the objectives of the Essential but also the specific performance behaviors that demonstrate achievement of the competency.

CUSN faculty have identified 12 doctoral competencies for direct patient care (see Table 3.1). Holmes, McAlpine, and Russell (2005) validate that "well-defined and user-friendly standards, components of standards, indicators of satisfactory accomplishment and scoring system . . . are essential elements for a reliable portfolio system" (81). Achievement of standards can be assessed either through screening (the standard is met or it isn't) or through evaluation. Case narratives involve components of both screening (Are the major elements of the narrative presentation included?) and evaluation (How well does the candidate explicate and provide evidence for clinical reasoning and decision-making?).

Evaluation of performance using competency-based methods is somewhat different from the use of traditional ranking systems, which look for a distribution of candidate performance. Dannefer and Henson (2007, p. 494) point out that portfolio use allows consideration of multiple sources and types of evidence and that the goal of this approach is to help students become reflective practitioners and continuous learners. The concept of competency-based evaluation is not a new one, appearing often in the literature during the 1970s and 1980s (see Carraccio et al., 2002, for a summary), and the evaluation method for case narratives uses this approach rather than one that stratifies or ranks candidate performance.

It is possible to identify the competency and its performance objectives in the narrative presentation by keeping a simple check sheet as to whether or not there is evidence of achievement (see Table 6.1).

For example, the second competency, requiring evaluation of a population or geographically based health risk using principles of epidemiology, clinical prevention, environmental health, and biostatistics, is evidenced by the narrative assessing a patient and family *at risk* for a condition—identifying the condition using epidemiological principles or environmental factors (e.g., the relative risk for asthma in an urban manufacturing district)—and/or assessing a patient and family *with* a condition (e.g., three of four young children with asthma and a grandmother with chronic obstructive pulmonary disease all living in crowded, substandard urban housing) and identifying related epidemiological or environmental factors operational in the situation. However, such an evaluation can take many pages and can become tedious and very linear or quantitative. The mentor or advisor checks to make sure major components are included and evaluates the quality of clinical reasoning and decision-making based on the mentor's or advisor's own clinical expertise and experience. Having several "gatekeepers" in the process of accepting a case narrative as meeting the standards identified—all five sources (the clinical mentor, peers, the case narrative advisor, the case narrative review committee, and the final portfolio evaluators)—provides a reasonable degree of inter-rater reliability when all levels are in agreement. If these sources are not in agreement, specific consensus-building conferencing is used for resolution.

Such a method does not necessarily recognize the differences in weights or relevance among the performance objectives or additional performance objectives, which may be important. This method may also miss the subtle nuances in the narrative that demonstrate the writer's sensitivity to individual and specific conditions in the situation. Although expert readers may and usually do recognize these nuances, it is sometimes difficult to identify how much weight the nuanced evaluation carried in the final evaluation. To quantify inter-rater reliability, it may be more reasonable and desirable to have an algorithm for scoring and codifying results. At CUSN, students are required to identify which performance objectives their narrative illustrates and the supporting evidence. This gives the candidate the opportunity to explain why a specific management expectation or standard of care or treatment may not apply in a particular situation and why she or he chose to take action that was counter to accepted evidence. The practice of nursing at this level, like the practice of medicine, is not always an "either/or," "apply or don't apply" situation. Furthermore, candidates are required to evaluate the nature and the weight of the evidence. Analyzing the process of the student's critical thinking and decision-making is as important as evaluating the achievement of performance objectives. This becomes an iterative process for the narrative sponsor as the cases are refined over the time of the residency and is also evident in the final case presentation to the narrative review committee and the portfolio reviewers.

Use of modern bioinformatics can assist in the process of evaluating the achievement of program competencies in a case narrative. Word pattern recognition using automated text categorization can provide a rapid assessment of key words and phrases that one would expect to find for a given competency. The principle is somewhat similar to the technology behind the well-known Turnitin program for detection of plagiarism. More sophisticated programs can incorporate machine learning, so that the program refines its search potential based on the types of documents and key words and phrases it is programmed to discover (Fabrizio, 2003). Either of these processes leaves more time for the reviewer to consider the integration of content explicated in the narrative and whether or not there is evidence of reflective and comprehensive practice.

Another use of bioinformatics employs a neural net program to combine raters' scores of a given portfolio. Several readers might evaluate the narrative cases and assign a score signifying how well the rater assesses the candidate in meeting the competencies explicated. The scores are entered into the neural net program, which then generates a "met competencies" or "did not meet competencies" score. Holmes et al. (2005) point out that there are several valid rating systems—pass/fail, go/no-go, and Likert-like scales. It is important to use a scale that does not elicit much, if any, emotional response from the candidates or evaluators. Holmes et al. suggest using whole numbers from 2 to 10, in two-digit inclinations. Having two inclinations between score points makes it easier to differentiate ratings, and a scale of 4 ("needs much improvement") to 10 ("exceeds standard"), with 8 being "meets standard," is fairly easy to use.

The rationale for using such a program rather than simply clinical mentors and experienced case narrative advisor evaluations is that expert judgments at some point are bound to vary. Although consensus conferencing may resolve differences of opinion, a neural net scoring system can accommodate these differences with an accuracy and validity of 97 percent. Neural network programs (Hanson & Marshall, 2001) are designed to mimic human cognition, which is multidimensional and chaotic (not linear). Cook et al. (2003) point out that the use of a specific neural network program derived from the case narrative competencies allows aggregate scores of raters to be considered *in toto* but also to be weighted according to both a predetermined and also evolving set of parameters, much like one might change an opinion based on new evidence. For example, it is possible that DNP competencies 1, 3, and 4 should carry more weight in case narrative evaluation than competencies 2 and 5. A neural network system can accommodate these weighted differences. Neural networks are data-driven support systems, as opposed to model-driven decision supports. Model-driven systems are designed to reproduce a specific expert opinion and do not accommodate new knowledge without significant reconfiguration. Data-driven systems are fluid and autodidactic to accommodate new data and patterns. Continued case narrative writing presents an opportunity to develop such a system tailored to the needs of the DNP student who is providing comprehensive care.

6.1 CUSN DNP Competencies for Direct Patient Care Residency Case Narrative Log

DNP students specializing in comprehensive care will demonstrate expertise in the provision, coordination, and direction of comprehensive care to patients, including those who present in healthy states and those who present with complex, chronic, and/or comorbid conditions, across clinical sites and over time. The DNP student will:

Domain (D) 1. Comprehensive Clinical Care

Competency	Competency Demonstrated	Performance Objectives (PO)	PO Demonstrated
Competency (C) 1		Performance Objective (PO)	
Evaluate patient needs based on age, developmental stage, family history, ethnicity, individual risk—including genetic profile—to formulate plans for health promotion, anticipatory guidance, counseling, and disease prevention services for healthy or sick patients and their families in any clinical setting.		A. Identify a potential genetic risk. B. Diagnose a genetic condition. C. Evaluate individual patient needs based on age, developmental stage, family history, ethnicity, and individual risk. D. Formulate a plan that addresses health promotion, anticipatory guidance, and/or disease prevention for the individual. E. Develop a plan that addresses health promotion, anticipatory guidance, and/or disease prevention for the family.	

(continued)

6.1 *(Continued)*

Domain (D) 1. Comprehensive Clinical Care

Competency	Competency Demonstrated	Performance Objectives (PO)	PO Demonstrated
Competency (C) 2		**Performance Objective (PO)**	
Evaluate population or geographically-based health risk utilizing principles of epidemiology, clinical prevention, environmental health, and biostatistics.		A. Assess the patient/ family *at risk* for a condition incorporating epidemiological principles and/or environmental factors that contribute to risk/incidence of disease. B. Assess the patient/ family *with* a condition incorporating epidemiological principles and/or environmental factors that contribute to risk/incidence of disease.	
Competency (C) 3		**Performance Objective (PO)**	
Formulate differential diagnoses, and diagnostic strategies and therapeutic interventions with attention to scientific evidence, safety, cost, invasiveness, simplicity, acceptability, adherence, and efficacy for patients who present with new conditions and those with ambiguous or		A. Formulate a differential diagnosis for a patient who presents with new undifferentiated signs and symptoms. B. Formulate a differential diagnosis for a patient who presents with ambiguous or incomplete data, complex illnesses, comorbid conditions, and potential multiple diagnoses. C. Discuss the rationale for the differential diagnosis. D. Discuss the rationale for the diagnostic evaluation with attention to scientific evidence, safety, cost, invasiveness, simplicity, acceptability, adherence, and efficacy.	

(continued)

6.1 CUSN DNP Competencies for Direct Patient Care Residency Case Narrative Log *(Continued)*

Domain (D) 1. Comprehensive Clinical Care

Competency	Competency Demonstrated	Performance Objectives (PO)	PO Demonstrated
Competency (C) 3		Performance Objective (PO)	
incomplete data, complex illnesses, comorbid conditions, and multiple diagnoses in all clinical settings.		E. Discuss the rationale for the therapeutic intervention with attention to scientific evidence, safety, cost, invasiveness, simplicity, acceptability, adherence, and efficacy.	
Competency (C) 4		Performance Objective (PO)	
Appraise acuity of patient condition, determine need to transfer patient to higher-acuity setting, coordinate, and manage transfer to optimize patient outcomes.		A. Assess the acuity of patient status. B. Determine the most appropriate treatment setting based on level of acuity. C. Formulate a transfer plan. D. Implement plan to transfer the patient to a higher level of care utilizing written and oral communication. E. Coordinate care during transition to the higher-acuity setting. F. Co-manage care in person, or G. Co-manage care through written and verbal instructions. H. Recommendations for patient disposition from the higher acuity location. I. Coordination of post-discharge care.	

(continued)

6.1 *(Continued)*

Domain (D) 1. Comprehensive Clinical Care

Competency	Competency Demonstrated	Performance Objectives (PO)	PO Demonstrated
Competency (C) 5		**Performance Objective (PO)**	
Evaluate and direct care during hospitalization, and design a comprehensive discharge plan for patients from an acute care setting.		A. Assess the acuity of patient's condition and determine the most appropriate inpatient treatment setting based on level of acuity. B. Actively participate in the admission process to the appropriate inpatient treatment setting. C. Actively co-manage patient care during hospitalization. D. Formulate plan for ongoing care to be provided in a subacute setting, such as a long-term care facility, rehabilitation facility, or home or community setting. E. Coordinate ongoing comprehensive care to be provided in a subacute setting, such as a long-term care facility, rehabilitation facility, or home or community setting.	
Competency (C) 6		**Performance Objective (PO)**	
Direct comprehensive care for patient in a subacute setting to maximize quality of life and functional status.		A. Assess the acuity of the patient's condition to determine the need for sub-acute, long-term care. B. Determine the most appropriate subacute or chronic care treatment setting based on level of acuity, functional status, and availability of formal and informal caregiver resources.	

(continued)

6.1 CUSN DNP Competencies for Direct Patient Care Residency Case Narrative Log *(Continued)*

Domain (D) 1. Comprehensive Clinical Care

Competency	Competency Demonstrated	Performance Objectives (PO)	PO Demonstrated
Competency (C) 6		Performance Objective (PO)	
		C. Coordinate ongoing comprehensive care provided in a subacute setting.	
		D. Initiate referral to other health care professionals while maintaining primary responsibility for patient care in a subacute setting.	
		E. Utilize consultant recommendations for decision-making while maintaining primary responsibility for care in a subacute setting.	
Competency (C) 7		Performance Objective (PO)	
Facilitate and guide the process of palliative care and/or planning end-of-life care by discussing diagnoses and prognosis, clarifying and validating patient desires and priorities, and promoting informed choices and shared decision-making by patient, family, and members of the health care team.		A. Facilitate and guide the palliative care process by discussing diagnoses and prognosis, clarifying and validating patient desires and priorities, and promoting informed choices and shared decision-making by the patient, family, and members of the health care team.	
		B. Facilitate and guide planning of end-of-life care by discussing diagnoses and prognosis, clarifying and validating patient desires and priorities, and promoting informed choices and shared decision-making by the patient, family, and members of the health care team.	

(continued)

6.1 *(Continued)*

Domain (D) 2. Interdisciplinary and Patient-Centered Communication

Competency	Competency Demonstrated	Performance Objectives (PO)	PO Demonstrated
Competency (C) 1		**Performance Objective (PO)**	
Assemble a collaborative interdisciplinary network, refer and consult appropriately while maintaining primary responsibility for comprehensive patient care.		A. Initiate referral to other health care professionals while maintaining primary responsibility for patient care. B. Accept referrals from other health care professionals and communicate consultation findings and recommendations to the referring provider and collaborative network. C. Utilize consultation recommendations for decision-making while maintaining primary responsibility for care. D. Evaluate outcomes of interventions. E. Provide ongoing patient follow-up and monitor outcomes of collaborative network interventions.	
Competency (C) 2		**Performance Objective (PO)**	
Coordinate and manage the care of patients with chronic illness utilizing specialists, other disciplines, community resources, and family, while maintaining		A. Coordinate care for a patient with chronic illness as the focus of care transitions across ambulatory, acute, subacute, and/or community settings. B. Co-manage care for a patient with chronic illness as the focus of care transitions across ambulatory, acute, sub-acute, and/or community settings.	

(continued)

6.1 CUSN DNP Competencies for Direct Patient Care Residency Case Narrative Log *(Continued)*

Domain (D) 2. Interdisciplinary and Patient-Centered Communication

Competency	Competency Demonstrated	Performance Objectives (PO)	PO Demonstrated
Competency (C) 2		**Performance Objective (PO)**	
primary responsibility for direction of patient care and ensuring the seamless flow of information among providers as the focus of care transitions across ambulatory to acute, sub-acute settings, and community settings.		C. Coordinate care for a patient with chronic illness utilizing specialists, other disciplines, community resources, and family. D. Direct care for patient with chronic illness and ensure the seamless flow of information among providers as the focus of care transitions across settings. E. Co-manage care for a patient with chronic illness utilizing shared decision-making and teaching. F. Co-manage care for a patient with chronic pain as the focus of care transitions across ambulatory, acute, subacute, and/or community settings.	

Domain (D) 3. Systems and Context of Care

Competency	Competency Demonstrated	Performance Objective	PO Demonstrated
Competency (C) 1		**Performance Objective (PO)**	
Construct and evaluate outcomes of a culturally sensitive, individualized intervention that incorporates shared decision-making and addresses the specific needs of a patient in context of family and community.		A. Assess culturally specific needs of patient in the context of family and community. B. Construct a culturally sensitive intervention to address the needs of the patient in the context of family and community. C. Evaluate outcomes of the intervention.	

(continued)

6.1 *(Continued)*

Domain (D) 3. Systems and Context of Care

Competency	Competency Demonstrated	Performance Objectives (PO)	PO Demonstrated
Competency (C) 2		**Performance Objective (PO)**	
Evaluate gaps in health care access that compromise optimal patient outcomes, and apply current knowledge of the organization and financing of health care systems to advocate for the patient and to ameliorate negative impact.		A. Identify gaps in access that compromise patient's optimum care. B. Identify gaps in reimbursement that compromise patient's optimum care. C. Demonstrate patient advocacy in the provision of continuous and comprehensive care. D. Apply current knowledge of the organization to ameliorate negative impact. E. Apply current knowledge of health care systems to ameliorate negative impact.	
Competency (C) 3		**Performance Objective (PO)**	
Synthesize the principles of legal and ethical decision-making and analyze dilemmas that arise in patient care, interprofessional relationships, research, or practice management to improve outcomes.		A. Synthesize ethical principles to address a complex practice dilemma. B. Apply ethical principles to resolve the dilemma. C. Synthesize legal principles to address a complex practice dilemma. D. Apply legal principles to resolve the dilemma.	

References

American Association of Colleges of Nursing (AACN). (2006). *The essentials of doctoral education for advanced nursing practice.* Retrieved August 31, 2009, from http://www/aacn.nche.edu/DNP/pdf/Essentials.pdf

Carraccio, C., Wolfsthal, S.D., Englander, R., Ferentz, K., & Martin, C. (2002). Shifting paradigms: From Flexner to competencies. *Academic Medicine, 77*(5), 361–367.

Cook, S.S., Kase, R., Middelton, L., & Monsen, R.B. (2003). Portfolio evaluation for professional competence: Credentialing in genetics for nurses. *Journal of Professional Nursing, 19*(2), 85–90.

Council for the Advancement of Comprehensive Care (CACC). (2003). *Competencies of a clinical nursing doctorate.* New York: Columbia University School of Nursing.

Dannefer, E.F., & Henson, L.C. (2007). The portfolio approach to competency-based assessment at the Cleveland Clinic Lerner College of Medicine. *Academic Medicine, 82*(5), 493–502.

Fabrizio, S. (2003). *Machine learning in automated text categorization: Advancements in information retrieval.* Paper presented at the 25th European Conference, Pisa, Italy.

Hanson, C.W., & Marshall, B.E. (2001). Artificial intelligence applications in the intensive care unit. *Critical Care Medicine, 29*(2), 427–435.

Holmes, D., McAlpine, R., & Russell, J. (2005). Use of neural net technology to quantify portfolio evaluations. In *Genetics nursing portfolios: A new model for the profession* (pp. 79–90). Washington, DC: American Nurses Association.

National Organization of Nurse Practitioner Faculties (NONPF) National Panel for NP Practice Doctorate Competencies. (2006). *Practice doctoral nurse practitioner entry-level competencies.* Retrieved August 31, 2009, from http://www.nonpf.com/NONPF2005/PracticeDoctorateResourceCenter/Competency-DraftFinalApril2006.pdf

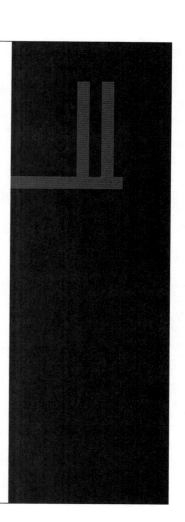

DNP Approach and Clinical Case Narratives in the Pediatric and Adolescent Population

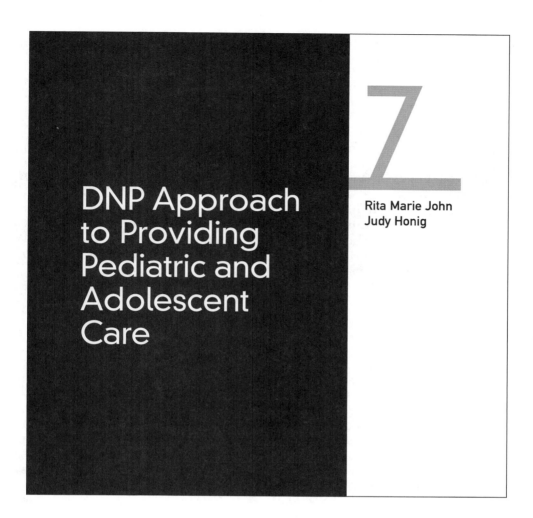

7

DNP Approach to Providing Pediatric and Adolescent Care

Rita Marie John
Judy Honig

The DNP who cares for a pediatric patient (DNP/PNP) assumes responsibility for the child's comprehensive care across settings and over time. As the complexity and chronicity of pediatric care issues increase and the settings in which care is delivered become more diverse, there is an acute need to provide families with coordinated, comprehensive, evidence-based, expert care. The DNP/PNP is educated to provide comprehensive family-centered evidence-based care to the pediatric patient. Building on the foundation of ambulatory pediatric primary care, the DNP in pediatrics expands the contextual boundaries and is accountable for the child's care in all settings, including the home, office, acute, and subacute settings. The DNP/PNP appraises the acuity of the patient's conditions and determines the setting that best optimizes the care.

The expanded DNP accountability is fostered during the DNP residency and is reflected in the case narratives. DNP/PNP clinical decision-making is reflective and deliberative. Clinical skills are enhanced by the broad underpinning of doctoral education. The support coursework includes ethical decision-making, epidemiology and environmental health, advances in clinical science, critical appraisal and application of research to practice, information technology for data retrieval, and decision support. The case narratives are the DNP's demonstration of this multifaceted, cognitive process.

This chapter focuses on the components of the comprehensive and interval history and complete physical examination needed to develop a differential diagnosis, assessment, and plan of care for pediatric patients. Comprehensive, family-centered, continuous care of pediatric patients is challenging and utilizes multiple skill sets. Pediatric patients are evaluated in the context of the family. The age and developmental status of the child, family history, and individual risks based on genetic profile are important components that need to be considered when providing care to children. The DNP/PNP formulates differential diagnoses and develops diagnostic strategies using evidence-based guidelines. The DNP/PNP communicates with the family in an open forum using shared decision-making.

HISTORY STYLE

A key element used to elicit a complete history is open communication. The DNP must eliminate any physical barriers between the practitioner and the patient. The DNP considers the setting in which the history is taking place and utilizes his or her skills of observation during the entire encounter to develop a complete assessment. With the use of electronic medical records, the provider needs to position the computer for maximum eye contact with the patient. In addition, the DNP minimizes barriers by refraining from typing while listening and paying close attention to the context of the history. Reviewing the concerns of the child and family prior to charting validates the DNP's understanding with the family and assures them that their issues are the priority. It is important that the DNP make every effort to obtain the most complete history because if it is terminated prematurely, the differential diagnoses may be limited (Heritage, Robinson, Elliott, Beckett, and Wilkes, 2007).

Beckman and Frankel's (1984) classic research points to the provider's interruption of initial concerns as one of the ways in which the focus of the history can be shifted from patient-centered to provider-centered. In this study, most physicians interrupted their patient within 18 seconds after the patient stated the reason for the visit. After interruption, patients did not resume their thoughts. Langewitz et al. (2002) reported that patients' responses to being asked what brought them to the clinic were brief and lasted only a minute and a half. Marvel et al. (1999) found that physicians (N = 29) interrupted patients after about 25 seconds. Recent research examining nurse practitioners' (NP) communication styles showed that nearly 70 percent of 53 NP-patient encounters involved provider-centered communications rather than patient-centered communications (Berry, 2009). An open communication style encourages dialog and conversation between the patient and provider. Such open communication is critical when caring for pediatric patients and their families. During the history, the DNP can frame open-ended questions such as "Do you have other concerns that you would like to discuss today?" to try to meet the patient's unmet concerns (Heritage et al., 2007) and help to encourage a more complete history. Probing questions are prompted by the child's past history, epidemiological and environmental factors, and the three-generational genogram. The components of a comprehensive history and interval history are outlined in the pediatric guidelines that can be found in the appendix.

HISTORY AND DEVELOPMENTAL STATUS

The specific focus and questions in a pediatric history are adjusted to the age of the patient. During infancy, there is an emphasis on perinatal, intrapartum, and postnatal history. The details of this early period help identify risk factors for psychological and physiological conditions. Family-centered care enables the DNP/PNP to meet the basic needs of the parents, enabling them to care for their infant. The DNP/PNP should focus considerable attention on the parents because meeting the needs of a new mother is critical to successfully parenting the very young infant. Allowing the infant to play with a toy while the guardian gives the history enables the DNP/PNP to watch the child at play while allowing the guardian to focus on the history.

As the child's language skills expand, information about the child's history should be obtained from the child. Communication between children and parents is different from communication with the adult who makes independent decisions about health. The DNP should provide the opportunity for the child to talk. Asking a child about home, school, and social life helps establish rapport and provides insight into psychosocial functioning.

The DNP can utilize time effectively during a visit with a school-age child by asking the child to draw a picture of his or her family or something that he or she wants to share. This picture can help the DNP gain insight from the child's perspective about his or her emotional and social status. During late childhood, the child may want to talk with the provider separately. By interviewing the child without the parent, the DNP helps facilitate the impending transition toward self-care during adolescence. During the adolescent years, it is imperative that the DNP provide for a private history interview. The DNP needs to assure the adolescent and the parents that the conversation between the adolescent and the DNP is private and confidential. It should be made explicitly clear that disclosure of the contents of the private meeting would only occur under the extreme circumstances of imminent danger, possible homicide, or suicide. The history needs to be directly obtained from the adolescent, in private, and the parent's history is obtained at the beginning or end of the visit.

The pediatric history is modified and depends upon the reason for the visit and the setting of the visit. However, fundamentally, during the history interview, the DNP collects information about the child's physical and emotional health, family, social situation, support systems, health habits, and sexuality.

PHYSICAL EXAMINATION

The developmental status of the child dictates the approach to the physical examination. Whereas the head-to-toe approach may be fine for the school-age child, younger children may be fearful of the examiner. Playing with the younger child can help build trust with the examiner. Keeping the child on the parent's lap and having fun distractions enables a complete exam to be performed. Listening for a song while looking in the ear or finding empty spots in the abdomen puts a child and parent at ease with the exam. Often, in the very young child, it is advisable to assess heart sounds before the child develops fear and cries. This allows critical parts of the exam to be completed more accurately. Some children may be impossible to examine because of their excessive fear. Role-playing at home with a medical kit may help these children to be more amenable to a physical exam. Keen observation of the child during the visit can provide important data about the child's general neurological and musculoskeletal status.

ASSESSMENT AND DIFFERENTIAL DIAGNOSIS

By using differential diagnosis, the DNP systematically synthesizes the data from the history and physical assessment using clinical science, causality, and probability. The DNP identifies all possible diagnoses and the most likely diagnosis while simultaneously excluding any life-threatening conditions. The differential diagnosis can be easily made or can be very challenging. This process provides the foundation for the final diagnosis and treatment.

A thorough and in-depth history and complete physical exam are important steps to developing a differential diagnosis. Careful review of the past medical history along with the presenting problem expands the differential diagnosis. In puzzling cases, consultation with a colleague or a subspecialist may help expand diagnostic possibilities. In addition, the use of an Internet-based decision support system such as Dxplain, Gideon, Lifecom, Visual Dx, and Isabel can assist the DNP to expand the differential conditions and formulate an appropriate plan for the presenting problem. These decision tools do not make a diagnosis but offer the DNP a list of possible diagnoses to consider based on age, gender, geographic area, symptoms, and signs. By asking open-ended questions, clarifying patient communications, and doing a thorough exam, the DNP assembles comprehensive subjective and objective data that will enable a thoughtful and sophisticated differential diagnosis and target a plan of care toward the most likely diagnosis.

PATIENT-CENTERED PLAN

The DNP plan for the child should include five key elements—diagnostics, therapeutic medications, referrals, patient education, and follow-up. The clinical decision-making for diagnostics should be based on evidence and include several factors, including the sensitivity and specificity of the diagnostic test, cost, radiation exposure, possible adverse effects, and which test is most specific for the most likely diagnosis. To conserve costs but optimize diagnosis, the DNP should develop a logical evidence-based plan for ordering diagnostic tests.

When ordering medication, the DNP should consider the evidence and rely on the highest level of evidence to support the medication of choice. In addition, the DNP should consider if generic drug treatment is available. Use of generic medication can help the patient conserve expenditures while decreasing the cost on the health care system. If a more expensive medication is needed and the patient is without insurance, it is important to give the patient information about prescription help from a variety of manufacturers.

Health education is an important part of the plan of care. The evidence on health-related reading materials suggests that easily understood handouts to enhance patients' understanding are lacking (Nielsen-Bohlman, Panzer, & Kindig, 2004). Inadequate health literacy is a hidden problem because many patients are afraid to admit their lack of understanding to health care providers (Baker et al., 1996; Parikh, Parker, Nurss, Baker, & Williams, 1996). It is important that the DNP use health-related reading materials that are culturally appropriate and geared to parents' and children's literacy level (Carmona, 2005; Flores, Abreu, & Tomany-Korman, 2005; Keller, Wright, & Pace, 2008; Pignone, DeWalt, Sheridan, Berkman, & Lohr, 2005; Nielsen-Bohlman et al., 2004). In general, education material needs to be evaluated for concepts of health literacy. In addition, the DNP must individualize the written and oral education to the level and the language of the patient and family.

The DNP assumes full accountability for the child's care across settings and over time and meets the child and family needs where care is warranted. The DNP/PNP incorporates knowledge of clinical and prevention science, evidence-based practice, information technology, genomics, advocacy and ethical decision-making, and principles of access and safety into the care of the pediatric patient. Using the multidimensional nursing paradigm that combines robust knowledge and reflective practice, the DNP/PNP provides comprehensive care to children from birth through adolescence.

References

Baker, D.W., Parker, R.M., Williams, M.W., Pitkin, K., Parikh, N.S., Coates, W., et al. (1996). The health care experience of patients with low literacy. *Archives of Family Medicine, 5*(6), 329–334.

Beckman, H.B., & Frankel, R. (1984). The effect of physician behavior on the collection of data. *Annals of Internal Medicine, 101,* 692–696.

Berry, J. (2009). Nurse practitioner/patient communication styles in clinical practice. *Journal for Nurse Practitioners, 5*(7), 508–515.

Carmona, R. (2005). Improving health literacy: Preventing obesity with education. *Journal of the American Dietetic Association, 105*(6)(Suppl. 1), S9–S10.

Flores, G., Abreu, M., & Tomany-Korman, S.C. (2005). Limited English proficiency, primary language at home, and disparities in children's health care: How language barriers are measure matters. *Public Health Reports, 120,* 418–430.

Heritage, J., Robinson, J., Elliott, M., Beckett, M., & Wilkes, M. (2007). Reducing patients' unmet concerns in primary care: The difference one word can make. *Journal of General Internal Medicine, 22*(10), 1429–1433.

Keller, D.L., Wright, J., & Pace, H.A. (2008). Impact of health literacy on health outcomes in ambulatory care patients: A systematic review. *Annals of Pharmacotherapy, 42*(October 2008), 1272–1281.

Langewitz, W., Denz, M., Keller, A., Kiss, A., Ruttimann, S., & Wossmer, B. (2002). Spontaneous talking time at start of consultation in outpatient clinic: Cohort study. *British Medical Journal, 325,* 682–683.

Marvel, M.K., Epstein, R.M., Flowers, K., & Beckman, H.B. (1999). Soliciting the patient's agenda, have we improved? *Journal of the American Medical Association, 281*(3), 283–287.

Nielsen-Bohlman, L., Panzer, A., & Kindig, D. (Eds.). (2004). *Health literacy: A prescription to end confusion.* Washington, DC: National Academies Press.

Parikh, N.S., Parker, R.M., Nurss, J.R., Baker, D.W., & Williams, M.V. (1996). Shame and health literacy: The unspoken connection. *Patient Education and Counseling, 27*(1), 33–39.

Pignone, M., DeWalt, D., Sheridan, S., Berkman, N., & Lohr, K. (2005). Interventions to improve health outcomes for patients with low literacy: A systematic review. *Journal of General Internal Medicine, 20,* 185–192.

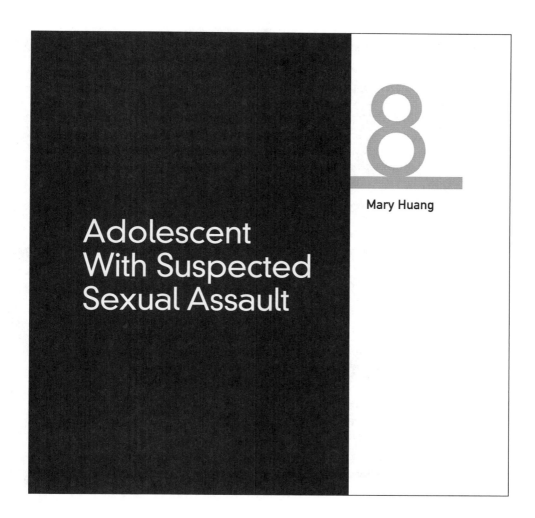

8

Mary Huang

Adolescent With Suspected Sexual Assault

The case describes the care I provided for a 13-year-old female with Medicaid insurance who was brought to a New York pediatric Level I trauma center by emergency medical services (EMS) for intoxication and possible sexual assault. The case narrative focuses on one encounter that occurred over a seven-hour period in the emergency department (ED). The case narrative demonstrates my ability to meet the following CUSN doctoral competencies for direct patient care:

DOMAIN 1, COMPETENCY 2

Evaluate population or geographically based health risk utilizing principles of epidemiology, clinical prevention, environmental health, and biostatistics.

PO A. Assess the patient/family *at risk* for a condition incorporating epidemiological principles and/or environmental factors that contribute to risk/incidence of disease.

DOMAIN 1, COMPETENCY 3

Formulate differential diagnoses, and diagnostic strategies and therapeutic interventions, with attention to scientific evidence, safety, cost, invasiveness, simplicity, acceptability, adherence, and efficacy for patients who present with new conditions and those with ambiguous or incomplete data, complex illnesses, comorbid conditions, and multiple diagnoses in all clinical settings.

PO A. Formulate a differential diagnosis for a patient who presents with new undifferentiated signs and symptoms.
PO C. Discuss the rationale for the differential diagnosis.
PO D. Discuss the rationale for the diagnostic evaluation with attention to scientific evidence, safety, cost, invasiveness, simplicity, acceptability, adherence, and efficacy.
PO E. Discuss the rationale for the therapeutic intervention with attention to scientific evidence, safety, cost, invasiveness, simplicity, acceptability, adherence, and efficacy.

DOMAIN 3, COMPETENCY 2

Evaluate gaps in health care access that compromise optimal patient outcomes, and apply current knowledge of the organization and financing of health care systems to ameliorate negative impact.

PO A. Identify gaps in access that compromise patient's optimum care.
PO C. Demonstrate patient advocacy in the provision of continuous and comprehensive care.
PO D. Apply current knowledge of the organization to ameliorate negative impact.
PO E. Apply current knowledge of health care systems to ameliorate negative impact.

ENCOUNTER CONTEXT

Encounter One (initial emergency department encounter)

DNP role: I am the DNP student and pediatric nurse practitioner seeing this patient for initial evaluation.

Identifying Information

Site: New York pediatric Level I trauma ED.

Setting: Pediatric ED.

Reason for encounter: Intoxication.

Informant: Patient, patient's friend, EMS, and mother.

Chief complaint: Patient complains of nausea and vomiting, dizziness, and headache. Patient admits drinking vodka with her friends approximately six hours ago but is unable to recall detailed events of the day.

History of Present Illness

As per EMS record, when EMS arrived on the scene, patient was sitting in the back seat of a truck of two women who stopped to help the patient and her friend. The patient and friend were found on the street, passed out in the snow. Soon after, the patient's biological mother arrived at the scene.

As per patient and her friend, they cut class today and had been drinking Smirnoff vodka with a couple of school friends at one of their homes. The patient passed out and was in a room with two male friends for approximately two hours while her friend was drinking with the other school friends in another room in the house. The patient was found by her friend several hours later with pants undone and shirt torn. Patient cannot recall details of what occurred in the room or whether there was sexual activity. Her friend states the two male friends told the other friends that they were in the room and had sex with the patient. Patient states that she did not shower, douche, brush her teeth, or change underwear or clothing after the alleged sexual assault.

Past Medical History (as per mother)

Perinatal history: No complications or infections.

Prenatal history: Mother admits receiving prenatal care.

Gestation: Full-term, 40 weeks.

Birth history: Normal spontaneous vaginal delivery with no complications; went home in two days.

Common childhood illness: None.

Illness: Denies.

Operations: Denies.

Hospitalizations: Denies.

Accidents: Denies.

Current medications: None.

Allergies: No known drug, food, or environmental allergies.

Immunizations: Up-to-date as per patient's mother.

Family History

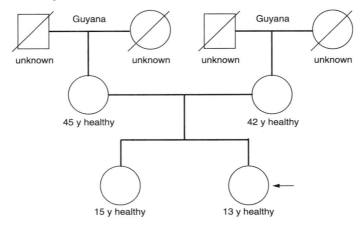

No consanguinity

Social History

- Household composition: Patient lives with her mother and 15-year-old sister. Parents are divorced. Father lives nearby and patient speaks to her father daily and visits with him every other weekend.
- Support systems: Patient has good relationship with paternal family, which includes a large extended family.
- Family relationship: Patient is very quiet and keeps to herself most of the time at home and at school. She does have many cousins that she is close to on her paternal side of the family.
- Cultural: Parents are from Guyana.
- Socioeconomic: Mother is currently unemployed and father works as an electrical engineer.
- After-school activities: Patient does not participate in after-school activities, as per mother, and is very shy and quiet.
- Family stresses: Parents have been divorced for the past six years. Mother states that the 15-year-old sister is very argumentative and disrespectful. The sisters are very different and not very close. Mother states their father "spoils" them by purchasing them whatever they want. Parents discipline patient by removing computer time and taking away her cell phone. Denies any physical punishment.

HEADSS (patient interviewed in private)

- Home: Patient lives with mother and older sister and visits with her father every other weekend. Father usually drives her to school in the morning and mother picks her up after school. Mother usually cooks at home, and patient eats well-balanced meals with occasional junk food, and she enjoys drinking soda.
- Family dynamics and relationships: See Social History.

- Education: Recent change in school from elementary to middle school. Patient is in the sixth grade and is enrolled in honor classes. She has never been in trouble in school and does not have any history of behavioral problems.
- School attendance: Rarely absent from school. Mother or father drives her to and from school every day.
- Grades: Grades averaging in the high 90s.
- Attitude about school relationships: She has met some new friends in her new school.
- Activities: She does not participate in any after-school activities, teams, or clubs.
- Spare time: She talks to her friends on the computer or goes out with her cousins.
- Physical activity: Plays with her cousins when the weather is nice outside.
- Drugs: Denies ever experimenting with drugs or using drugs regularly.
- Tobacco: Has tried smoking but does not smoke regularly.
- Alcohol: Has tried drinking before with friends, but this is the first time she has been intoxicated.
- History of harm to animals or others: Denies any history.
- Suicide ideation: Patient denies any prior suicidal ideation or attempts. She denies self-mutilating behaviors.
- Internet: Has own laptop computer. The only time there is restriction is when she is being punished.
- Chat rooms: Talks to her friends only. Denies talking to strangers or dating online or viewing violence or pornography.
- Violence: Denies any domestic violence in the home but admits her parents don't get along and argue.
- Sexuality: Patient denies having sexual intercourse in the past. Identifies herself as heterosexual.
- Gang: Denies any gang membership or having friends in gangs.

Review of Systems (as per mother and patient)

General: Has not been sick recently.

Skin: Denies rashes.

Head: No history of head injury.

Eyes: Denies wearing contacts or glasses.

Ears: Denies any hearing deficits.

Nose/sinus: Denies frequent cold, nasal discharge, nosebleeds, sinus pain.

Throat: Denies frequent tonsillitis/pharyngitis.

Dentition: Has braces and sees orthodontist every couple of months.

Neck: Denies stiffness or pain.

Respiratory: Denies cough at night or with activity or shortness of breath, TB.

Heart: Denies having murmur, palpitations, or chest pain.

Gastrointestinal: Denies frequent abdominal pain, was nauseous and vomited twice upon arrival, denies diarrhea or constipation history.

Genitourinary/reproductive: Denies having frequent urinary tract infections or vaginal discharge.

Female: First menstrual period (FMP) at 11 years old. Last menstrual period is reported as minimal amount two weeks ago. Complains of menstrual cramps with menses. Menses are irregular in frequency and amount. Denies any prior pregnancies.

Musculoskeletal: Denies muscle or joint pain, stiffness or backache.

Neurological: Denies fainting, seizures, weakness, numbness.

Hematological: Denies anemia or bruising easily.

Psychiatric: Denies anxiety, depression, mood swings, suicide attempts, violence.

Endocrine: Denies heat or cold intolerance, excessive sweating, excessive thirst, hunger, or polyuria.

Physical Examination

Vital signs: Temp 97.9°F oral; apical pulse 103; respirations 18; blood pressure 106/60; SaO_2 100% room air.

Growth: Weight 100 lb (25–50th percentile); height 62 inches (25–50th percentile); BMI 18.29.

General: Patient is drowsy but arousable. Cooperative and quiet during exam.

Skin: No ecchymosis or lacerations or lesions.

HEENT: Bilateral tympanic membrane grey with light reflex; pupils round, reactive to light; conjunctiva slightly injected; no oral lesions.

Lymph: No lymphadenopathy.

Neck: Supple, full range of motion with no tenderness.

Lungs: Bilaterally clear with good air exchange.

Breast: Tanner stage III/V.

Cardiovascular: S1S2 with no murmur heard; +2 capillary refill in four extremities.

Abdomen: Soft nondistended, nontender with no organomegaly.

Genitalia: Deferred at this time.

Anus: Deferred at this time.

Extremities: Full range of motion with 2+ deep tendon reflexes in all four extremities.

Spine: Midline with no tenderness.

Neurological: Speech slurred, gait unsteady, CN II–XII grossly intact.

Mental status: Oriented ×3; drowsy but arousable.

Thought processes: Appropriate for age and coherent.

Assessment

13-year-old Guyanese female brought to the pediatric ED by EMS for unsteady gait, slurred speech, amnesic episode, nausea, and vomiting due to alcohol intoxication and alleged sexual assault by two male friends. She is accompanied by her friend and mother. Based on the patient's history of drinking vodka during the day with classmates and her clinical presentation of unsteady gait, slurred speech, and nausea and vomiting, alcohol intoxication is the most likely diagnosis. Other possible causes for the patient's clinical presentation need to be explored with further laboratory toxicology testing **(D1, C3, PO A, C, D).**

ICD Codes

Nausea and vomiting: 787.01
Observation following alleged rape: V71.5
Idiosyncratic alcohol intoxication: 291.4

Plan

Laboratory Tests
CBC, basic metabolic panel, urine pregnancy, urine toxicology, and serum ethanol level **(D1, C3, PO D).**

Therapeutic Interventions
Intravenous insertion for fluid bolus of normal saline 1 L over 30 minutes **(D1, C3, PO E).**

The most frequent electrolyte disturbance found in this study was hypernatremia, with a prevalence of 41.3%. Rauchenzauner, Kountchev, Ulmer, Pechlaner, Bellmann, Wiedermann & Joannidis investigated acutely intoxicated patients in the ER who were probably still in the phase of increasing blood-alcohol levels, leading to suppression of antidiuretic-hormone release from the pituitary gland and consequent polyuria. The result would be a mild hypernatremia associated with lack of fluid intake due to intoxication. Chloride was elevated in 20.9% of our patients. The third most frequent electrolyte disturbance found in our study was hypermagnesemia. Investigations of the short-term effects of alcohol ingestion found an increase in serum-magnesium levels six hours after alcohol ingestion; this was attributed to transient hypoparathyroidism induced by alcohol ingestion. Hypermagnesemia may also reflect hypertonic dehydration, which would explain the highly significant correlation between magnesium, sodium and chloride. This study shows that in patients admitted to the ER for acute alcohol intoxication the pattern of electrolytes significantly differs from that seen in chronic alcohol abuse or in patients treated on a general ward, with hypernatremia being the predominant disturbance. This further indicates that hyperosmolar dehydration is the most frequent disturbance in acute alcohol intoxication and suggests that volume substitution is one of the most important first measures (Rauchenzauner, Kountchev, Ulmer, Pechlaner, Bellmann, Wiedermann & Joannidis, 2005).

Oxford Centre for Evidence-Based Medicine (CEBM), level 1b.

Family Education

As per mother's request and patient's consent, a sexual offense evidence collection kit will be performed. Both mother and patient are instructed to have very little contact and handling of clothing before sexual offense evidence collection is completed. Patient is asked to undress with a sheet beneath to catch debris for evidence submission. Mother is asked for permission to give up the patient's clothing for evidence submission and to have patient's father bring a change of clothing to wear for discharge to home **(D1, C3, PO E)**.

Patient Education

The patient is educated in private for preparation for a pelvic examination that includes an external genitalia examination or observing the external vaginal perineum area for signs of trauma or injuries. Because this will be the patient's first pelvic examination, the procedure, examination speculum, and what will be visualized during a pelvic or internal intravaginal examination are explained to the patient. Also discussed are the various laboratory tests that will be performed for detection of sexually transmitted infections. I reinforce to the patient that results of the laboratory tests for sexually transmitted infections are for medical purposes and will not be submitted into the sexual offense evidence kit.

The sexual offense evidence collection process is discussed with the patient. I inform the patient that the collection will be performed with all women clinicians and that the 12-step head-to-toe collection of evidence will be lengthy and must follow an orderly manner. I explain that some evidence collection will be uncomfortable, such as hair sample collection and pubic hair sample collection.

Referrals

Family is unable to be referred to pediatric ED social worker for family support and child safety risk assessment due to lack of availability of social worker, at this time. Therefore, I page the hospital director of social services to arrange for social work evaluation the following day on an outpatient basis **(D3, C2, PO A, C)**.

Patients who have been sexually assaulted will experience psychological trauma to one degree or another. The effects of this trauma may be more difficult to recognize than physical trauma. Every person has her own method of coping with sudden stress. When in crisis, patients can appear calm, indifferent, submissive, jocular, angry, or uncooperative and hostile toward those who are trying to help. It is important for the caregivers to understand that all of these responses are within the range of anticipated normal reactions. A judgment about the validity of the patient's account of the assault based on her demeanor can further traumatize the patient and hinder the collection of complete and objective data (NYSDOH, 2007).

CEBM, level 5.

Encounter Two (one hour later in the ED)

Patient states she is feeling less nauseated and dizzy and her headache is resolving. Patient is able to tolerate clear fluids without vomiting. Patient admits drinking vodka with her friends seven hours ago at her friend's house but still is unable to recall details of the entire day. Patient is unsure of type of violation and if sexual assault occurred. Patient is unsure of vaginal or anal contact or condom use.

Vital signs: Temp 98.4°F oral; apical pulse 106; respirations 22; blood pressure 114/62; SaO$_2$ 100% room air.

Physical Examination (performed by all-female emergency medicine fellow, pediatric resident, primary registered nurse, and myself)

General: Patient is alert but sleepy. Cooperative and quiet during exam.

Skin: No ecchymosis or lacerations or lesions.

Genitalia: Tanner IV staging, shaved pubic hair on mons, no lacerations at vaginal introitus, no lesions or erythema noted in external genitalia, slight whitish discharge on vaginal orifice, hymen membrane noted and intact with no laceration or blood. Internal exam deferred due to intact hymenal membrane.

Anus: No lesion, lacerations, or blood noted.

Laboratory result review: CBC, basic metabolic panel are within normal range. Urine pregnancy and toxicology tests are negative. Blood ethanol level is 176 mg/dL, normal is less than 10 mg/dL.

Alcohol test results from clinical, research, and forensic lab results are expressed in grams or milligrams of alcohol per fixed volume of fluid (100 mL of blood or serum) or per 210 L of air (for some breath test instruments). United States, breath testing instruments are calibrated to convert grams per volume of breath into milligrams of alcohol per 100 mL of blood (mg/dL) or grams per 100 mL (g%). Milligrams are easily converted to grams by dividing the value by 1,000, and g% is easily converted to mg/dL by multiplying the value by 1,000. A blood alcohol concentration (BAC) of

80 mg/dL is the same as 80 mg%, which is the same as 0.08%. If the labo-
ratory measures alcohol in serum, the results are not equal to whole-blood
test results. This may have important implications for scientists comparing
test results or in instances where such results are used as evidence in a
criminal or civil litigation. As alcohol is distributed throughout the water-
containing compartments of the body including the blood, serum alcohol
is not the equivalent of a BAC because serum contains more water than
the whole blood from which it is derived. Therefore, the concentration of
alcohol in whole blood is less than that of the serum in proportion to their
respective water contents. In other words, a hospital serum alcohol con-
centration will be higher than a whole BAC drawn from the same patient
at the same time.

When information about drinking is limited, the circulating alcohol
burden (CAB) is a useful measure of the total amount of alcohol "on board"
at the time of a blood or breath test. The CAB is independent of 2 variables,
rate of absorption and rate of elimination, and is therefore useful when
insufficient information is available to account for these variables. However,
CAB estimates assume that alcohol absorption is, for all practical purposes,
complete. Circulating alcohol burden may underestimate consumption in some
instances because about 80% of alcohol consumed is absorbed within about 30
minutes of the last drink. As CAB is the alcohol burden at a single moment in
time and does not account for elimination, it is a good estimate of minimum
alcohol consumption. In other words, the total alcohol intake will always be
greater than the CAB. The variables that affect absorption are complex and
may vary with beverage concentration, volume, presence or absence of food,
genetics, or other factors. Consistent with empirical studies, most medical
references describe the majority of alcohol as being absorbed within 20 to 30
minutes, with a maximum BAC occurring about 60 to 90 minutes after the last
drink. The accuracy of such estimates can be enhanced by using a range of
elimination rates and anthropometric formulas to estimate total body water.
Alcohol is distributed throughout the water-containing compartments of the
body, and all other factors being equal (e.g., absorption, elimination, weight),
the peak BAC produced by any dose will vary as a function of changes in the
ratio of muscle to fat. On average, men tend to be more muscular than women
and muscle contains more water than fat (Brick, 2006).

CEBM, level 5.

Assessment

Based on the patient's amnesic episode of the day's events and her inability to recall how her shirt was torn and pants unzipped and details of what
occurred when alone with two male friends, the risk of alleged sexual assault
needs to be considered, since the patient and her friends' accounts of sexual
activity are inconsistent. Forensic evidence needs to be collected for law
enforcement involvement, as per mother's request and patient's assent **(D1,
C3, PO A, C, D).**

Since the mid-1990s, there have been a growing number of unconfirmed reports of assailants surreptitiously using prescription and nonprescription drugs to induce disinhibition, sedation and amnesia to facilitate rape. This type of victimization is most commonly referred to as drug-facilitated sexual assault (DFSA). Although flunitrazepam, in particular, has been maligned as a "date rape drug," many other easily accessible substances have reportedly been used to facilitate sexual assault, including alcohol and alprazolam, chloral hydrate, gamma hydroxybutyrate, ketamine, lorazepam, ziploclone and zolpidem. Few studies have systematically measured the occurrence of drug-facilitated sexual assault. Because there is no agreed upon definition of the phenomenon, comparisons across studies are difficult. Rapes involving incapacitation were more likely to have occurred following time spent in a bar or at a party and were more likely to involve higher levels of drinking and self-reported intoxication. In this study, the reasons for suspecting DFSA were vague sensation that something is wrong (51.1%), woke to find clothing in disarray to unclothed (42.4%), reported by witness to have been seen in compromised circumstances, (16.3%) (DuMont, Macdonald, Rotbard, Asllani, Bainbridge, & Cohen, 2009).

CEBM, level 1b.

Plan

Alleged Sexual Assault

Laboratory Tests
The following tests are performed for baseline sexually transmitted infection (STI) status and will not be used as data for sexual offense evidence: trichomoniasis, bacterial vaginosis, gonorrhea, chlamydia cultures, Rapid Plasma Reagin Assay and acute hepatitis panel (hepatitis B core IgM antibody, hepatitis B surface antigen, hepatitis C antibody, and hepatitis A IgM antibody). HIV-1 antibody test (ELISA) counseling and consent are obtained before testing **(D1, C3, PO D, E).**

Laws in all 50 states strictly limit the evidentiary use of a survivor's previous sexual history, including evidence of previously acquired STIs, as part of an effort to undermine the credibility of the survivor's testimony. Trichomoniasis, BV, gonorrhea, and chlamydial infection are the most frequently diagnosed infections among women who have been sexually assaulted. Because the prevalence of these infections is high among sexually active women, their presence after an assault does not necessarily signify acquisition during the assault (CDC, 2006).

CEBM, level 5.

An initial examination should include the following procedures: testing for N. gonorrhoeae and C. trachomatis from specimens collected from any sites of penetration or attempted penetration. Culture or FDA-cleared nucleic acid amplification tests for either N. gonorrhoeae or C. trachomatis. NAAT offer the advantage of increased sensitivity in detection of C. trachomatis. Wet mount and culture of a vaginal swab specimen for T. vaginalis infection. If vaginal discharge, malodor, or itching is evident, the wet mount also should be examined for evidence of BV and candidiasis. Collection of a serum sample for immediate evaluation for HIV, hepatitis B, and syphilis (CDC, 2006).

CEBM, level 5.

Sexual Offense Evidence Collection Kit
This ED and the examiner do not have New York State Department of Health sexual assault forensic examiner (SAFE) or program designation; therefore, the sexual assault protocol as per New York State is followed step by step for the collection of sexual offense evidence. When all evidence and clothing are collected, the primary nurse locks the evidence in the designated sexual offense collection refrigerator until local law enforcement arrives to transport the evidence.

The Sexual Assault Reform Act (SARA) requires that, absent exigent circumstances, or unless the patient does not disclose a sexual assault at the time of triage, the sexual assault forensic examiner must meet the patient within 60 minutes of arriving at the hospital. In those rare circumstances when a sexual assault forensic examiner (SAFE) program does not have a sexual assault examiner available to perform the examination of the sexual assault patient, the hospital must ensure that the examination and associated treatment is provided in a manner that is consistent with Department standards (NYSDOH, 2007).

CEBM, level 5.

Accurately maintaining and accounting for the chain of custody of sexual offense evidence is essential for the evidence to be useful in a court of law. The "chain of custody" is a legal term describing the movement, location, and succession of people responsible for the evidence. In order to maintain the chain of custody, an evidence collection kit and the specimens it contains must be accounted for from the moment collection begins until the moment it is introduced in court as evidence. Each item of evidence must be labeled with the initials of everyone who handled it, the date, a description and source of the specimen, the name of the examiner, and the name of the patient. Evidence not included in the kit (e.g., clothing, photographs, etc.) must be individually packaged, sealed and labeled with a description of the item. Providers must have specific protocols in place to insure confidentiality and maintain the chain of custody of the evidence. Never leave the patient alone with the evidence. Under no circumstances is a patient, family member, or support person (e.g., advocate) allowed to handle or transport evidence after it has been collected. Maintaining the chain of custody during the examination is the sole responsibility of the examiner, and requires no outside assistance (NYSDOH, 2007).

CEBM, level 5.

Therapeutic Intervention

The prophylaxis treatment of sexually transmitted infection, including HIV-1 and pregnancy, is discussed with both mother and patient. Prophylactic treatment is provided to the patient for gonorrhea, chlamydia, trichomoniasis/bacterial vaginosis, and post-coital contraception (see the Medications list at the end of the chapter): ceftriaxone (Rocephin) 125 mg intramuscularly for gonorrhea, azithromycin (Zithromax) 1 g by mouth for chlamydia, metronidazole (Flagyle) 2 g by mouth to treat trichomoniasis, and levonorgestrel 0.75 mg, one tablet by mouth, then repeat in 12 hours for prevention of conception (CDC, 2006) **(D1, C3, PO E).**

> *Many specialists recommend routine preventive therapy after a sexual assault because follow-up of survivors of sexual assault can be difficult. The following prophylactic regimen is suggested as preventive therapy: postexposure hepatitis B vaccination, without HBIG, should adequately protect against HBV infection. Hepatitis B vaccination should be administered to sexual assault victims at the time of the initial examination if they have not been previously vaccinated. Follow up doses of vaccine should be administered 1–2 and 4–6 months after the first dose. An empiric antimicrobial regimen for chlamydia, gonorrhea, Trichomoniasis, and bacterial vaginosis. Emergency contraception should be offered if the post-assault could result in pregnancy in the survivor (CDC, 2006).*
>
> CEBM, level 5.

All prophylactic treatment is consented to and administered except the HIV-1 prophylaxis regimen as per mother's request and hepatitis B immune globulin and vaccine due to documented hepatitis B vaccination. Therefore, patient and mother are counseled to have HIV-1 antibodies rechecked on an outpatient basis with their primary pediatrician (Casey et al., 2006). The family is referred to their primary pediatrician for aftercare management and review of pending laboratory test results, monitoring for adverse reactions to prophylactic regimens, and monitoring of STI symptoms.

> *The CDC recommends that an RPR be rechecked at six weeks, three months, and six months and suggests that HIV post-exposure testing should be offered at the same intervals (Casey et al., 2006).*
>
> CEBM, level 5.

Counseling

Due to unavailability of social services for the family to provide counseling and support, I discuss with the parents possible changes the patient may experience, including withdrawal, nightmares, fear, anxiety, and psychosomatic symptoms that may be indicative of post-traumatic stress reactions. Upon arrival of the patient's father, both parents are counseled not to place blame or punish the patient but to inquire about the incident in a nonjudgmental manner. We discuss structures in the home to ensure the safety of their adolescents. Parents are recommended to discuss openly and honestly with the patient and her sister the safety house rules (Kellog, 2005). The parents are recommended to place parental censors on Internet access and set consistent expectations regarding curfew and meeting new peers **(D1, C2, PO A).**

The child should be reassured that what happened was not the child's fault and that he or she did nothing wrong. Children in whom sexual abuse is confirmed or suspected should be referred to a mental health professional for evaluation and counseling. The family of the victim may also need treatment and support to cope with the emotional trauma of their child's abuse.

(Kellog, 2005.)

Adolescents often know their perpetrators prior to the assault. Adolescents are most often raped by their peers; many of these patients have faced multiple assailants. For some adolescents, the assault may be their first sexual contact. Because sexual identity and body image are rapidly changing, the effects of a sexual assault can be particularly devastating. The adolescent patient may view the assault as a sexual encounter, rather than an act of violence, thereby distorting the image of a healthy sexual relationship. The psychological reactions of adolescent rape survivors are in many ways similar to those of adult survivors. However, these reactions may be intensified in the adolescent due to developmental concerns. Some of the critical effects may be: a destructive influence on emerging sexuality and sexual awareness; self-blame and guilt over the risk-taking behavior which may be perceived as having contributed to the victimization; fear of disclosure and repercussions, especially from family and peers; damage to sense of identity and self-esteem (e.g., self-doubt, loss of trust in one's own judgment, peer stigmatization); loss of autonomy and independence as a result of the assault (e.g., imposed curfew or other perceived punishment, family over-protectiveness); and, distrust of the protective nature of authority (NYSDOH, 2007).

CEBM, level 5.

Referrals

I inform both parents that the ED social worker will contact them tomorrow to discuss the incident and provide the family with community resource information for long-term support, investigation, and referral information so that the family can go to an outpatient rape crisis center for counseling **(D3, C2, PO C, D).**

Rape crisis counselor means any person certified by an approved rape crisis program as having satisfied the training standards set forth in section 206 of the Public Health Law, and who is acting under the direction and supervision of an approved rape crisis program. Rape crisis program means any office, institution or center, which has been approved, pursuant to subdivision 15 of section 206 of the Public Health Law, to offer counseling and assistance to clients concerning sexual offenses, sexual abuse or incest. The program must provide services to alleviate the immediate and long term negative physical and emotional effects of sexual assault and abuse. Services shall be accessible, confidential, provided without coercion, and available to individuals regardless of age, gender, race, ethnicity, sexual orientation, disability status, or ability to pay (NYSDOH, 2007).

CEBM, level 5.

I call the local police department precinct as per parents' request to file a report regarding the incident and to assist in the investigation of the event **(D3, C2, PO C, E).**

> *If a patient has not contacted law enforcement officers before arriving at a health care facility, she should be informed of the right to report the crime. Hospital personnel should not call the police and identify a sexual assault patient, absent a legal obligation to do so, or absent a patient's consent. It is the adult patient's choice whether or not to involve law enforcement personnel. If the patient so chooses, providers should assist her in contacting law enforcement officials (NYSDOH, 2007).*
>
> CEBM, level 5.

Encounter Three (seven hours after arrival in ED)

The patient and her parents are waiting for local police to arrive to file a sexual assault report and request an investigation regarding the incident. The patient tolerated a regular diet and is now sleeping in bed with family members at her bedside. I page the patient's primary pediatrician to discuss discharge and follow-up plans for the patient.

> *Upon admission of a patient who is an alleged sexual offense victim, the hospital shall seek patient consent for collection and storage of the sexual offense evidence and explain the specific rights of the patient and obligations of the hospitals . . . The hospital shall store the sexual offense evidence in a locked, separate and secure area for not less than thirty days unless the patient signs a statement directing the hospital not to collect and keep privileged evidence; such evidence is privileged and the patient signs a statement directing the hospital to surrender the evidence to the police before thirty days has expired; the evidence is not privileged and the police request its surrender before thirty days has expired; after thirty days from commencement of treatment, the refrigerated evidence shall be discarded and the clothes shall be returned upon the patient's request. The hospital shall designate a staff member to coordinate the required actions and to contact the local police agency and forensic laboratory to determine their specific needs and requirements for the maintenance of sexual offense evidence (NYSDOH, 2007).*
>
> CEBM, level 5.

> *Reporting to law enforcement: Reporting provides the criminal justice system with the opportunity to offer immediate protection to victims, collect evidence from all crime scenes, investigate cases, prosecute if there is sufficient evidence, and hold offenders accountable for crimes committed. Given the danger that sex offenders pose to the community, reporting can serve as a first step in efforts to stop them from reoffending. Equally important, reporting gives the justice system the chance to help victims address their needs, identify patterns of sexual violence in the jurisdiction, and educate the public about such patterns. It is recommended that service providers encourage victims to report due in part to the recognition that delayed reporting is detrimental to*

the prosecution and to holding offenders accountable. Victims need to know that even if they are not ready to report at the time of the exam, the best way to preserve their option to report later is to have the exam performed. Reporting requirements in sexual assault cases vary from one jurisdiction to another. Every effort should be made to facilitate treatment and evidence collection (if the patient agrees), regardless of whether the decision to report has been made at the time of the exam. Victims who are undecided about reporting who receive respectful and appropriate care and advocacy at the time of their exam are more likely to assist law enforcement and prosecution (U.S. Department of Justice, 2004).

CEBM, level 5.

COMPETENCY DEFENSE

Domain 1, Competency 2. Evaluate population or geographically based health risk utilizing principles of epidemiology, clinical prevention, environmental health, and biostatistics.

Defense. Domain 1, Competency 2, was met by assessing this patient at risk of drug-facilitated sexual assault. By obtaining a comprehensive history with recall bias and hesitancy to admit the truth from the patient and her friend regarding the day's events, such as being alone with two male peers for two hours and then found by her friend with her shirt ripped and her pants opened, a forensic evaluation for sexual assault was performed as per patient's mother's request for further investigation by law enforcement agency. I later counseled the parents about posttraumatic stress disorder (PTSD), adolescent home safety, and caring for their teenage daughter given the recent alcohol intoxication and possible sexual assault.

Domain 1, Competency 3. Formulate differential diagnoses and diagnostic strategies and therapeutic interventions with attention to scientific evidence, safety, cost, invasiveness, simplicity, acceptability, adherence, and efficacy for patients who present with new conditions and those with ambiguous or incomplete data, complex illnesses, comorbid conditions, and multiple diagnoses in all clinical settings.

Defense. Domain 1, Competency 3, was met with the assessment of sexual assault and the examination of trauma caused by sexual activity. In this case, the patient admitted to drinking alcohol but denied use of drugs during the day; urine toxicology was ordered to assess whether other substances were used to facilitate a sexual assault and to address concerns of physiological changes caused by stimulant or depressant substances.

Domain 3, Competency 2. Evaluate gaps in health care access that compromise optimal patient outcomes, and apply current knowledge of the organization and financing of health care systems to ameliorate negative impact.

Defense. Domain 3, Competency 2, was met when the unavailability of social services to provide the patient with optimum care was identified and I advocated for the director of social services to be paged to ensure contact with the family the following day so that they could be referred to the community sexual assault crisis center. I also contacted the police department.

Medications

Drug: Ceftriaxone Sodium (Rocephin)

Dose range: Gonorrhea, uncomplicated: 125 mg to 250 mg intramuscularly (IM) as a single dose.

Sexually transmitted infectious disease; prophylaxis—victim of sexual aggression: 125 mg IM as a single dose plus metronidazole 2 g orally as a single dose plus either azithromycin 1 g orally as a single dose or doxycycline 100 mg orally twice a day for 7 days.

Method of administration in this case: Intramuscular.

Mechanism of action: A bactericidal antimicrobial, inhibits bacterial wall synthesis of actively dividing cells by binding to one or more penicillin bind proteins (PBPs). These proteins are associated with the bacterial cell membrane and probably serve as synthesis. The result is formation of a defective cell wall that is osmotically unstable.

Clinical use: Gonorrhea.

Side effects
Common: Diarrhea, vomiting, transient increased liver enzymes.
Serious: Disorder of gallbladder, reversible erythema multiforme, hemolysis, immune-mediated immune hypersensitivity reaction, Stevens-Johnson syndrome, toxic epidermal necrolysis.

Drug: Metronidazole (Flagyl)

Dose range: Trichomoniasis: 2 g orally as a single dose or 250 mg orally 3 times daily or 375 mg orally twice daily for 7 days or 500 mg orally twice daily for 7 days.

Sexually transmitted infectious disease; prophylaxis—victim of sexual aggression: 2 g orally as a single dose plus ceftriaxone 125 mg IM as a single dose plus either azithromycin 1 g orally as a single dose or doxycycline 100 mg orally twice a day for 7 days.

Method of administration in this case: By mouth.

Mechanism of action: A nitroimidazole antibiotic. Metronidazole has a limited spectrum of activity that includes various protozoans and most Gram-negative and Gram-positive anaerobic bacteria. Metronidazole appears to selectively produce cytotoxic effects in anaerobes by a reduction reaction, depriving the organism of required reduction equivalents.

Clinical uses: Trichomoniasis, bacterial vaginosis.

(continued)

Side effects
Common: Abdominal discomfort, loss of appetite, metallic taste, nausea and vomiting, Jarisch Herxheimer reaction, ataxia, dizziness, headache, peripheral neuropathy, seizure, drug interaction with alcohol.
Serious: Leukopenia, ototoxicity, thrombocytopenia.

Drug: Azithromycin (Zithromax)

Dose range: Chlamydial infection: 1 g orally as a single dose.
Sexually transmitted infectious disease; prophylaxis—victim of sexual aggression: 1 g orally as a single dose or doxycycline 100 mg orally twice a day for 7 days, plus ceftriaxone 125 mg IM as a single dose plus metronidazole 2 g orally as a single dose.

Method of administration in this case: By mouth.

Mechanism of action: The antibacterial action of azithromycin is similar to that of erythromycin. Azithromycin inhibits messenger RNA-directed polypeptide and protein synthesis. It exerts this activity by binding at the 50 S ribosomal subunit.

Clinical uses: Gonorrhea, chlamydia, pelvic inflammatory disease.

Side effects
Common: Abdominal pain, diarrhea, nausea, vomiting, headache.
Serious: Allergic reaction (itching or hives, swelling in face or hands, swelling or tingling in mouth or throat, chest tightness, trouble breathing), blistering, peeling, red skin rash, palpitations, dark-colored urine, pale or black stools, severe diarrhea that may contain blood, vomiting within one hour after taking the medicine, jaundice.

Drug: Levonorgestrel (Plan B)

Dose range
Before menarche: Not indicated.

After menarche: 1 tablet (0.75 mg) orally as soon as possible within 72 hours after unprotected intercourse, followed by 1 tablet (0.75 mg) orally 12 hours after the first dose of 0.75-mg tablet.

Method of administration in this case: By mouth.

Mechanism of action: Oral levonorgestrel acts as an emergency contraceptive, principally by preventing ovulation or fertilization (by altering tubal transport of sperm and/or ova). In addition, it may inhibit implantation (by altering the endometrium). It is not effective once the process of implantation has begun. The major effect of low-dose levonorgestrel is the production of scanty, viscous cervical mucus, which retards sperm penetration.

(continued)

Clinical uses: Emergency post-coital contraception.

Side effects

Common: Weight gain, abdominal pain, altered appetite, diarrhea, nausea, vomiting, dizziness, headache, depression, breast tenderness, cyst of ovary. **Serious:** Severe stomach pain, fatigue, headache, nausea, vomiting or diarrhea.

Source: MICROMEDEX Healthcare Series (2009). DRUGDEX Drug Point.

References

Brick, J. (2006). Standardization of alcohol calculations in research. *Alcoholism: Clinical and Experimental Research, 30,* 1276–1287.

Casey, C., Vellozzi, C., Mootrey, G.T., Chapman, L.E., McCauley, M., Roper, M.H., Damon, I., & Swerdlow, D.L. (2006). Surveillance guidelines for smallpox vaccine adverse reactions. *Centers for Disease Control and Prevention Morbidity and Mortality Weekly Report, 55,* 1–16.

Centers for Disease Control and Prevention (CDC), Department of Health and Human Services. (2006). *Sexually transmitted diseases treatment guidelines 2006.* Retrieved December 20, 2008, from http://www.cdc.gov/std/treatment/

DuMont, J., Macdonald, S., Rotbard, N., Asllani, E., Bainbridge, D., & Cohen, M. (2009). Factors associated with suspected drug-facilitated sexual assault. *Canadian Medical Association Journal, 180,* 513–519.

Kellog, N. (2005). The evaluation of sexual abuse in children. *Pediatrics, 116,* 506–512.

New York State Department of Health (NYSDOH). (2007). *Protocol for the acute care of the adult patient reporting sexual assault.* Retrieved December 20, 2008, from http://www .health.state.ny.us/professionals/protocols_and_guidelines/sexual_assault/

Rauchenzauner, M., Kountchev, J., Ulmer, H., Pechlaner, C., Bellmann, R., Wiedermann, C.J., & Joannidis, M. (2005). Disturbances of electrolytes and blood chemistry in acute alcohol intoxication. *Middle European Journal of Medicine, 117,* 83–91.

U.S. Department of Justice, Office on Violence against Women. (2004). *A national protocol for sexual assault medical forensic examination adults/adolescents.* Retrieved May 30, 2009, from www.ncjrs.gov/pdffiles1/ovw/206554.pdf

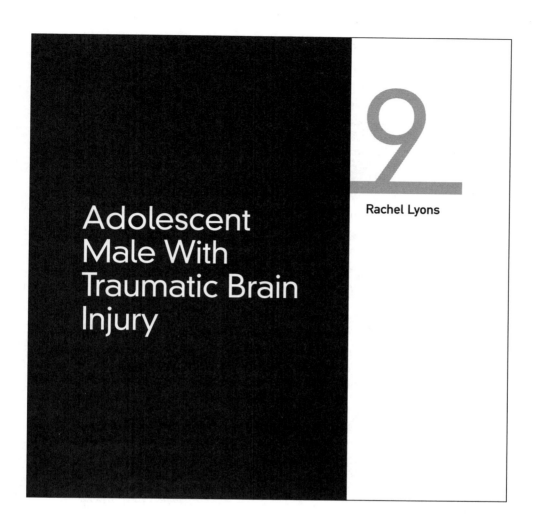

9

Rachel Lyons

Adolescent Male With Traumatic Brain Injury

This case demonstrates care I provided for a 12-year-old boy in the emergency department (ED) and in inpatient and outpatient settings. Care for this Medicaid-insured patient occurred during six encounters over a one-month period. The case narrative demonstrates my ability to meet the following Columbia University School of Nursing Doctoral Competencies for Comprehensive Direct Patient Care:

DOMAIN 1, COMPETENCY 3

Formulate differential diagnoses and diagnostic strategies and therapeutic interventions with attention to scientific evidence, safety, cost, invasiveness, simplicity, acceptability, adherence, and efficacy for patients who present with new conditions and those with ambiguous or incomplete data, complex illnesses, comorbid conditions, and multiple diagnoses in all clinical settings.

PO A. Formulate a differential diagnosis for a patient who presents with new undifferentiated signs and symptoms.

PO B. Formulate a differential diagnosis for a patient who presents with ambiguous or incomplete data, complex illnesses, comorbid conditions, and potential multiple diagnoses.

PO C. Discuss the rationale for the differential diagnosis.

PO D. Discuss the rationale for the diagnostic evaluation with attention to scientific evidence, safety, cost, invasiveness, simplicity, acceptability, adherence, and efficacy.

PO E. Discuss the rationale for the therapeutic intervention with attention to scientific evidence, safety, cost, invasiveness, simplicity, acceptability, adherence, and efficacy.

DOMAIN 1, COMPETENCY 4

Appraise acuity of patient condition, determine need to transfer patient to higher acuity setting, coordinate, and manage transfer to optimize patient outcomes.

PO A. Assess the acuity of patient status.

PO B. Determine the most appropriate treatment setting based on level of acuity.

PO C. Formulate a transfer plan.

PO D. Implement plan to transfer the patient to a higher level of care utilizing written and oral communication.

PO E. Coordinate care during transition to the higher acuity setting.

PO F. Co-manage care in person.

PO G. Co-manage care though written and verbal instructions.

PO H. Make recommendations for patient disposition from the higher acuity location.

PO I. Coordinate post-discharge care.

DOMAIN 1, COMPETENCY 5

Evaluate and direct care during hospitalization, and design a comprehensive discharge plan for patients from an acute care setting.

PO A. Assess the acuity of patient's condition and determine the most appropriate inpatient treatment setting based on level of acuity.

PO B. Actively participate in the admission process to the appropriate inpatient treatment setting.

PO C. Actively co-manage patient care during hospitalization.

PO D. Formulate plan for ongoing care to be provided in a subacute setting, such as a long-term care facility, rehabilitation facility, or home or community setting.

PO E. Coordinate ongoing comprehensive care to be provided in a subacute setting, such as a long-term care facility, rehabilitation facility, or home or community setting.

DOMAIN 3, COMPETENCY 1

Construct and evaluate outcomes of a culturally sensitive, individualized intervention that addresses the specific needs of a patient in the context of family and community.

PO A. Assess culturally specific needs of patient in context of family and community.
PO B. Construct a culturally sensitive intervention to address needs of patient in context of family and community.
PO C. Evaluate outcomes of the intervention.

DOMAIN 2, COMPETENCY 1

Assemble a collaborative interdisciplinary network, and refer and consult appropriately while maintaining primary responsibility for comprehensive patient care.

PO A. Initiate referral to other health care professionals while maintaining primary responsibility for patient care.
PO C. Utilize consultation recommendations for decision-making while maintaining primary responsibility for care.
PO D. Evaluate outcomes of interventions.
PO E. Provide ongoing patient follow-up, and monitor outcomes of collaborative network interventions.

ENCOUNTER CONTEXT

Encounter One (initial evaluation)

DNP role: I am the pediatric nurse practitioner and DNP resident seeing this patient for an initial ED evaluation.

Site: Urban academic medical center.

Setting: Pediatric Level 1 trauma center.

Reason for encounter: Child brought to ED by parents.

Informants: Parents and 12-year-old patient, who appear to be reliable historians.

Chief complaint: Headache and vomiting.

History of Present Illness

A 12-year-old male reports two days ago that he went to the park, four blocks from his home, to look for friends, but they were not in the park. He states that "nobody" was there; he heard "a fire cracker" and then "something sliced through my hair." He states that he did not know what it was, but he thought a rock hit him. The patient states that he touched his scalp, and there was a little blood in the area above his right ear. He ran home, went to his room, and slept for approximately one hour. He did not tell anyone he was hit by a "rock" in the park. He awoke from his nap feeling fine. He ate lunch and had no problems the rest of the day.

The following day, the patient awoke feeling sick: "my body was hot and I was sweating." His mother cooked rice and water, but he "threw it up." He reports he vomited five or six more times that day. Toward the end of the day he felt "dizziness," which he describes as feeling "like my head was spinning."

The next morning, he awoke with "dizziness" and right-sided headache, "like something's in my head." When asked what was in his head, he replies, "something like a rock." He vomited many times through the day. The vomiting and the headache got worse throughout the day. His head "felt like it was moving back and forth." If he stood up straight, he would fall to one side. His nausea improved throughout the day, and in the evening he told his mother that he had been hit by a rock in the park two days ago.

Past Health History

The patient fractured his left proximal humerus at age six after falling off a deck. This was treated with a sling and swathe. There have been no prior serious illnesses, hospitalizations, or surgeries. Birth history includes full-term, normal vertex presentation vaginal delivery without maternal or neonatal complications.

Current medications: None.

Allergies: No known drug, food, or environmental allergy.

Immunizations: Up-to-date.

Social History

Patient lives with his parents and his older brother. His parents are from Laos and Thailand. They reside in the second-story apartment house near the medical center. Both parents work during the day, and sometimes the father works in the evening as a delivery truck driver. The patient states he will begin seventh grade this fall, and his grades range between B's and C's. After-school time is mostly spent outdoors in the nearby park.

Cultural: The patient's parents speak only Hmong.

> *Traditionally, the Hmong believe that illnesses could have natural causes (e.g., spoiled food, exposure to the elements, fall, accident); these are treated with herbs, massage, cupping, or other nonspiritual methods (Helsel, Mochel, & Bauer, 2005).*
> Oxford Centre for Evidence-Based Medicine (CEBM), level 3.

Critical Appraisal

I requested the assistance of an interpreter to provide and incorporate culturally competent care and advocacy. As I assess this patient and his family, I am cognizant of their cultural beliefs (**Competency 7, PO A**).

Family History

There may be a maternal history of chronic headaches. It is difficult to elicit a definitive history of actual headaches, possibly because of the Hmong belief that illnesses could also have supernatural causes.

> . . . (e.g., lost souls, offended spirits, malevolent spirits); these tended to be more serious illnesses (Helsel, Mochel, & Bauer, 2005).

CEBM, level 3.

Review of Systems

Constitutional: The patient is an awake and alert male. The patient has had mild weight loss since his recent episodes of continued vomiting. The patient denies fever, but feels "sick all over" with the sensation that his head is moving "back and forth."

Head: States that he has been hit by a rock to the right side of his head two days prior and now has a cut above his right ear.

Eyes: Denies eye pain or visual disturbance.

Ears: Denies discharge or hearing loss, but does describe "dizziness" when attempting to ambulate.

Nose: Denies nasal discharge or congestion.

Neck: Denies lumps, bumps, or stiffness.

Throat: Denies difficulty swallowing or sore throat.

Cardiovascular: Denies chest pain.

Respiratory: Denies shortness of breath or wheezing.

Gastrointestinal: Denies constipation or diarrhea but has had multiple episodes of vomiting.

Genitourinary: Denies dysuria or hematuria.

Neurological: Complains about right-sided headache above his right ear. No complaints of lethargy or decrease in activity.

Musculoskeletal: Patient denies joint or muscle aches. Has not noticed any new lumps, bumps, or lesions.

Skin: No new rashes or bites noted.

Hematological: No history of easy bruising.

Immunological: Immunizations are up-to-date.

Psychological: Denies feeling unsafe at home or at school. Has no thought of harming self or others.

Physical Examination

General: Alert and oriented without distress.

Vital Signs: Heart rate 100, respiratory rate 22, blood pressure 115/70, temp 100.5°F, SaO_2 98% room air. Weight 36 kg.

Neurological: His Glasgow Coma Scale is 15.

HEENT: His pupils are equally round and reactive to light. Extraocular movements are intact. Visual fields are intact to confrontation. Fundoscopic exam reveals no evidence of papilledema. His face is symmetrical. His tongue and uvula are midline. His jaw is symmetrical. His motor and sensory exam on his face is intact. Examination of his head reveals a soft-tissue swelling above the right pinna that is very tender to palpation. There is also a crusted formation over the patient's right ear, embedded within his hair.

Respiratory: Breath sounds are clear and equal bilaterally without fremitus.

Heart: Heart rate is regular sinus rhythm, without rubs, clicks, or murmurs.

Gastrointestinal: Abdomen is soft, nontender, without masses and hyperactive bowel sounds.

Genitourinary: Circumcised penis with testes descended bilaterally. Tanner stage III.

Musculoskeletal: He has full range of motion to bilateral upper and lower extremities and neck.

Neurological: His motor exam is 5/5 power in upper and lower muscle groups. He has no pronator drift. Sensory exam is intact with the ability to distinguish two-point discrimination. Gait is slightly ataxic. Upper and lower deep tendon reflexes are +2. Abdominal reflexes are symmetric and present.

Skin: Overall slight pallor. Soft-tissue swelling above right pinna in hair with a crusted lesion 3 cm × 2 cm in same area. There are no other cutaneous lesions present.

Impression

Based on the history of being struck with a hard object to the back of the head, and physical examination findings of a soft-tissue swelling above right pinna with crusted lesion in same area, fever, dizziness, nausea, and vomiting, this patient is at risk for head trauma that is over forty-eight hours in time. Differential diagnoses taken into consideration include traumatic head injury, intracranial hemorrhage, intracranial hematoma, increasing intracranial pressure, headache, severe new-onset migraine, tension, thunderclap headache with postauricular lesion, and mastoid pain. Concern for traumatic brain injury will guide evaluation in this setting, with emergent CT scan of the head.

It is also unclear whether this patient's mother suffers from chronic headaches, which may be included in my differential diagnosis. There is literature that suggests that mild traumatic head injury may trigger episodes of migraine headaches.

> *Post-traumatic headaches as well as post-traumatic syndrome can occur in patients after mild, moderate, or severe traumatic brain injury. Most of the patients' symptoms clear within the first 3 to 6 months. The headaches fall into the category of chronic tension-type headache as well as headaches compatible with migraine and are treated in a similar fashion (Linder, 2007).*
>
> CEBM, level 5.

This patient may also coincidentally have a flu-like viral illness, causing his generalized malaise and emesis; however, this is considered less likely given history of head trauma.

ICD-9 Code: 432.9 Unspecified Intracranial Hemorrhage. 346.9 Unspecified Migraine. **(D1,C3, PO A, C).**

Plan

Therapeutics
IV with saline bolus and antiemetic ondansetron (Zofran) 5 mg intravenous (IV).

Diagnostics
Electrolyte panel, complete blood count (CBC), and CT scan of the head and brain.

> *The greatest risk to a patient with apparently minor traumatic brain injury (TBI) is an intracranial hematoma. The presence of this potentially fatal complication is often not apparent until clinical deterioration has occurred and recovery is endangered. Cranial computed tomography (CT) scanning has proven to be the most reliable diagnostic study for occult hematoma (Stein, Burnett, & Glick, 2006).*
>
> CEBM, level 2.

> *The precise mechanism of post-traumatic vomiting is unknown but it is likely that contact forces (impact) are less important than inertial forces (impulse)*

in its etiology. Whereas symptoms such as loss of consciousness and post-traumatic vomiting are induced by head motion, skull fracture depends on contact forces. In most injuries the two phenomena occur together (Stein, Burnett, & Glick, 2006).

CEBM, level 2.

Counseling and Education

I explain to the patient and family with a Hmong interpreter that a head CT scan will allow me to assess if there is any abnormality in the brain after this patient's injury, and the laboratory data will also support my diagnosis.

Working with Hmong people in medical settings raises a number of important cross-cultural health issues. For example, many Hmong people are apprehensive about the effects of invasive procedures. Specifically, patients may resist blood draws and lumbar punctures because tapping a finite amount of vital fluids can invite negative consequences. In addition, Hmong often fear operations because of the potential for impaired spiritual health. That is, souls may become frightened and leave the body during surgery, or the disfigured body may doom the soul to dissevered misery in the next reincarnation (Her & Culhane-Pera, 2004).

CEBM, level 5.

(D3, C1, PO B.)

Encounter Two

Diagnostic Test Results (35 minutes from initial evaluation)

Electrolyte panel and CBC were within normal limits.

I review the CT results with the pediatric radiologist. The CT scan reveals two metallic objects consistent with bullet fragments, one adjacent to the inner table of the mid right parietal calvarium measuring 3 mm in diameter, the other within the right occipital cortex medially measuring 6 mm in diameter. There is a beam hardening artifact from both bullet fragments, and a tiny density projects adjacent to the outer table of the calvarium that is probably a small bone chip at the same level. There is a minimally depressed calvarial fracture, presumably at the bullet entry site. There is overlying scalp swelling in that region consistent with what I assessed. There is also some posterior temporal lobe edema and air, presumably related to the bullet track because it could be followed from the entry site posteriorly and medially to the larger bullet fragment. There may be a small amount of right-sided tentorial subdural hemorrhage. There is no other intracranial hemorrhage, and there is very slight leftward midline shift without significant ventricular compression.

Diagnosis

Gunshot wound to head. ICD-9 Code: 873.0.

Plan

Counseling and Education
With the Hmong interpreter, I tell the family and patient that the blood tests are within normal limits; however, I am concerned about the CT scan. I explain that the injury sustained was due to a bullet and I need to contact local authorities, a primary care provider, a neurosurgery team, and our child protection team **(D2, C1, PO A).**

Critical Appraisal

I know it is important that the family understand that further intervention is needed. Utilizing the concept of the LEARN model, I am able to integrate my assessment with their cultural beliefs for a shared decision-making process:

- Listen with sympathy and understanding to the patient's perception of the problem
- Explain your perceptions of the problem
- Acknowledge and discuss the differences and similarities
- Recommend treatment
- Negotiate agreement

Source: Berlin & Fowkes, 2004

The traditional Hmong religious perspective addresses questions pertaining to the cycle of birth and death, wellness and disease. The World of the Light and the World of the Dark exist side by side, so the mostly unperceived, transparent spirit world permeates everyday reality. Disruption of harmony and balance between souls in the real world and spirits in the spirit world culminates in disease. When one of a person's three major souls wanders off, becomes lost, is ensnared by evil forces, or leaves the body to be reincarnated, then pain, suffering, and death will follow. Physicians should not underestimate the influence of a patient's family when strategizing about a care plan. Since Hmong belong to a patriarchal culture that values family-based decision making, patients often turn to relatives to decide courses of action, and male clan leaders may be consulted if a disease is serious and the treatment plan is perceived as dangerous. As a source of insight and support for the patient, the clan's primary responsibility is to the physical and spiritual health of family members (Her & Culhane-Pera, 2004).

CEBM, level 5.

Consultation
The family agrees to continue with the plan of care of contacting specialists and preparing for likely impending surgical intervention. I consult pediatric

neurosurgery and the child protection team. The child protection team is consulted because of the nature of this patient's diagnosis.

Critical Appraisal

Per our hospital policy, whenever there is a safety concern, whether it is in the home or in the community, the child protection team is contacted to aid in taking the history and to collaborate with law enforcement. The Child Protection Program Staff are experienced in working cooperatively with community physicians and agencies, law enforcement personnel, and the judiciary system to ensure the best outcome for children and their families.

I upgrade the patient's triage acuity and change to a trauma status as per our hospital protocol **(D1, C4, PO A, B)**.

I order phenytoin (Dilantin) to prevent any seizure activity that may occur due to injury. I also notify local law enforcement **(D1, C5, PO C)**.

Posttraumatic seizures contribute to secondary injury and have been observed to occur commonly in children with moderate to severe brain injury. Children differ from adults in exposures to injury, mechanisms of injury, and possibly in the pathophysiology of posttraumatic seizures. The child's brain reacts differently to an acute insult, with a higher rate of significant edema. Posttraumatic seizures may worsen ischemia and secondary injury by increasing cerebral metabolism and possibly by directly increasing intracranial pressure, contributing to poor outcomes. Prophylactic phenytoin has been shown to be effective in reducing early posttraumatic seizures in adults and may be effective in children as well (Young et al., 2004).

CEBM, level 1.

Neurosurgery Consultation (50 minutes since initial evaluation)

The patient is evaluated by the pediatric neurosurgery team and we collaboratively decide to admit this patient to the pediatric intensive care unit (PICU) after going to the operating room (OR) for bullet fragment removal. Since the gunshot penetrated the dura as noted on CT examination, the patient is scheduled for operative repair of the dura to prevent continued cerebral spinal fluid (CSF) leak **(D1, C5, PO A, B)**.

Counseling and Education (60 minutes since initial evaluation)

With the Hmong interpreter, I discuss the need for surgery to remove the bullet fragments. The family is anxious about surgery but understand that the bullet needs to be removed. The neurosurgeon obtains consent, and the patient is taken to the OR.

Encounter Three (inpatient day 1/postoperative day 1/POD1)

Patient has been transferred to PICU. When I visit, he is alone. He states that he no longer feels nauseated and is hungry.

Physical Examination

General: Asleep but easily arousable.

Vital signs: Temperature 98.9°F, heart rate 66, respiratory rate 18, blood pressure 103/62, SaO$_2$ 99% room air.

Neurological: Patient remains alert and oriented × 3. Normal facial sensation. 5/5 musculoskeletal strength in upper and lower extremities. Sensation along radial, medial, ulnar, brachial, and interosseous nerves intact.

HEENT: Head dressing is clean, dry, and intact. PERRL 3 mm bilaterally without evidence of papilledema. His face is without droop. His tongue and uvula are midline. His neck is supple without cervical lymphadenopathy. Left upper field unable to visualize my fingers during exam.

Cardiovascular: Heart rate is stable, without rub, click, or murmur. Peripheral pulses equal and strong +2.

Respiratory: Breath sounds are equal and clear bilaterally.

Abdomen: Soft nontender with bowel sounds in all four quadrants.

Genitourinary: Foley in place; urine output remains at > 1 cc/kg/hr.

Skin: Right parietal-temporal craniotomy dressing clean, dry, and intact.

Pain: Well controlled with morphine and/or acetaminophen with codeine. Rates his pain 1/10.

Fluids, electrolytes, and nutrition: D5 0.9 normal saline with 20 meq/Kcl/L at 1.5 times maintenance. Patient is tolerating clear liquids and may advance his diet as tolerated.

Intraoperative Report Review

The procedure included a right craniotomy for incision and debridement of wound. Some foreign bodies and what appeared to be scalp tissue were incorporated into the opening. A small projectile fragment was found in the epidural space that was sent to pathology. The patient tolerated the procedure well and was transferred to the PICU after recovering in the postanesthesia care unit (PACU).

Impression

Patient is stable status post craniotomy. He is comfortable and is almost completely pain-free. Testing his fields of gaze, I note a positive left-upper-field visual impairment that is a new finding post surgery and therefore will request ophthalmology consultation.

Plan

- Remove Foley catheter.
- Check electrolyte panel in the morning.
- Check phenytoin (Dilantin) level.
- Consult social work for discharge planning.
- Consult neurology regarding need to continue phenytoin (Dilantin).
- Consult ophthalmology for visual impairment.
- Docusate (Colace) 100 mg by mouth twice to prevent constipation secondary to opioid administration and change in diet.
- Continue with IV phenytoin (Dilantin) 100 mg twice daily for prophylaxis of seizure activity.
- Continue IV cefazolin (Ancef) 1 g three times daily for prevention of infection postoperatively.
- Continue with acetaminophen with codeine tablet orally every four hours for pain.
- Maintain intake and output.
- Continuous pulse oximetry, vital signs.
- Check weight daily.
- Physical therapy for gait training and transfers.

Encounter Four (child protection consultation)

Both the patient and his older sibling are interviewed by the child protection team. They both deny ever feeling unsafe or scared in the park or at home, ever being hit or punched or otherwise hurt in their home, or ever receiving any punishment for bad behavior or poor grades.

After the evaluation, the child protection team and I determine that there is no need for Department of Children, Youth and Families involvement as there is no concern of supervision or medical neglect. This child has suffered from a significant injury that may have long-term health effects. We also discuss the benefit of counseling services post discharge. I will discuss the counseling options with social work.

Encounter Five (inpatient day 2/POD2)

Patient is awake and alert playing video games. Pain is well controlled with acetaminophen with codeine. Patient is tolerating a regular diet. Patient has ambulated out of bed to the bathroom and the hallway with physical therapy and occupational therapy (PT/OT).

Physical Examination

Vital signs: Temp 99.0°F, heart rate 74, respiratory rate 20, blood pressure 106/74, SaO$_2$ 98% room air.

Neurological: Awake and alert × 3. Normal facial sensation and symmetry. Able to distinguish two-point discrimination.

HEENT: PERRL, EOM intact. Positive left-upper-field visual impairment. Tongue midline. Neck supple. No cervical lymphadenopathy and full neck range of motion.

Heart: Heart rate is regular, without rubs, clicks, or murmurs. Peripheral pulses equal and strong bilaterally in upper and lower extremities.

Respiratory: Breath sounds are equal and clear bilaterally with no adventitious sounds.

Abdomen: Soft nontender with bowel sounds in all four quadrants.

Genitourinary: Normal urine output.

Skin: Right parietal-temporal craniotomy dressing clean, dry, and intact.

Musculoskeletal: 5/5 musculoskeletal strength in upper and lower extremities.

PT/OT Consultation Note Review

They have assessed the patient as safe with functional mobility.

Laboratory Data Review

Phenytoin (Dilantin) level is 12 mcg/mL. Therapeutic range for children and adults: 10–20 mcg/mL. Electrolyte panel within normal limits.

Impression

12-year-old male remains stable status post craniotomy postoperative day two. He is comfortable and is almost completely pain-free. PT/OT consultation obtained, still awaiting neurology and ophthalmology consultation. Discharge planning is in process.

Plan

Await ophthalmology input for continued left-upper visual defect. Transfer to the general pediatric care unit.

Encounter Six (inpatient day 3/POD3)

The patient and his family are waiting in the room. I utilize a Hmong interpreter to explain that the patient is healing well and can be discharged home. He is ambulating without complaints of nausea, vomiting, or headache. Pain is well controlled with acetaminophen with codeine one tablet every four hours. Patient is tolerating a regular diet.

Physical Examination

General: Awake and walking in hallway giving me the "thumbs up" sign with a smile.

Vital signs: Temp 98.7°F, heart rate 70, respiratory rate 18, blood pressure 108/72, SaO$_2$ 99% room air.

Neurological: Patient remains alert and oriented × 3. Sensory and motor function along radial, medial, ulnar, brachial, axillary, and interosseous nerves intact. Gait is steady without ataxia.

HEENT: PERRL, EOM intact. Continued visual field deficit. Normal facial sensation and symmetry. Tongue midline.

Heart: Heart rate is stable, without rubs, clicks, or murmurs. Peripheral pulses equal and strong +2.

Respiratory: Breath sounds are equal and clear bilaterally.

Abdomen: Soft nontender with bowel sounds in all four quadrants.

Urinary: Normal urine output.

Skin: Right parietal-temporal craniotomy dressing clean, dry, and intact.

Musculoskeletal: 5/5 strength in upper and lower extremities.

Consultation Review

Neurology consultation: Neurologist assessed the patient and concluded that the patient would be maintained on phenytoin (Dilantin) for one week and scheduled for an outpatient EEG once the craniotomy incision healed to assess for any epileptogenic focus.

Ophthalmology consultation: Ophthalmologist assessed the patient's visual fields and found defects in right nasal and temporal fields. It was recommended that the patient have an outpatient MRI of the brain to better delineate the injury. The patient would also follow up in the eye clinic after discharge.

Impression

12-year-old male remains stable status post craniotomy postoperative day three preparing for discharge home. Pain is well controlled with acetaminophen with codeine one tablet every four hours. Patient is tolerating a regular diet. He is exhibiting no signs and symptoms of infection. Visual field defects have been assessed by ophthalmologist, and outpatient follow-up is indicated. Neurologist recommends continuing phenytoin (Dilantin) until EEG is obtained in outpatient to assess for epileptogenic focus.

Plan

Counseling

I speak with the patient and his family and explain that he will continue taking the phenytoin as per the neurologist's request for another seven days to reduce the potential of seizure activity and/or epilepsy.

Phenytoin or carbamazepine treatment reduces the risk of early seizures, but does not change late post-traumatic epilepsy or mortality. Therefore, treatment should not be maintained after acute neurological manifestations have resolved (Guerrini, 2006). Interestingly, there is evidence that post-traumatic psychogenic nonepileptic seizures have been described in children (Guerrini, 2006) and may be difficult to differentiate between postacute factors.

CEBM, level 5.

I explain they will receive close follow-up care with the specialists who provided care in the hospital. I explain that the visual changes he incurred post surgery may or may not be permanent and it is important to return to the ED if he develops headache, vomiting, or somnolence. The patient and his family verbalize an understanding with the interpreter.

Discharge home today with follow-up appointments in neurosurgery clinic and ophthalmology clinic within one week. Given that this patient has state Medicaid and clinics are usually not readily available, I call and schedule both appointments to ensure follow-up.

Pediatric health care providers' responsibilities to their pediatric patients are properly mediated by respect for parental autonomy and parental duties to advance the well-being of their children. In this manner caregivers integrate their duty to care for their primary patients and their prima facie duty to respect parental autonomy and family privacy—by forming therapeutic alliances with parents in the administration of medical treatment to their children. Nevertheless, whenever such alliances break down and parents refuse standard medical treatment for their children for whatever reason—thus denying those children primary goods meeting their basic interests—pediatric caregivers have a more fundamental responsibility to their pediatric patients and may override presumptive parental autonomy and family privacy in order to protect children's therapeutic interests. Thus, for pediatric caregivers, respect for parental autonomy and family privacy is constrained by considerations of children's basic welfare, or, to put it another way, the caregivers' positive duty of beneficence can trump the negative right of parental autonomy. Respect for parental autonomy is conditional on the parents' agreement to satisfy their children's basic medical needs (Twiss, 2006).

CEBM, level 5.

DISCHARGE INSTRUCTIONS

The patient is discharged to home with his parents. Follow-up with neurosurgeon in one week's time for wound check and staple removal. His dressing will remain on and will be removed by neurosurgery.

He will also follow up in two weeks with neurologist and discuss possible need for EEG after craniotomy heals to assess for any epileptic focus. Ophthalmologist will see this patient in the next week.

The patient may resume age-appropriate activity, including light exercise. Showering is permitted, but submerging wound under water is not. Diet is regular as tolerated. Dressing is to remain untouched until seen by neurosurgeon. I contact social work, requesting counseling services that the patient may need.

Discharge Prescriptions

Phenytoin (Dilantin) 75 mg by mouth three times daily.
Acetaminophen (Tylenol) with codeine 30 mg, one to two tablets by mouth every four to six hours as needed for pain.
Docusate sodium (Colace) 100 mg by mouth twice daily.

CASE ADDENDUM

I spoke with the patient's primary care provider, neurologist, neurosurgeon, and ophthalmologist one month after the patient was discharged. The patient was doing well at home, but occasionally had "bad dreams" that would awaken him at night. He attributed these to the events that took place after his injury. He is also afraid of walking alone and near the park. His wound continues to heal without signs of infection. Neurologically, he has had no seizures or complaints. His left visual field still remains slightly affected, and he will need an MRI in the near future **(D2, C1, PO D, E).**

Very little is known about the psychological outcomes of serious injury in children and adolescents. The association of risk factors for PTSD and incidence rates that have been studied in injured adults may be different in injured children and adolescents. A literature review suggests that developmentally sensitive assessment of symptoms after trauma may be more valid than the Diagnostic and Statistical Manual of Mental Disorders, Fourth Edition (DSM-IV) criteria, because symptoms of PTSD differ substantially between children and adults. These studies suggest that many children are underdiagnosed because of the utilization of current DSM-IV criteria. Because injury is the leading cause of death and morbidity in patients 19 years and younger and injury accounts for more hospitalizations and outpatient treatment than any other health condition, healthcare professionals need to be cognizant of the risk factors associated with PTSD in children for appropriate detection (McIntosh & Mata, 2008).

CEBM, level 3.

COMPETENCY DEFENSE

Domain 1, Competency 3. Formulate differential diagnoses and diagnostic strategies and therapeutic interventions with attention to scientific evidence, safety, cost, invasiveness, simplicity, acceptability, adherence, and efficacy for patients who present with new conditions and those with ambiguous or incomplete data, complex illnesses, comorbid conditions, and multiple diagnoses in all clinical settings.

Defense. This patient's differential diagnoses were essentially based on the history and physical. Clinical findings of ataxia, headache, and an old traumatic wound led me to obtain a diagnostic head CT scan, which ultimately led to the diagnosis of a gunshot wound to the head.

Domain 1, Competency 4. Appraise acuity of patient condition, determine need to transfer patient to higher acuity setting, coordinate, and manage transfer to optimize patient outcomes.

Defense. Based on trauma protocols, a gunshot wound to the head deems a heightened acuity and the involvement of subspecialty services such as neurosurgery.

Domain 1, Competency 5. Evaluate and direct care during hospitalization, and design a comprehensive discharge plan for patients from an acute care setting.

Defense. With the collaboration of inpatient specialists, formulating an outpatient plan was essential for the recovery of this patient. The input from each team member aided in the care during and after hospitalization. Without that team network, care would have been compromised. I was able to coordinate communication between these specialists so that comprehensive care was delivered.

Domain 3, Competency 1. Construct and evaluate outcomes of a culturally sensitive, individualized intervention that addresses the specific needs of a patient in the context of family and community.

Defense. Hmong culture roots its beliefs in naturopathic remedies for ailments that are likely caused from evil spirits. Understanding this concept allowed me to address my findings in a culturally sensitive way that underlined the urgency and importance of this diagnosis and the treatment needed. If I had not been able to recognize and communicate, this case might have turned out differently and shared decision-making would not have been achieved.

Domain 2, Competency 1. Assemble a collaborative interdisciplinary network, and refer and consult appropriately while maintaining primary responsibility for comprehensive patient care.

Defense. Collaborative care was needed with specialty services for this patient because he suffered visual acuity loss, an operation, and possible post-traumatic stress. I maintained primary responsibility while working with this team to provide comprehensive care for this child and his family.

Medications

Drug: Phenytoin (Dilantin)
Dose range
Loading dose: 15–20 mg/kg; based on phenytoin serum concentrations and recent dosing history.
(continued)

Maintenance dose: Same as IV maintenance dose per day listed previously. Divide daily dose into 3 doses per day when using suspension, chewable tablets, or nonextended release preparations.

Method of administration in this case: IV and PO.

Mechanism of action: Stabilizes neuronal membranes and decreases seizure activity by increasing efflux or decreasing influx of sodium ions across cell membranes in the motor cortex during generation of nerve impulses.

Clinical uses: Management of generalized tonic-clonic (grand mal), simple partial, and complex partial seizures; prevention of seizures following head trauma or neurosurgery.

Side effects
Common: Slurred speech, dizziness, drowsiness, lethargy, nausea, vomiting.
Serious: Heart block, bradycardia, Stevens-Johnson syndrome, coma, ataxia, dyskinesia.

Drug: Acetaminophen with Codeine (Tylenol)

Dose range

Codeine: 0.5–1 mg/kg/dose every 4–6 hours; maximum dose: 60 mg/dose.

Acetaminophen: 10–15 mg/kg/dose every 4–6 hours; do not exceed 5 doses in 24 hours; maximum dose for children ≥ 12 years: 4 g every 24 hours.

Method of Administration in this case: PO.

Mechanism of action: Inhibits the synthesis of prostaglandins in the central nervous system (CNS) and peripherally blocks pain impulse generation; produces antipyresis from inhibition of hypothalamic heat-regulating center; binds to opiate receptors in the CNS, causing inhibition of ascending pain pathways, altering the perception of and response to pain; causes cough suppression by direct central action in the medulla; produces generalized CNS depression. Caffeine (contained in some non-U.S. formulations) is a CNS stimulant; use with acetaminophen and codeine increases the level of analgesia provided by each agent.

Clinical uses: Relief of mild-to-moderate pain.

Side effects
Common: Nausea, vomiting, constipation.
Serious: Hepatic toxicity, respiratory depression, bradycardia, elevated intracranial pressure.

Drug: Cefazolin (Ancef)

Dose range

Infants and children: 25–100 mg/kg/day divided every 6–8 hours; maximum dose: 6 g/day.

Mild-to-moderately-severe infections: 25–50 mg/kg/day divided every 6–8 hours.

(continued)

Severe infections: 100 mg/kg/day divided every 6–8 hours.

Method of Administration in this case: IV.

Mechanism of action: Inhibits bacterial cell wall synthesis by binding to one or more of the penicillin-binding proteins and interfering with the final transpeptidation step of peptidoglycan synthesis resulting in cell wall death.

Clinical uses: Treatment of respiratory tract, skin and skin structure, urinary tract, biliary tract, bone and joint infections, and septicemia due to susceptible gram-positive cocci (except *Enterococcus*); some gram-negative bacilli, including *Escherichia coli*, *Proteus*, and *Klebsiella*, may be susceptible; perioperative prophylaxis; bacterial endocarditis prophylaxis for dental procedures.

Side effects
Common: Urticaria, transient elevation of ALT, AST, and alkaline phosphatase, diarrhea, nausea, vomiting.
Serious: Anaphylaxis, seizures, renal failure.

Drug: Docusate Sodium (Colace)

Dose range

6–12 years: 40–150 mg/day in 1–4 divided doses.

Adolescents and adults: 50–400 mg/day in 1–4 divided doses.

Method of Administration in this case: PO.

Mechanism of action: Reduces surface tension of the oil-water interface of the stool, resulting in enhanced incorporation of water and fat and allowing for stool softening.

Clinical uses: Stool softener in patients who should avoid straining during defecation and constipation associated with hard, dry stools; prophylaxis for straining (Valsalva) following myocardial infarction. A safe agent to be used in elderly; some evidence that doses < 200 mg are ineffective; stool softeners are unnecessary if stool is well hydrated or "mushy" and soft; shown to be ineffective used long-term.

Side effects
Common: Rash, diarrhea, abdominal cramping.
Serious: Intestinal obstruction.

Drug: Ondansetron (Zofran)

Dose range: Children 6 months to 18 years: 0.15 mg/kg/dose infused 30 minutes before the start of emetogenic chemotherapy, with subsequent doses administered 4 and 8 hours after the first dose.

Method of administration in this case: IV.

Mechanism of action: 5-HT^3 receptor antagonist. It works by blocking the action of serotonin, a natural substance that may cause nausea and vomiting.

Clinical uses: To prevent nausea and vomiting.

(continued)

Side effects
Common: Constipation, diarrhea, abdominal pain, flushing.
Serious: Weakness, musculoskeletal pain, tremor, twitching, ataxia, acute dystonic reaction (rare), hypokalemia (rare). (Taketomo, Hodding, & Kraus, 2008).

References

Berlin, E., & Fowkes, W. (1982). A teaching framework for cross-cultural health care. *Western Journal of Medicine, 139,* 934–938.

Guerrini, R. (2006). Epilepsy in children. *Lancet, 367,* 499–524.

Helsel, D., Mochel, M., & Bauer, R. (2005). Chronic illness and Hmong shamans. *Journal of Transcultural Nursing, 15,* 150–154.

Her, C., & Culhane-Pera, K.A. (2004). Culturally responsive care for Hmong patients. Collaboration is a key treatment component. *Postgraduate Medicine, 116,* 51–53.

Linder, S.L. (2007). Post traumatic headache. *Current Pain and Headache Reports, 11,* 396–400.

McIntosh, S., & Mata, M. (2008). Early detection of post traumatic stress disorder in children. *Journal of Trauma Nursing, 15,* 126–130.

Stein, S.C., Burnett, M.G., & Glick, H.A. (2006). Indications for CT scanning in mild traumatic brain injury: A cost-effectiveness study. *Journal of Trauma, Infection and Critical Care, 61,* 558–566.

Taketomo, C.K., Hodding, J.H., & Kraus, D.M. (2008). *Pediatric dosage handbook.* Hudson, OH: Lexi Comp.

Twiss, S.B. (2006). On cross cultural conflict and pediatric intervention. *Journal of Religious Ethics, 34,* 163–175.

Young, K.D., Okada, P.J., Sokolove, P.E., Palchak, M.J., Panacek, E.A., Baren, J.M., Huff, K.R., McBride, D.Q., Inkelis, S.H., & Lewis, R.J. (2004). A randomized, double-blinded, placebo-controlled trial of phenytoin for the prevention of early posttraumatic seizures in children with moderate to severe blunt head injury. *Annals of Emergency Medicine, 43,* 435–446.

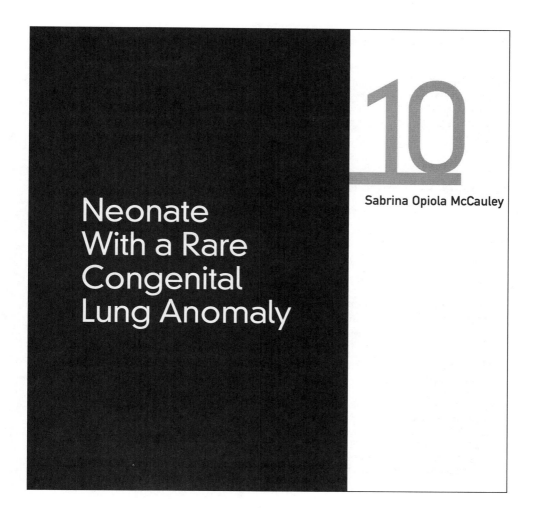

10

Sabrina Opiola McCauley

Neonate With a Rare Congenital Lung Anomaly

I have selected this case to document the comprehensive management of a pediatric patient diagnosed with a rare congenital lung anomaly, who presented with respiratory distress in the neonatal period. The patient was initially seen at an academic medical center and has commercial insurance. The following case focuses on three encounters that occurred over a one-month period in both inpatient and outpatient settings. This case narrative demonstrates my ability to meet the following Columbia University School of Nursing Doctoral Competencies for Comprehensive Direct Patient Care.

DOMAIN 1, COMPETENCY 1

Evaluate patient needs based on age, developmental age, family history, ethnicity, and individual risk including genetic profile to formulate plans for health promotion, anticipatory guidance, counseling, and disease prevention services for healthy or sick patients and their families in any clinical setting.

PO A. Identify a potential genetic risk.

PO C. Evaluate individual patient needs based on age, developmental stage, family history, ethnicity, and individual risk.

PO D. Formulate a plan that addresses health promotion, anticipatory guidance, and/or disease prevention for the family.

DOMAIN 1, COMPETENCY 3

Formulate differential diagnoses, diagnostic strategies, and therapeutic interventions with attention to scientific evidence, safety, cost, invasiveness, simplicity, acceptability, adherence, and efficacy for patients who present with new conditions and those with ambiguous or incomplete data, complex illnesses, comorbid conditions, and multiple diagnoses in all clinical settings.

PO A. Formulate a differential diagnosis for a patient who presents with new undifferentiated signs and symptoms.

PO C. Discuss the rationale for the differential diagnosis.

PO D. Discuss the rationale for the diagnostic evaluation with attention to scientific evidence, safety, cost, invasiveness, simplicity, acceptability, adherence, and efficacy.

DOMAIN 1, COMPETENCY 4

Appraise acuity of patient condition, determine need to transfer patient to higher acuity setting, coordinate and manage transfer to optimize patient outcomes.

PO A. Assess the acuity of patient status.

PO B. Determine the most appropriate treatment setting based on level of acuity.

PO D. Implement plan to transfer the patient to a higher level of care utilizing written and oral communication.

PO E. Coordinate care during transition to the higher acuity setting.

DOMAIN 1, COMPETENCY 5

Evaluate and direct care during hospitalization, and design a comprehensive discharge plan for patients from an acute care setting.

PO A. Assess the acuity of patient's condition and determine the most appropriate inpatient treatment setting based on level of acuity.

PO B. Actively participate in the admission process to the appropriate inpatient treatment setting.

PO C. Actively co-manage patient care during hospitalization.

PO D. Formulate plan for ongoing care to be provided in a subacute setting such as long-term care facility, rehabilitation facility, home, or community setting.

PO E. Coordinate ongoing comprehensive care to be provided in sub-acute setting such as long-term care facility, rehabilitation facility, home or community setting.

DOMAIN 2, COMPETENCY 1

Assemble a collaborative interdisciplinary network, refer and consult appropriately while maintaining primary responsibility for comprehensive patient care.

PO A. Initiate referral to other healthcare professionals while maintaining primary responsibility for patient care.

SUMMARY OF CARE PREVIOUSLY PROVIDED

Prenatal

The patient is a 3540 g Caucasian male newborn, product of a 41-week gestation to a 39-year-old gravida two, para one, AB one (VTOP), O+ mother. Mother received prenatal care, initiated at eight weeks gestation, with a private obstetrician. Prenatal course uncomplicated. Normal chorionic villus sampling reported. Maternal history and serologies negative (–GBS, –HIV, –HbsAG, –VDRL). Mother admitted in labor with spontaneous rupture of membranes 17 hours prior to delivery with clear fluid. Labor failed to progress past 9 cm, and a cesarean section was performed.

Delivery

Under controlled conditions, a 7-pound, 15-ounce (3540 g) male infant (Baby F) was delivered via Cesarean section. Apgar scores were nine at one minute, and nine at five minutes. Infant required no resuscitation at delivery and was transferred to the well baby nursery (WBN) for admission and routine care.

WBN

Baby F is a healthy male infant with normal newborn exam, as per nursing admission assessment. Pediatrician admission note absent, had not yet admitted newborn to WBN. Infant bathed and fed formula in the WBN by three hours of life without issue. Infant reported to have an increased respiratory rate and increased work of breathing by WBN nurse at six hours of life. I was called to evaluate infant at this time and reviewed history.

ENCOUNTER CONTEXT

Encounter One (part I—six hours of life: initial evaluation)

DNP role: I am a neonatal nurse practitioner (NNP) and DNP student evaluating this patient for initial consultation.

Identifying Information

Site: Academic medical center.

Setting: WBN.

Reason for encounter: Initial evaluation for respiratory status change, referral from staff nurse.

Informant: Information obtained from chart and parents.

Chief complaint: "Tachypnea and increased work of breathing" reported by nursing staff.

History of Present Illness

Baby F is a newborn Caucasian male presenting with respiratory distress exhibited by tachypnea, intercostal retractions, and grunting in the WBN at six hours of life.

> *Respiratory distress in newborn infants is manifested by signs including tachypnea, nasal flaring, intercostal retractions, audible grunting, and cyanosis, and occurs when pulmonary function is abnormal. This condition is common immediately after birth and is transient in most cases (Guglani & Ryan, 2008).*
> Oxford Centre for Evidence-Based Medicine (CEBM), level 5.

Past Medical History

Baby F is a 3540 g Caucasian male product of a 41-week gestation to a 39-year-old mother. Uncomplicated prenatal history, negative maternal medical history. Delivered via Cesarean section with Apgars of nine at one minute, and nine at five minutes.

Admitted to the WBN at 45 minutes of life, via transporter, in no distress. Infant received in WBN, pink and warm with temperature of 37°C.

Infant bathed at 60 minutes of life and fed 30 cc of formula without difficulty at 90 minutes of life. Infant transferred to an open crib, as per protocol.

Infant revaluated at three hours of life for feeding with stable temperature of 37°C and no noted distress. Infant fed and tolerated 20 cc of formula well at three hours of life and placed back in open crib. No parental interaction at this time.

At six hours of life, infant assessed for feeding and noted by RN to have an increased respiratory rate with increased work of breathing. At this time, the baby's temperature was stable at 37°C and respiratory rate assessed by RN was 74 bpm.

NNP called to evaluate infant by WBN RN at this time.

Medications: No current medications.

Allergies: No known food or medication allergies.

Immunizations: Parents refused Hepatitis B vaccine; no other immunization history at this time.

Family History

There is no consanguinity in this family.
The parents are both of English descent.

Family History

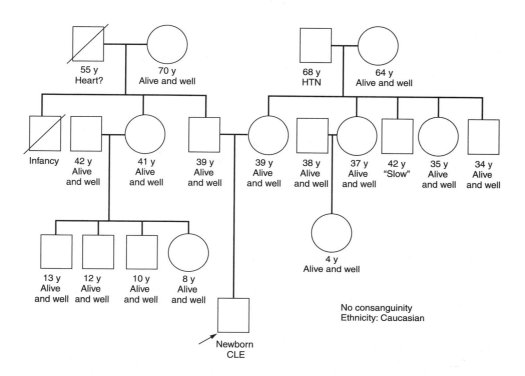

No consanguinity
Ethnicity: Caucasian

Social History

Baby F lives with his mother and father in a two-bedroom apartment. This is a planned pregnancy, and the parents have been married for two years. Father is currently employed; Mother is unemployed and is planning to stay home to be primary caretaker for Baby F.

Presently no family live in the United States, but the maternal grandmother has come to visit for one month after delivery and will be living with the family.

The parents are both Protestant but are currently not practicing.

Birth Weight	3540 g
Temperature	37° C
Heart Rate	132 bpm
Respiratory Rate	80 bpm
Blood Pressure	62/34

Weight	3450 g	50%
Head Circumference	35.5 cm	50%
Length	52 cm	50%

Physical Exam

General: Quiet-alert state, Caucasian newborn.

Head: Normocephalic; anterior fontanel open and flat; posterior fontanel open and flat; no bruit.

Eyes: Proper placement, set, and slant; +red reflex OU.

Ears: Appropriate placement and position.

Nose: Proper placement; nares bilaterally patent.

Throat: Tongue midline; no cleft; no masses; palate intact.

Neck: Supple; trachea midline; no masses; clavicles intact.

Lungs: Clear and equal bilaterally; intercostal retractions, grunting; no flaring; no apnea.

Cardiac: S1/S2 normal; well perfused; +pulses; capillary filling time brisk; I-II/VI murmur auscultated at left lower sternal border.

Gastrointestinal: Abdomen soft/flat, nontender, nondistended; bowel sounds present in four quadrants; umbilicus clamped and moist.

Genitourinary: Normal male testes descended bilaterally; meatus midline.

Anorectal: Patent, normal placement.

Spine: Straight, no dimples, no tufts.

Skin: Pink, intact, no lesions, smooth with visible veins.

Extremities: 10 fingers/10 toes; moving all extremities equally bilaterally.

Neuro: Positive grasp, moro, cry, suck reflexes active.

Ballard exam: 41 weeks, appropriate for gestational age (AGA).

Assessment/Impression

Baby F is a 41-week AGA newborn male with mild respiratory distress at six hours of life. The differential diagnosis based on increased work of breathing, retractions, grunting, and tachypnea includes transient tachypnea of the newborn (TTN), suspected neonatal sepsis, spontaneous pneumothorax, congenital cardiac lesion, and congenital cystic adenomatoid malformation (CCAM). Given the patient's symptoms, as well as maternal and delivery history, the most likely diagnosis at this time is TTN **(D1, C3,**

PO C; D1, C4, PO A). However, based on the known correlation between respiratory distress, neonatal sepsis, cardiac lesions, pneumothorax, and CCAM, further diagnostic testing needs to be done to exclude these diagnoses **(D1, C3, PO D).**

Transient tachypnea of the newborn (TTN) is a parenchymal lung disorder characterized by pulmonary edema resulting from delayed reabsorption and clearance of fetal alveolar fluid. TTN is thought to be a benign, self-limiting condition (Liem & Huq, 2007).

CEBM, level 2b.

Information about the method of delivery and associated complications may assist in diagnosis. TTN is a frequent cause of respiratory distress after cesarean delivery because mechanisms to reabsorb lung fluid have not been initiated (Jain & Dudell, 2006).

CEBM, level 5.

TTN presents within the first 6 hours of life, with tachypnea, retractions and grunting (Guglani & Ryan, 2008).

CEBM, level 5.

Neonatal early-onset sepsis continues to be a significant source of morbidity and mortality among newborns. Most early-onset neonatal GBS disease occurs in term infants born to mothers who have negative GBS screening cultures (Puopolo, 2008).

CEBM, level 5.

Incidence of spontaneous pneumothorax is highest during the neonatal period. This is most probably due to high transpulmonary pressure generated with the onset of breathing (Katar, Devecioglu, & Kervancioglu, 2006).

CEBM, level 1b.

Many newborns with congenital heart disease are symptomatic and identified soon after birth. Respiratory abnormalities may be a sign of congenital heart disease that must be distinguished from pulmonary disease. Persistent elevated respiratory rate or increased effort at rest merit further investigation (Wren & Reinhardt, 2008).

CEBM, level 2b.

Congenital cystic adenomatoid malformation is a rare developmental anomaly of the lower respiratory tract. Among CCAMs that are diagnosed after birth, approximately two-thirds present in the newborn period with respiratory symptoms. Typical signs include tachypnea, increased respiratory effort with grunting and retractions (Gardikis & Didilis, 2002).

CEBM, level 4.

Plan

- Admit infant to the neonatal intensive care unit based on clinical signs of respiratory distress **(D1, C4, PO A, B, D, E).**
- Obtain oxygen saturation and arterial blood gas (ABG) **(D1, C3, PO D).**
- Obtain CBC to examine for neonatal sepsis **(D1, C3, PO D).**

Many different aspects of the leukocyte count have been examined for their predictive value in diagnosing neonatal sepsis. The immature to total neutrophil ratio has been investigated as an early predictor of neonatal sepsis (Mohamed, Wynn, & Cominsky, 2006).

CEBM, level 4.

- Chest x-ray to evaluate for pneumothorax, CCAM, or sepsis **(D1, C3, PO D).**

The importance of tachypnea cannot be overemphasized in the recognition of infection. It is difficult to differentiate pneumonia in a fullterm infant from TTN. Chest x-ray may show increased peri-hilar markings with fluid in the interoblar fissures indicating TTN (Shiva, 2002).

CEBM, level 2b.

- Obtain blood culture and initiate antibiotic therapy to provide empiric coverage for neonatal sepsis **(D1, C3, PO D).**

Many infants are born infected or are from an infected environment. Blood cultures should be obtained. These infants should be started on Ampicillin and Cefotaxime or amnioglycoside (Gomella, Cunningham, Eyal, & Zenk, 2004).

CEBM, level 5.

- NPO with intravenous fluids of 10 percent dextrose and water (D10W) at 80 cc/kg/day **(D1, C3, PO D).**

Encounter One (part II—transfer and admit to NICU)
(D1, C4, PO B, D, E; D1, C5, PO C)

Transfer Summary

Infant transferred to the Neonatal Intensive Care Unit (NICU) at six hours of life, secondary to mild respiratory distress. Transported in room air via transporter in stable condition and placed in a heated isolette in NICU. Physical exam unchanged **(D1, C4, PO B, D, E).**

Admission

Temperature	36.2° C
Heart Rate	136 bpm
Respiratory Rate	88 bpm
Blood Pressure	72/40

CBC	
WBC	24 (9–34)
HCT	44 (40–65)
PLT	214 (150–450)
BANDS	23 (<3)
ABG	
pH	7.40
pCO2	31
pO2	81
BE	−4.7

Diagnostic Review

Chest x-ray: Good penetration, no rotation, left upper lobe hyperlucency with visible lung markings, slight right herniation across midline; mediastinal shift and right upper lobe collapse.

Congenital lobar emphysema (CLE) is a rare developmental anomaly of the lower respiratory tract that is characterized by hyperinflation of one or more of the pulmonary lobes (Stanton & Davenport, 2006).

CEBM, level 5.

Assessment

Baby F is a 41-week gestation male newborn at eight hours of life, with suspected congenital lobar emphysema based on chest x-ray findings of pathognomic left upper lobe hyperinflation with midline shift **(D1, C1, PO A; C3, PO A, C).**

The diagnosis of CLE often can be made from its characteristic appearance on a chest radiograph (Thakral & Maji, 2001).

CEBM, level 2b.

Plan

- Monitor respiratory status with oxygen saturation and respiratory rate.
- Obtain chest CT scan **(D1, C3, PO D)**.

CT may establish a diagnosis of CLE in infants with persistent respiratory distress (Rusakow & Khare, 2001).

CEBM, level 4.

- Consult surgery for possible thoracotomy for surgical management of CLE **(D2, C1, PO A)**.

The appropriate treatment of CLE in newborns with respiratory distress is surgical resection on the affected lobe (Choudhury & Chadha, 2007).

CEBM, level 1b.

- Consult social work for parental resources, insurance and financial concerns, and CLE support group information **(D2, C1, PO A)**.
- Consult cardiology to evaluate for anomalies **(D2, C1, PO A)**.

Cardiovascular anomalies are present in 14% of cases with CLE (Kravitz, 1994).

CEBM, level 5.

- Consult genetics for initial consultation and evaluation of genetic component of CLE **(D1, C1, PO A C; D2, C1 PO A)**.

There have been case reports of CLE in siblings and a report of an affected mother and daughter. This would suggest that inheritance plays a role, it is possible in some cases that the inheritance might be autosomal dominant with variable penetrance and expression.

(Roberts, Holland, Halliday, Arbuckle, & Cass, 2002).

CEBM, level 4.

- Continue antibiotic therapy.
- NPO with Intravenous fluids at 80 cc/kg/day.
- Monitor electrolytes at 24 hours of life and daily while NPO.
- Explain diagnosis and treatment plan to the parents, answer all questions, and provide emotional support.

Encounter Two (day of life 20, NICU)

Summary of Care Provided During Intervening Period

Baby F has been maintained in the NICU for the past 20 days. He was consulted by cardiology on day of life two and found to have a small two-millimeter patent ductus arteriosus, but otherwise normal cardiac anatomy and function requiring no treatment and no follow-up. A CT scan was performed on day of life three and revealed a hyperlucent, hyperextended left lobe with midline herniation, compression of the right lung, and mediastinal shift, thereby confirming his diagnosis of CLE. Surgery evaluated him and recommended lobectomy of the left upper lobe.

The NICU team decided to continue with nonsurgical/conservative treatment, due to his mildly symptomatic course. Genetics was consulted to address the possible genetic component of this rare anomaly of the lung. At this time no genetic testing has been performed on Baby F, at parents' request. He completed a 72-hour course of antibiotic therapy, and all blood work including blood culture, CBC, and electrolytes were within normal range.

Baby F's tachypnea resolved by day of life 14. No further episodes of respiratory distress have occurred. He slowly commenced bottle formula feeding starting on day of life 14 and advanced to full oral formula feedings with adequate calorie intake by day of life 19. His physical exam, growth, and development have been normal for gestational age. The parents have met with nurse practitioners and neonatologists on service daily and agree with the conservative treatment plan. Presently, Baby F is asymptomatic, and a social worker is arranging visiting nurse services with the parents in preparation for discharge.

Critical Appraisal

Although treatment for newborns diagnosed with CLE has historically meant thoracotomy, controversy remains regarding surgical incision at the time of diagnosis as opposed to conservative management of "watch and wait." After reviewing the literature and discussing options with the parents, the decision was made to continue with conservative management, which is reasonable in infants who have no or minimal symptoms.

Data on conservative management, although limited, does state that asymptomatic CLE may regress spontaneously, therefore observation is warranted (Laberge, Puligandla, & Flageole, 2005).

CEBM, level 2b.

NICU Progress Note: Day of Life 20

Weight	3854 g
Temperature	36.8° C
Heart Rate	136 bpm
Respiratory Rate	42 bpm
Blood Pressure	68/42

Respiratory: Lungs clear and equal bilaterally; no apnea, bradycardia, desaturation; no grunting, flaring, retractions; respiratory rate = 42, with oxygen saturations 99–100% in room air.

Infectious: Afebrile; blood culture negative to date; no current issues.

Cardiovascular: S1/S2 normal; well perfused; positive pulses; CFT brisk; no murmur auscultated.

Hematologic:

WBC	17 (9–34)
HCT	38 (40–65)
PLT	489 (150–450)
BANDS	2 (<3)

Metabolic: Infant feeding Similac 20 calorie/ounce formula 60 cc every three hours; total fluids 126 cc/kg/day, tolerated well; no emesis; abdomen soft with +bowel sounds; nontender, nondistended; passing stool; voiding 2.6 cc/kg/hour.

Neurologic: Grasp, cry, moro, suck reflexes present; infant is actively moving all extremities.

Impression: Full-term male infant on day of life 20 with congenital lobar emphysema, presently stable in room air preparing for discharge home with parents.

Plan

- Continue monitoring respiratory status.
- Feed Similac 20 calorie/ounce formula every three hours.
- Continue discharge planning and parental support.
- If stable, discharge home with parents in morning.
- Follow up with social work prior to discharge **(D1, C5, PO C, D, E)**.

Interval Note: Parental Discharge Planning Education Meeting in Hospital

I meet with Baby F's mother and father to discuss his potential discharge home. I begin the meeting by asking the parents whether they have any questions they want to ask. They respond "Not right now," and thank us for all that we have done.

I review Baby F's current improved health status and good prognosis regardless of the diagnosis of congenital lobar emphysema. I review the principal diagnosis, signs, and symptoms and the possibility he may need surgery in the future if he becomes symptomatic. I discuss outpatient follow-up care with their pediatrician that should be initiated within 48 hours of discharge and need for follow-up with surgery in one month **(D1, C5, PO D, E)**.

Encounter Three (day of life 30)

Setting: Outpatient office

DNP role: Primary care provider

Interim summary note: Baby F has been home after hospital discharge for nine days. He was seen by another provider in this office on day of life 21, one day post-discharge, for baseline assessment and weight check. His exam on that visit was normal, and he had no signs of respiratory distress. His parents were reported as "calm and happy to be home" during that visit. He received his first Hepatitis B vaccine in his left thigh. The next visit was scheduled for day of life 30, no communication with parents occurred in the interim.

Chief complaint: Parents state, "We are here for our baby's well-check." When asked, parents state, "No specific concerns at this time, just general sleeping and eating questions."

Activities of Daily Living

Nutrition: Infant taking formula 90–120 cc (three to four ounces) of formula from a bottle every four hours consistently. Burps well and no emesis reported.

Elimination: Infant is having 10 urine diapers/24 hours.

Stooling: Every diaper change; soft and yellow.

Developmental Base (observed during visit)

Motor: He is lifting and turning his head.

Language: He is making sounds and starting to mimic sounds.

Cognitive: He responds to sounds and follows parents' voices.

Social: He is starting to smile.

Milestones: He is tracking with his eyes and meets all appropriate milestones for age, as listed above.

Sleep (reported by parents): He sleeps in a bassinet next to his parent's bed in four-hour cycles during the day. He has slept for five hours at night, but parents wake him for feedings every four hours.

Mother states that he has no blankets or pillows in his bassinet, and sleeps swaddled in a "sleep sack" on his back.

Safety and Environmental Health

The family lives in a post-war apartment, which has been tested for lead during previous renovations and has been repainted in the past two years. The apartment has a smoke detector, but parents are not sure whether it has a carbon monoxide detector. There is no gun in the household. Parents deny smoking, and they have no pets at this time.

Weight	Head Circumference	Length
4029 g (8lbs, 14oz) 25–50%	37.25 cm 25–50%	56 cm 50%

Physical Exam

Vital Signs: Heart rate 122 bpm; respiratory rate = 32 bpm.

General: Active-alert state.

Head: Normocephalic; anterior fontanel open and flat; posterior fontanel open and flat.

Eyes: Proper placement, set, and slant.

Ears: Appropriate placement and position.

Nose: Proper placement; nares bilaterally patent.

Throat: Tongue midline; no cleft; no masses.

Neck: Supple; trachea midline; no masses; clavicles intact.

Lungs: Clear and equal bilaterally; no retractions; no grunting; no flaring; no apnea.

Cardiac: S1/S2 normal; well perfused; +pulses; capillary filling time brisk; no audible murmur.

Gastrointestinal: Abdomen soft/flat; nontender; nondistended; bowel sounds appreciated in four quadrants; passing soft yellow stools.

Genitourinary: Normal male testes descended bilaterally; meatus midline; intact foreskin.

Anorectal: Patent; normal placement.

Spine: Straight; no dimples; no tufts.

Skin: Pink; intact; no lesions; no rashes.

Extremities: 10 fingers/10 toes; moving all extremities × 4.

Neurological: Grasp, moro, cry, suck; rooting reflex; stepping reflex; fencing reflex; plantar grasp all present.

Impression

Baby F is a one-month-old male infant with congenital lobar emphysema diagnosed at birth, presently asymptomatic and managed conservatively with follow-up medical care. He is a healthy and vigorous infant, meeting all the age-appropriate milestones and thriving with active and involved parents.

Parental Teaching/Plan of Care

Parents will follow the CDC-recommended schedule for immunizations as discussed. Developmentally focused anticipatory guidance on growth and development, language development, and stimuli, as well as safety issues regarding accidents, sleep, sudden infant death syndrome (SIDS), signs and symptoms of illness, and household dangers are discussed. Anticipatory guidance provided for feedings and sleep-pattern changes.

We discuss the importance of reading to their infant, the importance of language stimulation through song and talking to him, and the impact this has on his future development. Future schedule of health promotion visits and immunizations are reviewed. I remind them that their next visit should be in one month, at two months of age, and tell them which immunizations will be administered. Parents demonstrate good understanding and are able to verbalize how to safely care for their baby and when the next visit will be.

We review CLE and what to watch for; parents are very knowledgeable about CLE and are able to verbalize appropriately. I advise them to call with any questions or concerns. Presently no follow-up appointments are planned with the surgeon. CLE is stable, and parents will continue to monitor and follow up for health promotion in one month **(D1, C1, PO D).**

Plan

- Health promotion appointment in one month.
- Immunize with second Hepatitis B vaccine today.
- Continue feedings every four hours during the day, and may feed on demand at night.
- Continue to observe for signs of respiratory distress/change related to CLE.
- Continue present infant care and encourage "tummy time."

Placing infants on their tummies helps to build and strengthen the muscles in the shoulders and neck as the infants attempt to hold their heads up and push themselves up so they can take in their surroundings (Chizawsky & Shannon, 2004).

CEBM, level 5.

Critical Appraisal

The immunization schedule used in this case follows the recommended immunization schedule for persons zero through eighteen years of age approved by the Advisory Committee on Immunization Practices, the American Academy of Pediatrics, and the American Academy of Family Physicians, as documented by the CDC in their 2009 immunization schedule guidelines. This is the standard immunization schedule followed in this practice unless an atypical immunization schedule is requested.

- Continue parental support and encourage calling with any questions or concerns.

The elements of a successful family-professional partnership are mutual commitment, respect, trust, open and honest communication, cultural competence and an ability to negotiate (Schor, 2003).

CEBM, level 5.

CASE SUMMATION

Baby F continues to be followed by the practice and is a happy and thriving baby boy. His CLE remains asymptomatic, and his parents plan on moving back to London in the next year.

COMPETENCY DEFENSE

Domain 1, Competency 1. Evaluate patient needs based on age, developmental stage, family history, ethnicity, and individual risk, including genetic profile, to formulate plans for health promotion, anticipatory guidance, counseling, and disease prevention services for healthy or sick patients and their families in any clinical setting.

Defense. Balancing management of this infant's complex diagnosis and possible genetic component, along with his routine health promotion and developmental needs, was challenging. Acting as a child's primary care provider from an early age, I feel it is imperative to promote a theme of family-centered care and not lose sight of the child behind the illness who must continue to thrive and meet his fullest potential. I was able to assess the family and child's needs in this case and have each encounter include routine health surveillance, parental concerns, encouragement, support, and practical guidance on growth, nutrition, and development. The possible genetic component of CLE was discussed with the parents, and referral to a genetic counselor was initiated. The parents were made aware of the possible autosomal-dominant inheritance pattern for CLE, and the fact that the course of treatment will not be changed based on the genetics. Family histories were reviewed, and an infant death of unknown etiology was identified, but at this time the parents do not wish to proceed with the genetic counselor appointment or the gene testing for themselves or their baby.

Domain 1, Competency 3. Formulate differential diagnoses, and diagnostic strategies and therapeutic interventions with attention to scientific evidence, safety, cost, invasiveness, simplicity, acceptability, adherence, and efficacy for patients who present with new conditions and those with ambiguous or incomplete data, complex illnesses, comorbid conditions, and multiple diagnoses in all clinical settings.

Defense. From my first meeting with Baby F, I carefully reviewed his symptoms and evaluated, based on evidence, which diagnosis best fit his clinical scenario, and what next step would guide his treatment. This was evident in my plan of care initiating in the WBN when I facilitated his transfer to the NICU, and continued as I ordered and implemented appropriate diagnostic tests and reviewed the results and the literature to formulate a safe and effective plan of care.

Domain 1, Competency 4. Appraise acuity of patient condition, determine need to transfer patient to higher acuity setting, coordinate and manage transfer to optimize patient outcomes.

Defense. I was able to act as this patient's primary care provider from initial evaluation in the WBN, where, after careful assessment of his condition, I made the decision to transfer him to the NICU. I coordinated and managed his transfer through both written orders and verbal communication with both the WBN staff and the NICU staff, while taking responsibility to notify the parents and the designated pediatrician about my diagnosis of respiratory distress, and communicate my initial differential and plan for intervention.

Domain 1, Competency 5. Evaluate and direct care during hospitalization, and design a comprehensive discharge plan for patients from an acute care setting.

Defense. I was the nurse practitioner responsible for facilitating and implementing transfer of the infant to the NICU, based on his clinical presentation and index of suspicion. I was responsible for his admission, inclusive of writing orders, drawing blood work, deciding upon and ordering appropriate diagnostic tests, coordinating care, and arranging for consultation with the appropriate specialists.

I was actively involved in this patient's care from admission until discharge, and was able to meet with the parents to discuss discharge planning and anticipatory guidance, and arrange outpatient follow-up care based on the patient's specific needs. I also provided the parents with a written discharge summary of Baby F's inpatient course for outpatient providers to reference.

Domain 2, Competency 1. Assemble a collaborative interdisciplinary network, refer and consult appropriately while maintaining primary responsibility for comprehensive patient care.

Defense. As this infant's primary care practitioner on day one of life when he was first diagnosed with CLE, I was able to initiate consultation with the pediatric surgeon. After this consultation, for which I was present and involved, along with the neonatologist on service, we were able to discuss the diagnosis, options, and recommendations as a team.

I also called and facilitated a cardiology, social work, and genetic consultation for this family. Communication among all members of this multidisciplinary health care team remained open, with all recommendations discussed and reviewed by myself along with the neonatologist in order to formulate the most appropriate plan of care for this patient.

References

Chizawsky, L., & Shannon, F. (2004). Tummy time preventing unwanted effects of the "Back to Sleep" campaign. *AWHONN, 9*(5), 382–387.

Choudhury, S.R., & Chadha, R. (2007). Lung resections in children for congenital and acquired lesions. *Pediatric Surgery, 23,* 851–855.

Gardikis, S., & Didilis, V. (2002). Spontaneous pneumothorax resulting from congenital cystic adenomatoid malformation: case report and literature review. *European Journal of Pediatric Surgery, 12,* 195–197.

Gomella, T.L., Cunningham, M.D., Eyal, F.G., & Zenk, K.E. (2004). *Neonatology Management, Procedures, on-Call Problems, Diseases, and Drugs* (5th ed.). New York: McGraw-Hill.

Guglani, L., & Ryan, R. (2008). Transient Tachypnea of the Newborn. *Pediatrics in Review, 29*(11), 59–65.

Jain, L., & Dudell, G.G. (2006). Respiratory transition in infants delivered by cesarean section. *Seminar in Perinatology, 30,* 296–298.

Katar, S., Devecioglu, C., & Kervancioglu, M. (2006). Symptomatic spontaneous pneumothorax in the term newborn. *Pediatric Surgery International, 22,* 755–758.

Kravitz, R.M. (1994) Congenital malformations of the lung. *Pediatric Clinics North America, 41*(3) June:453–472.

Laberge, J.M., Puligandla, P., & Flageole, H. (2005). Asymptomatic congenital lung malformations. *Seminar in Pediatric Surgery, 14*(1), 16–33.

Liem, J.J., & Huq, S.I. (2007). Transient tachypnea of the newborn may be an early clinical manifestation of wheezing symptoms. *Journal of Pediatrics, 151,* 29–32.

Mohamed, I.S., Wynn, R.J., & Cominsky, K. (2006). White blood cell left shift in a neonate: A case of mistaken identity. *Journal of Perinatology, 26,* 378–380.

Puopolo, K.M. (2008). Epidemiology of neonatal early-onset sepsis. *Neoreviews, 9*(12), 571–572.

Roberts , P.A., Holland, A.J., Halliday, R.J., Arbuckle, S.M., & Cass, D.T. (2002). Congenital lobar emphysema: Like father, like son. *Journal of Pediatric Surgery, 37*(5), 799–801.

Rusakow, L.S., & Khare, S. (2001). Radiographically occult congenital lobar emphysema presenting as unexplained neonatal tachypnea. *Pediatric Pulmonology, 32,* 246.

Schor, E.L. (2003). Report of the Task Force on Family Pediatrics. *Family Pediatrics, 111,* 1541–1571.

Shiva, F. (2002). Transient tachypnea of the newborn. *Medical Journal of Iran Hospital, 4*(2), 12–15.

Stanton, M., & Davenport, M. (2006). Management of congenital lung lesions. *Early Human Development, 82,* 289–291.

Thakral, C.L., & Maji, D.C. (2001). Congenital lobar emphysema: Experience with 21 cases. *Pediatric Surgery International, 17,* 88–91.

Wren, C., & Reinhardt, Z. (2008). Twenty-year trends in diagnosis of life-threatening neonatal cardiovascular malformations. *Archives of Childhood, Fetal and Neonatal Edition, 93,* 33–35.

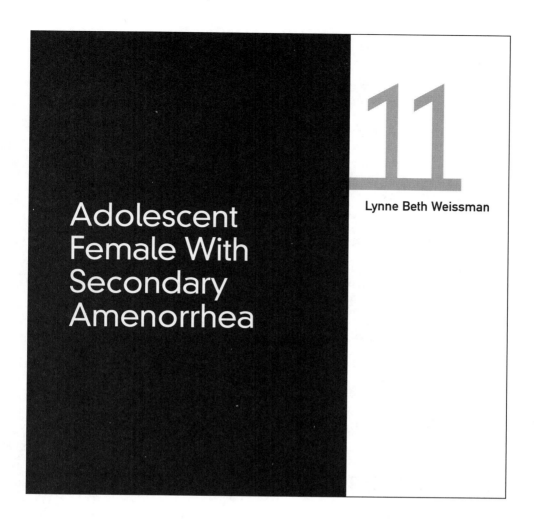

11

Lynne Beth Weissman

Adolescent Female With Secondary Amenorrhea

This case describes the care I provided for a 17-year-old adolescent female with Medicaid HMO insurance who presented for her yearly physical examination complaining of amenorrhea and fear of pregnancy (Patient B). The case narrative focuses on two encounters and one telephone consultation that occurred over a period of six weeks in the ambulatory care setting. This case narrative demonstrates my ability to meet the following Columbia University School of Nursing Doctoral Competencies for Comprehensive Direct Patient Care.

DOMAIN 2, COMPETENCY 1

Assemble a collaborative interdisciplinary network, refer and consult appropriately while maintaining primary responsibility for comprehensive patient care.

PO A. Initiate referral to other health care professionals while maintaining primary responsibility for patient care.

PO B. Accept referrals from other health care professions and communicate consultation findings and recommendations to the referring provider and collaborative network.

PO C. Utilize consultation recommendations for decision-making while maintaining primary responsibility for care.

PO D. Evaluate outcomes of interventions.

PO E. Provide ongoing patient follow-up and monitor outcomes of collaborative network interventions.

DOMAIN 3, COMPETENCY 2

Evaluate gaps in health care access that compromise optimal patient outcomes, and apply current knowledge of the organization and financing of health care systems to ameliorate negative impact.

PO A. Identify gaps in access that compromise patient's optimum care.

PO B. Identify gaps in reimbursement that compromise patient's optimum care.

PO C. Demonstrate patient advocacy in the provision of continuous and comprehensive care.

PO D. Apply current knowledge of the organization to ameliorate negative impact.

PO E. Apply current knowledge of health care systems to ameliorate negative impact.

DOMAIN 3, COMPETENCY 3

Synthesize the principles of legal and ethical decision-making and analyze dilemmas that arise in patient care, inter-professional relationships, research, or practice management to improve outcomes.

PO A. Synthesize ethical principles to address a complex practice dilemma.

PO B. Apply ethical principles to resolve the dilemma.

ENCOUNTER CONTEXT

Encounter One (initial evaluation)

DNP role: I am a pediatric nurse practitioner and DNP resident seeing this patient for annual comprehensive evaluation.

Identifying Information

Site: Ambulatory pediatric practice.

Setting: Primary care.

Reason for encounter: Annual comprehensive evaluation.

Informant: Seventeen-year-old African American female who appears to be a reliable informant.

Chief complaint: Patient reports, "My last period was two months ago. I am worried about being pregnant."

History of Present Illness

Patient B arrives unaccompanied to the office for her yearly physical examination. Her chief complaint is not getting her period for a few months and the possibility of pregnancy. Her last menstrual period was "two months ago." She has had unprotected intercourse over the past three months with the same partner. She has had only one partner. She denies nausea and vomiting. She complains of some breast tenderness.

She does not want her parents or boyfriend to know if she is pregnant. She wants to finish high school and go to college. She does not believe she could do this if she had a baby. She also believes her family would be judgmental and nonsupportive if she told them she was pregnant. She does not want to share decision-making with her boyfriend for fear he would leave her.

Medical History

Prenatal History: Patient B is the eldest of three children. She was the product of an uncomplicated pregnancy. Her mother started prenatal care during the first trimester. She was born via normal spontaneous vaginal delivery. It is not known whether medications were used during labor and delivery. There were no complications in the nursery, and the patient went home with her mother. She was breast-fed for the first three months, and then formula-fed for the rest of the year.

Childhood Illnesses (Chart Review):
- During the past year, Patient B has been seen for one episode of coughing, diagnosed as bronchitis, and treated with over-the-counter cough medication. Her symptoms resolved in approximately 10 days.
- Twenty-pound weight loss last year. The pediatrician checked thyroid function tests that were normal. Patient denies any increased stressors or use of drugs. She had been slightly overweight when she was younger and wanted to lose some weight. Her diet is not healthy, and she often skips breakfast. Her weight has remained stable for the past six months.
- Three episodes of viral pharyngitis over the past four years.
- One uncomplicated urinary tract infection treated with antibiotics.
- Grade I/VI functional heart murmur diagnosed at age seven.
- Positive Mantoux test after travel to an endemic country at age eight. Her chest x-ray was unremarkable. She was treated with INH (Isoniazid), 125 mg once daily, and Pyridoxine (vitamin B6), 50 mg daily, for nine months. She was seen in this office for side effects and liver function tests until the full course of treatment was completed.

- At age 14, she was seen with complaints of menorrhagia of two months' duration. According to the gynecologist's notes, the patient was diagnosed with dysfunctional uterine bleeding. A CBC demonstrated microcytic anemia. She was treated with oral contraceptive pills. The patient was seen by a hematologist two months later to rule out a bleeding disorder. A follow-up CBC demonstrated slight improvement of her anemia. A hemoglobin electrophoresis showed no evidence of thalassemia. She was treated with ferrous sulfate (Feosol) and followed for the next three months, at which time her anemia improved, and she was discharged from hematology. She was advised to continue iron therapy for at least three months. Patient B continued the ferrous sulfate (Feosol) for more than three months and the oral contraceptive pills for six months.

Hospitalizations: There are no recorded hospitalizations, accidents, or surgeries.

Medications: Past medications include Isoniazid (INH), pyridoxine (vitamin B6), ferrous sulfate (Feosol), and oral contraceptive pills. At present she is not taking any prescribed, over-the-counter, herbal, or homeopathic medications.

Allergies: There is no known history of medication, food, or environmental allergies.

Immunizations:

	1989	1990	1992	1993	1994	1995	1997	2004	2007	2008
DTaP	x	xx	x	x						
IPV	x	xx		x						
HiB			x							
HepA									x	x
HepB					xx	x				
MMR			x	x						
Varicella							x			x
Meningitis									x	
Td								x		
Tdap										
HPV										x

Current Health Status: Patient B states that she is currently healthy.

Family History

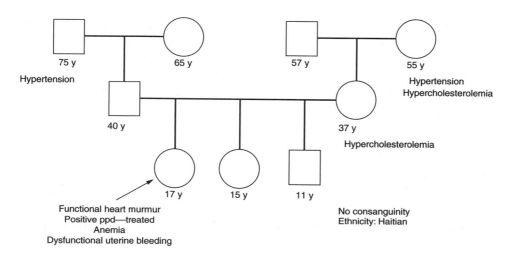

75 y
Hypertension

65 y

57 y

55 y
Hypertension
Hypercholesterolemia

40 y

37 y
Hypercholesterolemia

17 y

15 y

11 y

Functional heart murmur
Positive ppd—treated
Anemia
Dysfunctional uterine bleeding

No consanguinity
Ethnicity: Haitian

HEADS Assessment

Home

Patient B was born in Haiti and immigrated to the United States with her father and mother when she was two years old. She lives in a single-family-dwelling in suburban New York. The house is 15 years old and in good repair. Her household consists of her mother, father, and two younger siblings ages 15 and 11 years. She states that everyone gets along well. Her father works for the post office, and her mother is employed as a nurse in a local hospital. Her mother works the night shift so she can spend time with the family. When her mother is home, she is often busy with Patient B's younger siblings, keeping the house clean, and sleeping. Her family is economically "comfortable." Patient B states that she gets approximately eight hours of sleep most nights.

Patient B states that her relationship with her parents is good. Most of the punishment that she receives is related to missing curfew, and consists of grounding "for a while." Her parents have never hit her or her siblings, and issues are usually resolved through discussion.

Patient B states that although there are gangs in school, she and her friends are not a part of that group. She knows that there are drugs in school, but does not associate with those individuals who are involved with them.

Education and Employment

Patient B attends the local high school and is entering 12th grade. She has many friends. She is not involved in after-school activities because she works to have money to buy the "extras" that her parents cannot afford. She spends most of her money on CDs, clothes, and her cell phone bill.

Until this year, she was a "good" student who maintained a B average. This year, she failed science and the state science examination. She attended summer school to maintain eligibility to take the next science class. She is doing poorly in math. She enjoys languages and history, but finds science and math too hard.

Patient B would like to attend college out of state, but does not know what she would like to study. Her parents believe that since she is not doing well in school, she should attend the local community college until she decides on a major and improves her grade point average. She thinks that if she stays home, her parents will continue to treat her like a child, and she wants to make her own decisions.

Patient B works weekends for six hours at a clothing store in the local mall. She enjoys her work because she receives an hourly wage and a 10 percent discount on clothes she buys in the store. With the extra money she earns, she purchases CDs and clothes, and goes out with her friends.

Religion
Patient B is Roman Catholic and attends Mass on a regular basis with her family. She is not involved in church activities, except those in which her family participates. Her parents are strict and did not let her date until she was 17 years of age.

Family Stressors
Patient B has not been sleeping well, because she believes she is pregnant and feels very stressed. She thinks she will be less stressed when the pregnancy is terminated and she is able to resume her life. Patient B does not believe any family stressors exist at the present time because her family does not know about the pregnancy. She believes her parents would want her to have the baby. She feels that a baby would be too emotionally and financially stressful for herself and her family. She would have to rely on her parents to help her care for the infant. She believes she would not be able to finish school and would not have a career or a successful future. She does not think her boyfriend would help raise the infant.

Activities
Patient B enjoys being with her best friends, listening to music, and texting. She does not spend a lot of time watching TV, but spends most of her free time on the computer chatting with her friends. She denies talking with strangers via the Internet.

Drugs
B denies the use of recreational drugs, including marijuana, cocaine, huffing, snorting, skin popping, and mainlining. She states that although she goes to parties where alcohol is served, she has never had more than one beer a night and has never been intoxicated. She admits to smoking two to four cigarettes a week. She has no suicidal ideation. Up until this visit, she was a happy teenager. She is now concerned and sad about the possibility that she may be pregnant.

Nutrition

Patient B skips breakfast on weekday mornings because of lack of time. Lunch usually consists of a sandwich from the school cafeteria, with a bag of chips or pretzels and soda. Dinner is whatever her mother prepares and leaves for the family to eat. On days that Patient B eats at home, she eats with her siblings when they are available; otherwise, she eats alone. Her father usually eats dinner while watching TV. On days that she works, she purchases fast food, either a hamburger and fries or a slice of pizza with a soda. She states that she does not often snack, but uses the vending machines at school or buys coffee and donuts at work when she does.

Eighty percent of adolescents do not follow recommended dietary guidelines (Stephens, 2006).

CEBM, level 5.

Parents encourage their adolescent children at home by providing relatively controlled food choices. At the same time, teenagers ignore their parents' advice by making unhealthy food choices when on their own. Adolescents understand the healthiness of certain foods but have limited concern about the future. Their eating habits are characterized by frequent snacking, skipping meals, junk food consumption and consistently low intake of fruits and vegetables. (Bassett, Chapman, & Beagan, 2007).

CEBM, level 2b.

Sexual History and Gynecological Information (confidential)

Menarche: 13 years, 6 months. Periods every 30–31 days and last 6 to 7 days. She has no complaints of dysmenorrhea.

Last menstrual period: A little over two months ago.

Patient B states she has only one boyfriend and has become sexually active with him during the past three months. She has not used condoms or other methods of birth control. She denies oral sex. She has not seen a gynecologist since age 16, when she was told she no longer needed to take oral contraceptive pills for dysfunctional uterine bleeding. She states her mother was relieved because she felt that oral contraceptive pills promoted sexual promiscuity. She denies any history of sexually transmitted infections, although she states she has never been tested because she and her partner were virgins.

Review of Systems

General: She denies any weakness or fever but states that she has been a little more tired lately.

Skin: Denies any rashes, skin, or hair changes.

Head: Denies any trauma.

Eyes: Her last eye exam was one year ago. She wears contact lenses. She denies any irritation, dry eyes, discharge, or blurred vision.

Ears: Her last hearing test was almost one year ago. She denies any hearing difficulties. Her only exposure to loud noise is when she listens to her MP3 player. She states she does not frequently go to concerts where loud music is played.

Nose/sinuses: Denies frequent colds, nasal congestion, or nosebleeds.

Throat: Denies frequent episodes of sore throats or tonsillitis.

Dentition: Last dental exam was one year ago. She denies any tooth pain, bleeding gums, or difficulty chewing.

Neck: Denies any neck pain, swelling, or difficulty swallowing.

Respiratory: Denies any shortness of breath, coughing, or wheezing.

Heart: Denies any chest pain or palpitations.

Gastrointestinal: Denies any problems with diarrhea, constipation, or reflux. She has no nausea, vomiting, or abdominal pain.

Genitourinary/reproductive: See "History of Present Illness" and "Sexual History and Information." Patient B states she does not regularly perform breast self-examination.

Musculoskeletal: Denies muscle pain or stiffness, difficulty walking, back pain, or decreased range of motion.

Neurological: Patient B states she gets headaches approximately one to two times a month for the past year. Headaches occur when she skips meals and are relieved by acetaminophen (Tylenol). There is no relationship to her menstrual cycle. Headaches have not increased in frequency, intensity, or duration. She has no accompanying symptoms, including photophobia, phonophobia, auras, fainting, dizziness, or numbness in her extremities. There is no family history of migraines.

Psychiatric: Patient B denies mood swings, violence, or suicidal ideation. She states that she has many friends. She is anxious about the fact that she may be pregnant. She is concerned that her school grades have declined and she does not have sufficient time to study because of the hours she works.

Endocrine: Patient B states that she has no heat or cold intolerance, excessive sweating, or thirst.

Physical Examination

General: African American female who appears stated age. She is apprehensive and nervous.

Vital signs: Temp. 98.3° oral; BP 110/60; Pulse 68; Wt. 140.8; Ht. 66 1/4"; BMI 22.6.

Eyes: Conjunctiva clear; pupils equally round and reactive to light; extraocular movements intact; Fundi: no AV nicking. Vision: OU 20/25, OD 20/40 without glasses.

Ears: No tenderness, discharge, or lesions noted; ear canal with slight amount of cerumen bilaterally; tympanic membranes pearl color; light reflex and landmarks intact; hearing test: 25 decibel bilaterally.

Nose: Symmetric, no sinus tenderness, nasal obstruction, exudate, or inflammation.

Throat: Lips moist, teeth in good repair, tonsils 2+ with no crypts noted.

Neck: Full range of motion without pain; no lymph nodes palpated; thyroid non-palpable; no bruits auscultated.

Chest: Symmetric, respirations unlabored, no adventitious sounds.

Heart: Regular rate and rhythm, S1, S2, no murmur auscultated.

Breast: Symmetric in shape, no skin dimpling, no masses, slightly tender to touch; no nipple discharge.

Abdomen: Flat, bowel sounds active in all four quadrants. Non-palpable liver and spleen. No guarding or tenderness to palpation.

Pelvic: Deferred to gynecology as per institutional protocol.

Rectal: Deferred.

Musculoskeletal: Full range of motion. No tenderness to palpation. No edema noted. All extremities warm to the touch.

Peripheral vascular: No change in skin color or temperature. Radial, femoral, popliteal and dorsalis pedis pulses 2+ and equal bilaterally.

Neurologic: Cranial nerves II-XII intact. Brachioradialis, quadriceps, and ankle reflexes 2+ equal bilaterally. Toes are down going.

Diagnostic testing: Urine pregnancy test positive.

Assessment

17-year-old healthy African American female presents for comprehensive examination.

Her chief complaint is amenorrhea of two months duration. Patient is anxious that she may be pregnant and is concerned about family and social implications. Physical examination reveals breast tenderness; BMI is 22.6, which is acceptable percentile for age. Urine pregnancy test is positive. She had normal thyroid studies. The differential diagnosis for secondary amenorrhea includes pregnancy, stress, medication, chronic illness, low body weight, excessive exercise, thyroid malfunction, pituitary tumor, and early menopause. Based on the history and diagnostic testing, the most likely diagnosis is pregnancy. Gestational age is approximately eight weeks by dates.

Health concerns reevaluated today include:

- History of heart murmur: There was no evidence of a heart murmur on auscultation. This was most likely a functional murmur of childhood that has resolved.

- Anemia on previous lab has since resolved. Was most likely due to dysfunctional uterine bleeding; adequately treated with oral contraceptive pills and ferrous sulfate.

ICD-9 Codes (chronologically)

Heart murmur: inactive 785.2
Dysfunctional uterine bleeding: inactive 626.2
Anemia: inactive 285.9
Pregnancy: active V22.2

Plan

Health Maintenance

While examining Patient B, I instructed her in breast self-examination. She returned the demonstration accurately.

> *Despite the lack of definitive data for or against breast self-examination, breast self-examination has the potential to detect palpable breast cancer and can be recommended (Kearney & Murray, 2006).*
>
> Oxford Centre for Evidence-Based Medicine (CEBM), level 1a.

In discussing immunizations, Patient B elected to defer the HPV (GARDASIL) vaccine until her follow-up visit.

> *Federal law states that immunization from communicable diseases is in the public interest and may therefore be administered to minors without parental consent. If the HPV (GARDASIL) vaccine is seen as protection from a communicable disease then adolescents may consent. However, if the HPV (GARDASIL) vaccine is seen as part of routine medical care in which standard vaccines are provided adolescents would not be able to access the vaccine on their own because, by law, minors are not permitted to consent for their own general medical care. Instead, parental authorization would be required, as it is currently for other vaccines. Since precedence has been set by the minor treatment status regarding untreated STIs, it should not be problematic to extend these treatment statutes to adolescents who seek administration of the HPV (GARDASIL) vaccine without involvement of their parents (Farrell & Rome, 2007).*
>
> CEBM, level 5.

> *The Committee on Bioethics of the American Academy of Pediatrics concluded in their position paper that the "physician's responsibility to his/her child patient exists independently of parental desires and proxy consent." It is suggested that the role of the health care provider is to "do no harm" for the patient remains an important part of the physician-patient relationship (Diaz et al., 2004).*
>
> CEBM, level 5.

Counseling/Education

I discuss the following issues:

- Safe sex, including abstinence and condom use.
- Contraception for the prevention of subsequent pregnancies and sexually transmitted infections.
- Illicit drugs and alcohol use and abuse were discussed. I counseled her to never drive while under the influence of drugs or alcohol, as well as to never get into a car with an intoxicated driver. She was also advised to never pick up a beverage at a party that has been left unattended.
- Cigarette smoking. Because Patient B smokes a few cigarettes a week, we speak about the dangers of cigarette smoking and secondhand smoke effects. I ask whether she wants to quit and would like information and the phone number of the New York State Smokers' Quitline. At the moment, she does not see smoking as a problem.
- Seat belt usage. Although Patient B states that she wears a seat belt in the front seat, she often does not wear it while in the backseat.

Accidents, suicide and homicide are the leading causes of death among American adolescents. Additional morbidity and mortality is related to drugs, alcohol and tobacco use. Alcohol and drug use contribute to more than 40% of adolescent deaths from motor vehicle accidents. More than 75% of adolescents have used alcohol, and more than 25% have engaged in binge drinking. Tobacco use is also common in adolescents with 60% reporting to have at least used tobacco once. The five A's strategy (ask, advise, assess, assist and arrange) has been used for counseling for smoking cessation but can be used for other high-risk behaviors (Stephens, 2006).

CEBM, level 5.

- Stressors for adolescents include poor self-esteem, lack of support, and peer pressure. I advise her that there are many county agencies to which I can refer her to deal with stressors and lack of perceived support. I also inform her that she can contact me at any time to discuss problems she may be experiencing.

Parents and peers play a role in adolescent socialization, and superior outcomes are found among those adolescents who have high levels of support from their mothers, fathers, and friends. Deviant peers and unskilled parents have demonstrated a debilitating effect on adolescent adjustment. The source of support though may be less important than the fact that support is available (Laursen & Mooney, 2008).

CEBM, level 2b.

- I discuss getting extra help for math and science, such as speaking with her teachers about extra help in the morning or getting a student tutor on the weekend. I impress upon her the importance of coming forward if she feels depressed or unhappy so I can refer her for counseling or access the high school counselors.

Depression is a significant cause of morbidity in adolescents. In addition to suicide, depression is associated with disrupted interpersonal relationships and decreased quality of life. Adolescents often present with poor school performance, guilt, anger, irritability, and recurrent truancy (Stephens, 2006).

CEBM, level 5.

Primary care clinicians should evaluate for depression in adolescents at high risk, as well as those who present with emotional problems as the chief complaint. The primary care clinician should establish relevant links/collaboration with mental health services in the community (Zuckerbrot, Jensen, Stein, Laraque, & GLAD-PC Steering Group, 2007).

CEBM, level 5.

Pregnancy Counseling

I inform Patient B that everything she tells me would remain confidential. I let her know it is the policy of the office to only contact the patient to relate confidential information, including test results.

Some adolescents may not be aware of their confidentiality rights and need information in this instance. Teenagers are more likely to seek prompt follow-up and accept other health-promoting suggestions if they trust the source of the advice. Developing a written office confidentiality policy can help reassure adolescents (Stephens, 2006).

CEBM, level 5.

I discuss the options with Patient B. We talk about carrying to term and raising the infant herself with the support of her family, adoption, and termination of the pregnancy. We talk about support systems and disclosure to her family and boyfriend. She spoke of her inability to care for an infant and her personal desires to "remain single." I suggest that she speak with her parents while I am present. She believes her parents would be judgmental and see her as a disappointment. She fears they would make her carry to term and raise the infant. At the end of the conversation, I reassure her I would not divulge any information to her parents, but if she changed her mind I would be available to meet with her and her parents **(D3, C3, PO A, B)**.

A central role of the clinician is to promote communication between adolescents and their parents while preserving the adolescents' trust and participation in their health care. In the clinical setting assurance of confidentiality must be tailored to the adolescent's developmental stage. If a clinician is currently unable to provide confidential care to the extent allowed by local legislation, referral and assistance to the adolescent to access another appropriate site and clinician is warranted (Monasterio, Hwang, & Shafer, 2007).

CEBM, level 5.

Courts often want to preserve the family hierarchy, but they need to consider that doing so in cases of mandated parental involvement in minors' abortion decisions may preclude a minor from exercising her individual right to choose what she believes is the best course of action.

Minor consent laws and confidentiality limitations vary at the state level and translation of sexual health care principles into practice are influenced by the policies of the individual clinical site Individual clinic policies should be written from the standpoint of assuring access and confidentiality that is consistent with state legislation rather than a defensive posture of legal protection (Monasterio et al., 2007).

CEBM, level 5.

A majority of states require parental involvement in a minor's decision to have an abortion. In light of two U.S. Supreme Court rulings that prohibit parents from having absolute veto over their daughter's decision to have an abortion, many states require consent or notification of only one parent, usually 24–48 hours before the procedure. New York State allows a minor to consent to abortion (Diaz et al., 2004; Gutmacher Institute, 2008).

CEBM, level 5.

We discuss her long-term goals, including plans to finish high school and then attend college. She did not want to get married and raise an infant or share childrearing with her parents. She believes finishing school is the only way she would get ahead in life and not disappoint her parents.

The effect of a teenager's decision on her education . . . should be discussed so that her choices support her long-term goals. Studies suggest that early motherhood may be related to poorer educational outcomes and a greater risk of economic difficulties including being on welfare (Boden, Fergusson, & Horwood, 2008).

CEBM, level 2b.

Although Patient B knew she did not want to have a baby, she felt she was disappointing her parents and going against church teachings. We discuss the fact she is an adult who needs to make decisions that would facilitate achieving her long-term goals. We speak about the feelings that she may have post-abortion. She may feel a sense of guilt because the church does not sanction abortion, grief, and a sense of loss. Along with this she may also feel a sense of relief. These feelings are usually limited, but if needed after the abortion, I would refer her for counseling to help her deal with the feelings she might be experiencing.

Regardless of their religion, an unplanned pregnancy and choosing to terminate their pregnancy is an ethical, spiritual, religious, and developmental crisis that needs to be acknowledged by providers.

Anticipatory guidance may help reduce the chance of post-abortion difficulties. Because only 30–35% of women return for post-abortion appointments, some post-abortion counseling needs to occur at the pre-abortion visit. Women who report the greatest amount of self-knowledge prior to the abortion report having less emotional stress after abortion (Harris, 2004).

CEBM, level 2b.

Patient B decides to terminate the pregnancy, but not in this county. She does not want to use her family's medical insurance for fear that her parents will find out. She understands she will have to pay for this termination herself. She states she thinks she has enough money saved and does not want any help from her boyfriend. I provided the name and phone number of a physician at a clinic in an adjacent county who performs terminations of pregnancy on a fee-based sliding scale. I also made sure that she had a reliable friend to take her to the clinic. She says her best friend would take her and remain with her after the termination. She would have the termination on a day when she would let her parents know that she would be spending the night at her best friend's house.

> *Most abortions are provided at freestanding clinics and often these sites are difficult for adolescents to access due to their lack of knowledge. . . . details on transportation, hours of operation, and how to obtain an appointment can help increase a teenager's access to care (Dragoman & Davis, 2008).*
>
> CEBM, level 2b.

I inform Patient B of the importance of making an appointment in a timely manner to ensure that the termination would be performed during the first trimester. She relates fears about the safety of an abortion. We discuss the possibility of fever and excessive bleeding, as well as the fact that the medical risks for adolescents are usually low for first trimester terminations **(D2, C1, PO A)**.

> *There is a relationship between gestational age and safety of an abortion. The risk of morbidity and mortality increases with increased gestational age. However, the overall safety of abortion is comparable between older women and adolescents. Approximately 1–2 % of women may experience infection, hemorrhage, embolism, and complications of anesthesia (Dragoman & Davis, 2008).*
>
> CEBM, level 2b.

Contraception Counseling

I gave Patient B the names of gynecologists in the area who accept her insurance. I reassure her that I always refer young women at age 18 years of age for their first gynecologic visit. This way, she would have a reasonable explanation for her parents without informing them of the termination of her pregnancy **(D2, C1, PO A)**.

At this time, Patient B calls for an appointment at the clinic. I then schedule an appointment for a follow-up visit one week after the termination **(D2, C1, PO E)**.

> *Most adolescents who undergo abortion have minimal knowledge of contraception and need counseling. Contraceptive counseling should be integrated into abortion counseling (Dragoman & Davis, 2008).*
>
> CEBM, level 2b.

Encounter Two

One week after comprehensive evaluation, Patient B missed the follow-up appointment. I call, determine she is not in distress, and reschedule the appointment.

Encounter Three (three weeks after initial consultation)

The report from the physician who performed the termination revealed that Patient B was 11 weeks gestation when the termination was performed. Her blood test revealed that she was Rh+. She was given a prescription for Doxycycline (Vibramycin) 100 mg orally, twice a day for seven days. She was also asked to return for follow-up in two to three weeks, sooner if any problems develop.

Encounter Four (five weeks since initial comprehensive appointment and two weeks post-TOP)

Subjective

Patient B states she had forgotten about the appointment to see me one week after the termination. She reports she had terminated her pregnancy two weeks prior to this visit. She was accompanied by a close friend and did not have any problems, such as excessive bleeding or fever, following the procedure. She completed the antibiotic prescription. She had blood work to check for HIV and other STIs. She has not seen the physician for follow-up and did not yet have an appointment.

Studies have reported that pregnant adolescents were nearly twice as likely to have an STI compared to never pregnant peers (Truang et al., 2006).

CEBM, level 2b.

Patient B has not made a decision about future contraception. She does not want her parents to know that she has been sexually active. She fears that if she goes on the pill, they will find out. She also believes that she will gain "a lot of weight" if she goes on the pill. She does not want to use a method whereby she has to "put something in there."

The events of unplanned pregnancy and abortion influence adolescents to select contraceptive methods that are more effective at preventing pregnancy. Twenty-two percent of adolescents stated they intended to use condoms with spermicidal foam thereby combining contraceptive efficacy with STI prevention (Truang et al., 2006).

CEBM, level 2b.

Upon my asking about her feelings, she states a sense of relief but was having difficulty concentrating in school. She feels she has no one to talk to about the termination and feels "very alone." She also states that she is upset and depressed because she and her boyfriend were not getting along. She denies suicidal ideations, and has no plans to hurt herself or to use alcohol and drugs.

Physical Examination

Vital signs: Temp 99.1° oral; Pulse 68; BP 110/60

General: Alert and in no acute distress.

Lungs: Clear to auscultation without adventitious sounds.

Heart: RRR; no murmur, rubs, gallops.

Abdomen: Bowel sounds present in all quadrants; soft; non-tender to palpation.

Mental status: Appears distracted and detached.

Assessment

Seventeen-year-old African American female who recently terminated a pregnancy. At this time, she is having difficulty concentrating on school-work and feels sad. Consideration is given for the diagnosis of depression and grief. She has no suicidal or homicidal ideations, and symptoms are not present by time and quantity for a diagnosis of major depressive episode. Plan to address grief response, as patient does not have informal support system.

Contraception: Although not currently sexually active, she is aware she needs contraception but is unsure of what kind she would like to use. She is concerned about side effects and confidentially of oral contraceptives. She would like to explore the options with a gynecologist. Further counseling is indicated to resolve this, as patient does not have support from her family.

Plan

Counseling and Education
I inform Patient B that there are many different types of contraception, and an appropriate one for her could be found. I gave her the name and phone number of the local family planning clinic that works on a fee-based sliding scale and that would help her decide on a method of birth control that would best suit her needs. In the meantime, I also stress the need for condom use to prevent STIs and HIV. She states that she would definitely use a condom. She asks whether there was anything else that could prevent pregnancy. We talk about the use of spermicidal foam she can purchase without a prescription. Right now, Patient B feels that she does not want to have sex with anyone. We discuss the continued use of abstinence. She thought that abstinence would work for now, but she would still like to follow up with a gynecologist.

Status Post-TOP with Manifestation of Grief Response

I suggest counseling, and Patient B agrees. I provide her with a referral to the local mental health clinic. She agrees to call me if she has any difficulty getting an appointment or before then if she has any concerns regarding depression, suicidal ideations, or desires to use alcohol or drugs **(D2, C1, PO E).**

I emphasize the importance of a follow-up visit to get the results of her STI tests and before initiating intercourse again.

Most adolescents do not experience greater adjustment difficulties than older women following abortion in the short-term or long run. The absolute level of adjustment at post-abortion time has indicated that they are in no way experiencing psychological harm as a result of their choice to terminate an unwanted pregnancy . . . a woman's response to elective abortion is associated with a mixture of feelings. Women who are younger and unmarried, and who have strong religious convictions might be at higher risk for more intense emotions. Too often women are given the message to move on rather than grieve. Because abortion remains controversial and grief is a normal response, it is anticipated that support immediately after abortion will help prevent a more complicated grief process (Ferguson, Boden, & Horwood, 2007).

CEBM, level 2b.

Contraception (status post-termination of pregnancy and need for continued gynecologic care)

I refer Patient B to a gynecologist for continued care and additional counseling on birth control. The name, address, and phone number of a gynecologist who participates in her insurance plan are provided **(D3, C2, PO C).**

Most adolescents who undergo abortion have minimal knowledge of contraception and need counseling (Dragoman & Davis, 2008).

CEBM, level 2b.

The events of unplanned pregnancy and abortion influence adolescents to select contraceptive methods that are more effective at preventing pregnancy. Twenty-two percent of adolescents stated they intended to use condoms with spermicidal foam thereby combining contraceptive efficacy with STI prevention (Truang et al., 2006).

CEBM, level 2b.

Health Maintenance and Immunizations

I discuss the importance of receiving the HPV (GARDASIL) vaccine. A vaccine immunization information sheet is given. I inform her of the benefits and side effects of the vaccine. Patient B consents to the vaccine, and the vaccine is given. An appointment is scheduled for two months later to provide the second dose **(D3, C3, PO C, D).**

About 20 million people in the US are infected with HPV, and about 6.2 million more get infected each year. Most HPV infections don't cause symptoms and go away on their own. Each year about 10,000 women get cervical cancer. HPV is associated with several types of cancer and genital warts. More than 50% of sexually active men and women are infected with HPV at some point in their lives. There is no treatment for HPV infection. The vaccine includes 2 types of HPV that cause about 70% of cervical cancer and 2 types that cause about 90% of genital warts. The vaccine is recommended for girls age 11–12 years and for girls and women ages 13–26 who did not receive the vaccine when they were younger.

Centers for Disease Control and Prevention, 2007, p. 17.

Federal law states that immunization from communicable diseases is in the public interest and may therefore be administered to minors without parental consent. If the HPV (GARDASIL) vaccine is seen as protection from a communicable disease then adolescents may consent. However, if the HPV (GARDASIL) vaccine is seen as part of routine medical care in which standard vaccines are provided adolescents would not be able to access the vaccine on their own because, by law, minors are not permitted to consent for their own general medical care. Instead parental authorization would be required, as it is currently for other vaccines. Since precedence has been set by the minor treatment status regarding untreated STIs it should not be problematic to extend these treatment statutes to adolescents who seek administration of the HPV (GARDASIL) vaccine without involvement of their parents (Farrell & Rome, 2007).

CEBM, level 5.

The Committee on Bioethics of the American Academy of Pediatrics concluded in their position paper that the "physician's responsibility to his/her child patient exists independently of parental desires and proxy consent." It is suggested that the role of the health care provider is to "do no harm" for the patient remains an important part of the physician-patient relationship (Diaz et al., 2004).

CEBM, level 5.

CASE SUMMATION

Nine weeks after the initial narrative encounter, Patient B reports that she went for a follow-up appointment with the physician who performed the termination. She subsequently saw the gynecologist at a local clinic and is going to use oral contraception. She is being seen at the local mental health clinic and is feeling better. She is able to concentrate in school and is not worried about her relationship with her boyfriend. She has an appointment to come in for her second HPV (GARDASIL) vaccine in one month.

COMPETENCY DEFENSE

Domain 2, Competency 1. Assemble a collaborative interdisciplinary network, refer and consult appropriately while maintaining primary responsibility for comprehensive patient care.

Defense. Patient B had numerous issues needing to be addressed. It was my responsibility to refer her to appropriate resources for the termination of her pregnancy, as well as to community resources to ensure her mental health, and to school resources so she could accomplish her goals.

Domain 3, Competency 2. Evaluate gaps in health care access that compromise optimal patient outcomes, and apply current knowledge of the organization and financing of health care systems to ameliorate negative impact.

Defense. Patient B presented with the fear of pregnancy. Once it was determined that Patient B was pregnant and wished to terminate the pregnancy, it was up to me, as the primary care provider, to help her find a safe and anonymous way to proceed. Insurance coverage is an issue for adolescents because a Coordination of Benefits statement is sent to the holder of the insurance policy, thereby informing the family of the pregnancy and termination.

Domain 3, Competency 3. Synthesize the principles of legal and ethical decision-making, and analyze dilemmas that arise in patient care, interprofessional relationships, research, or practice management to improve outcomes.

Defense. Patient B was a sexually active pregnant adolescent who presented to the office. Although she was a minor who under usual circumstances would require parental consent for immunization, she was also at risk for developing HPV, a sexually transmitted disease. Since federal law states that sexually transmitted diseases can be treated without parental consent, HPV (GARDASIL) vaccine can be considered a "treatment" for HPV. Given that it is a provider's obligation to do no harm, my first responsibility is to my patient, independent of parental desire and consent.

Becoming a sexually healthy adult is a key developmental task of adolescents. As a primary care provider, it is my goal to supply resources and interventions to encourage healthy behaviors and outcomes of adolescent sexual behaviors. My goals were to be present through each step of her decision-making process regarding the termination, offering counseling referrals when she felt she could not cope, offering the HPV (GARDASIL) vaccine to keep her safe from a preventable sexually transmitted disease, and being open to answering all of her questions without passing judgment. Serving as the gatekeeper allowed me to provide comprehensive care to improve her outcome related to the pregnancy termination, and to aid prevention of cervical cancer.

Medications

Acetaminophen (Tylenol)

Dosing range: In 12-year-olds and greater: 325–650 mg every four to six hours, not to exceed 3 g daily.

Indications: INH adjunct to prevent neuropathy.

Side Effects
Common: Nausea, rash.
Serious: Hepatotoxicity, cholestasis, renal tubular necrosis, acute analgesic nephropathy, chronic anemia, hemolytic anemia, thrombocytopenia,

(continued)

pancytopenia, leukopenia, neutropenia, agranulocytosis, anaphylactic reaction, angioedema.

Doxycycline (Vibramycin)

Dosing range: 100 mg by mouth every 12 hours; duration varies based on indication.

Indications: Infections, bacterial.

Side Effects:
Common: Headache, nausea, dyspepsia, joint pain, diarrhea, URI symptoms, rash.
Serious: Tooth discoloration in patients less than eight years, photosensitivity, superinfection, Clostridium difficile-associated diarrhea, anaphylaxis, angioedema, lupus erythematosus, serum sickness-like reaction, vasculitis, pericarditis, hepatitis, autoimmune.

Ferrous sulfate (Feosol)

Dosing range: 325 mg by mouth two to three times daily.

Indications: Iron deficiency anemia.

Side Effects
Common: Dyspepsia, nausea, vomiting, diarrhea, constipation, dark stools.
Serious: May occur, but none reported.

HPV (GARDASIL) vaccine

Dosing range: 0.5 mL IM x3 at 0, 2, 6 mo.

Indications: Prevention of cervical, vulvar, and vaginal cancer caused by HPV types 16, 18; genital warts caused by HPV types 6, 11; and precancerous/dysplastic lesions of cervix, vagina, and vulva caused by HPV types 6, 11, 16, 18.

Side Effects
Common: Paresthesias, numbness, unsteady gait.
Serious: Anapylaxsis, bronchospasm, syncope, Guillain-Barre syndrome.

Isoniazid (Isonicotinic acid; INH)

Dosing range: 0–20 mg/kg by mouth or intramuscular daily for nine months; maximum dose: 300 mg/day.

Indications: Tuberculosis latent; to prevent progression of TB in PPD positive patients.

Side Effects
Common: Paresthesias, nausea, vomiting, epigastric discomfort, elevated liver transaminases, hypersensitivity reaction, pyridoxine deficiency.

(continued)

Serious: Agranulocytosis, aplastic anemia, thrombocytopenia, hepato-toxicity, optic neuritis, peripheral neuropathy, toxic psychosis, seizures, hypersensitivity.

Pyridoxine (vitamin B6)

Dosing range: 25–50 mg daily.

Indications: INH adjunct to prevent neuropathy.

Side Effects
Common: Paresthesias, numbness, unsteady gait.
Serious: May occur, none reported.

References

Bassett, R., Chapman, G.E., & Beagan, B.L. (2007). Autonomy and control: The co-construction of adolescent food choice. *Appetite, 50*, 325–332.

Boden, J.M., Fergusson, D.M., & Horwood, L.J. (2008). Early motherhood and subsequent life outcomes. *Journal of Child Psychology and Psychiatry, 49*(2), 151–160.

Centers for Disease Control and Prevention (2007). Quadrivalent human papillomavirus vaccine recommendations of the Advisory Committee on Immunization Practices (ACIP). *MMWR, 56*(No. RR-2), 1–19.

Diaz, A., Neal, W.P., Nucci, A.Y., Ludmer, P., Bitterman, J., & Edwards, S. (2004). Legal and ethical issues facing adolescent health care professionals. *The Mount Sinai Journal of Medicine, 71*(3), 181–185.

Dragoman, M., & Davis, A. (2008). Abortion for adolescents. *Clinical Obstetrics and Gynecology, 51*(2), 281–289.

Farrell, R.M., & Rome, E.S. (2007). Adolescents' access and consent to the Human Papillomavirus vaccine: A critical aspect for immunization success. *Pediatrics, 120*, 434–437.

Ferguson, D.M., Boden, J.M., & Horwood, L.J. (2007). Abortion among young women and subsequent life outcomes. *Journal of Adolescent Health, 39*(1), 6–12.

Gutmacher Institute (2008). State policies in brief: Parental involvement in minors' abortions. Retrieved September 1, 2009, from http://www.guttmacher.org/statecenter/spibs/index.html.

Harris, A.A. (2004). Supportive counseling before and after elective pregnancy termination. *Journal of Midwifery and Women's Health, 49*(2), 105–112.

Kearney, A.J., & Murray, M. (2006). Evidence against breast self-examination is not conclusive: What policymakers and health professionals need to know. *Journal of Public Health Policy, 27*(3), 282–294.

Laursen, B., & Mooney, K.S. (2008). Relationship network quality: Adolescent adjustment and perceptions of relationships with parents and friends. *American Journal of Orthopsychiatry, 78*(1), 47–53.

Levine, S.B. (2006). Dysfunctional uterine bleeding in adolescents. *Journal of Pediatric Adolescent Gynecology, 19*(49), 49–51.

Monasterio, E., Hwang, L.Y., & Shafer, M. (2007). Adolescent sexual health. *Current Problems in Pediatric Adolescent Health Care* (September), 302–325.

Pitkin, J. (2007). Dysfunctional uterine bleeding. *BMJ, 334*, 1110–1111.

Stephens, M.B. (2006). Preventive health counseling for adolescents. *American Family Physician, 74*, 1151–1156.

Truang, H.M., Kellogg, T., McFarland, W., Kang, M.K., Darney, P., & Drey, E.A. (2006). Contraceptive intentions among adolescents after abortion. *Journal of Adolescent Health, 39*, 283–286.

Zuckerbrot, R.A., Jensen, P.S., Stein, R.E., Laraque, D., & GLAD-PC Steering Group. (2007). Guidelines for adolescent depression in primary care (GLAD-PC): I. Identification, assessment, and initial management. *Pediatrics, 120*(5), e1299–e1312.

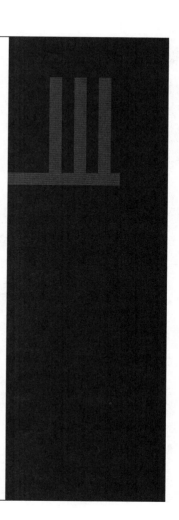

DNP Approach and Clinical Case Narratives in Chronic Care

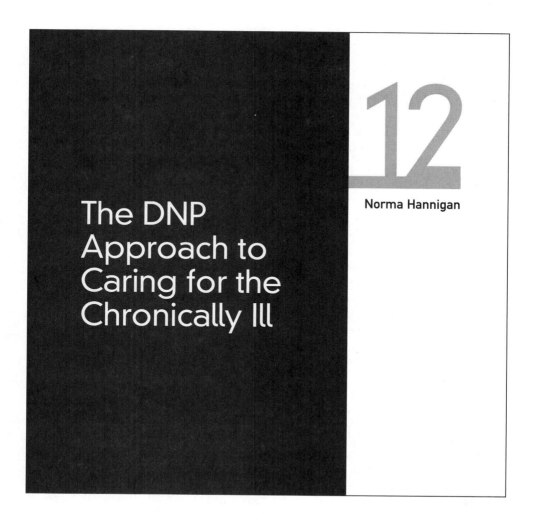

12

The DNP Approach to Caring for the Chronically Ill

Norma Hannigan

It's no longer a question of staying healthy. It's a question of finding a sickness you like.

Jackie Mason (1934–)

With twentieth-century advances in technology, and mass marketing of antibiotics and other lifesaving medicines, previously fatal diseases have metamorphosed into chronic illnesses. In the 1940s, chronic illness care, detection, and treatment became a priority in the United States; the first National Health Survey was conducted in 1957 to determine the extent of chronic disease (*About the National Health Interview Survey*, 2009). In 1992, the name of the Centers for Disease Control was amended to include "and Prevention" (*Announcement of CDC Name Change*, 1992), demonstrating a new focus on "addressing illness and disability before they occur." Of the top ten causes of death in the United States as of 2005, seven are chronic illnesses (*Chronic Disease Overview*, March 20, 2008).

As a nation we are currently focused on health care reform. It is well established that the U.S. health care delivery system is functioning poorly compared with health care delivery systems of other industrialized nations. It is the most costly system in the world, yet health care outcomes are not commensurate with expenditures. Chronic illness management is a major contributor to this dysfunction (Davis, et al, 2007; Anderson & Frogner, 2008; Nolte & McKee, 2008).

THE DOCTOR OF NURSING PRACTICE AND CHRONIC ILLNESS CARE

The doctor of nursing practice (DNP), with the expanded knowledge and skills necessary for provision of comprehensive care across settings and over time, is an expert clinician who views the patient in multiple contexts, interprets and analyzes health care choices, and engages the patient in a collaborative relationship. Because chronic illness may alternate with acute illness in the form of relapse, the DNP is prepared to address the needs of persons with chronic illness.

The Columbia University School of Nursing DNP faculty developed detailed, cognitively complex competencies that address the role of the DNP student in comprehensive care. DNP students demonstrate expertise in the provision, coordination, and direction of comprehensive care to patients, including those who present in healthy states and those who present with complex, chronic, and/or comorbid conditions, across clinical sites and over time. Domain 2, Competency 2, focuses on the DNP student role in management of chronic illness care. The DNP student coordinates and manages the care of patients with chronic illness, utilizing specialists, other disciplines, community resources, and family, while maintaining primary responsibility for direction of patient care and ensuring the seamless flow of information among providers as the focus of care transitions from ambulatory to acute or subacute settings and community settings.

The DNP student demonstrates this competency by

- Coordinating care for a patient with chronic illness as the focus of care transitions across ambulatory, acute, subacute, and/or community settings.
- Co-managing care for a patient with chronic illness as the focus of care transitions across ambulatory, acute, subacute, and/or community settings.
- Coordinating care for a patient with chronic illness, utilizing specialists, other disciplines, community resources, and family.
- Directing care for a patient with chronic illness and ensuring the seamless flow of information among providers as the focus of care transitions across settings.
- Co-managing care for a patient with chronic illness, utilizing shared decision-making and teaching.
- Co-managing care for patients with chronic pain as the focus of care transitions across ambulatory, acute, subacute, and/or community settings.

CHRONIC ILLNESS

Chronic illness is described (Lubkin and Larsen, 2002) as non-reversible illness continuing indefinitely; it may be viewed as a "mixed blessing," since it is usually a welcome alternative to death. The concept of chronicity can be applied regardless of the illness. Julie M. Corbin and Anselm Strauss developed the Illness Trajectory Model (1991) with its nine phases: pre-trajectory, trajectory onset, stable, unstable, acute, crisis, comeback, downward, dying. This model can be utilized by the DNP to provide a framework for educating patients and families about the experience of the chronic illness. Chronic illness may initially be new territory for the patient and family; the DNP can use the illness trajectory model as an anticipatory guidance tool.

Stigma plays an important role in the treatment of chronic illness because it affects the patient's self-perception (Saylor, 1990) and may affect the ability of the patient to participate in shared decision-making and self-care. Ideally, the DNP not only assists the patient to manage the disease but additionally assists with psychosocial issues, coping skills, and maintaining a sense of control.

BEHAVIORAL CHANGE

A major component of illness management is behavioral change. Management is accomplished in large part by behavioral changes. Prochaska et al. (1994), in their work on behavioral change for several different types of health concerns, refer to the Stages of Change model with five stages: pre-contemplation, contemplation, preparation, action, maintenance. As with any attempt to change behavior, relapse is a possible stage through which one may pass before achieving true maintenance. Understanding that relapse is an expected part of the disease trajectory with chronic disorders, the DNP is able to educate the patient regarding this expectation and support the patient and family during this phase. There are many tools available online to assess readiness for change, since recognizing this phase is integral to the process of changing behavior.

MOTIVATIONAL INTERVIEWING

In order to engage the patient in discussion of behavior change, motivational interviewing (MI) may be helpful: "Motivational interviewing represents a promising change-triggering alternative to direct persuasion and aggressive confrontation" (Rollnick & Miller, 1995). Major concepts are that people are generally ambivalent about change; most people will defy change imposed from outside (by the DNP, for example); exhorting or threatening will create resistance. Although most nurses are aware of using reflective technique and shared decision-making, this model is explicit in its purpose of decreasing ambivalence, and thus resistance, toward behavioral change on the part of the patient. The motivation comes from within the patient; it is the responsibility of the patient to resolve the ambivalence about the behavior change. Willingness or readiness to change is not static; nor is chronic illness. While, for some, the eliciting quality essential to motivational interviewing seems too slow a process, the experience of chronic illness is also a process over time. Rather than directing the patient to examine the behavior change itself, motivational interviewing seeks to direct a review of the ambivalence toward the change, so that the patient can come to his or her own conclusions when ready.

CHRONIC ILLNESS MANAGEMENT IN COMPREHENSIVE CARE

The majority of chronic illness management care will be done in an ambulatory or a subacute care setting. The Institute of Medicine (IOM) refers to primary care as "the provision of integrated, accessible health care services by clinicians who are accountable for addressing a large majority of personal health care needs, developing a sustained partnership with patients, and practicing within the context of family and community" (Institute of Medicine, 1994). In keeping with the Columbia University School of Nursing Doctor of Nursing Practice Competencies (2009), the DNP focuses on the integration of care across settings, sustaining partnerships with patients, families, communities, and colleagues. One of the primary goals of the DNP caring for chronically ill patients is to progressively evolve the provision of health care from the acute care model to the health promotion/disease prevention model of comprehensive care.

THE DNP UTILIZING THE CHRONIC CARE MODEL

"The care of chronic illnesses is often a poorly connected string of episodes determined by patient problems" (Rothman & Wagner, 2003). As the Institute of Medicine has indicated that primary care should be continuous, comprehensive, and coordinated, it behooves the DNP to insist that care not be carried out as a "poorly connected string of episodes" but rather as the product of a well-oiled comprehensive care machine.

The Chronic Care Model (CCM) was developed in order to improve the provision of primary care (Wagner, et al., 2001). The six elements of the CCM are:

- Health system—leadership that is on board with using the CCM is essential. The use of group visits can serve as an alternative to episodic visits that do not result in coordinated, comprehensive care. Community resources—partnering with other agencies that have the services the DNP or DNP's agency does not—can also improve access to care. Incentives should be provided based on quality of care; patient safety is incorporated into this part of the model.
- Delivery system design—incorporates delegating appropriate tasks to nonprofessional staff, use of case management, and provision of care that is clinically and culturally appropriate.
- Decision support—incorporating guidelines, flow sheets, reminders, and assessment tools into medical records, integrating specialty expertise into

primary care, sharing evidence-based guidelines with patients to promote participation in self-care.

- Clinical information systems—ready access to information on patients and populations, creating chronic illness registries, care coordination.
- Self-management support—emphasizes the patient's role in self-care, goal-setting, and problem-solving, as well as awareness of community resources to foster ongoing self-care.
- The community—encourages advocacy for policies that foster quality chronic illness care, use of community resources by clinicians and patients.

The DNP can incorporate the above guidelines into establishing the ideal kind of practice encouraged by the IOM.

THE PATIENT-CENTERED MEDICAL HOME

The patient-centered medical home (PCMH) model is described as comprehensive, first-contact, acute, chronic, and preventive care across the lifespan, delivered by a team of individuals that encompasses care coordination across multiple settings and clinicians (Rittenhouse & Shortell, 2009). This description is consistent with the DNP comprehensive care practice model. The American College of Physicians (ACP) has acknowledged that it would support pilot programs comparing leadership of PCMHs by nurse practitioners and physicians to augment the current evidence (American College of Physicians, 2009). It is essential that DNPs participate in pilot programs and regulatory discussion surrounding provision of comprehensive care for persons with chronic illness.

This is an exciting time for the doctor of nursing practice. Health care reform is the focus of the day; the DNP is perfectly poised to join in the political discussion and make the changes that our chronically ill health care system so desperately needs.

References

About the National Health Interview Survey. (2009). Retrieved August 17, 2009, from http://www.cdc.gov/nchs/nhis/about_nhis.htm.

American Association of Colleges of Nursing. (2006). *The Essentials of Doctoral Education for Advanced Nursing Practice.* Retrieved August 23, 2009, from https://www.aacn.nche.edu/DNP/pdf/Essentials.pdf.

American College of Physicians. (2009). *Policy monograph: nurse practitioners in primary care.* Retrieved August 23, 2009, from http://www.acponline.org/advocacy/where_we_stand/policy/np_pc.pdf.

Anderson, G., & Frogner, B. (2008). Health spending in OECD countries: obtaining value per dollar. *Health Affairs (Millwood), 27,* 1718–1727.

Announcement of CDC name change. (1992). *MMWR, 41*(43), 829–830. Retrieved August 17, 2009, from http://www.cdc.gov/mmwr/preview/mmwrhtml/00017962.htm.

Chronic Disease Overview (2008). Retrieved August 12, 2009, from National Center for Chronic Disease Prevention and Health Promotion, http://www.cdc.gov/nccdphp/overview.htm.

Corbin, J., & Strauss, A. (1991). A nursing model for chronic illness management based upon the trajectory framework. *Scholarly Inquiry for Nursing Practice, 4,* 155–174.

Davis, K., Schoen, C., Schoenbaum, S., Doty, M., Holmgren, A., Kriss, J., & Shea, K. (2007). *Mirror, Mirror on the Wall: An International Update on the Comparative Performance of American Health Care.* The Commonwealth Fund. Retrieved August 23, 2009, from http://www.

commonwealthfund.org/Content/Publications/Fund-Reports/2007/May/Mirror—Mirror-
on-the-Wall—An-International-Update-on-the-Comparative-Performance-ofAmerican-
Healt.aspx.

Institute of Medicine. (1994). *Defining Primary Care: An Interim Report*. National Academy of Sciences. Retrieved August 14, 2009, from http://books.nap.edu/openbook.
php?record_id=9153&page=15.

Lubkin, I., & Larsen, P. (2002). *Chronic Illness: Impact and Interventions*. Fifth edition. Sudbury,
MA: Jones and Bartlett Publishers, 4.

Nolte, E., & McKee, C. (2008). Measuring the health of nations: updating an earlier analysis.
Health Affairs (Millwood), 27, 58–71.

Prochaska, J., Velicer, W., Rossi, J., Goldstein, M., Marcus, B., Rakowski, W., et al. (1994). Stages
of change and decisional balance for twelve problem behaviors. *Health Psychology, 13*(1),
39–46.

Rittenhouse, D., & Shortell, S. (2009). The patient-centered medical home: will it stand the test
of health reform? *Journal of the American Medical Association, 301*(19), 2038–2040.

Rollnick, S., & Miller, W. (1995). What is motivational interviewing? *Behavioural and Cognitive
Psychotherapy 23,* 325–334.

Rothman, A., & Wagner, E. (2003). Chronic Illness Management: what is the role of primary
care? *Annals of Internal Medicine, 138*(3), 256–261.

Saylor, C. (1990). The management of stigma: redefinition and representation. *Holistic Nursing
Practice, 5*(1), 45–53.

Wagner, E., Austin, B., Davis C., Hindmarsh, M., Schaefer J., & Bonomi A. (2001). Improving
chronic illness care: translating evidence into action. *Health Affairs (Millwood) 20,* 64–78.

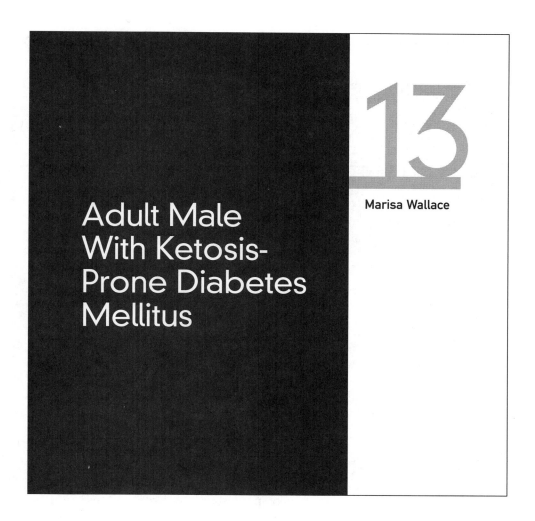

13

Marisa Wallace

Adult Male With Ketosis-Prone Diabetes Mellitus

I selected this case narrative to document consultative care I provided for a patient who required evaluation for an undifferentiated condition with a possible genetic component. I saw this Medicaid-insured patient once, at an urban medical center, prior to his discharge home. This case narrative demonstrates my ability to meet the following CUSN Doctoral Competencies for Comprehensive Direct Patient Care:

DOMAIN 1, COMPETENCY 1

Evaluate patient needs based on age, developmental stage, family history, ethnicity, individual risk, including genetic profile to formulate plans for health promotion, anticipatory guidance, counseling, and disease prevention services for healthy or sick patients and their families in any clinical setting.

PO A. Identify a potential genetic risk.
PO B. Diagnose a genetic condition.

PO C. Evaluate individual patient needs based on age, developmental stage, family history, ethnicity, and individual risk.

PO D. Formulate a plan that addresses health promotion, anticipatory guidance, and/or disease prevention for the individual.

DOMAIN 1, COMPETENCY 3

Formulate differential diagnoses, and diagnostic strategies and therapeutic interventions with attention to scientific evidence, safety, cost, invasiveness, simplicity, acceptability, adherence, and efficacy for patients who present with new conditions and those with ambiguous or incomplete data, complex illnesses, comorbid conditions, and multiple diagnoses in all clinical settings.

PO B. Formulate a differential diagnosis for a patient who presents with ambiguous or incomplete data, complex illnesses, comorbid conditions and potential multiple diagnoses.

PO C. Discuss the rationale for the differential diagnosis.

PO D. Discuss the rationale for the diagnostic evaluation with attention to scientific evidence, safety, cost, invasiveness, simplicity, acceptability, adherence, and efficacy.

PO E. Discuss the rationale for the therapeutic intervention with attention to scientific evidence, safety, cost, invasiveness, simplicity, acceptability, adherence, and efficacy.

DOMAIN 2, COMPETENCY 2

Coordinate and manage the care of patients with chronic illness utilizing specialists, other disciplines, community resources, and family, while maintaining primary responsibility for direction of patient care and insuring the seamless flow of information among providers as the focus of care transitions across ambulatory to acute, subacute settings, and community settings.

PO A. Coordinate care for a patient with chronic illness as the focus of care transitions across ambulatory, acute, subacute, and/ or community settings.

PO C. Coordinate care for a patient with chronic illness utilizing specialists, other disciplines, community resources, and family.

PO D. Direct care for patient with chronic illness and insure the seamless flow of information among providers as the focus of care transitions across settings.

PO E. Co-manage care for a patient with chronic illness utilizing shared decision-making and teaching.

ENCOUNTER CONTEXT

Encounter One (initial consult)

DNP role: FNP, member of diabetes inpatient team, and DNP student.

Identifying Information

Site: Urban academic medical center.

Setting: Inpatient hospital medical unit.

Reason for encounter: Consult requested by medical service for patient with difficult-to-control diabetes in preparation for discharge.

Informant: Chart review and patient who is a poor historian.

History of Present Illness

Mr. O is a 60-year-old Hispanic male with a history of diabetes (DM) found unresponsive at home by family. Emergency medical services (EMS) was called and upon arrival obtained fingerstick blood glucose (FSBG) of 34 mg/dl. Tonic-clonic seizures were also noted. EMS transferred Mr. O to the emergency department (ED), and he was subsequently admitted to neurological intensive care unit (NICU).

While in the NICU, Mr. O was treated with Dextrose 10% infusion; FSBG was monitored every one hour. Hypoglycemia persisted for more than 24 hours. His seizures were controlled with phenytoin (Dilantin). An intravenous insulin infusion was started once FSBG was greater than 200 mg/dl. Mr. O was transferred to a medical unit where glargine (Lantus) 15 units daily and lispro (Humalog) with meals were initiated. Blood glucose was acceptable on this insulin regimen, but suboptimal with FSBG ranging from 122–280 mg/dl. Repaglinide (Prandin) with meals was added, and lispro (Humalog) insulin with meals was discontinued. As a result, blood glucose levels became very elevated, ranging between 155 to 500 mg/dl. Consultation was requested of the inpatient DM team for discharge planning.

Diabetes History

The majority of this history was obtained through medical chart review. Mr. O is a poor historian.

At present, Mr. O denies weight changes, polydipsia, polyphagia, temperature intolerance, changes in hair and skin texture, urinary frequency, urgency, hesitancy, dysuria, hematuria, polyuria, nocturia, and incontinence of urine.

Time	Home Management	Hospitalization
1993	Diagnosed with Type 2 DM in 1993, presentation unclear. Treated with oral hypoglycemic agents for approximately five years.	
1998	Insulin initiated for questionable poor blood glucose control.	

(continued)

Time	Home Management	Hospitalization
2003 (time zero)	Hyperglycemia management included insulin lispro protamine/insulin lispro 75/25 (Humalog Mix 75/25) 40 units in AM, Glargine (Lantus) 20 units HS, and Pioglitazone (Actos)	Presented to hospital with first episode of diabetic ketoacidosis (DKA). For several days prior to his admission, he had stopped his insulin because he was having hypoglycemia. He was discharged home on insulin NPH (Novolin N) 30 units in AM and 20 units in HS, and Glipizide XL (Glucotrol XL) 5 mg daily in A.M.
2003 (six months)	Unclear home management. Regimen was most likely consistent with medication prescribed at time of discharge six months prior.	Presented to hospital in DKA, with no evidence of acute illness or severe stress provoking the DKA. Mr. O was discharged home on insulin NPH (Novolin N) 40 units in AM and 20 units HS.
2005 (24 months)	Home hyperglycemia management at that time was Glargine (Lantus) 60 units and Metformin (Glucophage) 500 mg q daily. Patient reported low FSBG in AM and high FSBG in PM on regimen.	Admitted for hypoglycemia. Discharge medications: insulin NPH (Novolin N) 30 units in AM and 15 units in HS, and Lispro (Humalog) with meals.
2006 (31 months)		Admitted for hypoglycemia. Discharge medications: insulin NPH/regular 70/30 (Novolin 70/30), Rosiglitazone (Avandia), and Glimepiride (Amaryl).
2006 (37 months)		Presented to hospital in DKA, with no evidence of acute illness or severe stress provoking the DKA. Discharge medication: insulin NPH/regular 70/30 (Novolin 70/30) 20 units in AM and 15 units HS.
2006 (38 months)		Readmitted for hypoglycemia. Discharge medications: Glargine (Lantus) 30 units q daily.

(continued)

Time	Home Management	Hospitalization
2006 (49 months)		Mr. O presented to the hospital in hyperosmolar hyperglycemic non-ketosis (HHNK). He was discharged home on Glargine (Lantus) 35 units, As an outpatient, Mr. O's Glargine (Lantus) dose was slowly increased to 50 units due to blood glucoses of 500 mg/dl, and Rosiglitazone (Avandia) 4mg q daily was added.
2007 (50 months)		Presents to hospital with hypoglycemia and seizures.

Medical History

- Diffuse Large B Cell Lymphoma diagnosed one year ago, status post four cycles of chemotherapy. Now in remission.
- Cardiomyopathy most likely secondary to chemotherapy with doxorubicin (Adriamycin). Last transthoracic echocardiogram done one month ago showed ejection fraction 40%. Followed by cardiologist.
- Diabetic retinopathy status post laser treatment. Last eye exam six months ago with no progression.
- DM with microalbuinuria treated with lisinopril (Prinivil).
- Hypertension treated with lisinopril (Prinivil). Blood pressure well controlled for past two years with recorded values ranging from 110–128/65–88.
- Dyslipidemia treated with atorvastatin (Lipitor) 40 mg orally in the evening. Last lipid panel one month ago: LDL 75, Triglycerides 152, HDL 36, total 140.
- Non-ST elevation myocardial infarction in 2006 with triple-vessel disease. Followed by cardiologist. Currently denies chest pain, orthopnea, dyspnea on exertion, postural nocturnal dyspnea, peripheral edema, leg cramps with walking a specific distance, or palpitations.
- Psoriasis. Currently denies rash, pruritus, dryness, non-healing wounds or lesions.

Home Medications (see also Medications list at the end of the chapter)

- Lisinopril (Prinivil) 5 mg orally daily.
- Digoxin (Digitek) 0.125 mg orally daily.
- Carvedilol (Coreg) 6.25 mg orally twice daily.
- Atorvastatin (Lipitor) 40 mg orally at bedtime.
- Aspirin (Ecotrin) 325 mg orally daily.
- Furosemide (Lasix) 40 mg orally daily.
- Glargine (Lantus) 50 units subcutaneously daily.
- Rosiglitazone (Avandia) 4 mg orally daily.

Family History

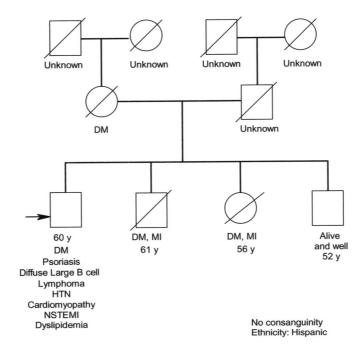

60 y
DM
Psoriasis
Diffuse Large B cell
Lymphoma
HTN
Cardiomyopathy
NSTEMI
Dyslipidemia

DM, MI
61 y

DM, MI
56 y

Alive
and well
52 y

No consanguinity
Ethnicity: Hispanic

Social History

Mr. O is a Hispanic unemployed former taxi driver who lives alone. He denies currently smoking. He stopped one year ago, but has a 40-pack-per-year history. He denies alcohol or illicit drug use. He is independent in his mobility, but has a home health attendant six hours a day, seven days a week, to help him with his activities of daily living, including cooking and shopping.

Review of Systems

Skin: See "Medical History."

Eyes: Denies changes in visual fields, blurred vision, floaters, glaucoma, or cataracts.

Respiratory: Denies chest pain, dyspnea, cough, or shortness of breath.

Cardiovascular: See "Medical History."

Gastrointestinal: Denies dysphagia, nausea or vomiting, diarrhea, or abdominal pain.

Endocrine: See "History of Present Illness."

Urology: See "History of Present Illness."

Peripheral vascular: See "Medical History."

Physical Examination

General: 60-year-old Hispanic male who appears stated age, minimally responsive, and is in no acute distress.

Vital signs: Pulse 90, respirations 18, blood pressure 125/67, height 167.6 cm, weight 64.5, BMI 23.

Neck: No enlarged lymph nodes or thyromegally appreciated.

Chest: Breath sounds are clear bilaterally, anteriorly, and posteriorly, without rales, rhonchi, wheezes, or rubs.

Heart: Regular rate and rhythm, S1, S2, no murmurs, rubs, or gallops.

Peripheral vascular: No cynanosis, clubbing, or edema. Decreased monofilament sensation bilateral plantar aspect of feet.

Labs	Patient Result	Normal Values
Cr	1.3	0.5–0.9 mg/dl
K	5.1	3.6–5.0 mM/l
AST	23	12–38 U/l
ALT	17	7–41 U/l
Urine microalbuminuria (UMA)	847	<30 ug/mg creatinine
C-peptide	<0.5	0.8 to 3.5
Glutamic acid decarboxylase	0.08	0.00 to 1.45
Islet cell autoantibodies	<1:4	<1:4
A1c	Now: 9.1	
	2007: 9.1	
	2003–2006: 7.9–11.9	4–6%

It is important to consider renal function when considering how to treat a patient with diabetes. Renal insufficiency contributes to abnormalities affecting glucose and insulin metabolism. While there is augmented hepatic gluconeogenesis, there is diminished renal gluconeogenesis. There is also decreased level of degradation of insulin in peripheral tissues. Exogenous insulin is primarily excreted by the kidney. As renal failure progresses, insulin clearance decreases, the half-life of insulin increases, and the overall requirements of insulin decline (Biesenbach et al., 2003).
Oxford Centre for Evidence-Based Medicine (CEBM), level 2b.

Since hepatic impairment can lead to reduced insulin metabolism and reduced hepatic gluconeogenesis, it is important to consider liver function in treating a patient with diabetes.

The normal rate of albumin excretion is less than 20 mg/day (15 µg/min); persistent albumin excretion between 30 and 300 mg/day (20 to 200 µg/min) is called microalbuminuria and, in patients with diabetes (particularly type 1 diabetes), is usually indicative of diabetic nephropathy unless there is some coexistent renal disease. Values above 300 mg/day (200 µg/min) are considered to represent overt proteinuria. Although these cut-offs defining normoalbuminuria, microalbuminuria, and overt proteinuria facilitate determining the risk for progression of nephropathy, the risk of developing overt diabetic nephropathy is probably linearly related to albumin excretion rates at all levels (Mogensen, 1990).

CEBM, level 5.

GAD and ICA are not generally recommended for diagnosis for diabetes. However, in order to distinguish between autoimmune diabetes and non-autoimmune diabetes, obtaining GAD and ICA, as well as a C-peptide appears to be the best for determining the type of diabetes a patient has (Balasubramanyam, 2006).

CEBM, level 5.

Impression

Mr. O is a 60-year-old Hispanic male with unclear type of diabetes with multiple episodes of DKA and hypoglycemia. Upon inquiry I find that Mr. O has a long history of diabetes and is familiar with the skills necessary for adequate measurement, and therefore has insight about his diagnosis of type 2 DM and its management. There is no reason to suspect that he gave himself too much insulin or is noncompliant with his DM management. Moreover, based on his laboratory results demonstrating negative GAD and negative C-peptide, a diabetes history of multiple admissions with DKA and hypoglycemia resulting from overdosing of basal insulin needs, family history, and ethnicity, he likely has what the American Diabetes Association (ADA) would classify as idiopathic DM, also known as type 1B DM from beta-cell dysfunction, and will need to be managed on subcutaneous insulin injections for blood glucose control. Mr. O's failing to take his oral hyperglycemic medications helps confirm this diagnosis **(D1, C1, PO C; D1, C3, PO B, C, D, E).**

Patients with idiopathic DM do not have the autoantibodies seen in type 1 DM, but are prone to ketoacidosis for unclear reasons. New evidence would classify Mr. O as having ketosis-prone DM type 1B (Maldonado et al., 2003) **(D1, C1, PO B; D1, C3, PO C).** His hypoglycemia likely resulted because his glargine dose was increased beyond his basal needs, rather than adding a bolus regimen to the patient's insulin regimen **(D1, C3, PO D, E).**

Critical Appraisal

In terms of interventions for Mr. O's DM management, it is important to attempt to classify more definitively what type of DM he has to help optimize his glycemic control. Since DKA is the most serious hyperglycemic emergency in patients with diabetes, it is important to isolate the reason why patients present in DKA. Generally there are precipitating factors that cause DKA. However, in recent years there have been an increasing number of cases of DKA without precipitating factors, and much attention has been given to attempt to describe these cases (Umiperrez, 2006). Clinical heterogeneity of certain presentations of diabetes in multiethnic populations has significant implications for diagnosis, classification, and management (Balasubramanyam, et al., 2006) **(D1, C1, PO A).**

CEBM, level 5.

The two broad categories of DM defined by the ADA are designated type 1 and type 2. However, for patients with type 1 DM, the most common reason for patients to present in DKA is subdivided into type1A and type1B (idiopathic) (ADA, 2009). Type 1A DM results from autoimmune β-cell destruction, as a result of a defect of an HLA allele, which leads to insulin deficiency. Individuals with type 1B DM lack an HLA genetic marker and immunologic markers indicative of an autoimmune destructive process of the β-cells. However, they develop insulin deficiency by unknown mechanisms and are ketosis prone. Recently, emerging data has shown that the ADA's definition of "idiopathic" diabetes is far too simplistic especially among non-Caucasian populations (Balasubramanyam, 2006). There is a high proportion of DKA in nonwhite adults that occurs in persons with type 2 DM (Balasubramanyam, Zern, Hyman, & Pavlik, 1999).

CEBM, level 5.

It is thought that there is a genetic susceptibility to ketosis prone DM, but it is not certain whether there are multiple genetic markers or just one major gene that leads to a defect in β-cell secretion (Mauvais-Jarvis et al., 2004). Ketosis-prone patients demonstrate that the presence or absence of islet cell autoantibodies or HLA susceptibility alleles are not necessarily the key determinants in β -cell function (Balasubramanyam et al., 2006). Ketosis-prone diabetes (KPD) is heterogeneous. Its causes could include novel β-cell functional defects. In order to improve outcomes of KPD patients, several studies have attempted to predict long-term β-cell function and insulin independence in patients with DKA. Of several methods to define KPD heterogeneity, the A β scheme is the most accurate in predicting long-term β-cell function and clinical outcomes (Balasubramanyam et al., 2006). A study done by an endocrinology group out of Baylor College of Medicine took 103 patients who presented with DKA and analyzed their β-cell function, β-cell autoimmunity, and HLA genotype. Maldonado et al., classified these patients into four Aβ groups, based on the presence of glutamic acid decarboxylase (GAD)65, GAD67, or islet cell autoantibodies (A+ or A-) and β-cell functional reserve (β+ or β-). It is believed that KPD comprises at least four etiologically distinct syndromes separable by autoantibody status, HLA genotype, and β-cell functional reserve. Novel, nonautoimmune, polygenetic causes of β-cell dysfunction are likely to underlie the A-β+ and A-β- syndromes (Maldonado et al., 2003).

CEBM, level 2b.

A Beta Symbol Scheme		
	β- (β-cell function -)	**β+ (β-cell function +)**
A+ (autoimmunity +)	KPD type 1A. These are A+β- patients. They have permanent and complete β-cell failure with serologic markers of islet cell autoimmunity and HLA genetic marker. They require lifelong exogenous insulin therapy. Usually lean build, no strong family history.	KPD type 2A. These are A+β+ patients. They have preserved β-cell function at the time of diagnosis but also have serologic markers of islet cell autoimmunity and HLA genetic marker. Some have a reversible form of β-cell dysfunction, characterized by prolonged preservation of β-cell function and ability to discontinue exogenous insulin therapy, while others have progressive β-cell failure and require lifelong exogenous insulin therapy. Usually obese, strong family history of T2DM, variant of LADA.
A- (autoimmunity -)	KPD type 1B. These are A-β- patients. They have permanent and complete β-cell failure but lack serologic markers of islet cell autoimmunity and lack HLA. They require lifelong exogenous insulin therapy. Usually non-obese, strong family history, non-white, may have variable insulin requirements.	KPD type 2B. These are A-β+ patients. They have preserved β-cell function and lack serologic markers of islet cell autoimmunity. The majority (especially if new onset) can discontinue exogenous insulin therapy. Usually a strong family history of Type 2 DM, obese, DKA at presentation but no recurrence, Flatbush; atypical DM; type 3 KPD.

Plan (D1 C1, PO D)

- HgA1c in three months that will be used, in addition to FSBG log book, to assess glycemic control.

Critical Appraisal

> Now that likely ketosis-prone type 1B DM has been the identified cause of Mr. O's multiple admissions, the goal is to reduce the number of admissions for DKA and hypoglycemia to zero. Once that goal has been achieved, the next goal will be that his HgA1c is less than 7%.

- Ophthalmology referral **(D2, C2, PO A).**

  ADA recommends an ophthalmology examination once a year to monitor for diabetic retinopathy (ADA, 2009).

  CEBM, level 5.

- Discharge patient on glargine (Lantus) 15 units subcutaneous daily and lispro (Humalog) six units with meals.
- Discontinue oral hypoglycemic agents. Since Mr. O has no beta-cell function, as evidenced by his near-negative C-peptide, there is little evidence to suggest that oral antihyperglycemic medications will be effective for DM management **(D1, C3, PO E).**
- DM self-management education reinforcement:
  - "Survival Skills": Diabetes education given to Mr. O regarding self-monitoring BG before each meal and before bed, target BG of 120–180 mg/dl, emergency BG values greater than 240 mg/dl each time a BG is checked for two consecutive days or one time BG greater than 400 mg/dl, basal versus bolus insulin-time-action profile of the two different insulins, reviewed hypoglycemic and hyperglycemic symptoms, prevention, and treatment, and consistent carbohydrate diet.
  - Education by hospital nutritionist and reinforced by me included exercise as tolerated, and the importance of following up with the inpatient diabetes nurse practitioner until seen by an endocrinologist at the diabetes center.
  - Written information given to Mr. O **(D2, C2, PO E).**

Teaching diabetes self management to hospitalized patients is a difficult and challenging task. Patients are hospitalized because they are ill, under increased stress, and in an environment that is not conducive to learning (ADA, 2009). They often have competing concerns related to their hospitalization, are being seen by many providers, and fundamentally, are not focused on learning all that there is to gain knowledge of appropriate diabetes self-management skills. Trying to teach everything there is to know about diabetes can be overwhelming to inpatients especially if diabetes is not the primary reason for admission. Since there are usually competing priorities, limited time, and an ill-conducive learning environment, the primary focus for diabetes self-management should be on those skills that are essential and sufficient for the patient to go home safely (Clement, 2004). Many clinicians refer to this as diabetes "survival skills" education. For patients who have a new diagnosis or have had little previous education, it generally means the following:

1. *Understanding the disease and its treatment*
2. *Understanding how to manage diabetes medications, including injecting insulin, with special emphasis on any changes made to a prior regimen*
3. *Understanding how to monitor blood glucose and target blood glucose values*
4. *Understanding how to recognize and treat high and low blood glucose*
5. *Understanding the importance of follow up care, when to contact their healthcare provider or go to the emergency department (Nettles, 2005).*

CEBM, level 5.

- Order visiting nursing service to reinforce DM self-management education **(D2, C2, PO E).**
- Follow-up appointment in one to two weeks at diabetes center. I called outpatient endocrinologist regarding inpatient management and outpatient instructions **(D2, C2, PO C, D).**
- **ICD-9 code:** 250.93 Diabetes with unspecified complication type 1 uncontrolled.

COMPETENCY DEFENSE

Domain 1, Competency 1. Evaluate patient needs based on age, developmental stage, family history, ethnicity, individual risk, including genetic profile to formulate plans for health promotion, anticipatory guidance, counseling, and disease prevention services for healthy or sick patients and their families in any clinical setting.

Domain 1, Competency 3. Formulate differential diagnoses, and diagnostic strategies and therapeutic interventions with attention to scientific evidence, safety, cost, invasiveness, simplicity, acceptability, adherence, and efficacy for patients who present with new conditions and those with ambiguous or incomplete data, complex illnesses, comorbid conditions, and multiple diagnoses in all clinical settings.

Defense. Competency 1 and Competency 3 were met because Mr. O has a strong family history with an ambiguous presentation of DM that indicated there was a risk for a potential genetic condition and a differential diagnosis needed to be formulated. Through comprehensive literature review and diagnostic tests, a diagnosis was made, and an appropriate management plan was formulated. The plan includes health promotion through a more appropriate understanding of his disease, and will likely improve his glycemic control.

Domain 2, Competency 2. Coordinate and manage the care of patients with chronic illness utilizing specialists, other disciplines, community resources, and family, while maintaining primary responsibility for direction of patient care and insuring the seamless flow of information among providers as the focus of care transitions across ambulatory to acute, subacute settings, and community settings.

Defense. Domain 2, Competency 2, was met because there needed to be a coordination of care among the hospital providers, such as the primary team, the social workers, the nurses, the nutritionist, and the outpatient endocrinologist, to ensure appropriate follow-up upon discharge home. A seamless transition of care was also met given that I was in contact upon Mr. O's discharge with the visiting nurse service as well as the endocrinologist.

Medications

Drug: Lisinopril (Prinivil)

Dose: 5 mg.

Method of administration in this case: By mouth daily.

Mechanism of action: ACE inhibition prevents the conversion of angiotensin I to angiotensin II, which is a potent vasoconstrictor. Decreased angiotensin II leads to decreased vasopressor activity and decreased aldosterone secretion leading to decreased blood pressure.

Clinical use: Lower blood pressure.

Side effects
Common: Hypotension, hyperkalemia, cough.
Serious: Angioedema, face, lips, throat; more frequent in black patients.

Drug: Digoxin (Digitek)

Dose: 0.125 mg.

Method of administration in this case: By mouth daily.

Mechanism of action: Digoxin inhibits sodium-potassium ATPase, which increases intracellular sodium concentration, leading to increased intracellular calcium concentration. This leads to positive inotropic action, reduced sympathetic response, and decreased renin-angiotensin system output.

Clinical use: Heart failure.

Side effects
Common: Diarrhea, loss of appetite, nausea and vomiting, headache, visual disturbance.
Serious: Cardiac dysrhythmia.

(continued)

Drug: Carvedilol (Coreg)

Dose: 6.25 mg.

Method of administration in this case: Twice a day by mouth.

Mechanism of action: Nonselective beta-adrenergic blocking agent with alpha 1-adrenergic blocking activity and no intrinsic sympathomimetic activity. The beta-adrenergic blocking activity of carvedilol decreases cardiac output, blunts the pressor effect of phenylephrine, causes vasodilation, and reduces peripheral vascular resistance.

Clinical use: Heart failure.

Side effects
Common: Bradyarrhythmia, hypotesion, peripheral edema, hyperglycemia.
Serious: Atrioventricular block, heart failure, Stevens-Johnson syndrome, aplastic anemia.

Drug: Atorvastatin (Lipitor)

Dose: 40 mg.

Method of administration in this case: By mouth at bedtime.

Mechanism of action: A synthetic lipid-lowering agent, inhibits HMG-CoA reductase and cholesterol synthesis in the liver and increases the number of hepatic LDL receptors on the cell surface to enhance uptake and catabolism of LDL, thus lowering plasma lipoprotein and cholesterol levels.

Clinical use: Lower cholesterol.

Side effects
Common: Increased liver enzymes.
Serious: Rhabdomyolysis.

Drug: Aspirin (Ecotrin)

Dose: 325 mg.

Method of administration in this case: By mouth daily.

Mechanism of action: Aspirin is a potent inhibitor of both prostaglandin synthesis and platelet aggregation.

Side Effects
Common: Indigestion, nausea, vomiting.
Serious: Gastrointestinal ulcer, angioedema, Reye's syndrome.

Drug: Furosemide (Lasix)

Dose: 40 mg.

Method of administration in this case: By mouth daily..

(continued)

Mechanism of action: Furosemide blocks the absorption of sodium and chloride in the proximal and distal tubules, as well as in the loop of Henle, causing an increase in urine output.

Clinical use: Diuretic.

Side effects
Common: Endocrine hyperuricemia, hypomagnesemia.
Serious: Orthostatic, thrombocytopenia.

Drug: Glargine (Lantus)

Dose: 50 units.

Method of administration in this case: Subcutaneous daily.

Mechanism of action: The primary action of insulin glargine is to regulate glucose metabolism. It lowers the blood glucose concentration by stimulating glucose uptake, especially by muscle and fat. It also inhibits hepatic glucose production, inhibits lipolysis in adipocytes, inhibits proteolysis, and enhances protein synthesis.

Clinical use: Diabetes mellitus type 1, individualized subcutaneous dose administered once daily at the same time every day.

Side effects:
Common: Injection site pain, lipodystrophy.
Serious: Immune hypersensitivity reaction.

Drug: Rosiglitazone (Avandia)

Dose: 4 mg.

Method of administration in this case: By mouth daily.

Mechanism of action: An insulin-sensitizing agent that primarily activates the peroxisome proliferator-activated receptor-gamma (PPAR(gamma)) nuclear receptors, enhancing peripheral glucose utilization and improving glycemic control.

Clinical use: Diabetes mellitus type 2. Adjunct: initial, 4 mg orally once daily or in two divided doses (morning and evening).

Black box warning: May cause or worsen congestive heart failure, is not recommended in patients with symptomatic heart failure, and is contraindicated in patients with established NYHA Class III or IV heart failure. Overall, the available data on the risk of myocardial ischemia is inconclusive.

Side effects
Common: Edema, weight gain.
Serious: Congestive heart failure, myocardial infarction, cholestatic hepatitis, pulmonary edema.

(continued)

Drug: Lispro (Humalog)

Dose: As directed.

Method of administration in this case: Subcutaneous with meals.

Mechanism of action: The primary activity of insulin lispro is to control the metabolism of glucose. Insulin lispro also acts in muscle and other tissues, except the brain, to increase intracellular transport of glucose and amino acids, promote anabolism, and inhibit protein catabolism. In the liver, insulin lispro promotes conversion of glucose to glycogen or fat, and inhibits gluconeogenesis.

Clinical use: Diabetes mellitus type 1, individualized per patient needs, given by subcutaneous injection.

Side effects
Common: Injection site pain, lipodystrophy.
Serious: Immune hypersensitivity reaction.

References

American Diabetes Association (2009). *Clinical Practice Recommendations 2009. Diabetes Care, 32*: Supplement 1.

Balasubramanyam, A., Zern, J.W., Hyman, D.J., & Pavlik, V. (1999). New profiles of diabetic ketoacidosis: Type 1 vs. type 2 diabetes and the effect of ethnicity. *Arch Intern Med, 159* (19), 2317–2322.

Balasubramanyam, A., et al. (2006). Accuracy and predictive value of classification schemes for ketosis-prone diabetes. *Diabetes Care, 29*(12), 2575–2579.

Balasubramanyam, A., Ramaswami, N., Hampe C., and Maldonado, M. (2008). Syndromes of ketosis-prone diabetes mellitus. *Endocrine Review, 29*(3), 292–302.

Biesenbach, G., Raml, A., Schmekel, B., and Eichbauer-Sturm, G. (2003). Decreased insulin requirement in relation to GFR in nephropathic type 1 and insulin-treated type 2 diabetic patients. *Diabetes Medicine, 20*(8), 642–645.

Clement, S., Braithwaite, S., Magee, M., Ahmann, A., Smith, E., Schafer, R., and Hirsch, I. (2004). Management of diabetes and hyperglycemia in hospitals. *Diabetes Care, 27*, 553–591.

Maldonado, M., et al. (2003). Ketosis-prone diabetes: Dissection of a heterogeneous syndrome using an immunogenetic and beta-cell functional classification, prospective analysis, and clinical outcomes. *The Journal of Clinical Endocrinology & Metabolism, 88*(11), 5090–5098.

Mauvais-Jarvis, F., et al. (2004). PAX4 gene variations predispose to ketosis-prone diabetes. *Human Molecular Genetics, 13*(24), 3151–3159.

Mogensen, CE. (1990). Prediction of clinical diabetic nephropathy in IDDM patients: Alternatives to microalbuminuria? *Diabetes, 39*(7), 761–767.

Nalini, R., et al. (2008). HLA class II alleles specify phenotypes of ketosis-prone diabetes. *Diabetes Care, 31*(6), 1195–1200.

Nettles, A. (2005). Patient education in the hospital. *Diabetes Spectrum, 18*(1), 44–48.

Umiperrez, G. (2006). Ketosis-prone type 2 diabetes. *Diabetes Care, 29*(12), 2755–2757.

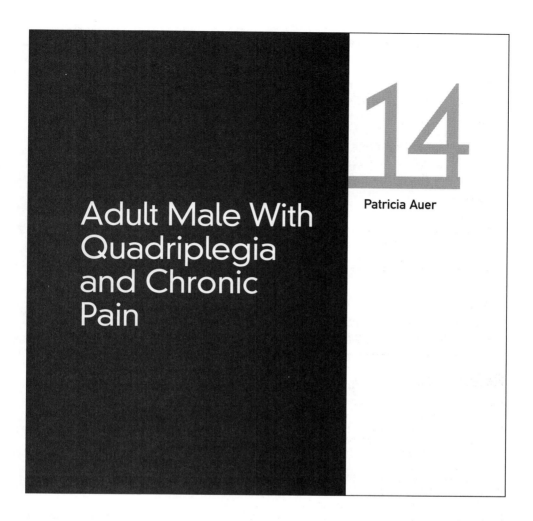

14

Patricia Auer

Adult Male With Quadriplegia and Chronic Pain

The case describes the care I provided for Mr. A, a 42-year-old homebound male with a C5 spinal cord injury. The patient's home health nurse referred this patient to me for home-based primary care because he had been unable to leave home to attend office appointments with his primary care physician (PCP) due to chronic pain for the past year. The patient is insured by Medicare and managed Medicaid insurance. The case narrative focuses on five encounters that occurred over a six-month period in the home setting. This case narrative demonstrates my ability to meet the following CUSN Doctoral Competencies for Direct Patient Care.

DOMAIN 2, COMPETENCY 1

Assemble a collaborative interdisciplinary network, refer and consult appropriately while maintaining primary responsibility for comprehensive patient care.

PO A. Initiate referral to other health care professionals while maintaining primary responsibility for patient care.

PO B. Accept referrals from other health care professions and communicate consultation findings and recommendations to the referring provider and collaborative network.

PO C. Utilize consultation recommendations for decision-making while maintaining primary responsibility for care.

PO D. Evaluate outcomes of interventions.

PO E. Provide ongoing patient follow-up and monitor outcomes of collaborative network interventions.

DOMAIN 3, COMPETENCY 2

Evaluate gaps in health care access that compromise optimal patient outcomes, and apply current knowledge of the organization and financing of health care systems to ameliorate negative impact.

PO A. Identify gaps in access that compromise patient's optimum care.

PO B. Identify gaps in reimbursement that compromise patient's optimum care.

PO C. Demonstrate patient advocacy in the provision of continuous and comprehensive care.

PO D. Apply current knowledge of the organization to ameliorate negative impact.

PO E. Apply current knowledge of health care systems to ameliorate negative impact.

ENCOUNTER CONTEXT

Encounter One (initial evaluation for home-based primary care)

DNP role: I am the family nurse practitioner and DNP resident seeing the patient to evaluate health care needs in a community based setting.

Identifying Information

Site: Rural neighborhood.

Setting: Patient's bedroom in a single-family home.

Reason for encounter: I am assuming primary care for this patient who was referred to me by the home health nurse. The request was verbal **(D2, C1, PO B).**

Informant: Patient and his brother. No records are available.

Time Zero

Patient states his chief complaint: "I hurt all the time."

History of Present Illness

Mr. A's past medical history is significant for a motor vehicle accident five years ago that resulted in a C5-level fracture and quadriplegia. Three years later, he developed a decubitus ulcer on the left buttock, ultimately requiring a surgical repair.

Today, Mr. A complains of constant, chronic pain in his left buttock, ranging from 3/10 when reclining to "greater than 10" when seated. This pain is concentrated around a decubitus ulcer that has been present for four months. The patient describes the pain as feeling "like a knife." Sometimes it is present in his groin and left leg. He has had another decubitus ulcer over the right trochanter for the past four months that is not painful.

These ulcers are treated with a silver-impregnated hydrofiber packing (Aquacel AG), daily, prescribed by the wound-care center at the local hospital. He has an alternating pressure mattress and takes zinc 50 mg orally, daily, for wound healing. He was also prescribed hydrocodone/acetaminophen (Vicodin) 5/500 mg, one to two tablets every 4 to 6 hours as needed, not to exceed eight tablets in 24 hours. Two months ago, he ran out of hydrocodone/acetaminophen (Vicodin) because he was unable to see his PCP, and the wound center would not prescribe controlled medication. He tried taking acetaminophen (Tylenol) and ibuprofen (Advil), but discontinued these because his pain was not relieved.

For the last four months, he has been treated at the wound center every one to two weeks. He states, "They don't do much anymore." It is very painful and difficult to attend these appointments. Pain prevents him from sitting in a wheelchair. He had an MRI last month, which was negative for "bone infection."

Mr. A also experiences intermittent pain due to muscle spasms in all four extremities, especially in his legs, left greater than right. The muscle spasm pain ranges from 5/10 to 8/10. This pain is precipitated when he is moved, but also occurs spontaneously. Spasms and the associated pain can sometimes be reduced by putting a limb in flexion. He has been prescribed baclofen 20 mg orally three times a day and 40 mg at bedtime, tizanidine (Zanaflex) four mg at bedtime, as well as gabapentin (Neurontin) 600 mg in the morning and at noon and 1200 mg at bedtime. He has had physical therapy in the past, but now his family and a female friend help him do daily range-of-motion exercises.

Medical History

Neurogenic bladder since neck injury, five years ago. He has an indwelling suprapubic catheter, which is changed monthly by the visiting nurse.

Deep vein thrombosis during hospitalization for neck injury, treated with a Greenfield filter and warfarin (Coumadin), with no recurrence.

Neurogenic bowel since his injury. He has never had a regular bowel routine "because nothing works." He takes docusate (Colace) 100 mg orally twice daily and bisacodyl five mg orally twice daily. He states that he has tried digital stimulation and enemas, but neither helps him evacuate, and he declines both steadfastly. He has a spontaneous bowel movement every three to seven days.

"Breathing problems" with upper respiratory infections have occurred since his injury. He has been prescribed albuterol (AccuNeb) nebulizer treatment every four hours as needed for dyspnea, when he has a "cold."

Surgical History

Appendectomy at age ten.
   Neck stabilization post-cervical fracture five years ago.
   Greenfield filter insertion five years ago.
   Stoma for suprapubic catheter five years ago.
   Flap procedure for decubitus closure left buttock two years ago.

Allergies

No known drug, environmental, food allergies.

Social History

Mr. A lives with his mother and father. His mother is his primary caregiver, and his brother, who lives across the street, has power of attorney for his health care. He also has a female friend who visits almost daily and assists with his care. A public health nurse comes to the home twice a week. She performs wound care, changes his suprapubic catheter, and draws blood for PT/INR.

He completed the 11th grade. He worked as a horse groomer until he became disabled five years ago. He never married. His 18-year-old daughter is pregnant and lives with her mother in a town about 40 miles from his home. She visits him occasionally. He is interested in sports and history, which he watches on television. He has stayed in bed for the past year due to intolerable pain when he sits up. When he has to go to medical appointments, his brother carries him from his bed to a van, lays him down on the backseat, and then carries him into the facility. He rarely leaves his small bedroom, which barely accommodates his hospital bed, a chest of drawers, and a large-screen television. He can see the front yard from his bed through a large window in his room. He wears no clothes, using towels and sheets to cover himself.

He has smoked one-half to one pack of cigarettes per day for 25 years. He does not drink alcohol or take illegal drugs. He says he eats only one meal a day and drinks a protein supplement about twice a week. He says he sleeps well at night but stays up late watching television and sleeps late in the morning.

Family History

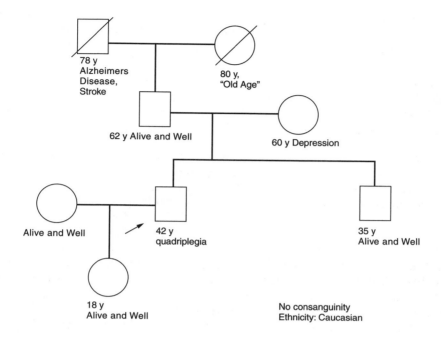

Review of Systems

General: He denies fatigue, fever, chills. He feels he has lost weight since he has been staying in bed, but has not been weighed since his injury. Previous weight 160 pounds. He admits he doesn't have much appetite.

Integumentary: See HPI. He denies rashes. He bruises easily.

Head: He denies headaches or dizziness.

Eyes: He denies itching, blurred vision, pain, or changes in visual acuity. He wears glasses.

Ears: He denies pain, discharge, tinnitus, or difficulty hearing.

Nose/sinuses: He denies pain, sneezing, sinusitis, frequent colds, discharge, or epistaxis.

Mouth/throat: Denies dental pain, sores, bleeding, or difficulty chewing. He has not been to the dentist since his injury. He denies sore throat, hoarseness, or voice changes.

Neck: He denies pain.

Respiratory: He admits to a non-productive cough, especially upon awakening in the morning. He denies dyspnea, hemoptysis, or wheezing.

Cardiovascular: He denies chest pain, palpitations, or peripheral edema.

Gastrointestinal: He doesn't have a good appetite, eats one meal a day at dinner. Denies dysphagia, heartburn, nausea, vomiting. He admits to abdominal cramping when he moves his bowels. He complains of chronic constipation and says his stools are hard when he passes them. He denies rectal bleeding or melena.

Genitourinary: He denies having problems passing urine through the suprapubic catheter. The catheter is changed every four weeks. The urine becomes full of sediment the week before it is changed but does not become clogged. He denies leakage or bleeding around the stoma. He denies pain or discharge from the penis or pain in the scrotum. He has an affectionate relationship with his female friend.

Musculoskeletal: See HPI.

Neurologic: See HPI. He is unable to initiate movement in his legs. He is able to lift his left arm from the bed, but has no grasp in the hand. His right arm has limited range of motion at the shoulder and some limited grasp with the hand. He denies seizures.

Endocrine: No polydipsia or polyphagia; no heat or cold intolerance.

Psychiatric: Denies depression, anxiety. He does not think he has any reason to take an antidepressant. He denies sleeping problems except when he has muscle spasms.

Physical Exam

Vital Signs: Blood pressure 88/60, heart rate 76, respiratory rate 16, temp 96.8°F. Height 5'8"; weight unknown.

General: Mr. A is a thin Caucasian male, reclining in bed, who is difficult to rouse from sleep at first. After he awakens, he is alert and oriented and responds appropriately.

Skin: No rashes. Two tunneling stage III decubitus ulcers. One ulcer is located over the right trochanter, 3 mm wide and 1 1/2 cm deep. The other ulcer is over the left ischial tuberosity and is 3 mm wide and 2 1/2 cm deep. These are packed with silver alginate packing. When packing is removed, there is minimal non-purulent drainage and no visible necrotic tissue. There is no erythema around the wounds.

Hair normal distribution and pattern.

Nails without clubbing, brisk capillary refill.

Head: Normocephalic, atraumatic. Face symmetric without involuntary movements.

Eyes: EOMs intact. No nystagmus. Conjunctivae clear, without discharge or crusting. Sclera white. PERRL. Fundi: disks sharp, no nicking. Unable to assess visual fields, due to patient's position in bed and inability to move.

Ears: Pinnae without lesions or tenderness. Canals clear. TMs pearly gray, landmarks intact. Whisper heard bilaterally.

Nose: No deformities. Nares patent, septum midline, without perforation.

Mouth: Mucosa and gingivae pink without bleeding. Teeth without apparent caries. Tongue protrudes midline. Pharynx without exudates. Gag present.

Neck: Without lymphadenopathy. Trachea midline. No JVD.

Chest: Respirations unlabored. Inspiratory effort increases during speech, with deeper expansion of thorax and flattening of abdomen. Lungs clear to auscultation, without adventitious sounds.

Heart: PMI at fifth intercostal space, mid-clavicle line, impulse without thrill or heave. Carotids without bruits. S1, S2 regular, without murmur or gallop. Peripheral pulses 2+ all extremities. No edema or erythema of extremities.

Abdomen: Flat, symmetric. Bowel sounds normoactive. No abdominal bruit. Abdomen soft, non-tender. No organomegaly or masses palpable.

Musculoskeletal: Lower extremities (LE): right LE extended, left LE contracted at rest at 45 degrees but can be passively extended to 120 degrees. Upper extremities (UE): strength 2/5 with spasticity; right UE active ROM abduction to 40 degrees with full flexion at elbow; left UE active ROM abduction to 20 degrees with flexion at elbow to 30 degrees. Muscle wasting present all extremities. Intermittent flexion muscle spasms of all extremities during the exam in response to tactile stimulation, level 3 on the Modified Ashworth Scale (Satkunam, 2003).

Neurologic: Alert, oriented, coherent thought. Cranial nerves II–XII intact.

Genitourinary: Suprapubic stoma without erythema or bleeding with urinary catheter in place, draining clear amber urine. Circumcised penis without lesions. No scrotal masses. No inguinal lymphadenopathy.

Rectal: No hemorrhoids.

Impression

42-year-old man with a history of C5 quadriplegia secondary to a motor vehicle accident five years ago with development of a decubitus ulcer three years later on the left buttock, surgically repaired with a flap procedure, who now has stage III tunneling decubiti over the left ischium and right trochanter. He now presents with constant, severe pain in the area of the decubitus in the left ischial area and intermittent severe, painful muscle spasms. He has been bedbound for the past year except for trips to the wound-care center secondary to pain. His physical examination is remarkable for the above-mentioned decubiti and muscle spasm of the extremities on tactile stimulation.

His left buttock pain is likely secondary to slow-healing wound. Osteomyelitis is unlikely given patient's report of recent MRI at wound center that showed no bone invasion. The patient's inability to sit secondary to pain severely impacts his quality of life and prognosis. His painful muscle spasms are secondary to spinal cord injury.

> *Pain after spinal cord injury is of two classes: Nociceptive, abnormal pain from stimulation of somatic or visceral nociceptors, or neuropathic, abnormal pain caused by a primary lesion or dysfunction in the nervous system (Hulsebosch, 2005).*
>
> Oxford Centre for Evidence-Based
> Medicine (CEBM), level 5.

ICD-9 Codes

707.05 Decubitus ulcer buttocks
729.5 Pain in limb
728.85 Spasm muscle

Plan

Therapeutic interventions
Hydrocodone/acetaminophen (Vicodin) 5/500 mg, orally one to two tablets every four to six hours as needed for pain.

> *Hydrocodone is a mild opioid agonist, indicated for moderate to moderately severe pain (Trescot et al., 2006).*
>
> CEBM, level 5.

> *The role of opiates in chronic, non-cancer pain is controversial, but proponents cite a relatively low incidence of abuse and the possibility of increased function with pain control (Atluri, S. et al., 2003).*
>
> CEBM, level 5.

Increase tizanidine (Zanaflex) to four mg twice daily by mouth to reduce muscle spasm.

> *Although the pathophysiology of spasticity in spinal cord injury is not completely understood, the basis of spasticity is thought to be an imbalance in*

the numerous excitatory and inhibitory influences on the pathway comprised of the muscle spindle, sensory neuron, and the alpha motor neuron. The patient is already taking a maximum dose of baclofen, which is a centrally acting GABA analogue and inhibits the muscle stretch reflex (Satkunam, 2003).

CEBM, level 5.

Tizanidine (Zanaflex) is an alpha2-adrenergic agonist which decreases excitatory input to alpha motor neurons. A recent Cochrane review assessing pharmacological interventions for spasticity concludes that tizanidine significantly reduces spasticity by Ashworth score, although has significant rates of adverse effects such as drowsiness (Taricco, Pagliacci, Telaro, & Adone, 2006).

CEBM, level 1a.

Decubitus ulcers: Continue packing three times a week with silver alginate (Aquacel AG) dressing.

This is a hydrofiber wound dressing impregnated with silver. When in contact with a moist wound, it interacts with exudates to form a soft gel that maintains a moist environment for healing without damage to healing tissues on removal. The silver is a bactericidal agent used to prevent infection (Hermans, 2006).

CEBM, level 5.

Tobacco use: Prescribe nicotine transdermal patches 21 mg/day for four weeks.
Calcium 500 mg orally with vitamin D 200IU three times a day, as patient at risk for osteoporosis.

Supplementation with calcium and vitamin D may contribute to calcium homeostasis after spinal cord injury (Jiang, Dai, & Jiang, 2006).

CEBM, level 5.

Counseling
I ask the patient to sign a controlled medication agreement (CMA), and he agrees.

The use of a written agreement between the prescriber and the patient at the outset of treatment with controlled substances outlining patient's responsibilities is advised (Atluri, S. et al., 2003).

CEBM, level 5.

Tobacco use: Patient interested in smoking cessation. He would like to try patches. I will evaluate for next dose at next appointment. I discuss administration of patch and the need to completely stop smoking or using any tobacco.

At risk for osteoporosis due to quadriplegia, long-term bed rest, and smoking history: I ask patient if he would be willing to have a DEXA scan. He says he will think about it in the future.

Osteoporosis is a common and serious complication of spinal cord injury and begins in the first months post-injury. It is thought to be a result of less mechanical force applied to the bone, blood circulation abnormalities distal to the lesion that affect bone cell differentiation, and hormonal deficiencies which all lead to increased bone resorption. It often leads to a higher frequency of fracture, especially in the distal femur or proximal tibia (Maimoun, Fattal, Micallef, Peruchon, & Rabischong, 2006).

CEBM, level 5.

Diagnostic tests

Comprehensive metabolic profile to monitor liver function because of long-term use of tizanidine (Zanaflex).

DVT prophylaxis: Continue warfarin (Coumadin) with PT/INR now to be sent to our office. The day this test is completed, the result goes to the covering provider, who orders the next dose and test, and the nursing staff calls the patient. CBC to monitor for anemia with long-term warfarin use.

Will request records from wound center to ascertain plan, previous cultures, and MRI result.

Referrals

Discuss possible physical therapy referral for evaluation of positioning, range-of-motion assessment and instruction, and consultation for any other modalities that might relieve pain and improve quality of life. Patient declines at this time.

Physical and occupational therapy are important in evaluation, goal setting and management with spasticity (Satkunam, 2003).

CEBM, level 5.

Decubitus ulcers: nutritional assessment and counseling through home health agency for adequate caloric and protein intake to promote wound healing **(D2, C1, PO A).**

Practice recommendations for prevention and treatment of pressure ulcers include maximizing nutritional status, including referral to and intervention by a dietitian who can provide assessment and development of a nutrition care plan that will enhance healing potential (Keast, Parslow, Houghton, Norton & Fraser, 2007).

CEBM, level 4.

A Cochrane Review of nutritional interventions for preventing and treating pressure ulcers concluded that there is inconclusive evidence that any nutritional supplementation contributes to healing of established pressure ulcers (Langer, Knerr, Kuss, Behrens, & Schlomer, 2007).

CEBM, level 1a.

Encounter Two (one month later; scheduled home visit)

Interval History

The wound center applied negative pressure wound therapy to the wound over Mr. A's right trochanter. Mr. A saw a dietician who discussed ways to improve protein intake, which he is implementing. She will continue to see him in follow-up.

His pain has improved and is stabile at 3/10. He is taking zero to four hydrocodone/acetaminophen (Vicodin) tablets over a 24-hour period. His muscle spasms have decreased since tizanidine (Zanaflex) was increased. They occur less frequently and are not as severe.

Has been using the nicotine patch, but still "smokes a few."

He denies nosebleeds, gums bleeding, urinary or rectal bleeding.

He continues to receive care from his mother and female friend. His daughter visited, and he is looking forward to the birth of his grandchild.

Physical Exam

Vital signs: Blood pressure 90/56, pulse 76, respiratory rate 20, temp 97.6°F.

General: Alert, oriented, appropriate affect.

Skin: Wound over left ischial tuberosity unchanged, still 3 mm wide and 21/2 cm deep with minimal non-purulent drainage and no visible necrotic tissue. Negative pressure wound therapy in place over other decubitus, draining sero-sanguinous fluid.

Lungs: Clear to auscultation, without adventitious sounds.

Cardiac: S1, S2 regular, rate without murmur.

Abdomen: Bowel sounds normoactive. Soft, non-tender, without organomegaly or masses.

Diagnostic Test Results

Result	Value	Normal Range
Glucose	83	65–99
BUN	10	7–22
Creatinine	0.7	0.7–1.2
Sodium	140	137–146
Potassium	4.0	3.5–5.1
Chloride	103	98–107
CO_2	29	21–32
Calcium	9.0	8.5–10.1
Total Protein	7.1	6.4–8.2
Albumin	3.3	3.4–5.0
Total Bilirubin	0.3	0.1–1.2
Alkaline Phosphatase	111	50–136
ALT	58	15–60
AST	22	14–36
WBC	6.5	4.8–10.0
RBC	4.84	4.0–5.1
Hgb	14.5	12.4–15.2
Hct	43.2	37–46
MCV	89.3	81–99
MCH	29.9	27–32
MCHC	33.5	32.5–35
Plts	232	130–350
PT	27.1	11.9–14.8
INR	2.6	<4

Record Review

Review of records from the wound center: There has been little progress in wound healing since the onset of treatment three months ago. At most visits, debridement of the tunneling wounds with a curette and forceps was done. At the initial visit, the surgeon reported the presence of necrotic tissue. An MRI was performed two months ago, and there was no osteomyelitis.

Impression

42-year-old man with a history of C5 quadriplegia secondary to a motor vehicle accident five years ago, with chronic pain secondary to decubitus ulcer and muscle spasms, who remains bedbound due to pain. Pain improved with use of hydrocodone/acetaminophen (Vicodin) and increase in tizanidine (Zanaflex). No increase in hepatic enzymes resulting from use of tizanidine (Zanaflex). PT/INR on target for DVT indication. Patient is using nicotine patch but continues to smoke.

ICD-9 Codes

707.05 Decubitus ulcer buttocks
729.5 Pain in limb
728.85 Spasm muscle

Plan

Therapeutic Interventions
Continue present treatment with hydrocodone/acetaminophen (Vicodin) and increased dose of tizanidine (Zanaflex).
Continue warfarin (Coumadin) at present dose.

Diagnostic Tests

PT/INR in one month.

Counseling
I counsel patient and his mother about measures to promote wound healing, assuming that he will then have much less pain and be able to tolerate sitting up in chair. Review need for improved protein intake and offloading of pressure at decubitus sites, as well as caution about friction. He agrees with this plan **(D2, C1, PO D).**

> *If a wound is not healing, the following possible elements should be considered: Risk factors, pressure reduction, nutrition, moisture/incontinence, friction and shear, mobility (Keast et al., 2007).*
>
> CEBM, level 4.

We discuss the danger of continuing to smoke while wearing the nicotine patch. He agrees to discontinue smoking while wearing patches. Continue nicotine patch 21 mg/day for two more weeks, then reduce to 14 mg/day for two weeks, then 7 mg/day for two weeks.

Encounter Three (two months later)

Interval History

The patient says he was nauseated and vomited once last week, was very lethargic for a day, had a non-productive cough, and then felt better. He denies shortness of breath, change in bowel pattern, fever, or chills.

Muscle spasms have increased in intensity and frequency, pain is rated 8/10 at times. The pain is concentrated around the decubitus ulcer. Sometimes it is present in his groin and left leg. The patient's friend asks about the use of pregabalin (Lyrica) for pain and muscle spasms.

Mr. A remains in bed, going only to the wound center by traveling in the back of his brother's van. The pain in his left buttock is relieved by hydrocodone/acetaminophen (Vicodin), which he takes as needed a few times a week. His pain is mainly controlled by position. He does not want to try to sit up. The negative pressure wound therapy was discontinued due to lack of progress with healing. The wound center referred the patient to a plastic surgeon for consideration of flap repair. The patient says he is unhappy with the consultation. He says that the surgeon "didn't even take the dressings off to look at the wounds and didn't seem to want to treat me." The wounds continue to be packed with silver alginate (Aquacel AG) dressing three times a week. The patient finished the nicotine patches and has resumed smoking.

Physical Exam

Vital signs: Blood pressure 94/60, pulse 64, respiratory rate 12, temp 97.4°F, SaO_2 98% room air.

General: Alert, responsive, angry affect.

Skin: The tunneling decubiti remain unchanged. The one over the right trochanter is 3 mm wide and 1 1/2 cm deep. The other, over the left ischial tuberosity, is 3 mm wide and 2 1/2 cm deep.

Ears: Canals clear, TMs pearly gray with landmarks intact.

Nose: Boggy, clear discharge.

Throat: Pharynx mildly injected, without exudates.

Neck: No adenopathy.

Lungs: Mild end-expiratory wheeze at right base. No crackles or egophony.

Cardiac: S1, S2 regular, without murmur.

Abdomen: Bowel sounds normoactive. Soft, non-tender, without organomegaly or masses.

Genitourinary: Suprapubic catheter draining clear, amber urine. Stoma free of discharge.

Extremities: Flexion muscle spasms of all extremities on examination, level 3 on the Modified Ashworth Scale (Satkunam, 2003).

Impression

42-year-old man with a history of C5 quadriplegia secondary to a motor vehicle accident five years ago, with chronic pain likely secondary to decubitus ulcer and muscle spasms. A component of central neuropathic pain cannot be ruled out, due to intermittent pain radiation into the left leg.

Central neuropathic pain below-level of the spinal cord injury occurs in der-matomes and often is described by spinal cord injured patients as legs hurting (Hulsebosch, 2005).

CEBM, level 5.

Patient describes vomiting over a single day and non-productive cough that has resolved. This was probably due to a viral illness.

Pain of muscle spasms has increased. This pain is likely secondary to viral illness. Other possible etiologies include urinary tract infection, constipation, or the presence of the decubiti. Urinary tract infection and constipation less likely, due to no indication from history and physical exam.

Decubiti are present but without change from previous exams.

Patient is distressed about lack of improvement of decubitus ulcers and limited consultation with plastic surgeon.

Tobacco use—relapse.

ICD-9 Codes

707.05 Decubitus ulcer buttocks
729.5 Pain in limb
728.85 Spasm muscle
786.2 Cough
787.03 Vomiting

Plan

Therapeutic Interventions

Use albuterol (AccuNeb) nebulizer every 4 hours as needed to relieve wheez-ing and coughing.

Change from gabapentin (Neurontin) to pregabalin (Lyrica) to see if there is improvement in chronic pain in buttock and effect on muscle spasms.

Central pain syndromes may be due to increased discharge of neurons in pain pathways. Therefore, the use of antiepileptic drugs is reasonable (Hulsebosch, 2005).

CEBM, level 5.

A Cochrane review of the subject found no evidence for clinically significant improvement in muscle spasms with gabapentin (Neurontin), among other medications (Taricco et al., 2006).

CEBM, level 1a.

Gabapentin (Neurontin) and pregabalin (Lyrica) are structurally related com-pounds that have efficacy in treating neuropathic pain due to an inhibitory effect on voltage-gated calcium channels. Pregabalin (Lyrica) has been shown to improve central neuropathic pain associated with spinal cord injury as well as improving anxiety and sleep (Siddall et al., 2006).

CEBM, level 1b.

Counseling

Patient should monitor temperature and call if elevated. If muscle spasms do not improve over the next week, patient should call, and I will order a urinalysis. We discuss effect of smoking on respiratory function, especially decreased chest expansion and long-term bedbound status, which increase risk for pneumonia. Patient doesn't want to discuss quitting smoking today, and we agree to discuss it at the next visit.

> *U.S. Preventive Task Force guidelines for smoking cessation recommend asking the patient about tobacco use, advising to quit, assessing willingness to quit, and arrange follow-up and support (U.S. Preventive Services Task Force, 2009).*
>
> CEBM, level 5.

The patient and I agree that I will call the plastic surgeon to speak with him about his impression.

Encounter Four (telephone conversation with plastic surgeon later that week)

I introduce myself as Mr. A.'s primary care provider and discuss the patient's disappointment with the consultation because the non-healing decubitus is the source of chronic pain that has kept him in bed for over a year, and he is hoping that surgery is the answer. I advise the surgeon that the patient did not understand all that was said, and I want to discuss the surgeon's impression to clarify the plan for ongoing treatment with the patient. The surgeon says that Mr. A's very small wounds would require very large, traumatic surgeries involving large graft sites. He could not guarantee that the tunneling wounds would not recur. He said he would perform the surgery if the patient still chooses to take the chance, but that would not be his advice. I thank the surgeon and inform him that I will speak with the patient, who will follow up if he wants to pursue surgery **(D3, C2, PO D)**.

Encounter Five (one month later)

Interval History

Patient reports a "90% reduction" in muscle spasms since gabapentin (Neurontin) was changed to pregabalin (Lyrica). He is no longer going to the wound center, since it is painful to travel and nothing seems to improve his wounds. He still spends all his time in bed because it is too painful to get up. He is still interested in quitting smoking. He is now smoking an average of one pack per day.

Physical Exam

Vital signs: Blood pressure 90/60, pulse 64, respiratory rate 14, temp 97.2°F.

General: Alert, responsive.

Skin: No change in decubiti. Wound over right trochanter 3 mm wide and 1 ½ cm deep. Wound over the left ischial tuberosity 3 mm wide and 2 ½ cm deep. Both have minimal non-purulent drainage and no visible necrotic tissue, both are packed with dressings.

Lungs: Clear to auscultation, without adventitious sounds.

Cardiac: S1, S2 regular, without murmur.

Abdomen: Bowel sounds normoactive. Soft, non-tender, without organomegaly or masses.

Extremities: Muscle spasticity level 2 on the Modified Ashworth Scale (Satkunam, 2003).

Impression

42-year-old man with a history of C5 quadriplegia secondary to a motor vehicle accident five years ago, with chronic pain secondary to decubitus ulcer and muscle spasms, who remains bedbound. Muscle spasms significantly improved with change to pregabalin.

Decubiti stable but without improvement.

Tobacco use, contemplating quitting.

ICD-9 Codes

707.05 Decubitus ulcer buttocks
729.5 Pain in limb
728.85 Spasm muscle
305.1 Tobacco use disorder

Plan

Therapeutic Interventions

Prescribe varenicline (Chantix) starter pack and teach Mr. A how to set a quit date.

> *Varenicline (Chantix) has been shown to be more effective as an aid to smoking cessation than bupropion or placebo (Gonzales et al., 2006).*
>
> CEBM, level 1b.

Diagnostic Tests

Culture and sensitivity of wounds to check for infection as a reason for non-healing.

Counseling

I relate my conversation with the plastic surgeon to the patient. He expresses his frustration that surgery seemed to be his only option. I suggest a consultation with a wound ostomy continence nurse therapist (WOCN). As there is no WOCN who consults with Mr. A.'s nursing agency, I will speak with the WOCN at the hospital **(D3, C2, PO A)**.

I discuss use of varenicline (Chantix) with patient. He is interested in using this medication to quit smoking.

Encounter Six (telephone consultation with WOCN at the hospital)

I describe Mr. A's history and wounds to the WOCN, as well as his present and past treatment. I tell her the wound culture did not have growth. She advises that because there has been no progress with silver alginate dressings (Aquacel AG), this intervention should be discontinued and therapy with wet-to-dry dressings using sterile gauze and saline should be initiated **(D3, C2, PO D)**.

> *As silver destroys Gram-negative bacteria, endotoxins are released that could contribute to the formation of biofilms and the production of matrix metalloproteases, thereby compromising tissue repair (Tomaselli, 2006).*
>
> CEBM, level 5.

Encounter Seven (telephone call to patient's mother, immediately following consult with WOCN)

I advise the patient's mother of my consultation and my plan to change the type of packing. I advise her that these dressings will have to be packed daily. She and Mr. A. agree that she will perform the dressing changes. I tell her that I will call the home health nurse to change the order, and that the home health nurse will bring the supplies, teach her how to do the dressings, and continue to visit every week to assess the wounds **(D2, C1, PO C)**.

Encounter Eight (two months later)

Interval History

The patient's mother reports that the wounds are much improved after changing the type of dressing. The patient reports that pain in the left buttock area has not improved, and that when he tries to sit up, the pain is "greater than a 10." The hydrocodone/acetaminophen (Vicodin) doesn't help at all, and he has therefore discontinued taking it. The patient's brother put him in his electric wheelchair when Mr. A's daughter brought her new baby to visit. He was able to sit in the wheelchair for less than a half hour because of pain, but he also discovered that the chair no longer worked and "did not really fit him anymore."

The patient has completely stopped smoking, and his appetite has improved a lot. He is now eating two to three meals a day.

Physical Exam

Vital signs Blood pressure 108/70, pulse 60, respiratory rate 16, temp 96.8°F.

General: Alert, with a cheerful affect.

Skin: Wound over right trochanter almost completely filled in with healthy tissue. Wound over left ischium has filled in to be 1 cm deep. Wounds packed with wet-to-dry dressings, saline, and gauze. On palpation around ischial wound, there is no tenderness. Pain that the patient identifies as severe pain on sitting can be reproduced on palpation around scar from previous decubitus left buttock that was repaired with flap.

Lungs: Clear to auscultation, without wheezing or crackles.

Cardiac: S1, S2 regular, without murmur.

Abdomen: Bowel sounds normoactive. Soft, non-tender, without organomegaly or masses.

Impression

42-year-old man with a history of C5 quadriplegia secondary to a motor vehicle accident five years ago. He developed a decubitus ulcer three years later on the left buttock, which was surgically repaired with a flap procedure. Mr. A presents with severe, chronic left buttock pain that prevents him from sitting up, and is not relieved with hydrocodone/acetaminophen. Physical exam is significant for severe pain on palpation of previous, healed decubitus site. Differential diagnosis includes chronic pain from healed decubitus site vs. pain from open, healing decubitus.

Decubiti, one healed, one significantly improved **(D2, C1, PO D)**.
Tobacco use—patient is not smoking.

ICD-9 Codes

707.05 Decubitus ulcer buttocks
729.5 Pain in limb

Plan

Therapeutic Interventions
Because pain is unrelieved with hydrocodone (Vicodin), trial of fentanyl (Duragesic) patch 25 mcg transdermally every three days. This should provide ongoing pain relief, and may allow Mr. A the freedom to change his position at will without specific premedication.

Fentanyl (Duragesic) is highly lipophilic and approximately 80 times more potent than morphine. It undergoes extensive metabolism in the liver, so administering it by transdermal patch avoids first-pass metabolism (Trescot et al., 2006).

CEBM, level 5.

Counseling

I instruct the patient and his mother that fentanyl patch should be applied to fatty rather than boney skin areas.

I congratulate the patient on not smoking.

Referrals

Order physical therapy evaluation of wheelchair fit and function **(D2, C1, PO A).**

Encounter Nine (telephone message from patient's mother)

The prescription for fentanyl (Duragesic) will require a prior authorization for insurance purposes **(D3, C2, PO B).** The patient is eager to try the medication and plans to buy a few patches himself.

Encounter Ten (authorization process)

The prescription was declined, and the insurer required that we instead try oxycodone (Percocet) and morphine. I prescribed both of these in succession. Each one provided limited relief of pain, but the patient became very nauseated after administration. I provided the insurer with this information and resubmitted the prescription for fentanyl. In the meantime, the patient tried a few fentanyl (Duragesic) patches with adequate pain relief, but couldn't continue to pay for the prescriptions. The resubmission was declined without explanation. I called the insurance company and asked to speak with the medical director. The insurance company said that the patient would have to sign a release, and they faxed the form, which the patient's mother picked up. After the signed form was returned, the company asked me for progress notes to document the need for this prescription, which I faxed. The fentanyl (Duragesic) was finally approved. This process took four weeks, including the trial periods of alternate medications **(D3, C2, PO C, E).**

Encounter Eleven (telephone conversation with home health nurse case manager)
(D2, C1, PO E)

The physical and occupational therapy consultations concluded that the patient needed a new electric wheelchair. The one he had was five years old and no longer met his needs. I provide a prescription and complete the required forms **(D2, C1, PO C).** The patient has a Hoyer lift, so that he can be transferred from the bed to the chair and back if his brother is not available to help.

CASE SUMMATION

The patient is looking forward to the delivery of his new electric wheelchair. He is feeling very hopeful about the decubiti healing and his achieving enough pain control to become more mobile. I intend to discuss the need for a DEXA scan. It is possible that osteoporosis may also be contributing to his pain.

COMPETENCY DEFENSE

Domain 2, Competency 1. Assemble a collaborative interdisciplinary network, refer and consult appropriately while maintaining primary responsibility for comprehensive patient care.

Defense. I accepted the referral from the public health nurse and assumed the role of primary care provider for this patient. I worked collaboratively with the public health nurse throughout the events of this narrative. I referred the patient for physical and occupational therapy evaluations to determine whether a new wheelchair was indicated. I consulted verbally with the WOCN and evaluated the outcomes of changing the patient's silver alginate (Aquacel AG) dressings to wet-to-dry dressings, and monitored the progress of his wounds. I consulted the plastic surgeon, discussed his recommendation with the patient, and developed an alternate plan of care based on this discussion.

Domain 3, Competency 2. Evaluate gaps in health care access that compromise optimal patient outcomes, and apply current knowledge of the organization and financing of health care systems to ameliorate negative impact.

Defense. I identified the gap in the patient's access to a wound ostomy continence nurse therapist and used my knowledge of the resources in the community to ameliorate this negative impact. I also identified the gap in reimbursement for a needed fentanyl (Duragesic) patch and applied my knowledge of the authorization process, including calling the medical director of the insurance company to ensure that this needed analgesic would be covered.

Medications

> ### Drug: Zinc sulfate (Orazinc)
>
> **Dose range:** 110 mg to 220 mg daily (25–50 mg elemental zinc) 3 times daily.
>
> **Method of administration in this case:** By mouth.
>
> **Mechanism of action:** Provides cytoprotection against reactive toxins, possibly through antioxidant activity, thereby increasing resistance to epithelial apoptosis (Lansdown et al., 2007).
>
> **Clinical uses:** Wound healing.
>
> *(continued)*

Side effects
Common: Diarrhea, nausea, vomiting, dizziness, restlessness.
Serious: Gastric ulcers.

Drug: Hydrocodone (Vicodin when combined with acetaminophen)

Dose range: 2.5 mg to 60 mg per 24 hour period; dosage may be limited by acetaminophen content.

Method of administration in this case: By mouth.

Mechanism of action: Binds to mu and kappa receptors in the central nervous system, resulting in decreased synaptic chemical transmission and inhibition of flow of pain sensations to higher centers (Trescot et al., 2006).

Clinical uses: Pain control.

Side effects
Common: Constipation, indigestion, xerostomia, diaphoresis dizziness, somnolence, ureteral spasm, urinary retention.
Serious: Respiratory depression, apnea.

Drug: Acetaminophen (Tylenol)

Dose range: Up to 4000 mg in 24 hours.

Method of administration in this case: By mouth.

Mechanism of action: Inhibits synthesis of prostaglandins in the central nervous system and blocks pain impulse generation in the periphery.

Clinical uses: Pain control.

Side effects
Common: Rash.
Serious: Hepatotoxicity, nephrotoxicity, pneumonitis.

Drug: Morphine sulfate

Dose range: Usual range 10 mg to 30 mg every 4 hours, but no ceiling.

Method of administration in this case: By mouth.

Mechanism of action: Binds to mu receptors in the CNS, causing inhibition of ascending pain pathways. This alters the perception of pain and response to pain (Trescot et al., 2006).

Clinical uses: Pain control.

Side effects
Common: Pruritus, bradycardia, hypotension, peripheral edema, rash, sweating, abdominal pain, constipation, xerostomia, diarrhea, headache, urinary retention, insomnia, paresthesia, somnolence, depression, fever.
Serious: Cardiac arrest, dyspnea, respiratory depression.

(continued)

Drug: Oxycodone hydrochloride (Percocet when combined with acetaminophen)

Dose range: Usual range 2.5 mg to 5 mg every 6 hours; dosage may be limited by acetaminophen content.

Method of administration in this case: By mouth.

Mechanism of action: Binds to mu and kappa receptors in the central nervous system, thereby decreasing the synaptic chemical transmission and inhibiting the flow of pain sensation to higher centers (Trescot et al., 2006).

Clinical uses: Pain control.

Side effects
Common: Lightheadedness, pruritus, constipation, nausea, vomiting, asthenia, somnolence, dizziness, sedation.
Serious: Hypotension, apnea, respiratory arrest, respiratory depression.

Drug: Fentanyl (Duragesic)

Dose range: As a patch changed every 72 hours, usual range 12.5 to 100 mcg/hr.

Method of administration in this case: Transdermal.

Mechanism of action: Binds with mu receptors in the central nervous system, resulting in decreased synaptic chemical transmission and inhibition of flow of pain sensation to higher centers (Trescot et al., 2006).

Clinical uses: Pain control.

Side effects
Common: Pruritus, site erythema, bradycardia, xerostomia, miosis, diaphoresis, constipation, nausea, vomiting, asthenia, confusion, dizziness, sedation, edema.
Serious: Cardiac dysrhythmia, chest pain, hypertension, hypotension, apnea, hypoventilation, respiratory depression, syncope, seizure.

Drug: Baclofen (Lioresal)

Dose range: 5 mg to 80 mg daily in 3 to 4 divided doses.

Method of administration in this case: By mouth.

Mechanism of action: Inhibits transmission of synaptic reflexes at the spinal cord, possibly by hyperpolarization of primary afferent fiber terminals.

Clinical uses: Treatment of muscle spasticity.

Side effects
Common: Nausea, vomiting, asthenia, dizziness, headache, somnolence, constipation, vertigo, insomnia, slurred speech, ataxia, hypotonia.
Serious: Seizure, syncope, withdrawal reactions with abrupt discontinuation.

(continued)

Drug: Tizanidine hydrochloride (Zanaflex)

Dose range: 4 mg to 36 mg/24 hours.

Method of administration in this case: By mouth.

Mechanism of action: As an alpha2-adrenergic agonist, decreases excitatory input to alpha motor neurons at the spinal cord level.

Clinical uses: Treatment of muscle spasticity.

Side effects
Common: Hypotension, xerostomia, asthenia, dizziness, somnolence.
Serious (rare): Hepatotoxicity, angina, heart failure, myocardial infarction, phlebitis, syncope, cellulites, gastrointestinal hemorrhage, leucopenia, thrombocytopenia, hepatitis, pulmonary embolism.

Drug: Gabapentin (Neurontin)

Dose range: 300 mg to 3600 mg daily in 3 divided doses.

Method of administration in this case: By mouth.

Mechanism of action: Binds to alpha2-delta subunit of calcium channels in the central nervous system, exerting an inhibitory effect on excitatory neurotransmitter release.

Clinical uses: Treatment of muscle spasticity and neuropathic pain.

Side effects
Common: Peripheral edema, fatigue, ataxia, dizziness, somnolence tremor, diarrhea, nausea, vomiting, xerostomia, constipation, nystagmus, blurred vision, infection.
Serious: Stevens-Johnson syndrome, seizure.

Drug: Pregabalin (Lyrica)

Dose range: 25 to 450 mg per day in 2 to 3 divided doses.

Method of administration in this case: By mouth.

Mechanism of action: Binds to alpha2-delta subunit of calcium channels in the central nervous system, exerting an inhibitory effect on excitatory neurotransmitter release.

Clinical uses: Treatment of muscle spasticity and neuropathic pain.

Side effects
Common: Edema, dizziness, somnolence, ataxia, headache, weight gain, xerostomia, tremor, blurred vision, diplopia, infection, accidental injury, chest pain, neuropathy, abnormal thinking, fatigue, confusion, euphoria, speech disorder, attention disturbance, incoordination, amnesia, pain, constipation, increased appetite, balance disorder, arthralgia, twitching.
Serious: Thrombocytopenia, acute renal failure.

(continued)

Drug: Warfarin (Coumadin)

Dose range: Usually 1 mg to 10 mg daily.

Method of administration in this case: By mouth.

Mechanism of action: Interferes with hepatic synthesis of vitamin K-dependent coagulation factors.

Clinical uses: Anticoagulation.

Side effects: Bleeding.

Drug: Bisacodyl (Dulcolax)

Dose range: 5 to 15 mg.

Method of administration in this case: By mouth.

Mechanism of action: Irritates smooth muscle of the intestine, thereby stimulating peristalsis and altering water and electrolyte secretion, increasing intestinal fluid accumulation.

Clinical uses: Neurogenic bowel.

Side effects
Common: Abdominal cramps, nausea, rectal burning, vertigo, vomiting.
Serious: Electrolyte and fluid imbalance.

Drug: Albuterol sulfate (Proventil)

Dose range: Usual range per nebulizer for adults, 0.083% solution over 5–15 minutes every 1–4 hours as needed.

Method of administration in this case: By nebulizer.

Mechanism of action: Acts on beta2-receptors in bronchial smooth muscle to produce relaxation.

Clinical uses: Bronchodilation.

Side effects
Common: Palpitations, nervousness, CNS stimulation, insomnia, dizziness, headache, tremor, paradoxical bronchospasm, diaphoresis.
Serious: Tachycardia, hypertension, hypokalemia.

Drug: Varenicline (Chantix)

Dose range: 0.5 to 2 mg daily.

Method of administration in this case: By mouth.

Mechanism of action: Partial agonist of neuronal alpha4B2 nicotinic receptors, which prevents nicotine stimulation of mesolimbic dopamine system.

Clinical uses: Aid to smoking cessation.

(continued)

Side effects
Common: Insomnia, headache, abnormal dreams, nausea, somnolence, flatulence, constipation, abnormal taste, dyspepsia, increased appetite.
Serious: Acute coronary syndrome, acute renal failure, arrhythmia, gastro-intestinal hemorrhage, intestinal obstruction, thrombocytopenia.

Drug: Nicotine patch

Dose range: 21 to 7 mg/day.

Method of administration in this case: Transdermal.

Mechanism of action: Stimulates autonomic ganglia and central nervous system, which provides replacement and weaning in nicotine addiction.

Clinical uses: Aid to smoking cessation.

Side effects
Common: Local erythema, local edema, rash, withdrawal symptoms, headache, palpitations, tachycardia, hypertension, nausea, hiccups, constipation, flatulence, diarrhea, paresthesias, arthralgia, chest discomfort, insomnia, abnormal dreams.
Serious: Risk of fetal harm.

Drug: Silver alginate dressing (Aquacel AG)

Dose range: NA.

Method of administration in this case: Wound application.

Mechanism of action: Provides moist wound bed and antimicrobial action against MRSA, resistant strains of Pseudomonas aeruginosa, and anaerobic wound pathogens (Tomaselli, 2006).

Clinical uses: Treatment of wounds and prevention of infection.

Side effects: Hypersensitivity to silver.

Source: (except where otherwise cited): *Lexi-Comp On Hand*, 2007.

References

Atluri, S., et al. (2003). Guidelines for the use of controlled substances in the management of chronic pain. *Pain Physician, 6,* 233–257.

Gonzales, D., et al. (2006). Varenicline, an alpha4beta2 nicotinic acetylcholine receptor partial agonist, vs sustained-release bupropion and placebo for smoking cessation: A randomized controlled trial. *JAMA, 296*(1), 47–55.

Hermans, M.H. (2006). Silver-containing dressings and the need for evidence. *American Journal of Nursing, 106*(12), 60–68.

Hulsebosch, C.E. (2005). From discovery to clinical trials: Treatment strategies for central neuropathic pain after spinal cord injury. *Current Pharmaceutical Design, 11*(11), 1411–1420.

Jiang, S.-D., Dai, L.-Y., & Jiang, L.-S. (2006). Osteoporosis after spinal cord injury. *Osteoporosis International, 17*(2), 180–192.

Keast, D.H., Parslow, N., Houghton, P.E., Norton, L., & Fraser, C. (2007). Best practice recommendations for the prevention and treatment of pressure ulcers: Update 2006. *Advances in Skin & Wound Care, 20*(8), 447–462.

Langer, G., Knerr A., Kuss O., Behrens J., & Schlome, G.J. (2007). Nutritional interventions for preventing and treating pressure ulcers. *Cochrane Database of Systematic Reviews 2003*(4).

Lansdown, A.B.G., Mirastschijski, U., Stubbs, N., Scanlon, E., & Agren, M.S. (2007). Zinc in wound healing: Theoretical, experimental, and clinical aspects. *Wound Repair & Regeneration, 15*(1), 2–16.

Lexi-Comp On Hand, retrieved 2007 from http://online.lexi.com.

Maimoun, L., Fattal, C., Micallef, J.P., Peruchon, E., & Rabischong, P. (2006). Bone loss in spinal cord-injured patients: From physiopathology to therapy. Spinal Cord, 44(4), 203–210.

Satkunam, L.-E. (2003). Rehabilitation medicine: 3. Management of adult spasticity. *Canadian Medical Association Journal, 169*(11), 1173–1179.

Siddall, P.-J., Cousins, M.J., Otte, A., Griesing, T., Chambers, R., & Murphy, T.-K. (2006). Pregabalin in central neuropathic pain associated with spinal cord injury: A placebo-controlled trial. *Neurology, 67*(10), 1792–1800.

Taricco, M., Pagliacci, M.C., Telaro, E., & Adone, R. (2006). Pharmacological interventions for spasticity following spinal cord injury: Results of a Cochrane systematic review. *Europa Medicophysica, 42*(1), 5–15.

Tomaselli, N. (2006). The role of topical silver preparations in wound healing. Journal of Wound, Ostomy, & Continence Nursing, 33(4), 367–378.

Trescot, A., et al. (2006). Opioid guidelines in the management of chronic non-cancer pain. *Pain Physician, 9*, 1–40.

U.S. Preventive Services Task Force (2009). *Counseling and interventions to prevent tobacco use and tobacco-caused disease in adults and pregnant women: U.S. Preventive Services Task Force reaffirmation recommendation statement.* Rockville, MD: Agency for Healthcare Research and Quality.

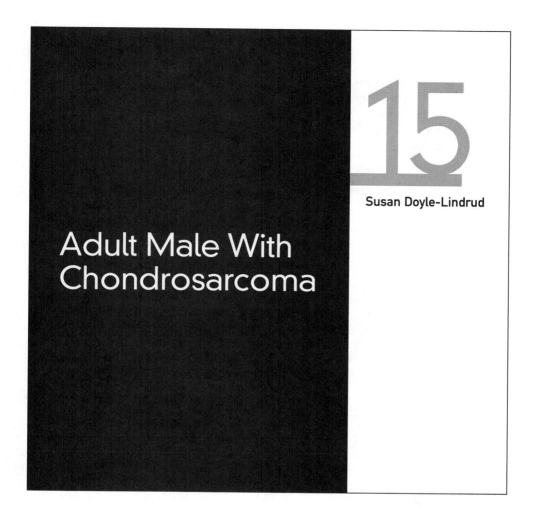

15

Susan Doyle-Lindrud

Adult Male With Chondrosarcoma

This case describes the care I provided for Mr. H, a 53-year-old male with commercial insurance who presented with a history of chondrosarcoma. Mr. H was interested in pursuing a clinical trial option due to the progression of his disease on standard regimens. This case narrative describes six encounters that occurred in a comprehensive cancer center over a period of two months. This case narrative demonstrates my ability to meet the following Columbia University School of Nursing Doctoral Competencies for Comprehensive Direct Patient Care.

DOMAIN 1, COMPETENCY 4

Appraise acuity of patient condition, determine need to transfer patient to higher acuity setting, coordinate, and manage transfer to optimize patient outcomes.

PO A. Assess the acuity of patient status.
PO B. Determine the most appropriate treatment setting based on level of acuity.
PO C. Formulate a transfer plan.

PO D. Implement plan to transfer the patient to a higher level of care utilizing written and oral communication.
PO E. Coordinate care during transition to the higher acuity setting.
PO F. Co-manage care in person.
PO G. Co-manage care through written and verbal instructions.

DOMAIN 1, COMPETENCY 1

Assemble a collaborative interdisciplinary network, refer and consult appropriately while maintaining primary responsibility for comprehensive patient care.

PO A. Initiate referral to other health care professionals while maintaining primary responsibility for patient care.
PO D. Provide ongoing patient follow-up and monitor outcomes of collaborative network interventions.

DOMAIN 3, COMPETENCY 2

Evaluate gaps in health care access that compromise optimal patient outcomes, and apply current knowledge of the organization and financing of health care systems to ameliorate negative impact.

PO C. Demonstrate patient advocacy in the provision of continuous and comprehensive care.
PO D. Apply current knowledge of the organization to ameliorate negative impact.

DOMAIN 1, COMPETENCY 7

Facilitate and guide the process of palliative care and/or planning end-of-life care by discussing diagnoses and prognosis, clarifying and validating patient desires and priorities, and promoting informed choices and shared decision making by patient, family, and members of the health care team.

PO B. Facilitate and guide planning end-of-life care by discussing diagnoses and prognosis, clarifying and validating patient desires and priorities, and promoting informed choices and shared decision making by patient, family, and members of the health care team.

DOMAIN 3, COMPETENCY 3

Synthesize the principles of legal and ethical decision-making and analyze dilemmas that arise in patient care, inter professional relationships, research, or practice management to improve outcomes.

PO A. Synthesize ethical principles to address a complex practice dilemma.

PO B. Apply ethical principles to resolve the dilemma.

ENCOUNTER CONTEXT

Encounter One (initial evaluation)

DNP Role: I am a DNP student and associate director of clinical research. I am evaluating this patient to determine eligibility for a Phase I clinical trial.

Identifying Information

Site: National Cancer Institute-designated comprehensive cancer center.

Setting: Medical oncology Phase I clinic.

Reason for encounter: Referral from patient's medical oncologist.

Informant: Patient and medical records. Mr. H is a 53-year-old male with a history of chondrosarcoma of the right lower extremity. He appears to be a reliable historian.

Chief complaint: Patient reports, "My medical oncologist has told me that he has no further treatment options available to me and recommends I come here to discuss clinical trial options."

History of Present Illness

Mr. H is a 53-year-old male with a history of chondrosarcoma of the right lower extremity. He comes to this cancer center seeking a medical opinion.

Mr. H developed a right foot pain in 2004. He was seen by an orthopedist who prescribed orthotics. The pain continued, and his primary care physician ordered an MRI of his right lower extremity. The MRI revealed an 8.7 × 5.8 × 7.9 cm mass, multilobular, of the right foot, extending into the calcaneus, with multiple lesions in the visualized distal tibia and fibula. A biopsy was positive for low-grade chondrosarcoma. He underwent a below-the-knee amputation (BKA) in 2005 by an orthopedic oncologic surgeon. Pathology from the BKA revealed a low-grade chondrosarcoma involving the metatarsals, tarsals, talus, calcaneus, tibia, and fibula. The tumor had penetrated the bone cortex to involve soft tissue in many sites. Proximal skin, soft tissue, blood vessel, and bone margins were negative for tumor.

Mr. H was followed over a nine-month period from surgery when he developed a palpable nodule at his amputation site. Biopsy of the mass revealed a recurrent chondrosarcoma. He has since been seen and treated by a medical oncologist. He received Ifosfamide (Ifex)/Epirubicin (Ellence) chemotherapy in 2006 for two months of therapy, which was discontinued for progression. This treatment was followed by Docetaxel (Taxotere)/Gemcitabine (Gemzar) chemotherapy. Mr. H developed pneumonitis, thought to be related to Gemcitabine (Gemzar), and the Gemcitabine (Gemzar) was discontinued after one month of treatment. He continued on Docetaxel (Taxotere) as a single agent for an additional five months; this was discontinued for progression of his disease.

Chondrosarcomas are the second most common primary malignant spindle cell tumor of the bone. They are generally slow growing, malignant tumors that are characterized by the formation of cartilaginous neoplastic tissue. They accounted for 3.6% of the annual incidence of all primary bone malignancies in the USA in 2006 (Chow, 2007). The five types of chondrosarcomas are central, peripheral, mesenchymal, differentiated and clear cell. The classic chondrosarcomas are central and peripheral and can arise as primary tumors or secondary to underling neoplasm (Pritchard, Lunke, Taylor, Dahlin, & Medley, 1980). One half of all chondrosarcomas occur in persons older than 40 years old, with the most common site being the pelvis (31%), femur (21%) and shoulder girdle (13%). Clinical presentation is related to site of disease, with local symptoms developing from mechanical irritation (Malawer, Helman, & O'Sullivan, 2005). The treatment of chondrosarcoma is surgical removal. Metastatic potential correlates with the histologic grade of the lesions. Marcove et al. (1972) reported on long-term follow-up of 113 patients with chondrosarcoma of the proximal femur and the pelvis. The survival rates in patients with grade I, II, or III lesions were 47%, 38%, and 15%, respectively; the overall survival rate was 52%. (Marcove et al., 1972), (Malawer et al., 2005).

Oxford Centre for Evidence-Based Medicine (CEBM), level 4.

Commonly used combination chemotherapy regimens for patients with soft tissue sarcoma include Ifosfamide/Epirubicin (Palumbo et al., 1999), and Docetaxel/ Gemcitabine (Leu et al., 2004).

CEBM, level 4.

Medical History

Chondrosarcoma diagnosed in 2004 (see HPI).
Gemcitabine pneumonitis in 2006 (see HPI).

Surgical History

Leg length discrepancy of his right leg, treated with leg-lengthening procedure in 1968, with long-term postoperative physical therapy and full recovery; no complications.
Right BKA in 2005.

Allergies

No known drug allergies. No known environmental or food allergies.

Medications

Prednisone (Sterapred) 10 mg by mouth daily, initiated with development of pneumonitis.

Transdermal fentanyl patch (Duragesic) 50 mcg every 72 hours.

Acetaminophen/oxycodone hydrochloride (Percocet) 5/325 mg by mouth, two to three tablets by mouth every four hours as needed for pain.

Albuterol (Proventil) meter-dosed inhaler as needed; initiated with development of pneumonitis.

Docusate sodium (Colace)/senna (Senokot) combination for constipation.

Family History

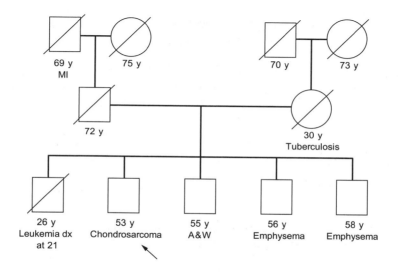

No consanguinity
Ethnicity: Caucasian

Social History

Mr. H is single and lives alone. He is a former dishwasher in a restaurant, on long-term disability for the past eight months.

Mr. H smoked two and a half packs of cigarettes per day for 10 years, discontinued in 1982. He has a history of marijuana use for 20 years, discontinued in 2004. He drinks one to two beers per week.

Mr. H lives in an apartment and has a neighbor and a few friends who come to visit several times a week. Mr. H is able to complete most activities of daily living on his own. He does have difficulty with shopping, and one of his friends accompanies him on these trips. He does not practice a religion, stating that he is not a spiritual person. He has no formal health care proxy or advanced directives.

Review of Systems

General: Fatigue on exertion, weight stable, denies fever, chills, or sweats.

Skin: Denies rash, pruriuis, lesions.

Head: Denies headaches, light-headedness, or head injury.

Eyes: Denies blurred or double vision; denies discharge or visual changes.

Nose: Denies congestion, sinus pain, or discharge.

Neck: Denies lumps, pain; denies sore throat, stiffness, or swelling.

Respiratory: Non-productive cough over the past week. He recently completed a three-day course of azithromycin (Zithromax). Shortness of breath on exertion improved with prednisone (Sterapred); has occasional wheezing.

Cardiovascular: Denies chest pain, palpitations, or edema.

Gastrointestinal: Constipation treated with daily docusate sodium (Colace) and senna (Senokot) with good results, appetite good, denies abdominal pain, denies diarrhea.

Genitourinary: Slow stream of urine when emptying his bladder. Denies nocturia, hematuria, dysuria, or frequency.

Musculoskeletal: Pain at his amputation site, described as a 6/10 on the pain scale (Appendix B). He also describes phantom pain of his right lower extremity. He is treated with fentanyl (Duragesic) 50 mcg patch every 72 hours and acetaminophen/oxycodone hydrochloride (Percocet) 5/325 mg, two tablets orally every four to six hours around the clock.

Neurologic: Denies history of seizure, fainting, denies any numbness, tingling of extremities, tremors, or paresis. Denies vertigo, loss of consciousness.

Psychologic: Denies depression, anxiety, and suicidal or homicidal ideations. He describes strong social support.

Physical Examination

Vital signs: Blood pressure 129/72, pulse 110, respiratory rate 16, temp 97.5°F. Weight 90 pounds. Height: 60.5 inches. BMI 15.

General: Well-appearing male, no acute distress.

Skin: Warm and dry, no rashes noted.

HEENT: Pupils equal, round, reactive to light and accommodation (PER-RLA); oropharynx pink, no lesions noted, no erythema.

Neck: Supple, no jugular venous distension, no adenopathy.

Chest: Clear to auscultation, no adventitious breaths sounds.

Heart: RRR, S1, S2 present, no S3 or S4, no murmurs, rubs, or gallops.

Gastrointestinal: Abdomen soft, not distended; bowel sounds present; no mass palpable; no hepatomegaly.

Musculoskeletal: Full range of motion of extremities; no pain to spine palpation.

Neurologic: Alert and oriented to person, place, and time; CN II–XII intact. Sensory: pin prick, vibration intact. Motor: 5/5 strength bilateral upper extremity and LLE. Cerebellar: finger to nose intact. DTRs 2 + bilateral upper extremities and left lower extremity.

Extremities: Right BKA with approximate 4" × 4" mass noted on inner aspect at amputation site; no erythema or skin breakdown; left leg with no clubbing, cyanosis, or edema; pulses intact.

Diagnostic Testing

Imaging: MRI of right lower extremity shows mass extending into the medial soft tissue, both anteriorly and posteriorly, with an additional mass noted laterally. Other lesions of the visualized distal right femur are noted, compatible with metastatic disease.

CT scan of the chest demonstrates improvement in the scattered areas of ground-glass abnormality of the lungs. Development within lungs of a more coarsened area, of either scarring or bronchiectasis.

Impression

Mr. H is a 53-year-old male with recurrent chondrosarcoma, status post right BKA. After initial recurrence, he received Iphosphamide (Ifex)/Epirubicin (Ellence). His disease continued to progress, and he was treated with Docetaxel (Taxotere)/Gemcitabine (Gemzar). Mr. H has no standard options available to him. He may qualify for a Phase I study that involves a histone deacetylase inhibitor that has shown antitumor activity on chondrosarcoma cell lines.

Inadequate pain control on current regimen, which includes four to five grams of acetaminophen (Tylenol) daily. The maximum adult dose of acetaminophen is four grams per day.

ICD-9 Codes:

171 Sarcoma
338.3 Pain

Discussion of Phase I Clinical Trial as Treatment Option

Mr. H comes to this cancer center, specifically the Phase I clinic, to discuss treatment options. He is eager to start a treatment as soon as possible. The medical oncologist and I review the purpose of a Phase I study with him. We explain to Mr. H that a Phase I trial is the first step in testing a new drug treatment in humans. These studies test the best way to give a new treatment—for example, by mouth, intravenous infusion, or injection—and the best dose. The dose is usually increased a little at a time in order to find the highest dose that does not cause harmful side effects. Because little is known about the possible risks and benefits of the treatments being tested, Phase I trials usually include only a small number of study volunteers.

We discuss a Phase I study for which Mr. H may be eligible, which involves a histone deacetylase inhibitor that has shown antitumor activity on chondrosarcoma cell lines (Sakimura et al., 2007). We review the drug, schedule, possible risks and benefits, and potential side effects of this medication. He is interested in pursuing this option.

The Phase I research nurse enters the room to review the consent form with Mr. H. The research nurse and I assess Mr. H's understanding of the clinical trial purpose and schedule, having him restate this information to us.

> *Histone acetylation and deacetylation play a key role in the regulation of chondrocytic differentiation. This has prompted investigators to look at the antitumor effects of histone deacetylatase (HDAC) inhibitors (Sakimura et al., 2007). Sakimura et al. examined the effects of a HDAC inhibitor, depsipeptide, on the growth of chondrosarcoma cell lines and the antitumor effect in vivo. Depsipeptide inhibited the growth of chondrosarcoma cell lines by inducing cell cycle arrest and/or apoptosis. In vivo studies and histologic analyses confirmed that depsipeptide significantly inhibited tumor growth and induced differentiation into the hypertrophic and mineralized state in chondrosarcoma cells.*
>
> Sakimura et al., 2007.

Plan

Education and Counseling
A copy of the consent form is given to Mr. H. He will contact the research nurse if he is interested in pursuing this clinical trial.

Diagnostic Tests
Radiology: A baseline evaluation for the trial will be scheduled, including an MRI of Mr. H's right lower extremity and a CT scan of the chest, abdomen, and pelvis to evaluate the extent of his disease, if he agrees to participate.

Laboratory: The research nurse, pending decision to participate, will coordinate baseline blood tests. This will include a CBC, comprehensive metabolic panel, liver function tests, and an EKG. All need to be within normal limits, as the drug being tested may cause pancytopenia, electrolyte abnormalities, elevated liver function, and prolonged QT interval.

Therapeutic Interventions

Pain not adequately controlled on current regimen. There is a concern about the amount of acetaminophen (Tylenol) he is taking. The maximum adult dose is four grams per day, and he is taking approximately four to five grams daily. Plan to increase the transdermal fentanyl (Duragesic) patch to 75 mcg every 72 hours, and change acetaminophen/oxycodone hydrochloride (Percocet) to oxycodone (Roxicodone). Patient is given a prescription for oxycodone (Roxicodone) 5 mg, one to two tablets orally every four hours as needed for pain, and again reminded to discontinue the acetaminophen/oxycodone hydrochloride (Percocet). We reviewed potential side effects of fentanyl (Duragesic) and oxycodone (Roxicodone). Mr. H is on a bowel regimen, and I reminded him that he should remain on this, as it will help with the constipating side effect of these medications.

Follow-up

Return to the Phase I clinic in one week.

Encounter Two (two weeks after initial visit)

Interim History

Mr. H had reviewed the consent form, discussed the schedule with the research nurse by phone, and decided to pursue this study. He states that since his last visit, his pain has persisted. He continues to have pain at the amputation site. He is applying transdermal fentanyl (Duragesic) 75 mcg patch every 72 hours and taking oxycodone (Roxicodone) 10 mg orally every six hours.

Diagnostic Testing

CT scan of the chest: Scattered patchy areas of air space consolidation and ground-glass attenuation seen throughout the lungs. Three pleural-based soft tissue masses, the largest measuring 2.5 × 2.0 × 2.9 cm, located in the right upper lobe; a 1.9 cm pleural-based mass in the left lower lobe and the right lower lobe.

CT scan of the abdomen and pelvis: Large, hypodense mass within the right inguinal region, measuring 4.9 × 6.5 × 4.8 cm, consistent with a necrotic lymph node.

MRI of the right lower extremity: Large multilobulated and multiloculated masses involving the tibia, and multifocal lesions within the femur. Posterior component of the mass measures 8.7 × 6.2 cm, and anterior component is 6.7 cm.

EKG: Sinus rhythm, rate 95; PR interval 0.08, QT_C 406 ms, right ventricular hypertrophy.

Laboratory Review

	Hematology	
	Value	Normal range/value
WBC	9.4 mm³	4–12 mm³
HGB	13.5 g/dl	12.0–16.0 g/dl
HCT	39.5 g/dl	37–47 g/dl
PLTS	346 mm³	140–440 mm³
	Chemistry	
Na	135 meq/l	136–145 meq/l
K	4.7 meq/l	3.5–5.0 meq/l
BUN	6 mg/dl	6–23 mg/dl
Creatinine	0.6 mg/dl	0.7–1.2 mg/dl
SGOT	15 u/l	12–45 u/l
SGPT	9 u/l	3–40 u/l
ALKP	94 u/l	37–107 u/l
Ca	9.1 mg/dl	8.6–10.4 mg/dl
Glucose	90 mg/dl	65–139 mg/dl

Impression

Mr. H has a history of metastatic chondrosarcoma, status post right BKA, status post-treatment failure with Ifosfamide (Ifex)/Epirubicin (Ellence) and Docetaxel (Taxotere)/Gemcitabine (Gemzar). With no standard option available, Mr. H is referred to our cancer center for a Phase I study. He is interested in pursuing this option, which will involve a randomized, partially blind placebo-controlled crossover study involving a histone deacetylase inhibitor. He is very eager to begin.

Staff Communication

The research nurse approaches me, hesitant to put Mr. H on study, stating, "I do not think he will be a good candidate; I have doubts as to whether he will be compliant. Phase I studies are complicated, and I am not sure he will understand the instructions."

I ask the nurse whether there had been something specific in her discussion with Mr. H that led her to believe he would have difficulty following instructions. She replies, "I just don't believe he is sharp enough."

Critical Appraisal

Mr. H is a patient with no other options. He is eager to participate, and has been able to reiterate the purpose of a Phase I study and the plan. Because of the complicated nature of these studies, he may require additional reinforcement of the schedule, but otherwise he is a good candidate, and I believe that we should give him the opportunity to participate.

Consultation

I discuss the research nurse's concerns and my rationale for enrolling this patient in the study with the medical oncologist, who agrees that we should enroll him in the study **(D3, C3, PO A, B)**.

Plan

Therapeutic Interventions

Pain: Increase transdermal fentanyl (Duragesic) patch to 100 mcg patch every 72 hours and continue oxycodone (Roxicodone) 10 mg by mouth every four hours as needed for pain. Prescription given.

Constipation: Continue senna (Senokot)/docusate (Colace) combination, two capsules orally twice daily, and add magnesium hydroxide (Phillips Milk of Magnesia) by mouth as needed.

Referral

Social worker for the Phase I group notified of patient, living conditions, and potential transportation issue. Mr. H relies on friends to bring him to the cancer center and has occasionally used a voluntary transportation service. Social worker will meet with Mr. H today to assist with transportation issues **(D2, C1, PO A)**.

Follow-up

Return to clinic in one week to initiate clinical trial. Mr. H has been given instructions to fast after midnight the day of treatment.

Referral

Clinical nutritionist to review dietary interventions to assist patient with gaining weight, as BMI is 15. Recommend nutritional supplement drinks at this time.

Third Visit Summary (one week later, 21 days after initial consultation)

Mr. H comes to the cancer center to initiate the study drug. Since his last visit, we have had a phone conversation about his pain. Due to his need for 10 mg oxycodone (Roxicodone) every three to four hours, his transdermal fentanyl (Duragesic) patch was increased to 150 mcg every 72 hours.

I am not available to see Mr. H for this visit. He is evaluated by the covering nurse practitioner. Mr. H states that even with the recent increase of the transdermal fentanyl (Duragesic) patch, he continues to have pain, 5 to 6/10 on the pain scale. He does not wish to further increase the dose on the transdermal fentanyl (Duragesic) patch, because, he states, "I think it may be making me light-headed." The nurse practitioner changes his regimen from transdermal fentanyl (Duragesic) 150 mcg patch to oxycodone slow release (OxyContin) 160 mg in AM, 80 mg in PM, for two days. If he tolerates this dose, he will increase the oxycodone slow release (OxyContin) to 160 mg every 12 hours. In addition, he was given instructions to take oxycodone (Roxicodone) 10 mg to 20 mg every three hours for pain as needed.

Prior to initiation of the study drug, the research nurse asks whether Mr. H has eaten since last evening. He states he had not eaten, but he did have some coffee the morning of the appointment. The study sponsor is contacted, and states that Mr. H must hold off on treatment today, and return in 24 hours. The research nurse notes "noncompliance" and reiterates a concern to the Phase I group about this patient's ability to follow instructions.

Encounter Four (24 hours later; 22 days after initial encounter)

Interim History

Mr. H returns to clinic the next morning. He states that he has not had anything to eat or drink since midnight, "not even coffee." He is not upset by the delay, and he feels badly that he made this mistake. He appears lethargic. He reports the concern that friends need money for gasoline to take him to the cancer center.

Review of Systems

General: He is tired, states that the change in medication has made him drowsy.

He slept fairly well last night, denies fever, chills, or sweats.

Skin: Denies rash, pruritus, lesions.

Head: Denies headaches, light-headedness, or head injury.

Eyes: Denies blurred or double vision, discharge, or visual changes.

Nose: Denies congestion, sinus pain, or discharge.

Neck: Denies lumps, pain, sore throat, stiffness, swelling.

Chest: Shortness of breath on exertion; intermittent cough, non-productive; denies wheezing.

Heart: Denies chest pain, palpitations, edema.

Gastrointestinal: Appetite good; denies abdominal pain or diarrhea. He has constipation, controlled with his bowel regimen.

Genitourinary: Slow stream of urine when emptying bladder. Denies nocturia, hematuria, dysuria, frequency.

Musculoskeletal: Pain at right amputation site improved, described as a 3/10 on the pain scale at this time.

Neurologic: Denies history of seizure, fainting, numbness, tingling of extremities, tremors, or paresis. Denies vertigo, loss of consciousness.

Psychological: Denies depression, states he has a good attitude and will "do what it takes" to try to treat his disease.

Physical Examination

Vital signs: Blood pressure 128/69, pulse 105, respiratory rate 16, temp 98.5°F. Weight 88 pounds.

General: Well-appearing male, no acute distress.

Skin: Warm and dry, no rash noted.

HEENT: PERRLA; oropharynx pink; no lesions noted; no erythema.

Neck: Supple; no jugular venous distension; no adenopathy.

Chest: Clear to auscultation; no adventitious breath sounds.

Heart: RRR, S1, S2 present; no S3 or S4; no murmurs, rubs, or gallops.

Gastrointestinal: Abdomen soft, not distended; bowel sounds present; no mass palpable, no hepatomegaly.

Musculoskeletal: Full range of motion of extremities; no pain to spine palpation.

Neurologic: Alert and oriented to person, place, and time; CN II-XII intact. Sensory: pin prick, vibration intact. Motor: 5/5 strength bilateral upper extremity and left lower extremity. Cerebellar: finger to nose intact. DTRs 2 + bilateral upper and left lower extremity.

Extremities: Right BKA with approximate 4" × 4" mass noted on inner aspect of amputation site, no erythema or breakdown, left leg with no clubbing, cyanosis, or edema.

Impression

Mr. H is a 53-year-old male with metastatic chondrosarcoma to the lung, right inguinal lymph node and amputation site, status post a right BKA, status post-treatment failure with Ifosfamide (Ifex)/Epirubicin (Ellence) and Docetaxel (Taxotere)/Gemcitabine (Gemzar). He now awaits initiation of a Phase I study with a histone deacetylase inhibitor.

He is having difficulty with transportation. Friends have been willing to drive him to the cancer center, but are requesting money for gasoline.

Plan

Diagnostic Laboratory Studies
Pharmacokinetic blood tests per protocol to assess drug absorption, distribution, metabolism, and elimination.

Therapeutic Interventions
Dosing of study drug by treatment nurse per study protocol.

Pain
Currently controlled on oxycodone slow release (OxyContin) 160 mg by mouth every 12 hours with oxycodone (Roxicodone) 20 mg orally every hours for rescue.

Counseling and Education
Mr. H may eat four hours post study drug administration

Referral
I contact the social worker for the Phase I study group. Social worker has been looking into eligibility for an American Cancer Society transportation grant and will come to discuss this with Mr. H **(D2, C1, PO D).**

Follow-up
Follow-up planned in one week, for placebo study drug administration.

Scheduled Visit (one week later, 29 days after initial consultation; telephone encounter)

Mr. H calls the research nurse the morning of his scheduled treatment, stating that his friend did not show up to bring him to the cancer center. He has been trying to call his friend but has been unable to reach him. He is not sure what he should do. The research nurse tells him she will get back to him, and communicates with the Phase I research team that once again Mr. H is "non-compliant." She would like to cancel part one, period two, and instead have him come back in two weeks for part two of the clinical trial. Several research nurses within the group agree with this plan.

As the primary objective of the study would not be met if he did not come in for the crossover visit, and the study allows a +/− three-day window, I recommend that the research nurse see whether she can arrange for him to come the following morning. I call the social worker and ask whether it is possible to assist with a car service using available transportation funds. This would also allow for an assessment of Mr. H and follow-up of his pain management. I call to discuss this plan with Mr. H, and he is very receptive. The social worker has the funds available for such a circumstance and assists with the arrangement of transportation **(D3, C2, PO C, D)**.

Encounter Five (one week and one day later, 30 days after initial consultation)

Interim History

Mr. H comes to the cancer center for drug administration, part one period two. I had spoken with him by phone, four days prior, about his pain. He states that he has had slightly worsening pain over the past few days. He has been taking the oxycodone slow release (OxyContin) 160 mg orally every 12 hours and oxycodone (Roxicodone) 20 mg by mouth every four hours. The pain is at the amputation site. He states that he has been "taking it easy" over the past week. He has had friends over, and they have helped him with shopping. He has been able to take care of himself, cook, and do his own laundry.

Review of Systems

General: He appears slightly lethargic, denies fever, chills, or sweats.

Skin: Denies rash, denies pruritus or lesions.

Head: Denies headaches, light-headedness, or head injury.

Eyes: Denies blurred or double vision, discharge, or visual changes.

Nose: Denies congestion, sinus pain, or discharge.

Neck: Denies lumps, pain, sore throat, stiffness, swelling.

Respiratory: Shortness of breath noted on exertion; non-productive cough, no wheezing.

Cardiovascular: Denies chest pain, palpitations.

Gastrointestinal: Appetite fair; denies abdominal pain, denies diarrhea. He has constipation controlled with his bowel regimen.

Genitourinary: Denies nocturia, hematuria, dysuria, frequency.

Musculoskeletal: Pain at his right amputation site continues. Pain described as a 5 to 6/10 on the pain scale. He has difficulty sleeping due to the pain.

Neurologic: Denies history of seizure, fainting, numbness, tingling of extremities or toes, tremors, and paresis. Denies vertigo, loss of consciousness.

Psychologic: Denies depression; states he continues to have a good attitude and has had good support from friends.

Physical Examination

Vital signs: Blood pressure 110/63, pulse 105, respiratory rate 18, temp 98.5°F. Weight 90 pounds.

General: Appears well, no apparent distress.

Skin: Warm and dry, pale-appearing, no rash noted.

HEENT: PERRLA, oropharynx pink, no lesions noted, no erythema.

Neck: Supple, no jugular venous distension, no adenopathy.

Chest: Clear to auscultation, no adventitious breath sounds noted.

Heart: RRR, S1, S2 present, no S3 or S4, no murmurs, rubs, or gallops.

Gastrointestinal: Abdomen soft, non-tender, not distended; positive bowel sounds, no mass palpable, no hepatomegaly.

Musculoskeletal: Full range of motion of bilateral upper extremities, no pain to spine palpation.

Neurologic: Alert and oriented to person, place, and time; CN II–XII intact. Sensory: pin prick, vibration intact. Motor: 5/5 strength bilateral upper extremity and left lower extremity. Cerebellar: finger to nose intact. DTRs 2 + bilateral upper and left lower extremity.

Extremities: Right BKA with approximate 4" × 4" mass noted on inner aspect of amputation site; no erythema or breakdown; left leg with no clubbing, cyanosis, or edema.

Laboratory Review

	Hematology	
	Value	Normal range/value
WBC	8.1 mm³	4–12 mm³
HGB	12.2 g/dl	12.0–16.0 g/dl
HCT	39.5 g/dl	37–47 g/dl
PLTS	374 mm³	140–440 mm³
	Chemistry	
Na	135 meq/l	136–145 meq/l
K	4.2 meq/l	3.5–5.0 meq/l
BUN	6 mg/dl	6–23 mg/dl
Creatinine	0.4 mg/dl	0.7–1.2 mg/dl
SGOT	19 u/l	12–45 u/l
SGPT	14 u/l	3–40u/l
ALKP	94 u/l	37–107 u/l
Ca	9.0 mg/dl	8.6–10.4 mg/dl
Glucose	95 mg/dl	65–139 mg/dl

Impression

Mr. H has a history of metastatic chondrosarcoma, status post right BKA, status post-treatment failure with Ifosfamide (Ifex)/Epirubicin (Ellence) and Docetaxel (Taxotere)/Gemcitabine (Gemzar), currently on a Phase I study. He is here today for part one, period two of the protocol. He is tolerating therapy without incident, although his pain has continued, requiring oxycodone (Roxicodone) rescue every four hours around the clock. I recommend to Mr. H that we schedule an appointment with the pain management service for an opinion regarding ways to improve his current regimen. Mr. H states that he would like to hold off right now, but will consider it in the future.

Plan

Laboratory
- Pharmacokinetic blood tests per study schedule.
- Dosing of the study drug today by treatment nurse per study protocol.
- Mr. H may eat at four hours post study drug administration.

Follow-Up
Patient scheduled to return to clinic in one week to initiate part two; continuous daily dosing of study drug.

Pain
Increase oxycodone slow release (OxyContin) to 200 mg by mouth every 12 hours, with continued oxycodone (Roxicodone) 20mg orally every hours as needed for rescue.

Constipation
Continue current bowel regimen.

Encounter Six (one week later; 37 days after initial consultation)

Interim History

Mr. H comes to the cancer center today for day one, part two of the study. He states that he has had a low-grade fever of 99.6°F over the past twenty-four hours, fatigue, and decreased appetite. He took small amounts of food and liquid last night and this morning. He denies nausea or vomiting, abdominal pain, or diarrhea. He has constipation controlled with his bowel regimen. He states that the increased dose of oxycodone slow release (OxyContin) has improved his pain, describing a rating of 4/10 on the pain scale.

Review of Systems

General: Denies chills or sweats.

Skin: Denies rash, pruritus, lesions.

Head: Denies headaches, light-headedness, or head injury.

Eyes: Denies blurred or double vision, discharge, or visual changes.

Nose: Denies congestion, sinus pain, or discharge.

Neck: Denies lumps, pain, sore throat, stiffness, swelling.

Respiratory: SOB on exertion without change; continued non-productive cough; denies wheezing.

Cardiovascular: Denies chest pain, palpitations, edema.

Gastrointestinal: See HPI.

Genitourinary: Denies nocturia, hematuria, dysuria, frequency.

Musculoskeletal: Pain at his right amputation site, pain described as a 4/10 on the pain scale.

Neurologic: Denies history of seizure, fainting, numbness, tingling of extremities, tremors, paresis, vertigo, loss of consciousness.

Psychologic: Denies depression, states that he continues to have a positive attitude. He continues to have support of friends.

Physical Examination

Vital signs: Blood pressure 110/64, pulse 110, respiratory rate 24, temp 100.0°F. Weight 86 pounds.

General: Fatigued, ill-appearing.

Skin: Warm and dry, no rash noted.

HEENT: PERRLA; oropharynx pink; no lesions noted; no erythema.

Neck: Supple; no jugular venous distension; no adenopathy.

Chest: Clear to auscultation; no adventitious breath sounds.

Heart: RRR, S1, S2 present; no S3 or S4; no murmurs, rubs, or gallops.

Gastrointestinal: Abdomen soft, not distended; bowel sounds present; no mass palpable, no hepatomegaly.

Musculoskeletal: Full range of motion of bilateral upper extremities; no pain to spine palpation.

Neurologic: Alert and oriented to person, place, and time; CN II–XII intact. Sensory: pin prick, vibration intact. Motor: 5/5 strength bilateral upper extremity and left lower extremity. Cerebellar: finger to nose intact. DTRs 2 + bilateral upper extremity and left lower extremity.

Extremities: Right below-the-knee amputation with approximate 4″ × 4″ mass noted on inner aspect of amputation site; erythema and warmth noted over mass; left leg with no clubbing, cyanosis, or edema.

Impression

Mr. H is a 53-year-old male with metastatic chondrosarcoma to the lung, right inguinal node and amputation site, status post a right BKA. He is here today for part two of the study protocol, involving initiation of continuous daily study drug. He has a low-grade fever, and warmth and erythema over the mass at his amputation site. The differential diagnosis includes cellulitis of his right lower extremity and pulmonary infection related to his cough.

Admission to solid tumor service is indicated for empiric treatment with intravenous antibiotics for cellulitis, and chest x-ray to evaluate for a pulmonary infection related to fever and cough (**D1, C4, PO A, B**).

Plan

Admit to the medical oncology; fellow notified.

Diagnosis: Right lower extremity cellulitis.

Condition: Stable.

Vital signs: Every 4 hours

Allergies: No known drug allergies.

Activity: Out of bed ad-lib.

Nursing: Notify for change in patient's status and/or temp > 101, HR > 100 or < 60, RR > 30 or < 10, SBP > 160 or < 100, DBP > 100 or < 60.

Diet: Regular.

IV: To heplock.

Medications: Cefazolin (Ancef) 1 g IV every eight hrs; oxycodone slow release (OxyContin) 200 mg orally every 12 hours; oxycodone (Roxicodone) 20 mg orally every three hours as needed.

Laboratory: CBC, comprehensive metabolic panel today, CBC daily. CBC to assess for infection, comprehensive metabolic panel as patient is on a Phase I study drug, with limited toxicity profile information in humans, may affect electrolytes/liver function test.

Radiology: Chest x-ray today to assess for possible pulmonary infection **(D1, C4, PO C).**

Hospital Course

A bed was not immediately available for Mr. H; therefore, I sent him to the emergency department (ED). I went with Mr. H to the ED and paged the fellow and resident to meet us there. I reviewed Mr. H's medical history and verified the plan of care with the fellow and resident **(D1, C4, PO D, E, F, G).** Cefazolin (Ancef) was initiated while Mr. H was in the ED. After four hours, he was admitted to the oncology floor. He responded well to the antibiotic. His fever and the warmth/erythema over the mass resolved. His chest x-ray revealed hilar mediastinal lymphadenopathy. During the hospitalization, he developed increasing dyspnea. The pulmonary service was called for consultation. A bronchoscopy was performed, and pathology revealed metastatic chondrosarcoma of the lung with pulmonary lymphangitic carcinomatosis.

The medical oncologist and I went to see Mr. H, and gave him the news of the spread of the tumor into his lungs. Mr. H was visibly upset by the news and was discouraged that the study drug was ineffective. He asked whether there are any additional therapies he could try. The medical oncologist advised the patient that there were no other therapies available, and that we should focus on making him comfortable. The oncologist and I initiated a discussion of hospice services, placing an emphasis on pain management and on skilled nursing care through an inpatient hospice facility. We explained that we would give Mr. H time to think about this option and would return to discuss this again the following day **(D1, C7, PO B).** That same day, the social worker met with Mr. H to evaluate his psychological state and offer assistance. In addition, pastoral services came to see him, although Mr. H declined this visit.

The following day, we returned to speak with Mr. H, who was receptive to inpatient hospice services. He thanked us for giving him the opportunity to participate in this study. Mr. H was transferred two days later to the hospice service, and within three weeks he died of his disease.

Interstitial spread of tumor through pulmonary lymphatics, also known as pulmonary lymphangitic carcinomatosis (PLC) constitutes 7% of pulmonary metastases. It is caused by spread of carcinoma to the pulmonary vasculature and lymphatics, often resulting in respiratory failure and cor pulmonale. It is usually noted in the late stages of malignancy and therefore indicates a poor prognosis. Tumors with a rich vascular supply and venous drainage appear more likely to metastasize to the lungs and include melanoma, renal cell carcinoma and sarcomas (Acikgoz et al., 2006; Molina & Valente, 2003).

CEBM, level 4.

COMPETENCY DEFENSE

Domain 1, Competency 4. Appraise acuity of patient condition, determine need to transfer patient to higher acuity setting, coordinate, and manage transfer to optimize patient outcomes.

Defense. Mr. H was an immunocompromised patient who came in for a routine visit and was found to have a fever and an area of soft tissue erythema. Clinical practice guidelines recommend that patients with signs of systemic toxicity or erythema that has progressed rapidly should be treated initially with parenteral antibiotics (Swartz, 2004). Utilizing evidence-based guidelines, I evaluated the acuity of Mr. H's condition, determined the need for hospital admission, and coordinated and managed his transfer to optimize outcomes.

Domain 2, Competency 1. Assemble a collaborative interdisciplinary network, refer and consult appropriately while maintaining primary responsibility for comprehensive patient care.

Defense. Mr. H had transportation issues to and from the cancer center due to his lack of financial resources, living alone, and his medical condition. I notified a social worker of these issues and asked her to provide assistance. I regularly updated the social worker as issues developed and was able to utilize available resources such as the American Cancer Society to assist Mr. H.

During the provision of care for this patient, I was approached by the research nurses with concerns about the patient's ability to comply with requirements. I acknowledged their concerns, communicated with the patient, formed my own opinion, and discussed the situation with the medical oncologist.

Domain 3, Competency 2. Evaluate gaps in health care access that compromise optimal patient outcomes, and apply current knowledge of the organization and financing of health care systems to ameliorate negative impact.

Defense. Mr. H was scheduled for a return study visit and a clinic evaluation but was unable to come in due to circumstances beyond his control. This clinical trial is a crossover study design. This visit was his crossover study visit. If he was unable to come, the primary objective of the study would not be met. I contacted the social work department and asked whether they had additional funds to arrange for a ride for Mr. H to our center. The department did have such funds. A car ride was arranged, and Mr. H was evaluated as planned.

Domain 1, Competency 7. Facilitate and guide the process of palliative care and/or planning end of life care by discussing diagnoses and prognosis, clarifying and validating patient desires and priorities, and promoting informed choices and shared decision making by patient, family and members of the health care team.

Defense. Mr. H was admitted to the hospital for a cellulitis of his right lower extremity. During the hospitalization workup revealed pulmonary lymphangitic carcinomatosis. The prognosis of this late-stage development is poor and leads to respiratory failure (Acikgoz et al., 2006; Molina & Valente, 2003). Mr. H had progressed through his current regimen, and it was time to discuss end-of-life planning. Both the medical oncologist and I explained the progression of his disease and that we did not have another treatment regimen to offer. We reviewed comfort care measures and described hospice services. We arranged with Mr. H and the discharge planner for admission to an inpatient hospice facility.

Domain 3, Competency 3. Synthesize the principles of legal and ethical decision-making and analyze dilemmas that arise in patient care, inter professional relationships, research, or practice management to improve outcomes.

Defense. Mr. H came to the cancer center for a clinical trial opportunity, as he had progressed on standard regimens and had no other options. Mr. H was eligible for a Phase I study, he understood the risks and benefits, and he wanted to participate. Legal standards for decision-making capacity for consent to treatment include the ability to communicate a choice, to understand the relevant information, to appreciate the medical consequences of the situation, and to reason about treatment choices (Appelbaum, 2007). Law and social practice accept a presumption of competence. It is presumed of any adult that he or she has sufficient decision-making capacity to make decisions for himself and to have these decisions respected by others (Buchanan & Brock, 1986).

Medications

Drug: Acetaminophen(Tylenol)/oxycodone hydrochloride (Percocet)

Dose range: Oxycodone 5 mg, acetaminophen 325 mg.

Method of administration in this case: 1–2 tablets orally every 6 hours as needed.

Mechanism of action: Acetaminophen is an analgesic and antipyretic drug. It is non-opiate and non-salicylate. Oxycodone hydrochloride, a semi-synthetic pure opioid agonist, has multiple actions similar in quality with those of morphine. It acts predominantly on the central nervous system (CNS) and organs composed of smooth muscle. Its principal actions in combination with acetaminophen are sedation and analgesia.

(continued)

Clinical uses: Chronic moderate to severe pain.

Side effects
Common: CNS depression, confusion, dizziness, drowsiness, headache, sedation, nausea, vomiting, constipation, respiratory depression, hepatotoxicity.
Serious: Respiratory depression.

Drug: Albuterol (Proventil)

Dose range: 2 puffs every 4–6 hrs as needed.

Method of administration in this case: Metered-dose inhaler.

Mechanism of action: A sympathomimetic amine, this is a beta-adrenergic agonist that selectively acts on the beta(2)-adrenergic receptors of intracellular adenyl cyclase, the catalyst for the conversion of adenosine triphosphate (ATP) to cyclic-3,′ 5′-adenosine monophosphate (cyclic AMP).

Clinical uses: Asthma, treatment and prophylaxis of exercise-induced asthma. Prophylaxis.

Side effects
Common: Nervousness, tachycardia, restlessness, tremor, cough, bronchospasm.
Serious: Angina, atrial fibrillation, supraventricular tachycardia.

Drug: Azithromycin (Zithromax)

Dose range: Mild to moderate respiratory tract, skin, and soft tissue infections—500 mg orally in a single loading dose on day 1, followed by 250 mg/day as a single dose on days 2–5.

Method of administration in this case: Oral.

Mechanism of action: Inhibits RNA-dependent protein synthesis at the chain elongation step; binds to the 50S ribosomal subunit resulting in blockage of transpeptidation.

Clinical uses: (oral, IV) Treatment of acute otitis media due to *H. influenzae*, *M. catarrhalis*, or *S. pneumoniae*; pharyngitis/tonsillitis due to *S. pyogenes*; treatment of mild to moderate upper and lower respiratory tract infections, infections of the skin and skin structure, community-acquired pneumonia, *Mycoplasma pneumoniae*, and *C. psittaci*; acute bacterial sinusitis.

Side effects
Common: Abdominal pain, anorexia, cramping, vomiting, rash, pruritus.
Serious: Acute renal failure.

Drug: Cefazolin (Ancef)

Dose range: Usual dosage range: I.M., I.V.: 1–1.5 g every 8 hours, depending on severity of infection. Maximum: 12 g/day.

(continued)

Method of administration in this case: 1 g IV every 8 hours.

Mechanism of action: Inhibits bacterial cell wall synthesis by binding to one or more of the penicillin-binding proteins, which in turn inhibits the final transpeptidation step of peptidoglycan synthesis in bacterial cell walls, thus inhibiting cell wall biosynthesis. Bacteria eventually lyse due to ongoing activity of cell wall autolytic enzymes (autolysins and murein hydrolases) while cell wall assembly is arrested.

Clinical uses: Treatment of respiratory tract, skin, genital, urinary tract, biliary tract, bone and joint infections, and septicemia due to susceptible gram-positive cocci (except enterococcus); some gram-negative bacilli including *E. coli*, *Proteus*, and *Klebsiella* may be susceptible; surgical prophylaxis.

Side effects
Common: Diarrhea, nausea, vomiting, abdominal cramps, anorexia, pseudomembranous colitis, oral candidiasis, rash, fever.
Serious: Toxic epidermal necrolysis.

Drug: Docetaxel (Taxotere)

Dose range: (IV) 100 mg/m^2 every 3 weeks.

Method of administration in this case: Intravenous.

Mechanism of action: Docetaxel is an antimitotic agent. It binds to free tubulin, then promotes the polymerization of tubulin into stable microtubules and inhibits microtubule disassembly, resulting in blockade of cellular mitotic and interphase functions and, consequently, in inhibition of cell division.

Clinical uses: Head and neck cancer, prostate cancer, bladder cancer.

Side effects
Common: Lethargy, alopecia, neurosensory event, fluid retention, fever, nausea, vomiting, myelosuppression.
Serious: Anaphylaxis, pulmonary edema, atrial fibrillation, deep vein thrombosis.

Drug: Docusate (Colace)

Dose range: 50–500 mg/day orally in 1–4 divided doses.

Method of administration in this case: Oral.

Mechanism of action: Reduces surface tension of the oil-water interface of the stool, resulting in enhanced incorporation of water and fat, allowing for stool softening.

Clinical uses: Stool softener in patients who should avoid straining during defecation and constipation associated with hard, dry stools; prophylaxis for straining (Valsalva) following myocardial infarction.

(continued)

Side effects
Common: Abdominal cramps, diarrhea.
Serious: Diarrhea.

Drug: Epirubicin hydrochloride (Ellence)

Dose range: 55 mg/m2 day 1 and day 2 every three weeks.

Method of administration in this case: Intravenous.

Mechanism of action: Epirubicin hydrochloride is an anthracycline anti-cancer agent with cytotoxic and antiproliferative properties. It intercalates between nucleotide base pairs with consequent inhibition of nucleic acid and protein synthesis, thus triggering DNA cleavage. It also prevents DNA helicase activity by inhibiting enzymatic separation of double-stranded DNA and interfering with the replication and transcription.

Clinical uses: Soft tissue sarcoma, bladder cancer, gastric carcinoma.

Side effects
Common: Lethargy, alopecia, nausea, vomiting, mucositis, myelosuppression.
Serious: Anaphylaxis, cardiomyopathy, myelodysplastic syndrome.

Drug: Fentanyl (Duragesic)

Dose range: 12.5 mcg/hr–100 mcg/hr.

Method of administration in this case: Transdermal patch. Apply to non-irritated and nonirradiated skin, such as chest, back, flank, or upper arm. Change every 72 hrs.

Mechanism of action: Opioid analgesics such as fentanyl bind with stereospecific receptors at many sites within the CNS to alter processes affecting both the perception of and emotional response to pain. Although the precise sites and mechanisms of action have not been fully determined, alterations in the release of various neurotransmitters from afferent nerves sensitive to painful stimuli may be partially responsible for the analgesic effects.

Clinical uses: Chronic moderate to severe pain, post-operative pain.

Side effects
Common: CNS depression, confusion, dizziness, drowsiness, headache, sedation, nausea, vomiting, constipation, xerostomia, dyspnea, respiratory depression, application-site reaction erythema.
Serious: Adult respiratory depression.

Drug: Gemcitabine hydrochloride (Gemzar)

Dose range: 675 mg/m2 on day 1 and day 8 every three weeks.

(continued)

Method of administration in this case: Intravenous infusion over 90 minutes every 3 weeks.

Mechanism of action: Gemcitabine is an antimetabolite of the pyrimidine analog type. Gemcitabine is cell cycle-specific for the S phase and for the G 1/S phase boundary of cell division. Activity occurs as a result of intracellular conversion to two active metabolites, gemcitabine diphosphate and gemcitabine triphosphate.

Clinical uses: Pancreatic cancer, metastatic breast cancer, ovarian cancer.

Side effects
Common: Nausea, vomiting, myelosuppression, elevation of transaminase.
Serious: Adult respiratory distress syndrome, anaphylaxis, arrhythmias.

Drug: Histone deacetylatase inhibitor (LBH589)

Dose range: 20 mg–40 mg.

Method of administration in this case: Oral dose tri-weekly.

Mechanism of action: Induce tumor cell growth arrest, differentiation or apoptosis in vitro and inhibit tumor growth in animals.

Clinical uses: Tumor growth inhibition and apoptosis.

Side effects
Common: Diarrhea, fatigue, thrombocytopenia, prolonged QTc.
Serious: Prolonged QTc, hypokalemia, bradycardia.

Drug: Ifosfamide (Ifex)

Dose range: 2.5 gm/m2 IV D1 to D4 every three weeks.

Method of administered in this case: Intravenous infusion every three weeks.

Mechanism of action: Ifosfamide is classified as an alkylating agent of the nitrogen mustard type. After metabolic activation, active metabolites of ifosfamide alkylate or bind with many intracellular molecular structures, including nucleic acids. The cytotoxic action is primarily due to cross-linking of strands of DNA and RNA, as well as inhibition of protein synthesis.

Clinical uses: Osteosarcoma, breast cancer, bladder cancer, germ cell tumor.

Side effects
Common: Myelosuppression, nausea, vomiting, alopecia, hematuria.
Serious: Acute renal failure, acidosis, cardiotoxicity.

(continued)

Drug: Magnesium hydroxide (Phillips Milk of Magnesia)

Dose range: 400 mg–1200 mg.

Method of administration in this case: Magnesium hydroxide 400 mg/5 mL: 5–15 mL as needed up to 4 times/day.

Mechanism of action: Antacid, laxative.

Clinical uses: Short-term treatment of occasional constipation and symptoms of hyperacidity, laxative.

Side effects
Common: Diarrhea, abnormal taste.
Serious: Diarrhea.

Drug: Oxycodone (Roxicodone)

Dose range: 5 mg.

Method of administration in this case: 1 tablet every three hours as needed for pain.

Mechanism of action: Narcotic analgesic; opiate analgesic.

Clinical uses: Management of moderate to severe pain.

Side effects
Common: Somnolence, dizziness, nausea, constipation.
Serious: CNS depressions, hypotension.

Drug: Oxycodone slow release (OxyContin)

Dose range: 10 mg, 15 mg, 20 mg, 30 mg, 40 mg, 60 mg, 80 mg, 160 mg.

Method of administration in this case: 2 tablets orally at bedtime daily, dose adjusted as needed.

Mechanism of action: Binds to opiate receptors in the CNS, causing inhibition of ascending pain pathways, altering the perception of and response to pain; produces generalized CNS depression.

Clinical uses: Management of moderate to severe pain when an analgesic is needed for an extended period of time.

Side effects
Common: Nausea, vomiting, sedation, dizziness.
Serious: CNS depression.

Drug: Prednisone (Sterapred)

Dose range: Initial: 5–60 mg/day orally.

(continued)

Method of administration in this case: Oral, one tablet daily.

Mechanism of action: An adrenocortical steroid with salt-retaining properties. It is a synthetic glucocorticoid analog, which is mainly used for anti-inflammatory effects in different disorders of many organ systems. It causes profound and varied metabolic effects, modifies the immune response of the body to diverse stimuli, and is also used as replacement therapy for adrenocortical deficient patients.

Clinical uses: Respiratory diseases, neoplastic diseases.

Side effects
Common: Hypertension, emotional instability, facial erythema, peptic ulcer, impaired wound healing.
Serious: Adrenal suppression, immunosuppression, myopathy.

Drug: Senna (Senokot)

Dose range: 8.6 mg.

Method of administration in this case: 2 tablets orally at bedtime daily.

Mechanism of action: Laxative, stimulant.

Clinical uses: Short-term treatment of occasional constipation.

Side effects
Common: Abdominal cramps, diarrhea, and nausea.
Serious: Diarrhea.

Source: Micromedex Health Care Series. Retrieved August 2, 2007, from http://thomsonhc.com Greenwood Village, CO: Thomson Micromedex.

References

Acikgoz, G., et al. (2006). Pulmonary lymphangitic carcinomatosis (PLC): Spectrum of FDG-PET findings. *Clin Nucl Med, 31*(11), 673–678.

Appelbaum, P.S. (2007). Assessment of patients' competence to consent to treatment. *N Engl J Med, 357*(18), 1834–1840.

Buchanan, A., & Brock, D.W. (1986). Deciding for others. *Milbank Q, 64*(Suppl 2), 17–94.

Chow, W.A. (2007). Update on chondrosarcomas. *Curr Opin Oncol, 19*(4), 371–376.

Leu, K.M., et al.(2004). Laboratory and clinical evidence of synergistic cytotoxicity of sequential treatment with gemcitabine followed by docetaxel in the treatment of sarcoma. *J Clin Oncol, 22*(9), 1706–1712.

Malawer, M.M., Helman, L.J., & O'Sullivan, B. (2005). Sarcomas of the bone. In V. DeVita, S. Hellman, & S.A. Rosenberg (Eds.), *Cancer: Principles & Practice of Oncology* (7th ed., pp. 1673–1676). Philadelphia: Lippincott Williams & Wilkins.

Marcove, R.C., et al. (1972). Chondrosarcoma of the pelvis and upper end of the femur: An analysis of factors influencing survival time in one hundred and thirteen cases. *Journal of Bone & Joint Surgery, 54*(3), 561–572.

Meisel, A. (1989). Presumption of competence. In W.L. Publications (Ed.), *The Right to Die* (pp. 207–208). New York: John Wiley & Sons.

Molina, D.K., & Valente, P.T. (2003). Lymphangitic spread of hepatocellular carcinoma. *Arch Pathol Lab Med, 127*(1), e11–e13.

Palumbo, R., et al. (1999). Dose-intensive first-line chemotherapy with epirubicin and continuous infusion ifosfamide in adult patients with advanced soft tissue sarcomas: A phase II study. *Eur J Cancer, 35*(1), 66–72.

Pritchard, D.J., et al. (1980). Chondrosarcoma: A clinicopathologic and statistical analysis. *Cancer, 45*(1), 149–157.

Sakimura, R., et al. (2007). The effects of histone deacetylase inhibitors on the induction of differentiation in chondrosarcoma cells. *Clin Cancer Res, 13*(1), 275–282.

Swartz, M.N. (2004). Clinical practice. Cellulitis. *N Engl J Med, 350*(9), 904–912.

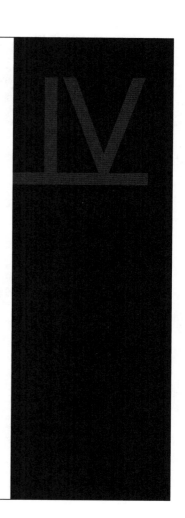

DNP Approach and Clinical Case Narratives in Mental Health Care

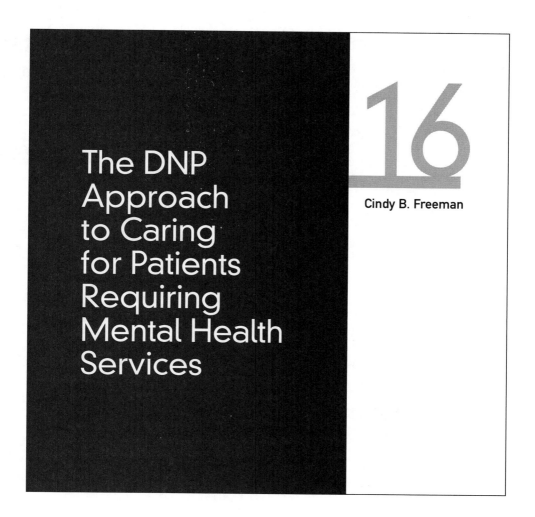

16

The DNP Approach to Caring for Patients Requiring Mental Health Services

Cindy B. Freeman

There is a severe shortage of mental health providers in parts of the United States and other wealthy countries, as well as in many low- and middle-income countries (Kaplan & Lake, 2008; Patel, 2009; WHO, 2009). Advanced practice nurses (APNs) educated in clinically focused doctor of nursing practice (DNP) programs are prepared to provide comprehensive, coordinated, safe, accessible, and high-quality care for patients in their areas of specialty with a general knowledge of primary care (Mundinger et al., 2009). Similar to other clinical doctoral programs, clinical DNP education is defining the standard for the future of advanced practice nursing (Mundinger, 2005). As DNPs who specialize in psychiatry and mental health (P/MH) educate the next generation of psychiatric nurses and nurse practitioners, our profession will increase the number of providers prepared to address the needs of children and adults with mental health issues (Kaye et al. , 2009).

Mental illnesses can result in debilitating, burdensome problems for patients, families, employers, communities, and government agencies. Psychiatric disorders affect all ages, genders, races, nationalities, and socioeconomic groups. Neuropsychiatric conditions constitute up to twenty-five percent of the worldwide burden of disease, with mental illnesses contributing to the majority of these conditions (Prince et al., 2007). Mental illness affects physical well-being, as well as emotional and cognitive states. The ability to integrate and derive meaning from the various components of human experience is seriously impacted by untreated psychiatric and mental illness.

Depression, one of the most frequently encountered mental illnesses, is ranked as the number-one cause of disability worldwide and considered the fourth highest contributor to the global disease burden by the World Health Organization (2009). Of the global population of nearly 7 billion, 120 million people are affected by depressive disorders yearly. One million of these individuals commit suicide (Nock et al., 2009). Depressive disorders are the second most common reason adults present to primary care providers (PCP) in the United States (Sharp & Lipsky, 2002). Some patients with psychiatric mental health diagnoses can be treated solely by the PCP, whereas other patients with complex psychiatric, mental health issues, or depression that is resistant to medication, require referral or consultation with a specialist P/MH provider (Schulberg et al., 1997). Integrated practice models are currently being developed in the primary care setting to address the need for P/MH care. P/MH APNs working in nurse-managed health centers address the needs of this vulnerable population and evaluate best practices (Roberts, Robinson, Stewart, & Wright, 2008).

P/MH DNP ROLE IN MANAGEMENT OF PATIENTS WITH COMPLEX CHRONIC COMORBID CONDITIONS

The P/MH DNP approaches the patient from multiple interconnected perspectives, with special attention to social, cultural, spiritual, and emotional parameters, as well as the biophysical context. The P/MH DNP also possesses the enhanced skills and expanded knowledge necessary to respond to the increase in prevalence and chronicity of emotional/psychological disorders.

Psychiatric patients present with serious chronic complex comorbidities and conditions often related to long-term medication management. The science of psychopharmacology and psychopharmacogenomics is growing rapidly. The care of the psychiatric patient invites a complex combination of astute assessment skills, diagnostic acumen, and broad understanding of multiple modalities of evidence-based treatment.

The DNP understands psychopharmacogenomics and integrates this knowledge into the therapeutic intervention. For example, the patient with chronic depression, diabetes type 2 (DM2), or hypertension (HTN) who is not responding well to antidepressant medications requires careful assessment of DM2 and HTN, including medications prescribed for their treatment. Understanding the genetic implications of variations in rates of drug metabolism provided by CYP450 studies is especially important when patients are being treated with antidepressant medications, as well as medications for other comorbid chronic conditions.

Accurate and appropriate CYP 450 tests, especially for CYP 2D6 in the case of psychotropics, can decrease the time necessary to assess patient response to a new psychotropic, as well as inform initial prescriptive decisions for that drug. Patients who are poor responders, with no CYP 2D6 enzyme, metabolize slowly or not at all. Thus, blood levels of the particular drug rise with subsequent doses and can cause a toxic reaction. Intermediate responders have a deficient amount of CYP 2D6 enzymes and take longer to metabolize a given dose; these patients may need slightly increased amounts or a different drug. Extensive or normal responders react as expected to a given dose, having an expected amount of CYP 450 enzyme. Ultra-rapid responders have more CYP 2D6, so as to make it seem that the patient is not responding to the medication. In such cases, a larger dose than normal is required to achieve the expected result (Flockhart, 2007).

The DNP with specialty certification in P/MH and boarded by the American Board of Comprehensive Care is ideally suited to expand the P/MH advanced practice nursing role by providing integrated specialty care for patients across clinical settings over time. Studies have shown correlations between mental illness and multiple chronic medical conditions, including cardiac disease (Lichtman et al., 2008), diabetes (Anderson et al., 2001), end-stage renal disease (Kimmel et al., 1998), cancer (Sharpe et al., 2004), Parkinson's disease (Langston, 2006), HIV/AIDS (Sadock & Sadock, 2007), and chronic pain (Blair et al., 2003). Any patients with multiple comorbidities requiring sustained lifestyle changes can benefit from the care perspective and interventions of the P/MH DNP for themselves and for their families. As a member of an interdisciplinary team providing care of patients with serious chronic illnesses, the P/MH DNP can address individual patient care issues that previously have not been identified.

Approximately one-half of cancer patients have emotional difficulties, including adjustment disorder, depression, anxiety, decreased life satisfaction, and loss of self-esteem (Sharpe et al., 2004). Cancer patients with advanced disease, prior psychiatric history, and poorly controlled pain are at most at risk for developing mental health related complications. End-of-life issues strongly impact resolution of these issues, and the DNP with P/MH specialty knowledge and skill can identify patients who require mental health services and incorporate these needs into the plan of care.

Adults with chronic kidney disease requiring dialysis may benefit from integrated DNP services. Mental health disorders observed in this patient population include affective disorders, substance use disorders, schizophrenia, psychoses, and personality disorders. These disorders account for a 1.5- to 3.0-times higher rate of hospitalization compared to patients with other chronic illnesses (Kimmel et al. 1998). When providing care for patients requiring dialysis, the DNP considers the physiologic etiology of presenting symptoms before making a psychiatric diagnosis. The DNP's ongoing relationship with the patient and team informs care when a patient requests to withdraw from dialysis. The DNP assists in determining whether there is underlying depression, dementia, uremia, or encephalopathy when determining whether the patient fully comprehends the consequences of withdrawing from dialysis.

The P/DNP can also contribute to the care of patients with degenerative neurologic diseases that affect the patient and informal caregivers. Parkinson's disease (PD), once considered a motor system disorder, is now recognized as disorder with neuropsychiatric and non-motor manifestations, including cognitive dysfunction, dementia, psychosis, hallucinations, depression, anxiety, sleep disturbances, and fatigue. The P/MH DNP can contribute to the care of the PD patient and family by providing education, coordinating services, and consulting for medication management (Langston, 2006).

THE DNP AND SYSTEMS OF CARE

Understanding systems of care and how to interact on behalf of the patient with mental health diagnoses among the multiple care providers and disciplines in the health system requires strong advocacy, collaboration, and intervention skills. In this capacity, the P/MH DNP initiates and accepts referrals from other members of the health care team (e.g., nurses, nurse practitioners, PAs, DNPs, and MDs) and other disciplines involved in care (e.g., human resource staff at place of employment, assisted living facility staff, or school counselors and teachers).

The care provided by the psychiatric DNP transcends boundaries of traditional practice settings. Care is provided in the setting that best suits the acuity of the patient's needs in the least restrictive environment possible. The P/MH DNP will have the knowledge and skills necessary to transition the patient across care settings as determined by the status of the patient's illness and need for monitoring. The P/MH DNP may admit the unstable patient to an emergency department for close monitoring and stabilization, and to the inpatient unit for continued diagnostic evaluation and management. The P/MH DNP can then provide follow-up care in the community or subacute setting such as a long-term care treatment facility.

In these settings, the P/MH DNP can contribute to the care of terminally ill patients by assisting the health care team in differentiating between a normal and appropriate reaction to dying, as opposed to a more serious psychiatric disorder, such as clinical depression. Among terminally ill patients, depression is correlated with decreased quality of life, greater difficulty treating the patient's illness, decreased compliance with the treatment plan, and earlier admission to inpatient or hospice care. Studies have found that depression is underdiagnosed and inadequately treated in the palliative care setting (Sharpe, et al., 2004).

With more psychiatric patients living in the community, the ongoing evaluation of psychiatric care needs through a continuous relationship with the patient is vitally important. Patient safety is paramount, as well as the safety of people in the patient's environment and support system. The DNP who specializes in the provision of psychiatric mental health care blends the art and science of nursing and medicine, using a comprehensive, patient-centered approach to provide successful and thoughtful evidence-based care with positive patient outcomes.

References

Anderson, R.J., Freedland, K.E., Clouse, R.E., & Lustman, P.J. (2001). The prevalence of comorbid depression in adults with diabetes: A meta-analysis. *Diabetes Care, 24,* 1069.

Blair, M.J., Robinson, R.L., Katon, W., & Koenke, K. (2003). Depression and pain comorbidity: A literature review. *Arch Intern Med 163*(20), 2433–2445.

Flockhart, D.A. (2007). Drug interactions: Cytochrome P450 drug interaction table. Indiana University, School of Medicine. http://medicine.iupi.edu/clinpharm/ddis/table.asp Accessed October 13, 2009.

Kaplan, J., & Lake, M. (2008). Exposing medical students to child and adolescent psychiatry: A case-based seminar. *Academic Psychiatry, 32*(5), 362–365.

Kaye, L., Warner, L., Lewandowski, C., Greene, R., Acker, J., & Chiarella, N. (2009). The role of nurse practitioners in meeting the need for child and adolescent psychiatric services: A statewide survey. *Journal of Psychosocial Nursing, 47*(3), 34–40.

Kimmel, P.L., Thamer, M., Richard, C.M., & Ray, N.F. (1998). Psychiatric illnesses in patients with end-stage renal disease. *American Journal of Medicine, 105*(3), 214–221.

Langston, J.W. (2006).The Parkinson's complex: Parkinsonism is just the tip of the iceberg. *Annals of Neurology, 59(4),* 591–596.

Lichtman, J.H., Bigger, J.T., Blumenthal, J.A., et al. (2008). Depression and coronary heart disease. *Circulation, 118,* 1768–1775.

Mundinger, M., Starck. P., Hathaway, D., Shaver, J., & Woods, N. (2009). The ABCs of the doctor of nursing practice: Assessing resources, building a culture of clinical scholarship, curricular models. *Journal of Professional Nursing, 25*(2), 69–74.

Mundinger, M. (2005). Who's who in nursing bringing clarity to the doctor of nursing practice. *Nursing Outlook, 53*(4), 173–176.

Nock, M., Hwang, I., Sampson, N., et al. (2009). Cross-national analysis of the associations among mental disorders and suicidal behavior: Findings from the WHO world mental health surveys. *PLoS Medicine, 6*(8). Retrieved October 10, 2009, from: www.plosmedicine. org.

Patel, V. (2009). The future of psychiatry in low- and middle-income countries. *Psychological Medicine, 39*(11), 1759–1762.

Prince, M., Patel, V., Saxena, S., Maj, M., Maselko, J., Phillips, M., & Rajman, A. (2007). No health without mental health. *The Lancet, 370*(9590), 859–877.

Roberts, K.T., Robinson, K.M., Stewart, C., & Wright J. (2008). Integrated mental health practice in a nurse managed health center. *The American Journal for Nurse Practitioners, 12*(10), 33–44.

Sadock, B.J., & Sadock, V.A. (2007). *Kaplan & Sadock's Synopsis of Psychiatry: Behavioral Sciences/Clinical Psychiatry* (10th ed.). Philadelphia: Lippincott Williams & Wilkins.

Sharp, L., & Lipsky, M. (2002). Screening for depression across the lifespan: A review of measures for use in primary care settings. *American Family Physician, 66*(6). Retrieved October 10, 2009, from: http://www.aafp.org/afp/20020915/1001.html.

Sharpe, M., Strong, V., Allen, K., et al. (2004). Major depression in outpatients attending a regional cancer centre: screening and unmet treatment needs, *British Journal of Cancer, 90,* 314–320.

Schulberg, H.C., Block, M.R., Madonia, M.J., et al. (1997). The "usual" care of major depression in primary care practice. *Archives of Family Medicine, 6*(4), 334–339.

WHO Initiative on depression in public health (2009). Geneva. Retrieved October 10, 2009, from http://www.who.int/mental_health/management/depression/definition/en/print.html.

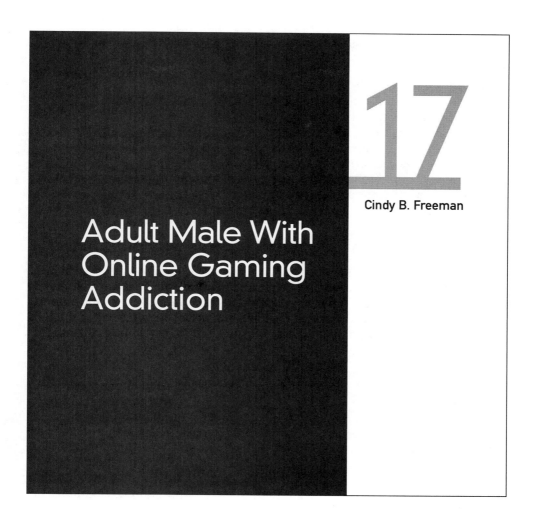

17

Cindy B. Freeman

Adult Male With Online Gaming Addiction

I chose this case because it addressed a newly recognized psychiatric problem associated with controversy, not only in what to call it and how to categorize it, but also in how to treat it. Online gaming addiction, as a subtype of Internet addiction disorder, is currently treated as a subtype of impulse control disorders such as pathological gambling. The case narrative focuses on seven encounters that occurred over a period of six months in the outpatient private psychiatric setting for a commercially insured patient. This case narrative demonstrates my ability to meet the following Columbia University School of Nursing (CUSN) doctoral competencies for comprehensive direct patient care.

DOMAIN 1, COMPETENCY 1

Evaluate patient needs based on age, developmental stage, family history, ethnicity, and individual risk, including genetic profile, to formulate plans for health promotion, anticipatory guidance, counseling, and disease prevention services for healthy or sick patients and their families in any clinical setting.

PO A. Identification of a potential genetic risk.

PO B. Diagnosis of a genetic condition.

PO C. Evaluate individual patient needs based on age, developmental stage, family history, ethnicity, and individual risks.

PO D. Formulate a plan that addresses health promotion, anticipatory guidance, and/or disease prevention for the individual.

PO E. Develop a plan that addresses health promotion, anticipatory guidance, and/or disease prevention for the family.

DOMAIN 1, COMPETENCY 3

Formulate differential diagnoses and diagnostic strategies and therapeutic interventions with attention to scientific evidence, safety, cost, invasiveness, simplicity, acceptability, adherence, and efficacy for patients who present with new conditions and those with ambiguous or incomplete data, complex illnesses, comorbid conditions, and multiple diagnoses in all clinical settings.

PO A. Formulate a differential diagnosis for a patient who presents with new undifferentiated signs and symptoms.

PO B. Formulate a differential diagnosis for a patient who presents with ambiguous or incomplete data, complex illnesses, comorbid conditions, and potential multiple diagnoses.

PO C. Discuss the rationale for the differential diagnosis.

PO D. Discuss the rationale for the diagnostic evaluation with attention to scientific evidence, safety, cost, invasiveness, simplicity, acceptability, adherence, and efficacy.

PO E. Discuss the rationale for the therapeutic intervention with attention to scientific evidence, safety, cost, invasiveness, simplicity, acceptability, adherence, and efficacy.

ENCOUNTER CONTEXT

Encounter One (day 1)

DNP role: I am a certified mental health nurse practitioner, doctor of nursing practice (DNP) resident, and member of the faculty at the University of Texas-Houston School of Nursing.

Identifying Information

Site: Ambulatory care.

Setting: Psychiatric private practice.

Reason for encounter: Evaluation for depression.

Demographics: Patient is a 26-year-old Caucasian male. The patient lives with his parents and works part-time with his mother at a local grocery store. He received an honorable discharge from the military six months ago. He completed two years of college and is currently attending classes at a community college.

Chief complaint: Feels depressed.

History of Present Illness

Patient has been having trouble concentrating, feels depressed (rated 7 on scale of 1 to 10), feels he has no emotions, and feels isolated. Problems are increased at night when family is sleeping.

Patient's mother accompanies him to the office and reports he spends almost all his time isolated in his room, playing an online computer game. She reports he is irritable when disturbed or called to eat meals with family. The patient does not see this as an issue.

The patient reports he has been experiencing insomnia, racing thoughts, anxiety, and panic attacks for an extended period. He reports he feels less anxiety when alone and playing the computer game. The game is *Lineage*, a massively multiplayer online role-playing game (MMORPG).

History of Psychiatric Illness

The patient was in the military for nine years and had planned to make it his career. Patient describes himself as having always been prone to having little social interaction. Patient reports he started playing online role-playing games during the period he was in the military. He tended to isolate himself for extended periods, which eventually led him to be asked to leave the military, although he did receive an honorable discharge. He describes his current playing time as 8 to 12 hours daily, mostly in the evenings and at night.

Medical History

The patient has a history of migraines. He reports he has had them periodically since age 12. The most recent migraine was six months ago. He describes them as mild and is able to treat them effectively by taking ibuprofen (Advil) 600–800 mg and staying in a dark room for a few hours.

A study by Beghi et al. (2007) showed the presence of a depressive episode present in 59.9% of migraine sufferers and 69.6% of those suffering from migraine and tension headaches. Comorbid anxiety was reported in 18.4% of those with migraines alone and with migraines and tension headache. This comorbidity is very interesting for many reasons. The most significant comorbidity in this case being that drugs, including serotonin reuptake inhibitors and anticonvulsants, used to treat mood disorders can also be useful in migraine prophylaxis (Ramadan, 2007).

Oxford Centre for Evidence-Based Medicine (CEBM),
levels 2b (Beghi et al.), 3a (Ramadan).

Current medications: Over-the-counter ibuprofen (Advil) for migraines 600–800 mg by mouth as needed.

Allergies: No known drug allergies.

Family psychiatric history: Both parents suffer from depression; two maternal aunts have bipolar disorder, and one maternal aunt has social phobia.

Social history: The patient lives with his parents and works part-time at a local grocery store. He received an honorable discharge from the military six months ago. Patient had no significant combat or traumatic experience. He has completed two years of college. He denies recreational drug use, reports minimal alcohol use. He denies any history of physical or sexual abuse.

Mental Status Examination

Patient is a 26-year-old Caucasian male whose appears his stated age. Patient is awake, alert, and oriented to person, place, time, and situation. He is groomed and dressed appropriately for the situation. He makes minimal eye contact. Patient exhibits steady gait and has firm handshake. No psychomotor agitation or retardation is noted. All movements are voluntary and purposeful. Speech is of normal rhythm and volume with minimal stammering noted. Behavior is friendly and cooperative. His stated mood is anxious, and affect is congruent. He denies any hallucinations, delusions, or paranoia. His thought processes are logical and goal-directed. He denies any current suicidal or homicidal ideations. His memory is intact in all measures. He is of above-average intelligence and is currently enrolled in college courses. Insight into his situation is currently limited because he does not recognize the problems created by the amount of time he spends playing the online game. His judgment is also limited by his insight. The patient is a reliable historian.

> *A formal mental status examination is part of a comprehensive patient evaluation and is used to evaluate a range of mental functions at a precise moment in time. A patient's thought processes are assessed by noting the coherence of speech as to how logically their brain is making associations. Assessing thought content includes a patient's preoccupations, phobias, delusions, hallucinations and suicidal or homicidal ideation (Mueller, Kiernan, & Langston, 2000).*
>
> CEBM, level 5.

Review of Systems

General: Denies fever, fatigue, weight loss.

Skin: Denies rashes, lesions.

Head: Denies trauma, pain.

Eyes: Denies eye pain, redness, excessive tearing, visual disturbance, glaucoma, or cataracts.

Ears: Denies hearing loss, discharge, tinnitus, vertigo, pain, or infection.

Nose: Denies nasal discharge or itching, hay fever, nosebleeds, or sinus trouble.

Mouth and throat: Denies chewing problems, sore tongue, sores in mouth, dry mouth, frequent sore throats, hoarseness, or bleeding gums.

Neck: Denies lumps, swollen glands, goiter, or neck pain.

Chest and cardiovascular: Denies chest pain, extremity edema.

Respiratory: Denies cough, shortness of breath.

Gastrointestinal: Denies nausea, vomiting, or diarrhea.

Genitourinary: Denies dysuria, hematuria, or incontinence.

Neurologic: Denies headache, weakness, seizures, or paralysis.

Musculoskeletal: Denies history of trauma, injury, or falls.

Hematologic: Denies history of anemia, easy bruising, or prolonged bleeding from small cuts.

Immunologic: Last Td 2005 while in military.

Endocrine: Denies thyroid problems, heat or cold intolerance, excessive sweating, or excessive thirst or hunger.

Physical Examination

Vital signs: Heart rate 87, respiratory rate 16, temp 98.3°F, blood pressure 128/68, height 5'11", weight 170 lb., BMI 23.7.

The body mass index (BMI) is an accepted method of calculating a person's weight status. It is a ratio of height to weight and takes into consideration that taller people have more tissue than shorter people. A BMI > 25 increases your chances of an early death and is the current definition of overweight, while BMI > 30 is the definition of obesity (NIH, 1998).

CEBM, level 5.

Vital signs, a medical history and review of systems can show the clinician's attention to the interplay between physical and mental symptoms and disorders. It may provide the clinician with valuable information as to the cause of mental status changes and any physical handicaps or limitations the patient may have (Flynn & Mueller, 2000).

CEBM, level 5.

Telephone consultation with the patient's primary care provider (PCP) supports the patient's claim of overall good health. Except for his history of migraines, there are no physical impairments, and recent laboratory data are unremarkable.

A complete physical examination of each patient would be optimal in psychiatric practice. However, most outpatient psychiatric clinicians do not have the time, adequate examination rooms and equipment. In lieu of this, collaboration among health care providers is essential for quality patient-centered care (Lewin, Skea, Entwhistle, Zwarenstein, & Dick, 2009).

CEBM, level 3a.

Clinical Impression

The patient is a 26-year-old male who presents with trouble concentrating, significant depression, anhedonia, social isolation, anxiety, irritability, insomnia, and excessive amount of time spent in MMORPG. The examination is remarkable for anxious and depressed affect congruent with stated mood, as well as limited judgment and insight into his current situation. He has a positive family history of mood and anxiety disorders.

Consultation with PCP reveals no remarkable findings on physical examinations or laboratory tests. Patient's diagnosis of migraines is confirmed to be moderate and long–standing, with a maternal migraine history as well. Possible causes of the patient's symptoms include the following:

- Major depressive disorder, recurrent and severe, as evidenced by difficulty concentrating, anhedonia, depressed mood, irritability, anxiety, insomnia, and social isolation.
- Bipolar disorder, type II, with most recent episode depressed as evidenced by difficulty concentrating, anhedonia, depressed mood, irritability, anxiety, insomnia, and social isolation. Although bipolar disorder is less likely in this patient because he has no known history of manic or hypomanic behaviors as of this time, his positive family history for mood disorders necessitates that providers and family be vigilant for the symptoms indicating a switch to a manic episode.

The fact that mental illness can run in families is not new (Jones, Kent, Paul, & Craddock, 2001; Meiser, Mitchell, McGirr, Van Herten, & Schofield, 2004). The evidence suggests that the genetic basis of bipolar disorder is complex and involves an interaction of multiple genes and environmental factors (Craddock & Forty, 2006; Maier, Zobel, & Wagner, 2006; Schulze, Hedeker, Zandi, Rietschel, & McMahon, 2006).

CEBM, levels 3a (Jones et al., Meiser et al.), 5 (Craddock & Forty).

- Generalized anxiety disorder, as evidenced by difficulty concentrating, irritability, and insomnia.
- Impulse control disorder not otherwise specified, as evidenced by excessive time spent playing online games with irritability when disturbed while playing. He also has decreased anxiety when playing games and appears to have little control over the amount of time he plays.

Differential Diagnoses

Axis I: Major depressive disorder, recurrent, severe. Impulse control disorder, not otherwise specified.

Other Axis Diagnoses
Axis II: Deferred.

Axis III: Migraines.

Axis IV: Career, family, mental illness.

Axis V: Global assessment of functioning (GAF) current 60, highest in past year 60 **(D1, C1, PO A, B, C; D1, C1, PO A, B, C).**

Initial Treatment Plan

I discuss the rationale for the diagnoses, indicated laboratory studies, and treatment options, including medications and psychotherapies, with the patient and his mother. They agree with the following plan **(D1, C3, PO D, E).** (See Medications list at the end of the chapter for information on all medications.)

- Because patient does not present in imminent danger to self or others, he will be treated in the least restrictive environment, which at this time is the outpatient setting.
- Start citalopram (Celexa) 20 mg orally in the morning. Prescription written: citalopram (Celexa) 20 mg one tablet orally in the morning; dispense 30 tablets with no refills.
- Start clonazepam (Klonopin) 0.5 mg orally three times a day with breakfast, lunch, and dinner. Patient may take 1/2 dose if he feels too drowsy to function safely. Prescription written: clonazepam (Klonopin) 0.5 mg one tablet orally three times a day, as needed; dispense 90 tablets with no refills.
- Start zolpidem (Ambien) 10 mg at bedtime as needed for insomnia. Prescription written: zolpidem (Ambien) 10 mg one tablet orally at bedtime as needed for insomnia; dispense 30 tablets with no refills.
- Patient to schedule follow-up appointment in this office in two weeks.
- Individual psychotherapy is recommended, and a list of local cognitive behavioral therapy (CBT) providers is given to the patient.
- Laboratory studies: complete blood count (CBC), comprehensive metabolic profile (CMP), thyroid panel, urinalysis. and urine toxicology screen.

(D1, C1, PO C, D, E.)

As with other addictions or dependencies, the most effective treatments have been a combination of psycho-pharmacology and psychotherapy. Cognitive Behavioral Therapy (CBT) and twelve-step programs have also shown promise (Wieland, 2005). Selective serotonin reuptake inhibitors (SSRIs), and

*atypical antipsychotic medications, alone and in combination have had thera-
peutic effects in published clinical trials and case studies in the treatment
of this and other impulse control disorders (Atmaca, 2007; Koran, Bullock,
Hartson, Elliott, & D'Andrea, 2002).*

CEBM, levels 5 (Wieland), 3b (Atamaca), 4 (Koran et al.).

*CBT has been recognized as beneficial treatment and antidepressants as
likely to be beneficial for Generalized Anxiety Disorder. Benzodiazepines are
recognized as needing to weigh the risks versus the benefits of treatment for
GAD (Gale, 2002).*

CEBM, level 5.

Encounter Two (one week after initial evaluation)

Diagnostic test review, patient not seen. The results of the CBC, CMP, thyroid
panel, and urinalysis are within normal ranges. The urine toxicology screen
is negative for amphetamines, barbiturates, benzodiazepines, cannabinoids,
cocaine, opiates, and phencyclidine.

*There are no laboratory tests available at this time to provide for the
diagnosis of a mental illness. Evaluation of thyroid function to rule out thyroid
abnormalities and other tests to rule out infectious processes are necessary
because the problematic symptoms may resolve with treatment of the underlying condition. Other medical conditions may need to be addressed concurrent
with the psychiatric symptoms. The current use of psychoactive substances
can also account for the presence of psychiatric symptoms and needs to be
evaluated (Flynn & Mueller, 2000).*

CEBM, level 5.

Encounter Three (two weeks after initial appointment)

Setting: Outpatient psychiatric private practice.

Encounter context: Medication evaluation.

Interval history: The patient reports a decrease in depression and anxiety.
He continues to experience intermittent anxiety attacks, but they occur less
frequently and are less severe. He continues to have a lack of motivation. He
is isolating himself and spending excessive amounts of time, at least eight
hours daily, playing online games. He denies excessive drowsiness with the
clonazepam (Klonopin) 0.5-mg dose. He has used zolpidem (Ambien) 5 out
of 15 nights since last office visit. He has not attempted to contact any of the
CBT providers as of this time. He does state he intends to do this. The patient
has had no further migraines.

Clinical impression: 26-year-old male with recurrent major depressive
disorder, anxiety, and impulse control disorder presents alone for this

office visit. Patient is partially responding to current medication regimen. He continues to demonstrate significant intermittent anxiety attacks, amotivation, and social isolation, and he plays his online game the equivalent of full-time employment. He has avoided contacting a therapist.

Plan

- Laboratory results are discussed with the patient, and he is advised of no abnormal findings.
- Because patient does not present imminent danger to self or others, he will be treated in the least restrictive environment, which at this time is the outpatient setting.
- Increase citalopram (Celexa) 40 mg to target depressive symptoms, impulse problems, and anxiety. Prescription written: citalopram (Celexa) 40 mg one tablet in the morning by mouth. Dispense 30 tablets with no refills.

    According to Stahl (2005), many patients have a better response to the 40-mg dose than to the 20-mg dose.

    CEBM, level 5

- Continue scheduled clonazepam (Klonopin) until dosing on citalopram manages depression and anxiety attacks are controlled. No new prescription needed.
- Continue zolpidem (Ambien) for insomnia on an as-needed basis. No new prescription needed.
- Patient to have scheduled appointment with therapist by next office visit in one month.
- Patient to continue monthly medication checks in this office.
- Patient may also be seen on an as-needed basis if problems arise.

Encounter Four (one month later; six weeks after initial appointment)

Setting: Outpatient psychiatric private practice.

Encounter context: Medication evaluation.

Interval history: 26-year-old male with recurrent major depressive disorder, anxiety, and impulse control disorder has met with CBT provider on two occasions with satisfactory results. Therapist has contacted me by phone to discuss the patient's progress. Therapist stated that although he has never treated a patient for online game addiction, he agrees that CBT will be effective with this patient. E-mail or phone contact was weekly arranged between therapist and me to closely monitor patient progress.

Patient reports he now sees his involvement in online game as excessive. He has reduced his gaming time to two hours in the evenings. He is spending more time with his family, and his grades have gone from B's to A's. He has not experienced any anxiety attacks in two weeks. He feels the medications have been helpful. He states he would like to take as few medications as possible. He has been needing zolpidem only one to two times weekly. The patient has had no further migraines.

Clinical impression: The patient has been treatment compliant and reports benefit from both medication and CBT. His anxiety appears to be managed by citalopram at this time, so clonazepam can be tapered to as-needed use only.

Plan

- Because patient does not present an imminent danger to self or others, he will be treated in the least restrictive environment, which at this time is the outpatient setting.
- Continue with citalopram (Celexa) 40 mg because the patient has begun to experience a decrease in symptoms of depression, anxiety, and computer game-playing. Prescription written: citalopram (Celexa) 40 mg one tablet by mouth in the morning; dispense 30 tablets with no refills.
- Patient to taper clonazepam (Klonopin) 0.5 mg as needed for breakthrough anxiety. No new prescription needed.
- Patient will continue zolpidem (Ambien) on an as-needed basis for insomnia. No new prescription needed.
- Patient to continue CBT.
- Patient to continue monthly medication checks in this office.
- Patient may also be seen on an as-needed basis if problems arise.

Encounter Five (one month later; 10 weeks after initial appointment)

Setting: Outpatient psychiatric private practice.

Encounter context: Medication evaluation.

Interval history: Patient has kept all CBT appointments. All correspondence between providers has been positive. Both parents accompany patient to this office visit. Patient and his parents are pleased with his progress. He is no longer playing online game every day and never for more than one hour a day. Because symptoms have been well controlled, patient has tapered himself off clonazepam (Klonopin) and is sleeping at least eight hours nightly without sleep agents. The patient has had no further migraines.

Clinical impression: 26-year-old male with recurrent major depressive disorder, anxiety, and impulse control disorder has been treatment compliant. He has shown insight into his disorders and is progressing well.

Insight is defined as the degree to which a patient is self-aware and able to understand their illness. It is both intellectual and emotional (Sadock & Sadock, 2002).

CEBM, level 5.

Plan

- Because patient does not present an imminent danger to self or others, he will be treated in the least restrictive environment, which at this time is the outpatient setting.
- Continue with citalopram (Celexa) 40 mg because patient has continued to experience a decrease in symptoms of depression, anxiety, and computer game-playing. Prescription written: citalopram (Celexa) 40 mg one tablet by mouth in the morning; dispense 90 tablets with no refills.
- Patient will continue clonazepam (Klonopin) 0.5 mg as needed for breakthrough anxiety. Prescription written: clonazepam (Klonopin) 0.5 mg as needed for breakthrough anxiety; dispense 30 tablets with no refills.
- Patient will continue zolpidem (Ambien) as needed for insomnia. Prescription written: zolpidem (Ambien) 10 mg one tablet orally at bedtime as needed for insomnia; dispense 30 tablets with no refills.
- Patient to continue CBT.
- Patient to schedule medication checks every three months in this office.
- Patient may also be seen on an as-needed basis if problems arise. Refills on clonazepam (Klonopin) and zolpidem (Ambien) may only be obtained by contact with provider.

Encounter Six (three months later; 22 weeks after initial appointment)

Setting: Outpatient psychiatric private practice.

Encounter context: Medication evaluation.

Interval history: Patient has completed CBT. He has not experienced any significant problems with mood, anxiety, or sleep. He has made several friends in classes, been to the movies three times, and attended one outdoor concert. He plays online game less than one hour weekly. The patient has had no further migraines.

Clinical impression: 26-year-old male with recurrent major depressive disorder, anxiety, and impulse control disorder whose insight and compliance with treatment have assisted patient in regaining his prior level of functioning.

Plan

- Because patient does not present imminent danger to self or others, he will be treated in the least restrictive environment, which at this time is the outpatient setting.
- Continue with citalopram (Celexa) 40 mg because patient has continued to experience a decrease in symptoms of depression, anxiety, and computer game-playing. Prescription written: citalopram (Celexa) 40 mg one tablet by mouth in the morning; dispense 90 tablets with one refill.
- Patient may continue clonazepam (Klonopin) 0.5 mg as needed for breakthrough anxiety. No new prescription needed.

- Patient will continue zolpidem (Ambien) as needed for insomnia. No new prescription needed.
- Patient to schedule medication checks every six months in this office.
- Patient may also be seen on as-needed basis if problems arise. Refills on clonazepam (Klonopin) and zolpidem (Ambien) may only be obtained by contact with provider.

Encounter Seven (six months later; 46 weeks after initial appointment)

Setting: Outpatient psychiatric private practice.

Encounter context: Medication evaluation.

Interval history: Patient has continued to do well. He completed all coursework available in the community college environment and plans to attend the university in the fall. He intends to major in education. The patient has not played online games in three months. The patient has had no further migraines.

Clinical impression: 26-year-old male with recurrent major depressive disorder, anxiety, and impulse control disorder whose insight and compliance with treatment have assisted patient in regaining his prior level of functioning.

Plan

- Because patient does not present an imminent danger to self or others, he will be treated in the least restrictive environment, which at this time is the outpatient setting.
- Continue with citalopram (Celexa) 40 mg. Prescription written: citalopram (Celexa) 40 mg one tablet by mouth in the morning; dispense 90 tablets with one refill.
- Patient may continue clonazepam (Klonopin) 0.5 mg orally as needed for breakthrough anxiety. No prescription needed.
- Patient will continue zolpidem (Ambien) as needed insomnia. No prescription needed.
- Patient to schedule medication checks every six months in this office.
- Patient may also be seen on as-needed basis if problems arise. Refills on clonazepam (Klonopin) and zolpidem (Ambien) may only be obtained by contact with provider.

Critical Appraisal

This case provided an opportunity to put recent research results into practice. The use of selective serotonin reuptake inhibitors (SSRIs) to treat impulse control disorders such as pathological gambling has been reported by several studies. It is interesting to note that the same medication used for the patient's depression can also be effective for migraine prevention.

The phenomenon of Internet Addiction came into focus in 1995 when New York Psychiatrist Ivan Goldberg described it, as a joke to a group on psychiatrists he communicated with online (Goldberg, 1995). The concept was presented by Young at the 1996 American Psychological Association's 104th annual convention. While Goldberg and others believe the problem to be a symptom, not a disease (I. Goldberg, personal communication, March 11, 2007), Young (1996, 2004) and colleagues advocate the inclusion of Internet Addiction Disorder as a new diagnosis in the next edition of The Diagnostic and Statistical Manual of Mental Disorders published by the American Psychiatric Association (DSM-V) expected in 2011 (see American Psychiatric Association, 2000).

CEBM, level 5.

A review by Widyanto & Griffiths (2006) reported treatment recommendations from case studies only. Another review by Dell'Osso et al. (2006) discusses some treatment options for compulsive-impulsive Internet usage disorder along with other impulse control disorders and some treatment options from clinical trials. Research in this area is still in the preliminary stage (Charlton & Danforth, 2007).

CEBM, levels 4 (Widyanto & Griffiths, Charlton & Danforth), 5 (Dell'Osso et al.).

Mental health providers are seeing more and more patients with similar presenting complaints. Whether the psychiatric symptoms precede the MMORPG use or are a consequence of it, the result is the same. Game players who spend excessive amounts of time in virtual worlds have symptoms in common with other addicts. They may get restless or irritable if they are not able to play. They have likely sacrificed time for family, social and work relationships (Aboujaoude, Koran, Gamel, Large, & Serpe, 2006). They spend more and more time playing, and they may totally lose track of the time, entering a "zone" as a flow experience. In a flow experience hours may seem like seconds. Those who experience these flow experiences are more prone to addiction (Chou & Ting, 2003). They may lie about or misrepresent time spent playing. They may lose interest in other activities and continue to play despite the negative consequences caused by MMORPGs. According to Yee (2002) over 40% of players consider themselves addicted to MMORPGs and 4.8–30% have made unsuccessful attempts to stop playing.

CEBM, levels 3b (Aboujaoude et al.), 4 (Chou & Ting), 5 (Yee).

As with other addictions or dependencies, the most effective treatments have been a combination of psycho-pharmacology and psychotherapy. Cognitive Behavioral Therapy (Christensen, Orzack, Babington, & Patsdaughter, 2001) and twelve-step programs have also shown promise (Wieland, 2005). Selective serotonin reuptake inhibitors (SSRIs), and atypical antipsychotic medications, alone and in combination have had therapeutic effects in published clinical trials and case studies in the treatment of this and other impulse control disorders (Atmaca, 2007; Koran et al., 2002). Other treatment options studied for impulse control disorders include lithium and mood stabilizers, opioid antagonists, tricyclic antidepressants, selective serotonin and nor-epinephrine reuptake inhibitors, benzodiazepines and the norepinephrine dopamine reuptake inhibitor, bupropion (Wellbutrin) and beta blockers (Dell'Osso et al., 2006).

CEBM, levels 5 (Christensen et al., Wieland), 4 (Koran et al.).

COMPETENCY DEFENSE

Domain 1, Competency 1. Evaluate patient needs based on age, developmental stage, family history, ethnicity, and individual risk, including genetic profile, to formulate plans for health promotion, anticipatory guidance, counseling, and disease prevention services for healthy or sick patients and their families in any clinical setting.

Defense. This competency was met by making Axis I–V diagnoses, identifying the genetic basis for mental illness, and making an individualized treatment plan with participation of the patient and family, including patient education, medications, and recommendations for cognitive behavioral therapy.

Domain 1, Competency 3. Formulate differential diagnoses and diagnostic strategies and therapeutic interventions with attention to scientific evidence, safety, cost, invasiveness, simplicity, acceptability, adherence, and efficacy for patients who present with new conditions and those with ambiguous or incomplete data, complex illnesses, comorbid conditions, and multiple diagnoses in all clinical settings.

Defense. This competency was met by making the differential diagnosis using scientifically based diagnostic strategies and making an individualized treatment plan with participation of the patient and family, for a previously undiagnosed patient with complex illnesses, comorbid conditions, and multiple diagnoses.

Medications

Medications used in this case by class:

Antidepressants

Drug: Citalopram (Celexa)

Dose range: 20–60 mg/day.

Method of administration in this case: By mouth.

Mechanism of action: Selective serotonin reuptake inhibitor.

Clinical uses: Depression, generalized anxiety disorder.

Side effects
Common: Apathy, anxiety, agitation, confusion, dry mouth or increased saliva, flatulence, insomnia or hypersomnia, tremors, sweating, nausea,

(continued)

dyspepsia, vomiting, diarrhea, dizziness, headache, sexual dysfunction, tremor, asthenia, flu syndrome, anxiety, anorexia.
Serious: Rash, hyponatremia, increased depression, suicidal ideation, serotonin syndrome, extrapyramidal symptoms, mania, seizures, syndrome of inappropriate antidiuretic hormone (SIADH), altered platelet function, priapism, anaphylaxis, hypoglycemia, hyponatremia.

The selective serotonin reuptake inhibitors, like citalopram (Celexa), are FDA approved for the treatment of depression (Stahl, 2005). Published clinical trials have also shown them effective in the treatment of impulse control disorders (Koran et al., 2002). Antidepressants are also recognized as effective treatment for generalized anxiety disorder (Gale, 2002).

Anxiolytics

Drug: Clonazepam (Klonopin)

Dose range: Anxiety, 0.25–2.00 mg two to three times daily.

Method of administration in this case: By mouth.

Mechanism of action: Binds to benzodiazepine receptors, enhances gamma-aminobutyric acid (GABA) effects.

Clinical uses: Anxiety, panic, seizure prophylaxis.

Side effects
Common: Depression, anxiety, confusion, memory impairment, diarrhea, constipation, ataxia, drowsiness, fatigue, weakness, headache, dry mouth, sleep changes, rash, slurred speech, visual changes, dysuria, hypotension.
Serious: Physical and psychologic dependence, respiratory depression, hepatotoxicity, depression, suicidality, leukopenia, eosinophilia, thrombocytopenia.

Benzodiazepines are widely prescribed and provide the most effective relief available for acute anxiety (Lydiard, 2005; Rosenbaum, 2004). According to Pollack (2004), benzodiazepines are prescribed because of their efficacy, tolerability, rapid onset of action, and use in treating antidepressant-induced activation. Anxiolytics such as clonazepam are used to treat anxiety acutely, whereas antidepressants produce cumulative changes in brain chemistry to treat chronic anxiety. Tricyclic antidepressants, selective serotonin reuptake inhibitors, serotonin norepinephrine reuptake inhibitors, and dopamine 1-A agonists are all recognized as effective treatment for anxiety. The use of a benzodiazepine to treat insomnia or anxiety at the initiation of treatment along with an antidepressant is sometimes warranted, but the benzodiazepine should be discontinued once the antidepressant becomes effective to decrease the likelihood of dependence (Kingsbury, Yi, & Simpson, 2001). Because of the possibility of dependence, Stahl (2005) recommends using the lowest dose for the shortest amount of time when prescribing benzodiazepines. The longer half-life of clonazepam (Klonopin) may decrease the potential for withdrawal symptoms when discontinuing regular dosing (Nardi & Perna, 2006).

(continued)

Sedative Hypnotics

Drug: Zolpidem (Ambien)

Dose range: 5–10 mg at bedtime.

Method of administration in this case: By mouth.

Mechanism of action: Produces CNS depression by binding to GABA receptors.

Clinical uses: In the immediate release form, is FDA approved for the short-term treatment of insomnia (Stahl, 2005).

Side effects

Common: Depression, drowsiness, dizziness, lethargy, back pain, allergic reactions, diarrhea, constipation, sinusitis, pharyngitis, flu syndrome, dry mouth, rash.

Serious: Hallucinations, complex sleep-related behaviors, physical and psychologic dependence, anaphylaxis, aggressive behavior, amnesia.

Ambien (Zolpidem), in the immediate release form, is FDA approved for the short-term treatment of insomnia (Stahl, 2005).

References

Aboujaoude, E., Koran, L., Gamel, N., Large, M., & Serpe, N. (2006). Potential markers for problematic Internet use: A telephone survey of 2,513 adults. *CNS Spectrums, 10, 750–755.*

American Psychiatric Association. (2000). *The diagnostic and statistical manual of mental disorders text revised* (4th ed.). Washington, DC: American Psychiatric Publishing, Inc.

Atmaca, M. (2007). A case of problematic Internet use successfully treated with an SSRI-antipsychotic combination. *Progress in Neuro-Psychopharmacology and Biological Psychiatry* (in press, corrected proof). Retrieved April 7, 2007, from http://www.sciencedirect.com/science/article/B6TBR-4MV0MCN-4/2/98ec0144af429a648a46d57e2f823dec

Beghi, E., Allais, G., Cortelli, P., D'Amico, D., De Simone, R., d'Onofrio, F., Genco, S., Manzoni, G., Moschiano, F., Tonini, M., Torelli, P., Quartaroli, M., Roncolato, M., Salvi, S., & Bussone, G. (2007). Headache and anxiety-depressive disorder comorbidity: The HADAS study. *Neurological Sciences, 28,* S217–S219.

Benazzi, F. (2003). Diagnosis of bipolar II disorder: A comparison of structured versus semi-structured interviews. *Progress in Neuro-Psychopharmacology and Biological Psychiatry, 27,* 985–991.

Charlton, J., & Danforth, I. (2007). Distinguishing addiction and high engagement in the context of online game playing. *Computers in Human Behavior, 23,* 1531–1548.

Chou, T., & Ting, C. (2003). The role of flow experience in cyber-game addiction. *CyberPsychology and Behavior, 6*(6), 663–675.

Christensen, M., Orzack, M., Babington, L., & Patsdaughter, C. (2001). Computer addiction: When monitor becomes control center. *Journal of Psychosocial Nursing and Mental Health Services, 39*(3), 40–47.

Craddock, N., & Forty, L. (2006). Genetics of mood disorders. *European Journal of Human Genetics, 14,* 660–668.

Dell'Osso, B., Altamura, A., Allen, A., Marazziti, D., & Hollander, E. (2006). Epidemiologic and clinical updates on impulse control disorders: A critical review. *European Archives of Psychiatry and Clinical Neuroscience, 256*(8), 464–475.

Flynn, F., & Mueller, J. (2000). Physical examination and laboratory evaluation. In Goldman, H. (Ed.), *Review of general psychiatry* (5th ed.). Retrieved November 9, 2006, from http://online.statref.com/document.aspx?fxid=177&docid=37

Gale, C. (2002). Generalised anxiety disorder. In Godlee, F. (Ed.), *Clinical evidence (mental health).* London: BMJ Publishing. Retrieved May 19, 2007, from http://www.clinicalevidence.com/ceweb/conditions/meh/1002/1002.jsp

Ghaemi, S., Ko, J., & Goodwin, F. (2002). "Cade's disease" and beyond: Misdiagnosis antidepressant use, and a proposed definition for bipolar spectrum disorder. *Canadian Journal of Psychiatry, 47*, 125–134.

Goldberg, I. (1995). Internet addiction. Retrieved February 20, 2007, from http://www.psycom.net/iasg.html

Jones, I., Kent, L., Paul, M., & Craddock, N. (2001). Clinical implications of psychiatric genetics in the new millennium—Nightmare or nirvana? *Psychiatric Bulletin, 25*, 129–131.

Kingsbury, S., Yi, D., & Simpson, G. (2001). Psychopolypharmacy: Rational and irrational polypharmacy. *Psychiatric Services, 52*(8), 1033–1035.

Koran, L., Bullock, K., Hartson, H., Elliott, M., & D'Andrea, V. (2002). Citalopram treatment of compulsive shopping: An open label study. *Journal of Clinical Psychiatry, 63*(8), 704–708.

Lewin, S., Skea, Z., Entwhistle, V., Zwarenstein, M., & Dick, J. (2009). Interventions for providers to promote a patient-centered approach in clinical consultations. *Cochrane Database of Systematic Reviews, 4*. Retrieved January 31, 2010, from http://www.mrw.interscience.wiley.com/cochrane/clsrev/articles/CD003267/frame.html

Lydiard, R. (2005). The challenge of managing the complex clinical course of generalized anxiety disorder. *PsychCME Program for Continuing Medical Education*. Raleigh, NC: Duke University Medical Center.

Maier, W., Zobel, A., & Wagner, M. (2006). Schizophrenia and bipolar disorder: Differences and overlaps. *Current Opinion in Psychiatry, 19*(2): 165–170.

Meiser, B., Mitchell, P., McGirr, H., Van Herten, M., & Schofield, P. (2004). Implications of genetic risk information in families with a high density of bipolar disorder: An exploratory study. *Social Sciences and Medicine, 60*, 109–118.

Mueller, J., Kiernan, R., & Langston, J. (2000). The mental status examination. In Goldman, H. (Ed.), *Review of general psychiatry* (5th ed.). Retrieved November 9, 2006, from http://online.statref.com/document.aspx?fxid=17&docid=37

Nardi, A., & Perna, G. (2006). Clonazepam in the treatment of psychiatric disorders: An update. *International Clinical Psychopharmacology, 21*, 131–142.

National Institute of Health (NIH). (1998). *Clinical guidelines on the identification, evaluation and treatment of overweight and obesity in adults: The evidence report* (NIH publication No. 98–4083). Washington, DC: U.S. Government Printing Office. Retrieved November 12, 2006, from http://www.nhlbi.nih.gov/guidelines/obesity/ob_gdlns.pdf

Pollack, B. (2004). Efficacy of and concerns about benzodiazepines and their alternatives for anxiety disorders. In J. Rosenbaum (chair), Using benzodiazepines in clinical practice: An evidence based discussion (Academic Highlights). *Journal of Clinical Psychiatry, 6*, 1565–1574. Retrieved November 4, 2006, from http://www.psychiatrist.com/private/cme/newcme/6511/article3.htm

Ramadan, N. (2007). Current trends in migraine prophylaxis. *Headache, 47*, S52–S57.

Rosenbaum, J. (2004). Benzodiazepines: Then and now. In J. Rosenbaum (chair), Using benzodiazepines in clinical practice: An evidence based discussion (Academic Highlights). *Journal of Clinical Psychiatry, 65*, 1565–1574. Retrieved November 4, 2006, from http://www.psychiatrist.com/private/cme/newcme/6511/article3.htm

Sadock, B., & Sadock, V. (2002). *Kaplan & Saddock's synopsis of psychiatry: Behavioral sciences/clinical psychiatry* (9th ed.). New York City: Lippincott Williams & Wilkins.

Schulze, T., Hedeker, D., Zandi, P., Rietschel, M., & McMahon, F. (2006). What is familial about familial bipolar disorder? Resemblance among relatives across a broad spectrum of phenotypic characteristics. *Archives of General Psychiatry, 63*(12), 1368–1376.

Stahl, S. (2005). *Essential psychopharmacology: The prescriber's guide*. New York: Cambridge University Press.

Widyanto, L., & Griffiths, M. (2006). Internet addiction: A critical review. *International Journal of Mental Health, 4*, 31–51.

Wieland, D. (2005). Computer addiction: Implications for nursing psychotherapy practice. *Perspectives in Psychiatric Care, 41*(4), 153–161.

Yee, N. (2002). *Ariadne: Understanding MMORPG addiction*. Retrieved March 11, 2007, from http://www.nickyee.com/hub/addiction/home.html

Young, K. (1996). *Internet addiction: The emergence of a new clinical disorder*. Paper presented at the 104th annual meeting of the American Psychological Association, Toronto.

Young, K. (2004). Internet addiction: A new clinical phenomenon and its consequences. *American Behavioral Scientist, 48*(4), 402–415.

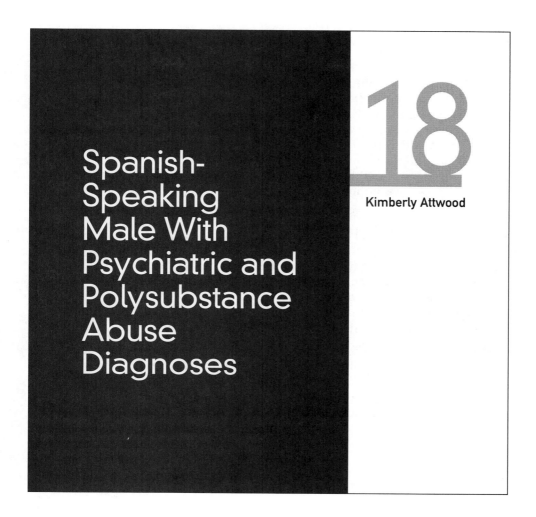

18

Spanish-Speaking Male With Psychiatric and Polysubstance Abuse Diagnoses

Kimberly Attwood

The following case study addresses the initial comprehensive management and follow-up for a patient who presents with symptoms consistent with bipolar disorder, mixed episodes, and polysubstance abuse. This case narrative describes care provided for this Medicaid-insured patient during the initial evaluation and three follow-up visits over a period of two months. Care was provided at a community mental health clinic with referral for acute hospitalization.

The case study addresses the following Columbia University School of Nursing comprehensive doctoral competencies for direct patient care.

DOMAIN 1, COMPETENCY 1

Evaluate patient needs based on age, developmental stage, family history, ethnicity, and individual risk, including genetic profile, to formulate plans for health promotion, anticipatory guidance, counseling, and disease prevention services for healthy or sick patients and their families in any clinical setting.

PO A. Identify a potential genetic risk.

PO B. Diagnose a genetic condition.

PO C. Evaluate individual patient needs based on age, developmental stage, family history, ethnicity, and individual risk.

PO D. Formulate a plan that addresses health promotion, anticipatory guidance, and/or disease prevention for the individual.

PO E. Develop a plan that addresses health promotion, anticipatory guidance, and/or disease prevention for the family.

DOMAIN 1, COMPETENCY 3

Formulate differential diagnoses and diagnostic strategies and therapeutic interventions with attention to scientific evidence, safety, cost, invasiveness, simplicity, acceptability, adherence, and efficacy for patients who present with new conditions and those with ambiguous or incomplete data, complex illnesses, comorbid conditions, and multiple diagnoses in all clinical settings.

PO B. Formulate a differential diagnosis for a patient who presents with ambiguous or incomplete data, complex illnesses, comorbid conditions, and potential multiple diagnoses.

PO C. Discuss the rationale for the differential diagnosis.

PO E. Discuss the rationale for the therapeutic intervention with attention to scientific evidence, safety, cost, invasiveness, simplicity, acceptability, adherence, and efficacy.

ENCOUNTER CONTEXT

Encounter One (initial outpatient comprehensive evaluation)

DNP role: I am the nurse practitioner and DNP resident evaluating this patient.

Identifying Information

Site: Community mental health clinic.

Setting: Private office.

Context: Referral to this practice was first generated when the patient was 16 years old. He has received intermittent mental health services for nine years. He was referred to adult mental health services when he was discharged by his child psychiatrist.

Name: Juan (pseudonym).

Age: 25 years old.

Gender: Male.

Informant: Patient.

Reliability: Semireliable historian.

Chief complaint: "I got a lot of mood swings and keep fighting with people. I've been throwing a lot of things at home and I put a hole in the wall. The bitch kicked me out."

History of Present Illness

Juan is a 25-year-old married Hispanic male who presents today to assume adult mental health services. He is well known to the community mental health clinic because he has been treated by the child psychiatrist intermittently since age 16. His prior diagnoses include attention deficit hyperactivity disorder (ADHD) and intermittent explosive disorder (IED). At present, he is being treated with sustained-release bupropion (Wellbutrin SR) with alprazolam (Xanax) as needed.

Juan admits to long-standing mood lability, alternating between periods of depression and rage. He describes being easily agitated, often to the point of damaging his property. He has been involved in several street fights in the past month but has never been arrested. He describes feeling unmotivated and anhedonic. He persistently argues with his wife and finds taking care of their six children to be exhausting. He is not sleeping at night, sometimes being awake for up to 72 hours followed by episodes of sleeping for nearly 24 hours.

Juan was expelled from the local public school at the age of 16 due to interpersonal problems with both teachers and peers. He was receiving special education services for an undiagnosed learning disability. He describes himself as a "slow learner."

Juan admits to smoking tetrahydrocannabinol (THC), also known as marijuana. He has smoked it on a daily basis since the age of 12. His daily usage has ranged from one to three "blunts" per day. He drinks two to three glasses of alcohol per day and smokes approximately one-half pack of cigarettes per day, with a pack history of 15 years.

Juan feels helpless and hopeless in regards to his personal living situation. He has been unemployed since 2006 and feels that he "has no purpose in life" except taking care of his children while his "lazy bitch sits on the couch." He rates his current depression as an 8 on the 1–10 scale.

Medical History

Medications: Juan is currently taking sustained-release bupropion (Wellbutrin SR) 150 mg by mouth per morning and alprazolam (Xanax) 0.5 mg by mouth up to two times per day, as needed for anxiety.

Allergies: The patient has an allergy to shellfish. He denies any medication allergies.

Surgeries: The patient had an appendectomy at age eight.

Medical hospitalizations: The patient had one medical hospitalization for the aforementioned appendectomy.

Psychiatric hospitalizations: Juan was hospitalized for five days after a suicide attempt in 2007. He attempted to cut his throat with a knife.

Emergency department visits: The patient was taken to the emergency department (ED) twice in 2007 and once in 2008 for anxiety and rage-related symptoms.

Trauma: The patient sustained a laceration to his neck after his suicide attempt.

Transfusions: The patient denies any history of transfusion.

Illnesses: The patient's past illnesses include ADHD and IED. He has a self-reported history of Parkinson's disease. He denies any follow-up with neurology. He receives no ongoing treatment for the disease.

Routine health maintenance: The patient receives infrequent care from his primary care provider. He maintains follow-up at the local family practice clinic. He believes his last visit was in 2000. He has not seen a dentist since he was in high school. He is uncertain regarding his vaccination status.

Family History

Juan maintains contact with his mother, father, and five siblings. He has three brothers and two sisters. He describes his oldest brother as "sick in the head." He denies knowledge of a more specific psychiatric diagnosis, although he reports that this brother is currently incarcerated after he "chased the mailman down the street with a butcher knife." His second brother has a diagnosis of depression, and his third brother has a diagnosis of bipolar disorder. His older sister is "sick in the head" and is incarcerated in federal prison for attempted murder. His younger sister has no known psychiatric problems. The patient reports that all of his siblings and his mother use marijuana on a regular basis. In fact, their mother provided it to them when they were children.

The patient's mother has a history of alcohol abuse and sex addiction. She worked as a prostitute for many years during Juan's childhood.

The patient's father has no history of mental illness and does not use marijuana. He has congenital unilateral deafness and a prior wrist fracture requiring metal hardware.

Juan's maternal grandmother suffocated her twin brothers as a child. His maternal uncle is currently incarcerated for decapitating an individual after hitting the victim with his car. No additional family history is known by the patient.

Psychosocial History

Stressors and support: The patient identifies interpersonal, vocational, financial, and familial stressors. His support system includes his family members, wife, and children.

Abuse history: He reports physical and mental abuse by his parents during his childhood. He indicates that his parents would hit him with a leather belt whenever angry with him. Further, they would tell him that he was "stupid" and "worthless." He denies any history of sexual abuse.

Lifestyle risk factors: The patient utilizes street drugs of unknown quality. He maintains a high-fat diet, engages in no formal exercise, and does not seek routine preventive medical care.

Legal history: Juan was permanently expelled from school due to his poor impulse control and irritability. He denies any arrests or warrants and has never been incarcerated.

Caffeine use: The patient drinks one cup of coffee in the morning and occasionally has a soda in the afternoon.

Diet and exercise: Juan enjoys rice, beans, and plantains. He does not engage in formal exercise, although his only means of transportation is walking.

Patient profile: Juan is a 25-year-old Hispanic male with a ninth-grade education. He lives in a single-room apartment with his wife of five years and their six children. Specifically, they have three children together and his wife has three children from a prior relationship. He reports having no personal assets. He was last employed in 2006 as a construction worker. His family currently receives welfare funding, food stamps, and cash assistance in the amount of approximately $500 per month.

Review of Systems

General: Denies weakness, fatigue, fever, or chills. He denies any changes in his weight or appetite.

Skin: Denies any rashes, lumps, sores, pruritus, or dryness. He denies any changes in hair, nails, or moles. He reports having cystic acne since his early teens.

HEENT:

Head: Denies any headaches, injuries, syncope, or lightheadedness.
Eyes: No change in vision. The date of his last eye exam is unknown. He denies excessive tearing, double or blurred vision, or scotoma.
Ears: Denies hearing problems, tinnitus, vertigo, otalgia, infections, or discharge.
Nose and sinuses: Denies frequent colds, nasal discharge, epistaxis, or sinusitis.
Throat: Last dental appointment was when he was in high school. He is missing several teeth and reports persistent tooth pain. He denies sore throat, dry mouth, or hoarseness.

Neck: Denies swollen glands, goiter, lumps, pain, or stiffness in neck.

Breasts: Denies any lumps, pain, discomfort, or discharge.

Respiratory: He denies cough, hemoptysis, dyspnea, or wheezing. He denies any history of asthma, pneumonia, or tuberculosis.

Cardiovascular: He denies any history of hypertension, murmurs, chest pain, or palpitations. He has no history of edema or orthopnea.

Gastrointestinal: He denies any history of dysphagia, dyspepsia, or nausea. He usually has one formed brown stool every day. He denies constipation, diarrhea, hemorrhoids, or pain with defecation. He has no history of blood in the stools or black, tarry stools. He has no history of hepatitis, cholecystitis, or jaundice.

Urinary: He voids approximately three to four times per day; he denies nocturia, hematuria, polyuria, urgency, or dysuria. His urinary stream is normal, and he denies any hesitancy. He denies flank pain or a history of renal calculi, ureteral colic, suprapubic pain, or incontinence.

Genital: He denies history of hernia; no discharge from or sores on penis. No testicular masses or scrotal pain. He is currently sexually active. He denies past or present impotence. He denies risk of HIV or other sexually transmitted diseases. He denies prostituting or receiving services from prostitutes. Denies any problems with libido; denies anorgasmia. He denies pain upon ejaculation.

Peripheral vascular: He denies intermittent claudication, leg cramps, varicose veins, clots, or edema in the calves, legs, or feet. He denies any change in color of fingertips or toes in cold weather.

Musculoskeletal: He denies any muscle or joint pain, stiffness, arthritis, gout, or backache. He has not sustained any traumatic injuries.

Psychiatric: See "History of Present Illness" and relevant family and social history.

Neurologic: He denies any history of traumatic brain injury. Specifically, he denies any history of blackouts, seizures, paralysis, or weakness. He reports a possible personal history of Parkinson's disease but denies pursuing any follow-up. He was not taking any prescription medications at the time of symptom presentation; however, he admits to using various street drugs at the time of symptom onset. He reports paresthesia and numbness in his bilateral hands of unknown duration.

Hematologic: He denies any history of easy bruising or bleeding. He has never had a transfusion.

Endocrine: He denies polydipsia, polyphagia, and polyuria. He denies any thyroid problems, heat or cold intolerances, excessive sweating, or change in shoe or glove size.

Physical Examination

The patient was referred to his primary care provider (PCP) for a comprehensive physical examination. The patient has consistently refused to see his PCP, asserting "I'm not going there. They all look at me like I'm a crook."

Psychiatric Mental Status Examination
(performed by myself)

Appearance: Juan appears disheveled and unkempt. His clothing is visibly dirty. He has severe facial acne. He is malodorous. His appearance is consistent with his stated age. He is dressed in season- and gender-appropriate attire.

Reliability: He appears to be a reliable historian.

Speech: Juan fluently speaks both Spanish and English, alternating between the two languages. His speech is pressured but understandable and spontaneous. He is very talkative throughout the interview.

Mood and affect: He is cooperative and engaged in the interview. He appears anxious, and his mood is apathetic. He does not maintain eye contact. His affect is flat but congruent with thought content. He describes his mood as angry and anxious.

Psychomotor activity: There is no evidence of tics or twitches. He is restless throughout the interview, often wringing his hands and tapping his legs. There is no evidence of psychomotor retardation.

Thought process: Juan's thought content is coherent, although he has an abundance of ideas. His thinking appears goal-directed, and he responds to questions appropriately.

Thought content: Juan appears paranoid and preoccupied at times. He perseverates on his relationship with his wife. He believes he is at risk for being "gunned down" due to multiple shootings in his area.

Cognitive functions: The Folstein Mini Mental State Exam was utilized in the following assessment.

Attention and concentration: Juan is alert, oriented to person, place, and time, and appropriately responsive to environmental stimuli. He demonstrates the ability to concentrate on topics of interest, but specific measurements (including counting backwards by 7) are compromised by intellectual function.

Memory (immediate, recent, remote recall): Juan is able to repeat "apple, penny, and glove" after several minutes and again at 30 minutes. He is able to discuss historical events with accuracy.

Calculations: Juan is not able to perform simple calculations. Specifically, when purchasing an item for 50 cents, he is unable to determine the refund if he supplied a one dollar bill.

Abstractions: When ask to describe the statement "people in glass houses shouldn't throw stones," Juan replies, "Don't worry about other people's business or they will come after you."

Verbal commands: Juan was able to follow directions, including picking up a piece of paper in his right hand, folding it in half, and placing it on the floor. He correctly named a pencil and was able to repeat the statement, "no ifs, ands, or buts."

Writing commands: Juan is able to write his name but indicates he is not able to read or write in either English or Spanish. He is able to copy intersecting pentagons.

Insight: Juan acknowledges his illness and need for help. He identifies that he is avoiding his wife because of concerns that he could harm her if she provokes him.

Judgment: When asked how he would respond if he found a stamped, addressed envelope in the street, Juan indicates he would take it to the post office. If he was in a room filled with smoke, he would "get the hell out."

Database

Laboratory data: Laboratory testing was completed on site, prior to my appointment with the patient. Results including complete blood count, basic metabolic profile, thyroid stimulating hormone, and lipid profile were within normal ranges.

Urine drug screen: Positive for THC.

Impression

The diagnosis of a chronic psychiatric disorder can be complicated by concurrent substance abuse. Although marijuana abuse does not typically qualify a patient for a drug rehabilitation program, it is associated with withdrawal symptoms when abruptly discontinued. Examples of withdrawal symptoms include irritability, anxiety, decreased quality and quantity of sleep, and decreased food intake (Haney, 2005). Health care providers must consider that abrupt cessation of use may be the result of financial constraints rather than a desire to stop using the drug.

Juan reports paresthesia and numbness in his bilateral hands of unknown duration. Numbness is associated with the use of "wet," a combination of marijuana, phencyclidine, and embalming fluid (Modesto-Lowe & Petry, 2001). Although not considered in the original differential diagnosis, this finding might be significant during the course of Juan's care. Particularly if a neurologic cause can be excluded, it may be suggestive of chronic wet use.

It is not uncommon for bipolar disorder to be diagnosed in early adulthood. Because the diagnosis requires knowledge of the patient's history, a diagnosis of bipolar disorder tends to evolve over time. Thus, the symptoms consistent with intermittent explosive disorder may have been an early indication of bipolar disorder.

A review of Juan's family history reveals the propensity for multiple psychiatric disorders. He has one sibling with a known history of bipolar disorder. However, bipolar disorder cannot be excluded for several of his family members, because they have either not been formally diagnosed or Juan is not aware of the diagnosis. This fact supports the importance of encouraging patients to review their histories with their family members.

Using the previous information as a guide, Juan will be encouraged to seek genetic counseling for his children **(D1, C1, PO A).**

Twin studies exploring the genetic relationship of bipolar disorder have identified that it is among the most heritable of medical disorders. However, the search for specific gene involvement has been complicated by the paucity of animal studies, the limited understanding of the associated pathogenesis, and the overall genetic complexity of the disorder. It is currently accepted that the genetic liability of bipolar disorder is the result of many genes being affected in a small way. The polygenicity of the disorder correlates with the need for studies with very large sample populations (Barnett & Smoller, 2009).

Oxford Centre for Evidence-Based Medicine (CEBM), level 2b.

Bipolar I disorder often starts with depression, although most patients experience both depression and mania (Sadock & Sadock, 2007). Using the DSM-IV-TR criteria, the patient meets the following qualifications for bipolar I disorder, mixed episode: ". . . a manic episode and . . . a major depressive episode nearly every day during at least a one week period, the mood disturbance is sufficiently severe to cause marked impairment in occupational function or in usual social activities or relationships with others, and the symptoms are not due to the direct physiological effects of a substance or medical condition" (American Psychiatric Association, 2000).

CEBM, level 5.

The following diagnoses are established based upon the criteria outlined in the *Diagnostic and Statistical Manual of Mental Disorders, 4th edition, Text Revision* (DSM-IV-TR) (American Psychiatric Association, 2000).

Assessment

Axis I: As follows:

1. Bipolar I disorder, most recent episode mixed (ICD-9: 296.6) **(D1, C1, PO B; D1, C3, PO B).**
2. Polysubstance dependence (ICD-9: 309.81) **(D1, C3, PO B).**
3. Attention deficit hyperactivity disorder by history (ICD-9: 314.01).

Axis II: Learning disorder not otherwise specified (ICD-9: 315.9).

Axis III: Questionable history of Parkinson's disease.

Axis IV: Limited familial/spousal support, marital conflict, financial constraints, and limited vocational and educational achievement.

Axis V: Global assessment of functioning (GAF) 45.

Initial Plan (week 1)

- Continue sustained-release bupropion (Wellbutrin SR) 150 mg by mouth every morning.
- Discontinue alprazolam (Xanax) and begin clonazepam (Klonopin) 0.5 mg by mouth every 12 hours.

- Begin extended-release valproate (Depakote ER) 250 mg by mouth at bedtime for seven days, then increase to 500 mg by mouth at bedtime.
- Begin aripiprazole (Abilify) 5 mg by mouth at bedtime for 14 days, then increase to 10 mg by mouth at bedtime.
- Check serum Depakene level in one month.
- Increase frequency of cognitive behavioral therapy to twice weekly one-hour sessions.
- Patient should return to office for medication reevaluation in seven days, and sooner if symptoms worsen. He should schedule follow-up visits with psychiatric nurse practitioner (NP) on days when he is not receiving psychotherapy.
- Implement metabolic syndrome screening protocol **(D1, C1, PO D).**
- Patient should contact crisis hotline if symptoms worsen. Alternatively, he can contact 911 or go directly to the local ED. The number for the local crisis hotline is programmed into the patient's mobile phone **(D1, C1, PO D).**
- Education
    - Laboratory monitoring is required as part of treatment plan.
    - Monitor for signs of hyperglycemia, including ketoacidosis.
    - Patient should monitor his weight and report changes in appetite.
    - Patient should report suicidal or worsening symptoms of depression or mania.
    - Patient should monitor for worsening mood and call our office immediately for an appointment.
    - Patient should not stop medications abruptly because he may experience symptoms of withdrawal.
    - Patient should not consume alcohol or drugs while taking psychotropic medications.
    - Patient should take medications only as prescribed. Taking more than is ordered may result in accidental overdose or death.
    - Once the patient has received prescriptions from the pharmacy, he should return to our office. The NP's assistant will organize the medications for him **(D1, C1, PO D).**

- Refer for Spanish-speaking intensive case manager (ICM) **(D1, C1, PO D).**
- Patient should attend bipolar disorder support group and encourage wife to attend spouse support group **(D1, C1, PO E).**
- Patient should pursue follow-up with PCP and neurology once ICM services are in place.
- Patient should contact local shelter for emergency housing.

Bipolar disorder is a chronic condition that is associated with frequent recurrence and relapse. While mood stabilizers are thought to improve the overall course of the disease, they rarely result in long-term remission. As such, polypharmacy is often necessary for the effective management of bipolar disorder. The implementation on current mood stabilization with antipsychotic therapy is considered the most effective approach (Lin, Mok, & Yatham, 2006).

Aripiprazole is indicated in the treatment of acute and maintenance treatment of manic and mixed episodes associated with bipolar I disorder.

Similarly, it is approved as adjunctive therapy to either lithium or valproate for the acute treatment of manic or mixed episodes. Similar to other second generation antipsychotic agents, patients should be assessed for hyperglycemia and evidence of metabolic syndrome (Bristol-Myers Squibb, 2008) **(D1, C3, PO E).**

Valproate has demonstrated safety and efficacy in the treatment of bipolar disorder. Evidence suggests that it is particularly useful in mixed mania and/or comorbid substance or alcohol abuse. Valproate's rapid onset of action has made it particularly useful in acute mania (Lennkh & Simhandl, 2000). The spectrum of efficacy is greatest for valproate when compared to other mood stabilizers (Bowden, 2003) **(D1, C3, PO E).**

For individuals with bipolar disorder, treatment with antidepressant agents can result in a switch in mood polarity. Specifically, the addition of an antidepressant can result in the transition to a hypomanic or manic state. Bupropion is associated with a lower risk of mood polarity changes, making it a good option for the individual with bipolar disorder (Leverich et al., 2006). Satisfactory mood stabilization is necessary for all patients with bipolar disorder who are prescribed antidepressant agents (Goodwin et al., 2008) **(D1, C3, PO E).**

CEBM, level 2b (Leverich et al., 2006).

The benefits of cognitive behavioral therapy (CBT) for individuals with bipolar disorder have been questioned. Specifically, a recent meta-analysis of quality studies exploring the efficacy of CBT identified that it was not effective in preventing relapse (Lynch, Laws, & McKenna, 2009).

CEBM, level 2b.

Critical Appraisal

Although the efficacy of cognitive behavioral therapy in preventing symptom relapse has not been proven, there are other practical benefits for offering this service to patients. For example, in the case of Juan, he has limited support from family and friends. The psychotherapist can be an additional source of support. Similarly, when a patient is experiencing acute symptomatology, frequent encounters with the patient can promote early intervention and, as a result, decrease the need for acute hospitalization **(D1, C3, PO E).**

Encounter Two (one-week follow-up appointment)

Chief complaint: "I'm doing a little better. I'm sleeping better at night and it seems like my mind is clearer. I've been staying out of trouble."

Assessment: The patient is alert and oriented to person, place, and time. His thinking appears logical and he denies any hallucinations. His depression is identified as a 5 on the 1–10 scale. He is sleeping approximately six hours per night and feels well rested during the day. He denies any impulsive behavior and has avoided any verbal or physical altercations with others. He remains estranged from his wife and children and has been living in the cemetery for the past week because there is no space available in the local shelters. He is attempting to arrange temporary housing with a friend of the family. He is taking his medications as directed and denies any side effects. He also denies homicidal and suicidal ideations and is able to contract for safety.

Juan appears unkempt and malodorous. His clothing remains visibly dirty. His affect is brighter at this visit, and his eye contact is improved. Speech is clear, articulate, and understandable. He brings his medications with him and has the appropriate number of pills remaining. He has attended all scheduled psychotherapy appointments.

Impression: Juan is a 25-year-old Hispanic male with bipolar I disorder, most recent episode mixed, polysubstance dependence, attention deficit hyperactivity disorder by history, with marital conflict, financial constraint, and limited vocational and educational achievement. Since last appointment depression is improving. He appears to be responding well to the current treatment plan. He is cognizant of the need to arrange temporary housing.

Plan (week 2)

- Continue medications as outlined.
- Continue twice weekly cognitive behavioral therapy.
- Patient should continue to wait for ICM services to become available. His name has been placed on the waiting list.
- Return to the office in one week for reexamination.

Encounter Three (one week after last appointment; two weeks since intake)

The patient did not arrive for his appointment today. Attempts to reach him were not successful. The patient has also not attended his past two psychotherapy sessions. Office staff will continue to attempt to reach him.

Encounter Four (four weeks after initial visit)

Chief complaint: Juan arrives with his father, who states, "We need your help. Juan is passing through something, and I'm afraid he's gonna die."

History of present illness: Juan arrives at the clinic for an unscheduled visit accompanied by his father. His father indicates that Juan was found in the street last night by a friend of the family. He was disoriented and "acting strange." The family friend subsequently took Juan to his parents' home. The last contact family members had with Juan was five days prior to the event.

According to his father, Juan was staying with a friend. Juan had attempted to contact his father five days prior in request of money. He appeared "normal" and "in a good mood." It is uncertain what has transpired since that day.

Review of systems: Deferred; Juan is unable to participate in the review of systems.

Psychiatric Mental Status Examination (performed by myself)

Appearance: He appears unkempt and malodorous. He is unshaven, and his clothing is covered in mud.

Reliability: He is a poor historian. He is unable to recall prior visits to the clinic and has no recollection of his medication regimen. He is not able or willing to discuss the events occurring in the past day.

Speech: Juan is speaking exclusively in Spanish and does not respond to commands or questions in English. His speech is mumbled, yet pressured and off-topic.

Mood and affect: His mood is labile. He demonstrates episodes of anger, refusing to sit in the chair in the office. His affect is consistent with his labile mood. He demonstrates poor eye contact and appears to ignore all external interaction.

Psychomotor activity: Movement is hyperactive and bizarre. He is walking with a shuffling gait and walks into the office chair several times. Subsequently, he turns the chair onto its side and proceeds to walk forward.

Thought process: His thinking is incongruent and off-topic. He does not respond to questions.

Thought content: Juan believes he is being followed by the "Illuminati" because he has knowledge of gang-related activity. He is seeing "all those dead people; there are a ton of them right here in this room." Reports he sold "rat poison instead of heroin" and is now "paying the price" by having the individuals who died "return to haunt him." He perseverates on this topic, and attempts to redirect him are unsuccessful.

Juan's father is not aware of his ingestion of any substances or medications. His father reviews the contents of his pockets and identifies only his mobile phone.

Juan's anger continues to escalate. He raises his voice, speaking to a presence in the room. Security is called for assistance, and "911" is called by office personnel. Local police officers and ambulance crew arrive within several minutes. Juan is restrained and taken to the local ED.

Interim Communication (one day following previous events)

Telephone contact with the attending psychiatrist at the local hospital reveals that Juan tested positive for tetrahydrocannabinol (THC) and phencyclidine (PCP). All other laboratory data were normal.

Juan's father contacted the hospital with pertinent information. He had received a visit from the friend Juan was staying with over the past week. The friend indicates that he and Juan were smoking "wet" throughout the day and "this may have something to do with it." This information was consistent with the findings identified on the previous drug screen.

> *Wet refers to the combination of marijuana, phencyclidine, and embalming fluid. Also known as illy, wet sticks, amp, and fry, it is sold on the streets as super-marijuana. It is purported that embalming fluid enhances the absorption of both marijuana and phencyclidine by slowing the rate at which the marijuana burns. There is no available evidence to suggest that these medications are synergistic (Modesto-Lowe & Petry, 2001).*
>
> *Embalming fluid is typically composed of a number of ingredients, including formaldehyde, methanol, ethyl alcohol or ethanol, and other solvents. To improve the taste, mint or parsley may be added (Modesto-Lowe & Petry, 2001).*
>
> *The clinical picture associated with wet use has been documented primarily by emergency medicine providers. Consistent with the symptoms associated with PCP use, wet induces hallucinations, psychomotor agitation, impaired judgment, and intermittent violence. Cognitive deficits are often noted and may persist. While the acute symptoms typically subside in 24 to 36 hours, the long-term effects of wet are unknown (Elwood, 1998; Modesto-Lowe & Petry, 2001).*

CEBM, level 3b.

Critical Appraisal

Knowledge of current drug use patterns is essential for the psychiatric health care provider. Awareness of the presenting signs and symptoms and the associated side effects will expedite diagnosis and treatment. Further, health care providers can inform the patient of the risks associated with specific drug use.

COMPETENCY DEFENSE

Domain 1, Competency 1. Evaluate patient needs based on age, developmental stage, family history, ethnicity, and individual risk, including genetic profile, to formulate plans for health promotion, anticipatory guidance, counseling, and disease prevention services for healthy or sick patients and their families in any clinical setting.

Defense. I was able to formulate an appropriate treatment plan addressing Juan's needs. I identified various pertinent stressors that may influence the treatment protocol, including limited family support, unemployment, and limited health literacy. As a result, the treatment regimen was simplified to enhance adherence, and the patient was encouraged to return to the office for assistance in preparing his medications according to the established schedule. Further, a referral for a Spanish-speaking intensive case manager was made. Due to the propensity for metabolic complications associated with second-generation antipsychotic agents, the metabolic syndrome screening protocol was implemented. The patient was provided with information regarding the local crisis hotline service and was assisted in programming the number into his mobile phone. After a comprehensive family history was compiled, it became evident that multiple family members had a psychiatric disorder, including depression, bipolar disorder, and substance abuse. Although limited information was available in regards to specific psychiatric disorders, the legal status of several family members suggests a possible mood or impulse control disorder. Finally, information was given in regards to the support group for the patients diagnosed with bipolar disorder and their family members. This would promote awareness of the disease process, including signs of an exacerbation, and may promote adherence to the therapeutic regimen.

Domain 1, Competency 3. Formulate differential diagnoses and diagnostic strategies and therapeutic interventions with attention to scientific evidence, safety, cost, invasiveness, simplicity, acceptability, adherence, and efficacy for patients who present with new conditions and those with ambiguous or incomplete data, complex illnesses, comorbid conditions, and multiple diagnoses in all clinical settings.

Defense. Juan's diagnoses were formulated using the *DSM-IV* criteria for bipolar I disorder, most recent episode mixed, and polysubstance abuse. Given his presenting symptoms, I identified that a polypharmacologic regimen would be essential to control his symptoms. The available evidence supports the efficacy of mood stabilization with antipsychotic therapy. Specifically, valproate was identified as an appropriate agent for use in the patient with mixed mania and comorbid substance abuse. Similarly, aripiprazole is indicated in the treatment of acute and chronic mixed and manic episodes in patients with bipolar I disorder. Because Juan presents with a history of depressive symptoms, antidepressant therapy must be considered. However, the addition of an antidepressant must be done with caution because of the risk of causing a switch in mood polarity. Bupropion has been associated with a lower risk for mood polarity switch, making it an ideal option for Juan. Although the literature does not consistently support the efficacy of cognitive behavioral therapy, it was identified as an important component of Juan's treatment regimen.

Medications

Drug: Bupropion (Wellbutrin SR)

Dose range: 150–300 mg/day.

Method of administration in this case: By mouth.

Mechanism of action: Antidepressant with nonadrenergic, dopaminergic, and stimulant-like properties.

Clinical uses: Depression and smoking cessation.

Side effects
Common: Headache, insomnia, upper respiratory complaints, and nausea.
Serious: Seizures (Biovail Corporation, 2008).

(continued)

Drug: Alprazolam (Xanax)

Dose range: 0.5–2.0 mg two to four times daily.

Method of administration in this case: By mouth.

Mechanism of action: Benzodiazepine anxiolytic agent thought to modulate gamma-aminobutyric acid (GABA) neurotransmission in the amygdala.

Clinical uses: Anxiety, insomnia.

Side effects
Common: Orthostasis, conduction defects, reflex tachycardia, anticholinergic effects.
Serious: Ventricular arrhythmias, potentially lethal in overdose.

Drug: Clonazepam (Klonopin)

Dose range: 0.5–2.0 mg twice daily.

Method of administration in this case: By mouth.

Mechanism of action: Benzodiazepine anxiolytic agent thought to modulate GABA neurotransmission in the amygdala.

Clinical uses: Anxiety.

Side effects
Common: Hypotension, impaired memory, tremor, fatigue.
Serious: Respiratory depression, potentially lethal in overdose.

Drug: Extended-Release Valproate (Depakote ER)

Dose range: Starting dose of 250–750 mg/kg followed by titration to therapeutic level while monitoring serum blood levels.

Method of administration in this case: By mouth.

Mechanism of action: Anticonvulsant agent with mood-stabilizing properties.

Clinical uses: Manic phase of bipolar disorder, mixed or dysphoric mania, rapid cyclers, history of recurrent manic episodes, or comorbid substance abuse.

Side effects
Common: Gastrointestinal upset, thrombocytopenia, increased transaminase levels, hair loss, tremor, weight gain, sedation.
Serious: Fatal hepatic toxicity.

Drug: Aripiprazole (Abilify)

Dose range: 2–30 mg daily.

(continued)

Method of administration in this case: By mouth.

Mechanism of action: Unknown; efficacy thought to be mediated through a combination of partial agonist activity at D2 and 5-HT 1a receptors and agonist activity at 5-HT 2a receptors.

Clinical uses: Control of schizophrenia, bipolar I disorder, and as adjunctive therapy to antidepressants for major depressive disorder.

Side effects

Common: Metabolic abnormalities (including hyperglycemia, insulin resistance, and dyslipidemia), weight gain, somnolence, tardive dyskinesia, orthostatic hypotension, leucopenia, neutropenia, agranulocytosis, seizures or convulsions, cognitive and/or motor impairment.

Serious: Neuroleptic malignant syndrome, increased suicidality, increased mortality in elderly patients with dementia-related psychosis (Bristol-Myers Squibb, 2008).

References

American Psychiatric Association. (2000). *Diagnostic and statistical manual of mental disorders (DSM-IV-TR)* (4th ed.). Washington, DC: American Psychiatric Publishing.

Barnett, J., & Smoller, J. (2009). The genetics of bipolar disorder. *Neuroscience, 4.*

Biovail Corporation (2008). Wellbutrin. Retrieved May 20, 2009, from http://www.biovail.com/local/files/ProductsInfo/us_wellbutrinXL.pdf

Bowden, C. (2003). Acute and maintenance treatment with mood stabilizers. *International Journal of Neuropsychopharmacology, 6,* 269–275.

Bristol-Myers Squibb. (2008). *Abilify (aripiprazole): US full prescribing information including black box warnings.* Retrieved May 20, 2009, from http://www.abilify.com/hcp/bipolar-disorder-efficacy.aspx#studydesign

Elwood, W. (1998). *TCADA research brief: "Fry": A study of adolescents' use of embalming fluid with marijuana and tobacco.* Houston: Texas Commission on Alcohol and Drug Use.

Goodwin, G., Anderson, I., Arango, C., Henry, C., Mitchell, P., Nolen, W., Vieta, E., & Wittchen, H. (2008). ECNP consensus meeting. Bipolar depression. *European Neuropsychopharmacology, 18,* 535–549.

Haney, M. (2005). The marijuana withdrawal syndrome: Diagnosis and treatment. *Current Psychiatric Reports, 7,* 360–366.

Lennkh, C., & Simhandl, C. (2000). Current aspects of valproate in bipolar disorder. *International Clinical Psychopharmacology, 15,* 1–11.

Leverich, G., et al. (2006). Risk of switch in mood polarity to hypomania or mania in patients with bipolar depression during acute and continuation trials of venlafaxine, sertraline, and bupropion as adjuncts to mood stabilizers. *American Journal of Psychiatry, 163,* 1642–1643.

Lin, D., Mok, H., & Yatham, L. (2006). Polytherapy in bipolar disorder. *CNS Drugs, 20,* 29–42.

Lynch, D., Laws, K., & McKenna, P. (2009). Cognitive behavioural therapy for major psychiatric disorders: Does it really work? A meta-analytical review of well-controlled trials. *Psychological Medicine, 29,* 1–16.

Modesto-Lowe, V., & Petry, N. (2001). Recognizing and managing "illy" intoxication. *Psychiatric Services, 52,* 1660.

Sadock, B, & Sadock, V. (2007). *Kaplan and Sadock's synopsis of psychiatry: Behavioral science/clinical psychiatry* (10th ed.). Philadelphia, PA: Lippincott Williams & Wilkins.

Stahl, S. (2008). *Stahl's essential psychopharmacology: Neuroscientific basis and practical applications* (2nd ed.). New York: Cambridge University Press.

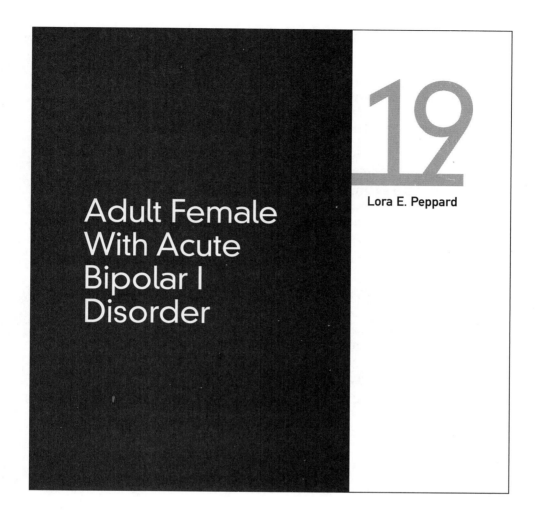

19

Adult Female With Acute Bipolar I Disorder

Lora E. Peppard

This case describes the care I provided for Ms. C, a 59-year-old female with Medicaid insurance who presented to the hospital in an acute manic episode. The case narrative focuses on five hospital encounters that occurred over a period of five days while Ms. C was admitted to the inpatient psychiatric service. This case narrative demonstrates my ability to meet the following Columbia University School of Nursing (CUSN) doctoral competencies for comprehensive direct patient care.

DOMAIN 1, COMPETENCY 3

Formulate differential diagnoses and diagnostic strategies and therapeutic interventions with attention to scientific evidence, safety, cost, invasiveness, simplicity, acceptability, adherence, and efficacy for patients who present with new conditions and those with ambiguous or incomplete data, complex illnesses, comorbid conditions, and multiple diagnoses in all clinical settings.

PO A. Formulate a differential diagnosis for a patient who presents with new undifferentiated signs and symptoms.

PO B. Formulate a differential diagnosis for a patient who presents with ambiguous or incomplete data, complex illnesses, comorbid conditions, and potential multiple diagnoses.

PO C. Discuss the rationale for the differential diagnosis.

PO D. Discuss the rationale for the diagnostic evaluation with attention to scientific evidence, safety, cost, invasiveness, simplicity, acceptability, adherence, and efficacy.

PO E. Discuss the rationale for the therapeutic intervention with attention to scientific evidence, safety, cost, invasiveness, simplicity, acceptability, adherence, and efficacy.

DOMAIN 1, COMPETENCY 5

Evaluate and direct care during hospitalization, and design a comprehensive discharge plan for patients from an acute care setting.

PO A. Assess the acuity of patient's condition and determine the most appropriate inpatient treatment setting based on level of acuity.

PO B. Actively participate in the admission process to the appropriate inpatient treatment setting.

PO C. Actively co-manage patient care during hospitalization.

PO D. Formulate plan for ongoing care to be provided in a subacute setting, such as a long-term care facility, rehabilitation facility, or home or community setting.

PO E. Coordinate ongoing comprehensive care to be provided in a subacute setting, such as a long-term care facility, rehabilitation facility, or home or community setting.

DOMAIN 2, COMPETENCY 1

Assemble a collaborative interdisciplinary network, and refer and consult appropriately while maintaining primary responsibility for comprehensive patient care.

PO A. Initiate referral to other health care professionals while maintaining primary responsibility for patient care.

PO D. Evaluate outcomes of interventions.

PO E. Provide ongoing patient follow-up, and monitor outcomes of collaborative network interventions.

DOMAIN 2, COMPETENCY 2

Coordinate and manage the care of patients with chronic illness, utilizing specialists, other disciplines, community resources, and family, while maintaining primary responsibility for direction of patient care and ensuring the seamless flow of information among providers as the focus of care transitions across ambulatory to acute, subacute, and community settings.

PO A. Coordinate care for a patient with chronic illness as the focus of care transitions across ambulatory, acute, subacute, and/or community settings.

PO B. Co-manage care for a patient with chronic illness as the focus of care transitions across ambulatory, acute, subacute, and/or community settings.

PO C. Coordinate care for a patient with chronic illness utilizing specialists, other disciplines, community resources, and family.

PO D. Direct care for patient with chronic illness and ensure the seamless flow of information among providers as the focus of care transitions across settings.

PO E. Co-manage care for a patient with chronic illness utilizing shared decision-making and teaching.

ENCOUNTER CONTEXT

Encounter One (initial evaluation)

DNP role: I am the attending nurse practitioner and DNP resident assuming responsibility of care for this patient.

Identifying Information

Site: Urban academic hospital.

Setting: Inpatient medical psychiatric floor.

Reason for encounter: Psychiatric evaluation.

Informant: Patient.

Chief complaint: "Everything from the past is coming up. I can finally talk about it. I need to talk about it."

History of Present Illness (HPI)

Ms. C is a 59-year-old divorced African American female with a past psychiatric history significant for multiple psychiatric hospitalizations for treatment of bipolar disorder. She presents with severely pressured speech, flight of ideas, impulsivity (spending $200 of money she did not have at a thrift store, stealing from department stores), anxiety, decreased need for sleep (one to two hours per night), and command auditory hallucinations of male voices telling her to harm herself. Her symptoms started approximately three weeks ago when Ms. C stopped taking her medications. The symptoms have been gradually increasing in severity since that time. Ms. C reports she ordered her medications through an online pharmacy and has not received them yet, resulting in her relapse. She lives in a senior citizen community and has been isolating from her two daughters and one son while volunteering up to 12 hours per day at the senior center.

Ms. C's oldest daughter, who brought Ms. C to the emergency department (ED), visited her mother the day of admission to discover that her mother had barricaded herself in the house and created mazes with furniture. Ms. C initially refused to let her daughter in the house, which is very uncommon behavior for her. The daughter reports that it also appeared as if Ms. C had not eaten for a few days, because there was not any food or remnants of food in the house. Ms. C denies any drug or alcohol use, suicidal or homicidal ideation, and any visual hallucinations.

Past Psychiatric History

- Multiple psychiatric hospitalizations in the past for treatment of bipolar disorder. First hospitalization was in her late twenties. She has been hospitalized at a state hospital twice before. Her last hospitalization was "several years ago" per daughter's report.
- Multiple suicide attempts by overdose beginning in her late twenties. Last suicide attempt was "over ten years ago."
- Connected with a core service agency and regularly sees a psychiatrist and case manager at this facility.
- Ms. C denied any type of physical, sexual, or emotional abuse in her past until her current hospitalization, during which she is now reporting extensive sexual abuse by her mother's boyfriend when she was six years old.

Past Substance Abuse History

- Reports drinking alcohol "a very long time ago" with "no problems now." Family and Ms. C report last alcohol use was many years ago.
- Denies any other history of or current drug use.

Past Medical History

- No known drug allergies.
- Hypertension managed with triamterene/hydrochlorothiazide (Dyazide) 37.5/25.0 mg daily.

Medications

Quetiapine (Seroquel) 25 mg by mouth daily in the morning and 75 mg by mouth at the hour of sleep.

Lamotrigine (Lamictal) 100 mg by mouth at the hour of sleep.

Triamterene/hydrochlorothiazide (Dyazide) 37.5/25.0 mg by mouth daily.

Divalproex sodium (Depakote) 750 mg by mouth twice daily.

Family History

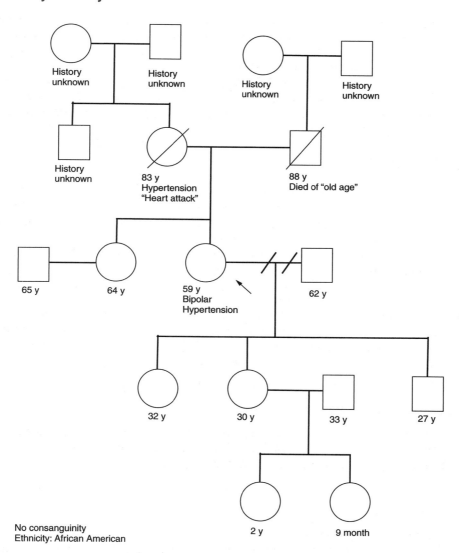

History
unknown

History
unknown

History
unknown

History
unknown

History
unknown

83 y
Hypertension
"Heart attack"

88 y
Died of "old age"

65 y

64 y

59 y
Bipolar
Hypertension

62 y

32 y

30 y

33 y

27 y

2 y

9 month

No consanguinity
Ethnicity: African American

Social and Developmental History

Ms. C reports a normal labor and delivery followed by reaching all developmental milestones at an appropriate age. She reports having a good relationship with her parents and her older sister growing up. Her mother and father divorced when she was five years old. She continued living with her mother, who went through "a few" boyfriends before staying single. Ms. C had a large group of friends throughout school and graduated high school with good grades. She maintained contact with her father. After high school, Ms. C began work as a secretary and remained in this position for 11 years before her first psychiatric hospitalization, when she was diagnosed with bipolar disorder. Shortly thereafter, she married her husband and had two daughters and one son. She was married for 20 years before her husband "couldn't handle me anymore" due to frequent relapses of her mental illness, and they divorced. Ms. C began volunteering at the local senior citizen center when she was in her early fifties and now lives in the senior citizen community. She denies any legal issues and reports frequent visits with her family. She enjoys spending time with her two granddaughters, ages nine months and two years old.

Review of Systems

General: Reports "a few pounds" weight loss due to not eating adequately during manic episode over past three weeks.

Skin: Reports no rashes or other changes, warm, dry.

HEENT: Denies history of head injury. Denies blurred vision, hearing difficulty, tinnitus, vertigo, infections, difficulty swallowing. Reports all teeth intact and gums in good condition. Last dental visit three months ago.

Neck: Denies lumps, pain, goiter, or swollen glands.

Respiratory: Denies cough, wheezing, shortness of breath.

Cardiovascular: Denies chest pain or palpitations.

Gastrointestinal: Reports appetite is fair, bowel movement every one to two days. Denies diarrhea or abdominal pain.

Urinary: Denies any pain on urination or blood in urine. Reports normal frequency.

Genital: Denies infections. Denies pain.

Peripheral vascular: Denies history of phlebitis or leg pain.

Musculoskeletal: Denies back or joint pain.

Neurologic: Denies fainting, seizure history, motor or sensory loss. No memory deficits noted.

Hematologic: Denies bleeding or anemia.

Endocrine: Denies thyroid trouble or temperature intolerance. Denies symptoms or history of diabetes.

Psychiatric: See History of Present Illness.

Physical Examination

General: Ms. C is 5 feet, 6 inches tall, of average muscle build, 160 pounds, BMI 25.8, poor hygiene and grooming. She was casually dressed, and she was able to lie flat without discomfort.

Vital signs: Blood pressure 120/78, heart rate 88, respiratory rate 20, temp (oral) 98.0°F, pain 0 on a scale of 0–10.

Skin: Warm and dry with good color.

HEENT: Hair of average texture. Scalp without lesions or evidence of trauma. Normocephalic. Vision 20/20 in each eye. Visual fields full by confrontation. Conjunctiva pink, sclera white. Pupils constrict and are round, regular, and equally reactive to light. Extraocular movements intact. Small amount of wax in both ears. Tympanic membrane gray with good cone of light. Acuity good to whispered voice. Weber midline. Pink mucosa in nose, septum midline. No sinus tenderness. Oral mucosa pink. Dentition good. Tongue midline. Tonsils present. Pharynx without exudates.

Neck: Supple, no lymphadenopathy. No thyromegaly. No carotid bruits. No jugular venous distention.

Lungs: Clear to auscultation bilaterally. Vesicular with no adventitious sounds.

Cardiac: Regular rate and rhythm. S1, S2, no murmur.

Abdomen: Soft, nontender, no organomegaly. Bowel sounds present in all quadrants.

Extremities: Normal range of motion. No edema.

Neurologic: Alert and oriented to person, place, time, and situation. Cranial nerves II–XII intact. No motor or sensory deficits. Reflexes normal. No cerebellar findings. Gait steady.

Mental Status Exam

Ms. C is alert and oriented in all spheres. She appears disheveled and is not wearing makeup. She has a very poor attention span and concentration with extremely pressured speech. She describes her mood as "pitiful," related to her ruminating thoughts of multiple episodes of sexual abuse in the past. Affect labile. Ms. C would burst into a gospel song one minute and would be sobbing the next minute while speaking rapidly about "holding all of the past inside me." Impulsive and strange behaviors, as described in HPI. Ms. C has been spending money she does not have and shoplifting, which daughters describe as "common" behaviors for Ms. C when she is manic. She denies visual hallucinations. Command auditory hallucinations instructing Ms. C to harm herself. Possible delusional content of multiple incidences of sexual abuse in the past, which daughters and son report Ms. C has never mentioned before. Flight of ideas at times. Very difficult to direct or redirect Ms. C into a sequential thought process. Unable to complete further thought process assessment because of Ms. C's inability to concentrate and manic state. Appetite: "I don't know. I haven't had time to think about it." Sleeping at most two to three hours per night over the past three weeks. Reports difficulty staying asleep due to racing thoughts and "needing to help the senior citizens." No evidence of obsessions and compulsions. Short-term and immediate memory intact. Long-term memory influenced by current manic state. Insight into condition and judgment at this time poor, as evidenced by Ms. C's not caring for herself by not eating and barricading herself in her house.

Laboratory Data

Complete blood count (CBC), comprehensive metabolic panel (CMP), and thyroid-stimulating hormone (TSH) are all within normal limits. Urinalysis (UA), urine pregnancy test (UHCG), and urine drug screen (UDS) were negative. Divalproex sodium (Depakote) level is 0 µg/mL.

The American Psychiatric Association (2000) prohibits the diagnosis of a psychiatric condition before all possible contributing general medical conditions are ruled out. Laboratory data assist in identifying general medical conditions, which often present with psychiatric symptoms.

CEBM, level 5.

A CBC is useful for determining if a patient is suffering from an infection or anemia. A CMP assists in revealing any nutritional, electrolyte, or glucose abnormalities in addition to giving an overview of how a person's kidneys and liver are functioning. A TSH level explains if too much or too little Thyroid Stimulating Hormone is being produced, both of which can cause psychiatric symptoms. A UA combined with a CBC rules out the possibility of a Urinary Tract Infection, and a UDS detects substances such as marijuana and cocaine within the body. All substances can induce mood, anxiety, and psychotic symptoms (Corbett, 2000).

CEBM, level 5.

Ms. C is unable to report whether or not she had reached menopause, making a urine pregnancy test necessary. A positive pregnancy test would heavily influence the appropriateness of pharmacologic treatment and medication choices.

Many psychotropic medications are teratogenic and place the fetus at risk of harm if taken by the mother (Stahl, 2008).

CEBM, level 5.

A divalproex sodium (Depakote) level of 0 µg/mL indicates that Ms. C has not been taking her medication for at least a few days.

A Divalproex Sodium (Depakote) level between 50 µg/mL and 100 µg/mL is usually required to achieve antimanic effects when a patient is experiencing an acute manic episode. Trough plasma drug levels up to 100 µg/mL are generally well tolerated (Stahl, 2008).

CEBM, level 5.

Psychiatric Impression

Ms. C is a 59-year-old African American divorced female who has struggled with bipolar I disorder since her late twenties and has suffered from a mix of depressive and manic symptoms since that time. Her last psychiatric hospitalization was ten years ago, and she is well established in the community at a core service agency. She is usually adherent with her therapeutic regimen. She utilizes an online pharmacy to fill her prescriptions and experienced a three-week break in her daily medication routine when she forgot to fill her prescriptions on time. She began to relapse into a manic episode, which increased in severity over the three-week period. Her oldest daughter found Ms. C barricaded in her house and brought her into the hospital for treatment. Ms. C is an intelligent, compassionate woman who has a very close relationship with her two daughters and son. Both Ms. C and her family report that she does extremely well and can live independently when stable on her medication.

Ms. C presents with classic bipolar I disorder symptoms. A diagnosis of schizoaffective disorder, bipolar type, is less likely because Ms. C has never experienced any delusional content or psychotic symptoms while not in a severe manic or depressive episode. Both Ms. C and her family report that the disorganized thought process and delusional content surface only when Ms. C is manic, thereby excluding a schizoaffective diagnosis (**D1, C3, PO A, B, C**).

Diagnosis According to DSM-IV-TR

Axis I: Bipolar I disorder, recurrent, severe, most recent episode manic with psychotic features (296.4).

Axis II: None.

Axis III: Hypertension (401.9).

Axis IV: Unemployed, lives alone in senior citizen community.

Axis V: Global assessment of functioning on admission: current 30, highest in past year 65.

The DSM is produced by the American Psychiatric Association and is used as the standard diagnostic tool for psychiatry. According to the most recent revision of the DSM (2000), the DSM-IV-TR, Axis I represents clinical disorders and other conditions warranting clinical focus. Axis II is reserved for personality disorders and mental retardation. Axis III describes general medical conditions. Psychosocial stressors or environmental problems are listed on Axis IV, and Axis V is a score, which rates the patient's global assessment of functioning from 0 to 100 (100 being superior).

CEBM, level 5.

Plan

Mania or Mood Instability

- Voluntary admission to inpatient psychiatry where a safe environment will be provided in addition to group, individual, and milieu therapy **(D1, C5, PO A, B, C).**
- Discuss the risks, benefits, and alternatives to restarting divalproex sodium (Depakote) 750 mg by mouth twice a day, lamotrigine (Lamictal) 25 mg by mouth at bedtime, quetiapine (Seroquel) 25 mg by mouth daily in the morning and 75 mg by mouth at the hour of sleep, and triamterene/hydrochlorothiazide (Dyazide) 37.5/25.0 mg by mouth daily (see Medications list at the end of the chapter for indications) **(D1, C3, PO D, E).**

Lamotrigine (Lamictal) has received a black box warning for life threatening skin reactions including Stevens-Johnson Syndrome and Toxic Epidermal Necrolysis. It is therefore usually dosed at 25 mg daily for the first 2 weeks, titrated up to 50 mg daily for another two weeks, and then titrated up to a minimum target dose of 100 mg daily for antidepressant and mood stabilization effects. Divalproex Sodium (Depakote) inhibits the metabolism of Lamotrigine (Lamictal) and raises Lamotrigine (Lamictal) plasma levels (Stahl, 2008).

CEBM, level 5.

Because Ms. C has been effectively treated on the current dose of lamotrigine (Lamictal) and divalproex sodium (Depakote) for many months without any reports of a rash, I will not make any changes at this time. However, I will educate Ms. C on the potential side effect of a rash and ask her to please notify me or her outpatient provider at the first sign of a rash.

Lamotrigine (Lamictal) co-administered with Divalproex Sodium (Depakote), Lithium (Eskalith), an atypical antipsychotic, or a selective serotonin reuptake inhibitor, in the treatment of bipolar disorder was well tolerated in an 8- to 16-week preliminary trial of 1305 patients diagnosed with bipolar disorder (Bowden, Edwards, & Evoniuk, 2008).

CEBM, level 2b.

Diagnostic Studies

- Check Ms. C's divalproex sodium (Depakote) level and hepatic panel in 72 hours and adjust medication if necessary to reach a therapeutic level between 50 and 100 µg/mL **(D1, C3, PO D, E).**

Divalproex Sodium (Depakote) is metabolized primarily by the liver, and patients should be monitored for hepatotoxicity, especially when initiating treatment or titrating the dose upward (Stahl, 2008).

CEBM, level 5.

- Order a fasting lipid profile and plasma glucose because Ms. C is being continued on quetiapine (Seroquel), an atypical antipsychotic. Order vital signs twice daily **(D1, C3, PO D).**

Quetiapine (Seroquel), an atypical antipsychotic, may increase the risk for diabetes and dyslipidemia. The exact mechanism of weight gain and increased incidence of diabetes and dyslipidemia with atypical antipsychotics is unknown. Quetiapine (Seroquel) also has the potential to cause orthostatic hypotension, usually during initial dose titration (Stahl, 2008).

CEBM, level 5.

- Therefore, I will monitor her vital signs twice daily, get a baseline lipid profile and plasma glucose, and treat accordingly **(D1, C3, PO D).**

Glassman (2005) emphasizes the importance of assessing a patient's baseline medical condition and their risk of cardiovascular disease before starting antipsychotic medication.

CEBM, level 3a.

- Monitor weight **(D1, C3, PO E).**

Education and Coping (D2, C2, PO C, E)

- Educate Ms. C on the symptoms of her illness and mental health basics, such as adequate nutrition, hydration, exercise, and relaxation. Discuss course of illness and prognosis if managed with therapeutic interventions, and assess patient's understanding of and agreement with the information.
- Schedule a family meeting with Ms. C's two daughters and son to provide education about Ms. C's illness and answer any questions they may have.

Brown, M., Goldstein-Shirley, J., Robinson, J., and Casey, S. (2001) conducted a study on the effects of a multi-modal intervention of daylight, exercise, and vitamins on women's mood. Fifty-three women in the intervention group were instructed to walk outside during daylight hours for 20 minutes 5 days per week, maximize their exposure to commonly available indoor and *outdoor light in all aspects of their life, and take a daily vitamin tablet containing thiamine (B_1) 50 mg, pyridoxine (B_6) 50 mg, riboflavin (B_2) 50 mg, folic acid 400 mg, selenium 200 mcg, and vitamin D 400 IU. The supplements and their doses were based on randomized, controlled trials according to the authors of the study. The placebo group received a placebo vitamin daily. Both groups improved significantly in mood, self-esteem, and general sense of well-being, but the intervention group improved significantly more in all outcomes. Women in the intervention group reported decreased tension and anger, decreased depression, increased self-control, vitality and positive well-being.*

CEBM, level 1b.

- Through individual counseling and group therapy, discuss with Ms. C the appropriate steps to take if she is unable to gain timely access to her medications or begins experiencing manic or depressive symptoms.

Baldesserini, Perry, and Pike (2007) discuss the following factors as being associated with treatment nonadherence in patients diagnosed with Bipolar Disorder: comorbid alcohol dependence, younger age, greater number of affective symptoms, medication side effects, treatment side effects, comorbid obsessive-compulsive disorder, and recent mania or hypomania. They also found that patient reported rates of nonadherence were several-times higher than physician-estimated rates, even when the criteria involved included major defaulting by patients as well as missing occasional doses.

CEBM, level 2c.

Support and Follow-up
- Contact Ms. C's case manager and psychiatrist.
- After stabilization of Ms. C's acute situation, arrange outpatient follow-up with her core service agency, which will provide case management, counseling, and medication management services **(D2, C1, PO A; D2, C2, PO A, B).**

ICD 9 code: Bipolar I disorder, recurrent, severe, most recent episode manic with psychotic features (296.4).

Encounter Two (inpatient day 2)

Staff report that Ms. C slept two hours and was up socializing and expressing her vocal talent throughout the night. She also made several phone calls to multiple family members and elaborately discussed her beliefs about her former sexual abuse. Upon exam, Ms. C's speech remains extremely pressured and her mood extremely labile as evidenced by her excitement to see me followed instantly by tears while voicing a flight of ideas. She reports that she is tolerating the medications well, and she denies any suicidal ideation or auditory hallucinations.

I contact Ms. C's daughter, who is very open to the idea of a family meeting when Ms. C's condition stabilizes. I also contact Ms. C's outpatient providers, who are aware of her admission and say they can see her immediately after discharge (D2, C1, PO A; D2, C2, PO D).

ICD 9 code: Bipolar I disorder, recurrent, severe, most recent episode manic with psychotic features (296.4).

Encounter Three (inpatient day 3)

Staff report that Ms. C slept for six hours and was slightly more redirectable. They note she is able to ask for water when she is thirsty and sit quietly in her room for periods of time. Upon exam, Ms. C is able to engage in a much more logical conversation and reports feeling significantly better. She continues to deny suicidal ideation or auditory hallucinations. She states, "Whew. I forgot what it feels like to sleep." Speech remains moderately pressured. She is able to perform serial sevens and abstractions, and is of average intelligence with a good fund of knowledge. She voices remorse over calling so many family members and worrying them the day before with her many claims of former abuse. She also begins to question these ideas of former abuse, but continues to report that one incidence of being sexually abused as a child was correct (D2, C1, PO D).

Ms. C welcomes a family meeting, but she is afraid to face her family after what she had done the day before. We discuss how the family meeting would be a time to share and process the impact of symptoms like those she experienced the day before, and Ms. C began preparing what she would like to say to her family the next day.

I contact Ms. C's oldest daughter, and a family meeting is arranged for the following day (D2, C2, PO F).

ICD 9 code: Bipolar I disorder, recurrent, severe, most recent episode manic with psychotic features (296.4).

Encounter Four (inpatient day 4)

Staff report that Ms. C slept for seven hours and is able to attend to her activities of daily living without direction. They note a marked improvement in their conversations with her as well as her well-groomed appearance. Upon exam, Ms. C has slightly pressured speech but is redirectable and does not interrupt people when they are speaking. She denies any psychotic symptoms, and her thought process is clear, logical, and goal-directed. Her mood is "much more steady" with a bright affect. She continues to deny suicidal ideation or auditory hallucinations. She has organized her thoughts about what she wants to share with her family at the meeting (D2, C1, PO D).

A family meeting is held with Ms. C's two daughters and son. Ms. C's family voiced their concern for Ms. C and stressed how necessary it was for her to remain on her medication without any gaps in treatment. Ms. C apologized to her family for her behaviors, and her family kindly accepted this apology. Ms. C brought up the instance of abuse in her past, and she and her family discussed how Ms. C could continue to talk through the topic with her outpatient providers. Ms. C stated, "I just feel so much better now that it's out in the open." The family appeared cohesive and supportive, and there was a very warm and gentle dynamic among all of them. Various responsibilities were delegated to the family members, and frequent visitations were arranged as Ms. C recovered so that she could return to live independently. Education about bipolar disorder was provided for the family, and they were given the opportunity to ask questions. Discharge is planned for the following day provided Ms. C is able to maintain her progress **(D1, C5, PO D, E; D2, C2, PO C).**

ICD 9 code: Bipolar I disorder, recurrent, severe, most recent episode manic with psychotic features (296.4).

Encounter Five (inpatient day 5)

Ms. C awoke after her third night of six or more hours of sleep and reported feeling ready for discharge. Her mood is stable, speech is of normal rate and volume, and there is no evidence of psychosis. Her divalproex sodium (Depakote) level is 62 µg/mL. Her lipid profile, fasting blood glucose, hepatic panel, and blood pressure are all within normal limits **(D2, C1, PO D).**

Education on Ms. C's medications is reinforced, and she recites the information back and voices understanding. When discussing how Ms. C will remember to take her medications, she decides she is going to purchase a weekly pill holder and ask her oldest daughter to call her every Sunday and remind her to fill her holder with her medications for the week. When her oldest daughter arrives to pick Ms. C up, Ms. C talked with her about this plan, and the daughter agreed it would be beneficial. Ms. C's daughter reports that she would make sure Ms. C made it to her outpatient appointment the next day. She also confirms that an appointment with Ms. C's primary care provider had been made for Ms. C the following week **(D1, C5, PO D, E; D2, C2, PO C).**

ICD 9 code: Bipolar I disorder, recurrent, severe, most recent episode manic with psychotic features (296.4).

CASE SUMMATION

I call Ms. C's oldest daughter two days later to follow up, and she reports that Ms. C is continuing to improve and her outpatient providers are very supportive of Ms. C during Ms. C's visit with them. She also confirms that Ms. C gave her outpatient providers her most recent medication list from her hospitalization. **(D1, C5, PO E.)**

COMPETENCY DEFENSE

Domain 1, Competency 3. Formulate differential diagnoses and diagnostic strategies and therapeutic interventions with attention to scientific evidence, safety, cost, invasiveness, simplicity, acceptability, adherence, and efficacy for patients who present with new conditions and those with ambiguous or incomplete data, complex illnesses, comorbid conditions, and multiple diagnoses in all clinical settings.

Defense. Ms. C presented in a classic manic state with psychotic symptoms. The existence of psychotic symptoms outside of mania or depression warranted a potentially different medication regimen such as higher doses of an antipsychotic. Therefore, it was necessary to rule out schizoaffective disorder, bipolar type, to formulate the most appropriate treatment plan for Ms. C.

Domain 2, Competency 2. Coordinate and manage the care of patients with chronic illness utilizing specialists, other disciplines, community resources, and family, while maintaining primary responsibility for the direction of patient care and ensuring the seamless flow of information among providers as the focus of care transitions from ambulatory to acute, subacute, and community settings.

Defense. Education for Ms. C, her family, and her outpatient providers was imperative to reduce her risk of relapse in the future. Ms. C identified her family as her greatest support and requested their assistance in her recovery by listening, sharing in the decision-making process, and coordinating outpatient care in both behavioral health and primary care.

Domain 1, Competency 5. Evaluate, direct care during hospitalization, and design a comprehensive discharge plan for patients in acute care settings.

Defense. I assessed Ms. C for admission to the psychiatric unit, managed and coordinated her care during the hospitalization, and communicated with community resources, providers, and family to ensure appropriate follow-up and continuity of care after discharge.

Domain 2, Competency 1. Assemble a collaborative multidisciplinary network and refer patients appropriately while maintaining primary responsibility for comprehensive patient care.

Defense. Ms. C has a history of several relapses in her condition when she does not consistently take her medication. Although her core service agency is comprehensive in nature, arranging appropriate family observation and following up with Ms. C via telephone after discharge were additional interventions required in Ms. C's case to increase the likelihood of Ms. C maintaining stability outside of the hospital.

Medications

> ### Drug: Divalproex Sodium (Depakote)
>
> **Dose range:** 1,200–1,500 mg/day.
>
> **Method of administration in this case:** By mouth.
>
> **Mechanism of action:** Mood stabilizer that blocks voltage-sensitive sodium channels and increases brain concentrations of gamma-aminobutyric acid (GABA) by an unknown mechanism.
>
> **Clinical uses:** Acute mania and mixed episodes.
>
> **Side effects**
> **Common:** Dizziness, drowsiness, nausea, weight gain.
> **Serious:** Hepatotoxicity, pancreatitis.
>
> ### Drug: Lamotrigine (Lamictal)
>
> **Dose range:** 100–200 mg/day.
>
> **Method of administration in this case:** By mouth.
>
> **Mechanism of action:** Mood stabilizer that blocks voltage-sensitive sodium channels and inhibits release of glutamate and aspartate.
>
> **Clinical uses:** Maintenance treatment of bipolar I disorder.
>
> **Side effects**
> **Common:** Headaches, dizziness, insomnia, benign rash.
> **Serious:** Rare serious rash, rare multiorgan failure associated with Stevens-Johnson syndrome, rare blood dyscrasias.
>
> ### Drug: Quetiapine (Seroquel)
>
> **Dose range:** 150–800 mg/day.
>
> **Method of administration in this case:** By mouth.
>
> **Mechanism of action:** Atypical antipsychotic and mood stabilizer that blocks dopamine 2 receptors and serotonin 2A receptors.
>
> **Clinical uses:** Schizophrenia, acute mania.
>
> **Side effects**
> **Common:** May increase risk for diabetes and dyslipidemia, dizziness, sedation, dry mouth, constipation, weight gain, orthostatic hypotension.
> **Serious:** Hyperglycemia, rare neuroleptic malignant syndrome, rare seizures, increased risk of death and cerebrovascular events in elderly patients with dementia-related psychosis.
>
> *(continued)*

Drug: Triamterene/Hydrochlorothiazide (Dyazide)

Dose range: 37.5/25.0 mg, 1 to 2 capsules per day.

Method of administration in this case: By mouth.

Mechanism of action: Diuretic and antihypertensive drug product that combines natriuretic and antikaliuretic effects; hydrochlorothiazide component blocks the reabsorption of sodium and chloride ions; triamterene component exerts its diuretic effect on the distal renal tubule to inhibit the reabsorption of sodium in exchange for potassium and hydrogen ions.

Clinical uses: Hypertension, edema.

Side effects
Common: Nausea or vomiting, dizziness, headache, stomach pain.
Serious: Hyperkalemia, metabolic or respiratory acidosis, acute renal failure.

Source: Stahl, 2008; Wilson, Shannon, & Stang, 2003.

References

American Psychiatric Association. (2000). *Diagnostic and statistical manual of mental disorders* (4th ed., text revision). Washington, DC: American Psychiatric Association.

American Psychiatric Association. (2002). *Practice guidelines for the treatment of psychiatric disorders.* Washington, DC: American Psychiatric Association.

Baldesserini, R.J., Perry, R., & Pike, J. (2007). Factors associated with treatment nonadherence among US bipolar disorder patients. *Human Psychopharmacology,* December.

Bowden, C.L., Edwards, S., & Evoniuk, G. (2008). Open-label, concomitant use of lamotrigine and other medications for bipolar disorder. *CNS Spectrum, 13*(1), 75–83.

Brown, M., Goldstein-Shirley, J., Robinson, J., & Casey, S. (2001). The effects of a multi-modal intervention trial of light, exercise, and vitamins on women's mood. *Women and Health, 34*(3), 93–112.

Corbett, J.V. (2000). *Laboratory tests and diagnostic procedures.* Upper Saddle River, NJ: Prentice Hall.

Glassman, A.H. (2005). Schizophrenia, antipsychotic drugs, and cardiovascular disease. *Journal of Clinical Psychiatry, 66*(Suppl 6), 5–10.

Stahl, S.M. (2008). *Essential psychopharmacology: The prescriber's guide.* Cambridge: Cambridge University Press.

Wilson, B.A., Shannon, M.T., & Stang, C.L. (2003). *Nurses drug guide 2003.* Upper Saddle River, NJ: Prentice Hall.

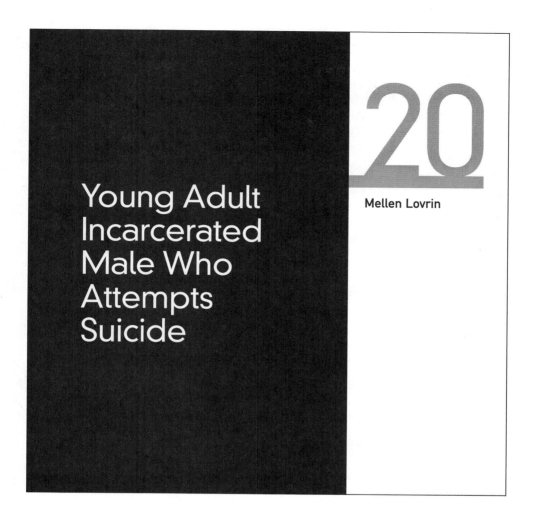

20

Young Adult Incarcerated Male Who Attempts Suicide

Mellen Lovrin

This case was chosen because it presents a psychiatric case narrative requiring emergency treatment following a patient's suicide attempt by hanging while incarcerated. The case narrative is based on a single emergency department (ED) admission with a 20-year-old male patient who was brought for evaluation. The narrative demonstrates my ability to meet the following Columbia University School of Nursing (CUSN) doctoral competencies for comprehensive direct patient care.

DOMAIN 1, COMPETENCY 3

Formulate differential diagnoses and diagnostic strategies and therapeutic interventions with attention to scientific evidence, safety, cost, invasiveness, simplicity, acceptability, adherence, and efficacy for patients who present with new conditions and those with ambiguous or incomplete data, complex illnesses, comorbid conditions, and multiple diagnoses in all clinical settings.

PO A. Formulate a differential diagnosis for a patient who presents with new undifferentiated signs and symptoms.

PO B. Formulate a differential diagnosis for a patient who presents with ambiguous or incomplete data, complex illnesses, comorbid conditions, and potential multiple diagnoses.

PO C. Discuss the rationale for the differential diagnosis.

PO D. Discuss the rationale for the diagnostic evaluation with attention to scientific evidence, safety, cost, invasiveness, simplicity, acceptability, adherence, and efficacy.

PO E. Discuss the rationale for the therapeutic intervention with attention to scientific evidence, safety, cost, invasiveness, simplicity, acceptability, adherence, and efficacy.

DOMAIN 3, COMPETENCY 2

Evaluate gaps in health care access that compromise optimal patient outcomes, and apply current knowledge of the organization and financing of health care systems to ameliorate negative impact.

PO A. Identify gaps in access that compromise patient's optimum care.

PO B. Identify gaps in reimbursement that compromise patient's optimum care.

PO C. Demonstrate patient advocacy in the provision of continuous and comprehensive care.

PO D. Apply current knowledge of the organization to ameliorate negative impact.

PO E. Apply current knowledge of health care systems to ameliorate negative impact.

ENCOUNTER CONTEXT

Encounter One (initial encounter)

DNP role: I am a certified mental health nurse practitioner and doctor of nursing practice (DNP) resident evaluating this patient for an initial psychiatric evaluation.

Identifying Information

Site: Psychiatric ED.

Setting: Suburban community hospital.

Reason for encounter: Initial evaluation following suicide attempt while incarcerated.

Informant: Patient accompanied by corrections officer. Patient appears to be a reliable historian.

Demographics: Patient is a 20-year-old, single African American male who previously lived at home with his mother. He has a graduate equivalency diploma (GED) and has no intention of returning to school. He is unemployed and currently incarcerated for possession of stolen property. The patient has Medicaid insurance. Patient was transported to the hospital ED by ambulance following a suicide attempt by hanging while in jail. Patient complains of neck pain to ED staff.

Chief complaint: Neck pain and suicide attempt by hanging while in jail.

History of Present Illness

This is a 20-year-old inmate who was brought to the ED after attempting suicide, by hanging, in his cell today. He was discovered by a prison guard, who called 911.

The patient was previously evaluated in the ED and hospitalized three weeks ago after an apparent hanging with a bed sheet in the jail. According to the police report, he "was depressed and tried to kill himself." Patient has a recent past history of heroin dependence and withdrawal and of benzodiazepine dependence and withdrawal, for which he was treated during his hospitalization three weeks ago. At that time, the patient was admitted to a medical unit and placed on a telemetry monitor. He was found to have periods of bradycardia and atrial arrhythmias, which were monitored during his hospitalization. After being on the medical unit for one week, the patient was discharged back to the county jail.

Since discharge two weeks ago, he reports feeling sad, tired, short-tempered, and hopeless. He is having difficulty sleeping, is not hungry, his mind wanders during the day, and he is getting into physical and verbal altercations. He feels life is not worth living and he has recurrent thoughts of death.

Past medical history: He is HIV-positive, has never taken medication, and has no history of AIDs-defining illness.

Review of systems: The ED physician examined the patient and reported that the patient's neurologic, cardiovascular, pulmonary, genitourinary, endocrine, and hematopoietic review of systems was unremarkable. The patient describes periodic skin rashes and complains of neck pain, as noted in the History of Present Illness.

Physical examination (performed by ED staff): Vital signs were blood pressure 114/68, pulse 65. Physical examination for head, eyes, ears, nose, and throat (HEENT), cardiac, pulmonary, gastrointestinal, and neurologic systems was unremarkable.

Laboratory data: Complete blood count (CBC) and comprehensive metabolic panel were reported to be within normal limits.

Allergies: No known drug allergies.

Psychiatric consultation: The patient, an inmate at a nearby jail, allegedly tried to hang himself for the second time in three weeks. The patient, a 20-year-old African American male, was found hanging by the neck with a bed sheet. The patient reports a history of depression eight months ago, for which he was hospitalized for two weeks. He was treated with an antidepressant and a sleeping pill, names not recalled. The patient also reports a recent history of heroin, "Xanax," and marijuana abuse. The patient reports feeling depressed and that "life is not worth living." He discusses his suicide attempt three weeks ago and states he will continue to try to kill himself until he is successful.

Medications: None.

Family history: Mother has inoperable colon cancer. Father is in jail; patient has had no contact with him for "many years."

Social history: Patient is an inmate. He is awaiting trial for alleged charges of stolen property. He smokes less than one pack of cigarettes per day. He has a history of substance abuse and dependence on heroin, cocaine, crack, and alcohol. The patient reports that he currently has a girlfriend with whom he is in regular contact.

Mental Status Examination

The patient presents as a young, healthy, well-nourished African American male who appears his stated age. He is alert and oriented to person, place, and time. Initially the patient is uncooperative with the interview, but he later agrees to speak to me and complete the psychiatric interview.

His speech is coherent, though simplistic. His thought processes are clear and goal-directed. He denies auditory and visual hallucinations. He denies homicidal ideation. Recent and remote memory is intact. Mood is dysthymic; affect is congruent with mood. The patient describes feeling suicidal and reports that he will continue to attempt suicide by hanging if he is returned to jail. His insight is fair and judgment is poor. The patient has been incarcerated for the past 90 days and is awaiting trial.

He states he does not believe I am able to help him and is surprised I am willing to spend time with him. He notices that everyone who works in the ED is white, and he expects me to be uninterested in trying to help him because he is black, in handcuffs, and HIV-positive.

Clinical Impression and Interventions

The patient describes the following symptoms, which have been present most of the day, nearly every day for the past eight months, and which are consistent with a *DSM-IV-TR* diagnosis of major depressive disorder, severe, recurrent: sadness, anhedonia as expressed by his inability to enjoy most or all activities, insomnia, hypophagia, irritability, decreased energy, decreased ability to concentrate, hopelessness and worthlessness, and recurrent thoughts of death.

The patient has made two serious suicide attempts in the past three weeks and is at high risk for another attempt. The patient has been accused of stealing property, which was found in his garage. He has a history of impulsivity, substance dependence and abuse, aggressiveness as demonstrated by repeated physical fights, and reckless disregard for the safety of self and others, thus meeting *DSM-IV-TR* criteria for antisocial personality disorder.

The patient denies history of decreased need for sleep or other symptoms of hypomania or mania. The patient has a recent history, within the past month, of heroin and benzodiazepine dependence and withdrawal and of marijuana abuse. The patient thus meets *DSM-IV-TR* criteria for substance dependence (heroin, benzodiazepine) and substance abuse (marijuana) **(D1, C3, PO A, B, C)**.

Diagnostic criteria for major depressive disorder, substance abuse and dependence, and antisocial personality disorder are described within the DSM-IV-TR.
   Oxford Centre for Evidence-Based Medicine (CEBM), level 5.

DSM-IV-TR Diagnoses

Axis I: Major depressive disorder, recurrent, severe, substance abuse (marijuana); substance dependence (benzodiazepine, heroin).

Axis II: Antisocial personality disorder.

Axis III: Mild heart murmur, HIV-positive.

Axis IV: Severe, incarcerated, awaiting trial.

Axis V: 50, suicide attempt.

Suicide epidemiology: Suicide took the lives of 30,622 people in the United States in 2001 (CDC 2004). Suicide rates are generally higher than the national average in the western states and lower in the eastern states and midwestern states (CDC 1997). In 2002, 132,353 individuals were hospitalized following suicide attempts; 116,639 were treated in emergency departments and released (CDC 2004). In 2001, 55% of suicides were committed with a firearm (Anderson & Smith, 2003; CDC, 1985, retrieved 2/6/2007).

* Groups at Risk: Males: suicide is the eighth leading cause of death for all U.S. men (Anderson & Smith, 2003). Males are four times more likely to die from suicide than females (CDC 2004). Suicide rates are highest among Whites and second highest among American Indian and Native Alaskan men (CDC 2004). Of the 24,672 suicide deaths reported among men in 2001, 60% involved the use of a firearm (Anderson & Smith, 2003). Suicide is the third leading cause of death among young people ages 15 to 24. In 2001, 3,971 suicides were reported in this age group (Anderson & Smith, 2003). Of the total number of suicides among ages 15 to 24 in 2001, 86% (n = 3,409) were male and 14% (n = 562) were female (Anderson & Smith, 2003).*

* A study published in 2004 provided statistical evidence that psychiatric-related emergency department visits, those reflecting any of 3 common psychiatric International Classification of Diseases, Ninth Revision codes for a suicide attempt, increased 15% nationwide, from 3.7 million in 1992 to 4.3 million in 2000, representing 5.4% of all ED visits. In a national survey of 340 emergency physicians conducted by the American College of Emergency Physicians (ACEP), 67% of respondents said mental health services had declined in their community during the previous year, and 60% reported increased pressure on the front line, particularly because psychiatric patients consume*

provider attention, increase patient boarding, and forced ambulance diversions. Between 1997 and 2001, there were an average of 412,000 annual ED visits for suicide attempts and self-inflicted injuries, accounting for 1% of all ED visits. Approximately 70% of all nonfatal self-inflicted injuries treated in the ED are the result of a suicide attempt (Baraff, Janowicz, & Asarnow, 2006).

Suicidal behavior in jail: In most countries, the incidence of suicidal behavior in correctional institutions is higher than in the population at large. In one study, the majority of suicide completers died by hanging; most attempted suicides were performed impulsively by cutting wrists. The incarceration of alcohol and/or drug abusers was a complicating issue (Kerkhof & Bernasco, 1990). Hanging is a common method of committing suicide. In the UK, 1558 suicides by hanging were recorded in 2000 with a male-to-female ratio of approximately 6:1. In the U.S., hanging is the third most common method of suicide after firearms and drugs (Hanna, 2004). Factors related to suicide in New York state prisons are as follows: Mental illness, anxiety, agitation, behavioral change, stressors, history of substance abuse, and non-African-American were important risk factors in several studies (Way, Miraglia, Sawyer, Beer, & Eddy, 2005; Matschnig, Fruhwald, & Frottier, 2006).

CEBM, level 5.

Plan

- Reassure patient that I wish to listen to him to try to understand his needs, regardless of his status.
- Assess for suicidality.
- Place on one-to-one watch, close observation.
- Plan for follow-up care within the context of patient's involuntary status, both as an inmate and following a suicide attempt.
- Request for inpatient hospitalization. I telephone the attending psychiatrist and convey request for admission because of severe depression and suicidality.
- Patient education: I instruct the patient on the need for safe sex practices given his diagnosis of HIV. The patient says he understands the need to use condoms during sex. Patient states he is in a relationship with a woman who is HIV-negative and has shared with her his HIV status.

HIV in correctional facilities: *Approximately 70% of all jail inmates, in 1998, were characterized as being regular drug users, or were incarcerated for committing a drug offense. Inmates who inject drugs are at elevated risk for HIV and AIDS because major risk factors include injection drug use, sharing needles, and/or having unprotected sex, especially with persons who are injection users. The demographic profile of HIV-positive individuals diagnosed in correctional facilities differs from that of other HIV-positive individuals, with more injection drug users, African Americans and younger individuals in jails and prisons than in the HIV positive population outside of corrections (Lyons, Goldstein, & Kiriazes, 2006).*

Epidemiology of HIV/AIDS in correctional facilities: The National Commission on Correctional Health Care estimates that HIV infection rates in jails range between 1.2% and 1.8%, which is between four and five times the U.S. prevalence. Prison rates are higher, with high rates particularly in the northeast. The Centers for Disease Control (CDC) estimates that each year approximately 25% of all people with HIV, 29% of people with hepatitis C, and 16% with hepatitis B pass through a correctional facility.

The CDC has funded voluntary correctional testing and counseling programs in 45 states and municipalities, and the number of tests in this program increased 194% between 1992 and 1998 (Lyons et al., 2006).

CEBM, level 4.

Encounter Two (several hours later in the ED)

- I am called by hospital administration. My request for inpatient admission is denied. Since the patient is incarcerated, he is not entitled to inpatient hospitalization at this community hospital, which is not equipped with a secure psychiatric unit. Because of his inmate status, he will not be permitted to remain in this hospital unless he needs further medical attention. The ED physician's medical evaluation of the patient did not identify a reason for medical admission.
- I inform the patient that it is not possible for him to remain in the ED or the community hospital. The patient pleads with me to admit him to the medical or the psychiatric unit.
- I call the medical director and nurse at the prison and am advised that the only way for him to be admitted to a secure psychiatric facility is to have him return to the jail, where another psychiatric evaluation will be performed, and then he could be transferred to a state facility if it is deemed necessary.
- I discuss the information I received from the medical director and nurse at the prison with the patient. He becomes upset and says he will continue to try to kill himself if I send him back to the jail. I inform him that I have no choice but will request he be placed on one-to-one observation in jail until such time as he can be evaluated for transfer to a state facility.
- I telephone the medical director, nurse, and supervisor at the prison to discuss the plan for the patient, as well as to request one-to-one observation for the patient when he returns to his cell.
- I speak with the correctional officers who escort the patient.

Impression

20-year-old incarnated African American male who has made two serious suicide attempts in the past three weeks and is at high risk for another attempt. Upon being informed that admission to this hospital is being declined, the patient expresses plan to continue to attempt suicide until successful.

Critical Appraisal

I believe the patient would have had closer observation and more humane treatment if he had been directly transferred from this facility and admitted to the state hospital, which has a secure, locked unit where patients who have legal considerations and co-occurring mental illness can be treated.

Plan

- I order quetiapine (Seroquel) 200 mg for anxiety and agitation. The patient has a recent history of benzodiazepine withdrawal from alprazolam three weeks earlier, eliminating the possibility of administering a benzodiazepine for anxiety.
- Discharge medications
  - Fluoxetine (Prozac) 20 mg once daily.
  - Quetiapine (Seroquel) 200 mg twice daily for insomnia or anxiety.
- Discharge patient to the care of guards and return him to the county prison.
- One-to-one close observation status in county prison requested (**D3, C2, PO C, D**).
- Follow-up with mental health services in the county upon discharge from jail, and provide telephone numbers for county services.

COMPETENCY DEFENSE

Domain 1, Competency 3. Formulate differential diagnoses and diagnostic strategies and therapeutic interventions with attention to scientific evidence, safety, cost, invasiveness, simplicity, acceptability, adherence, and efficacy for patients who present with new conditions and those with ambiguous or incomplete data, complex illnesses, comorbid conditions, and multiple diagnoses in all clinical settings.

Defense. Using the *DSM-IV-TR*, this patient meets criteria for major depressive disorder, recurrent and severe. Given his comorbidity of substance abuse (marijuana) and substance dependence (heroin and benzodiazepines), it was important to consider the possibility of a substance-induced mood disorder; however, since his depressive symptoms occurred before onset of substance use, he meets criteria for both major depressive disorder as well as substance use and substance dependence disorders. Taking into account that this patient has multiple Axis I and Axis II disorders, it is critical that he continue to receive psychiatric treatment following hospitalization and throughout the time he serves in prison. Therapeutic interventions are based on the evidence that suicide rates are higher for male patients who have attempted suicide in the past, incarcerated individuals, and those with a co-occurring substance abuse history.

Domain 3, Competency 2. Evaluate gaps in health care access that compromise optimal patient outcomes, and apply current knowledge of the organization and financing of health care systems to ameliorate negative impact.

Defense. Given the patient's involuntary status as an inmate and his serious suicide attempt, special consideration must be given to his right for adequate follow-up treatment. He was denied admission to this hospital because it was not a secure unit; however, this decision does not address his need for close observation and appropriate psychiatric care. This patient would benefit from intensive individual supportive psychotherapy, group therapy, and assessment for response to psychotropic treatment. The difficulty of ensuring adequate follow-up care for an inmate after discharge from an ED is one of the clinical issues that has raised ethical issues for me as well.

Although I contacted the supervisor at the prison, I felt that there were gaps in this patient's care for which I was unable to provide sufficient interventions. I requested he be transferred to a secure mental health facility; however, once he was discharged from the ED, I was no longer able to manage his care. I felt it was important to document my treatment decisions and recommendations and include them in his discharge summary.

Medications

Drug: Fluoxetine (Prozac)

Dose: 20 mg.

Method of administration in this case: Oral.

Mechanism of action: Selective serotonin reuptake inhibitor (SSRI). In the absence of pharmacologic manipulation, the reuptake of 5-HT into the presynaptic nerve terminal typically leads to its inactivation. Fluoxetine, by blocking the reuptake process, acutely enhances serotonergic neurotransmission by permitting 5-HT to act for an extended period of time at synaptic binding sites. A net result is an acute increase in synaptic 5-HT. Placebo-controlled, double-blind trials have established the superiority of fluoxetine over placebo (Kasper et al., 1992). Statistically significant reductions from baseline in the Hamilton Rating Scale for Depression (Ham-D) score have been seen as early as the second week of treatment; however, the rate of response to any SSRI are highly individualized. Although fluoxetine is perceived as "activating," considerable evidence supports its utility in depression with anxious features (Schatzberg & Nemeroff, 2004).

Side effects: Nausea, insomnia, weakness.

Drug: Quetiapine (Seroquel)

Dose: 200 mg twice daily.

Method of administration in this case: Oral.

(continued)

Mechanism of action

Quetiapine for schizophrenia: Second-generation antipsychotic or atypical antipsychotic, quetiapine is a dibenzothiazepine derivative. It received approval by the U.S. FDA in September 1997 for the treatment of schizophrenia. Quetiapine has low to moderate affinity for dopamine-2 (D2) receptors and moderate to high affinity for serotonin-2 (5-HT2) receptors. Inhibition of serotonin activity in the nigrostriatal dopaminergic pathway results in greater activity of A9 dopamine (DA) cells, which is believed to override the blockade of D2 receptors and prevent extrapyramidal side effects (EPS). The lack of substantial or sustained increase in prolactin is likely less due to 5-HT inhibition than to the low D2 affinity of quetiapine (Schatzberg & Nemeroff, 2004).

Quetiapine for anxiety symptoms: Treatment for resistant unipolar depression includes augmentation of antidepressant therapy with a nonantidepressant drug, including the atypical antipsychotics. Olanzapine (Zyprexa) in combination with fluoxetine is safe and effective in patients with bipolar depression and those with fluoxetine-resistant unipolar depression. Risperidone (Risperdal) is effective in combination with fluvoxamine (Luvox), paroxetine (Paxil), or citalopram (Celexa) in treat-resistant unipolar depression, with reported remission rates of 61 to 76 percent. Ziprasidone (Geodon) and aripiprazole (Abilify) augmentation of various SSRIs has been reported to be effective in refractory unipolar depression in open-label studies. Data on use of quetiapine or clozapine (Leponex) as augmentation therapy for depression or anxiety are not yet available (Nemeroff, 2005).

Quetiapine monotherapy: Shows efficacy in treating anxiety symptoms in bipolar I depression; however, studies are still needed to show efficacy in unipolar depression (Hirschfeld, Weisler, Raines, & Macfadden, 2006).

Can we thus extrapolate from this study the applicability of prescribing quetiapine for anxiety in patients with unipolar depression? It is common practice in the ER setting for psychiatrists and psychiatric nurse practitioners to prescribe atypical antipsychotic medication both for anxiety and for sleep, particularly for patients for whom benzodiazepines are not appropriate, such as mentally ill, chemically addicted patients or patients with a history of benzodiazepine dependence.

Most psychiatrists and other physicians routinely prescribe medication for off-label use. Kramer & McCall (2006) suggests seven steps that psychiatrists and other health care providers can use to reduce risk to both the patient and themselves when considering prescribing a medication for off-label use: (1) Be familiar with evidence-based findings and guidelines. (2) Clarify your rationale for off-label prescription. (3) Obtain second-opinion consultation if indicated. (4) Perform risk-benefit analysis. (5) Obtain informed consent from patient or appropriate surrogate. (6) Document steps 1 through 5 in the patient's record. (7) Monitor for known and unexpected adverse advents.

(continued)

Quetiapine and insomnia: Patients with neurologic disorders commonly experience sleep dysfunction and psychiatric disorders. The most common sleep dysfunction is insomnia, which is a primary symptom in 30 to 90 percent of psychiatric disorders. Insomnia and fatigue are prominent symptoms of anxiety disorders and major depression, including patients who are treated but have residual symptoms. Anxiety and depressive disorders account for 40 to 50 percent of all cases of chronic insomnia. Sedative hypnotic agents are the most studied agents to treat insomnia, particularly those that are active through the benzodiazepine receptor-GABA complex, such as benzodiazepines, eszopiclone (Lunesta), zaleplon (Sonata), and zolpidem (Ambien). Although there has been insufficient research on the use of atypical antipsychotic agents in severe insomnia, psychiatrists use quetiapine, olanzapine, or other agents to lessen agitation that disrupts sleep onset or maintenance (Becker, 2006).

Side effects: Dry mouth, sedation, somnolence, constipation, dizziness, abdominal pain, postural hypotension, weight gain, lethargy, hyperglycemia.

References

American Psychiatric Association. (2000). *Diagnostic and statistical manual of mental disorders* (4th ed., text revision). Washington, DC: Author.

Anderson, R.N., & Smith, B.L. (2003). Deaths: Leading causes for 2001. *National Vital Statistics Reports 2003, 52*(9), 10–86.

Baraff, L.J., Janowicz, B.A., & Asarnow, J.R. (2006). Survey of California emergency departments about practices for management of suicidal patients and resources available for their care. *Annals of Emergency Medicine, 48*(4), 452–458.

Becker, P.M. (2006). Treatment of sleep dysfunction and psychiatric disorders. *Current Treatment Options in Neurology, 8*(5), 367–375.

Centers for Disease Control and Prevention (CDC). (1985). National Center for Injury Prevention and Control. *Suicide surveillance, 1970–1980.* Retrieved February 6, 2007, from www.cdc.gov

Hanna, S.J. (2004). A study of 13 cases of near-hanging presenting to an accident and emergency department. *INJURY, International Journal of the Care of the Injured, 35,* 253–256.

Hirschfeld, R.M., Weisler, R.H., Raines, S.R., & Macfadden, W.; for the BOLDER Study Group. (2006). Quetiapine in the treatment of anxiety in patients with bipolar I or II depression: A secondary analysis from a randomized, double-blind placebo-controlled study. *Journal of Clinical Psychiatry, 67*(3), 355–362.

Kasper, S., Fuger, J., Moller, H.J. (1992). Comparative efficacy of antidepressants. *Drugs, 43* (Suppl 2:11–22; discussion 22–3).

Kerkhof, A.J., & Bernasco, W. (1990). Suicidal behavior in jails and prisons in the Netherlands: Incidence, characteristics, and prevention. *Suicide and Life Threatening Behaviors, 20*(2), 123–137.

Kramer, S.I., & McCall, W.V. (2006). Off-label prescribing: 7 steps for safer, more effective treatment. *Current Psychiatry, 5*(4), 14–28.

Lyons, T., Goldstein, P., & Kiriazes, J. (2006). HIV in correctional facilities: Role of self-report in case identification. *AIDS Patient Care and STDs, 20*(2), 93–96.

Mahoney, J.S., Carlson, E., & Engebretson, J.C. (2006). A framework for cultural competence in advanced practice psychiatric and mental health education. *Perspectives in Psychiatric Care, 42*(4), 227–237.

Matschnig, T., Fruhwald, S., & Frottier, P. (2006). Suicide behind bars—an international review. *Psychiatrische Praxis, 33*(1), 6–13.

Nemeroff, C.B. (2005). Use of atypical antipsychotics in refractory depression and anxiety. *Journal of Clinical Psychiatry, 66*(Suppl 8), 13–21.

Sadock, B.J., & Sadock, V.A. (2003). *Kaplan and Sadock's synopsis of psychiatry. Behavioral sciences/clinical psychiatry* (9th ed.). Philadelphia: Lippincott Williams & Wilkins.

Schatzberg, A.F., & Nemeroff, C.B. (2004). *The American Psychiatric Publishing textbook of psychopharmacology* (3rd ed.). Washington, DC: American Psychiatric Publishing.

Way, B.B., Miraglia, R., Sawyer, D.A., Beer, R., & Eddy, J. (2005). Factors related to suicide in New York state prisons. *International Journal of Law Psychiatry, 28*(3), 207–221.

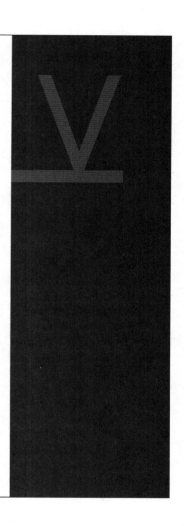

DNP Approach and Clinical Case Narratives in Adult Care

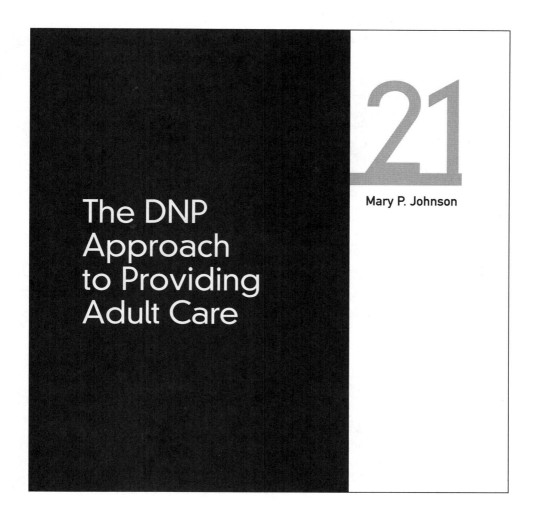

21

Mary P. Johnson

The DNP Approach to Providing Adult Care

THE NEED FOR COMPREHENSIVE CROSS-SITE CARE FOR ADULTS

The DNP provides comprehensive, cross-site care to adult patients, a role not always associated with advanced practice nursing. With the changing demography and advances in clinical care and in innovative diagnostic and treatment strategies, care of late adolescent, adult, and geriatric age groups increasingly blends, continuing to evolve and become more complex. This invites and requires coordination of comprehensive, cross-site chronic and acute care for this expanded age demographic.

As the population ages, patients are living with multiple comorbidities and serious illnesses. Multiple comorbidities carry overlapping and interacting treatments and often require extensive use of specialists and subspecialists. This can result in conflicts and gaps in treatment regimens.

Never has the need for a comprehensive, cross-site provider been more acute. Patients are navigating a complicated health care system. Assistance and advocacy can be fragmented or nonexistent. The DNP in adult care must be expert at coordinating the services and ensuring that the patient's status and record are communicated effectively, accurately, and in a timely fashion. The DNP oversees and manages the elaborate systems of care. The DNP must be a facilitator in directing care across settings (inpatient, ambulatory, rehabilitation, and long-term care) and in effectively transitioning patients from one level of care to another as indicated by patient need. The stability, acuity, and complexity of the patient's health status determine where care is best provided.

DNP APPROACH IN THE ACUTE CARE SETTING

The DNP manages and co-manages care in the emergency department (ED) and other acute care settings to provide the patient with continuity of care. The DNP strives to ensure that the inpatient teams of providers are in synchrony and that all aspects of patient care are addressed.

DNPs treat patients with complex comorbid conditions in specialty services such as acute coronary service, stroke service, liver transplant, cardiac surgery, orthopedics, and neurosurgery. Their educational preparation is ideally suited to provide comprehensive, coordinated care for patients who often have five or more specialist clinicians caring for their organ-specific conditions.

Hospital Admission

When admitting the patient to the hospital, in the acute care setting the DNP demonstrates effective communication with all involved parties, which has a significant impact on the patient's experience and eventual outcome. All team members need to be included in communication at the time of hospital admission. This includes the patient's primary care provider, specialty consultants, the hospital team members, informal caregivers, and family members who the patient requests receive information. By giving advance notice to the providers who need to be involved in the patient's hospital stay and discharge, the patient receives optimal care in a timely manner.

Hospital Admission Note

The DNP may write the hospital admission note, which includes the standard sections of a comprehensive history and physical examination. It should include all pertinent information about the patient, presented in a logical and organized format.

The chief complaint (CC) is the patient's stated reason for coming to the hospital. A direct quote should be used when possible. It is important to note discrepancies between the patient's reason for admission and what the provider believes is the reason for admission. A discrepancy could unveil several issues, including patient confusion, possible psychiatric disorder, or simply poor communication among providers regarding the rationale for hospital admission. It is important to remember that open, honest communication regarding diagnoses and treatment plans must be provided to the patient throughout the hospital course.

The history of present illness (HPI) should flow as a chronologic narrative that begins with the onset of the current problem and describes how the problem has subsequently evolved. The medical history section lists the current medical problems that may now be stable, past medical problems not already discussed in the HPI, and the patient's medications, allergies, surgeries, hospitalizations, and blood transfusions. Travel history should also be included if relevant. Psychosocial history includes questions about finance, family, career, lifestyle, and stressors. This section can include habits such as tobacco, alcohol use, illicit drug use, nutrition and physical activity. The review of systems provides the opportunity to elicit information about general health status not reported in the previous section, as the information does not directly pertain to the patient's reason for hospitalization.

The admission physical examination is completed according to institutional protocol and patient level of acuity. This is followed by the impression, which succinctly describes the database, differential diagnoses, reason for excluding specific diagnoses, the primary diagnosis, and rationale. If the primary diagnosis is unclear, the potential diagnoses and plan to further elucidate a final diagnosis are presented. The plan of care is derived from the impression and includes diagnostic testing, treatments, medications, specialty consultations, and therapeutic goals.

Hospital Discharge

Comprehensive care requires a plan for hospital discharge that provides continuity of care by bridging the gap between hospital and home. The DNP combines advanced understanding of health care systems with expert knowledge regarding the patient's medical condition and social support system to ensure a seamless transition from hospital to home, long-term care, and/or rehabilitation setting. Studies have shown reduced length of stay and overall cost of hospitalization as well as a decrease in hospital readmissions when nurse practitioners are involved in the management of hospitalized patients (Christmas et al., 2005; Kaluski et al., 2008; Naylor, 2004; Wood & Hurley, 2007).

Discharge needs should be anticipated throughout the hospitalization. Evaluation of patient's home environment and support networks are a key part of this. The DNP reinforces the need for early and thorough education throughout the hospital stay. For example, the patient placed on insulin for the first time requires extensive diabetes education throughout the hospitalization with continuous reinforcement of cognitive and psychomotor skills.

Many topics need to be discussed on the day of discharge, such as follow-up appointments and prescriptions. The DNP addresses as many self-care issues as possible prior to the day of discharge. In particular, any tasks the patient or family member will need to perform, such as dressing changes, drainage tube management, and injections, are taught and reinforced prior to the day of discharge. This allows for return demonstration of skill to ensure proper technique and adequate time to provide appropriate support services as needed when the patient returns home.

Social workers are employed in most large urban hospitals and are invaluable members of the team. As part of the referral network, DNPs notify social workers when there is any indication that the patient may need skilled nursing and home health care services upon discharge home. In other situations, the DNP is responsible for coordinating services that will be required in the ambulatory setting. The DNP is responsible for ensuring that the appropriate services have been arranged prior to discharge and completes the discharge summary. DNPs view patients in the context of their illness, environment, and social networks. Patient discharge is approached as a process that can make a significant difference in patient outcomes, well-being, and cost reduction.

Discharge Summary Note

The discharge note is an important document. It is an invaluable resource during the patient's post-hospitalization office visits. Since some ambulatory care providers may not have been involved in the patient's hospital care, the discharge summary serves as a source of accurate data as to what happened during the hospitalization. A formal discharge note is usually required for any admission longer than 24 hours. A guide for the discharge summary note is included in Appendix F.

DNP APPROACH TO PREVENTIVE HEALTH CARE FOR ADULTS

In addition to the increase in complexity and comorbidities, many health problems stem from genetic predisposition, environmental, and lifestyle choices. The DNP conducts a complete health, behavioral, and risk assessment. Utilizing motivational interviewing and shared decision-making, the DNP works with the patient to develop a strategy directed toward primary, secondary, and tertiary prevention (Woolf, Jonas, & Kaplan-Liss, 2008).

Primary prevention refers to measures taken to prevent illness or injury. Preventive care may include examinations and screening tests tailored to an individual's age, health, and family history (Woolf et al., 2008). A detailed health risk assessment is performed by the DNP during a comprehensive evaluation, often in the setting of an annual evaluation. This provides opportunity for identification of the risk associated with genetics and lifestyle, as well as for patient counseling and education to minimize risk and enhance health.

Secondary prevention activities are aimed at early disease detection, thereby increasing opportunities for interventions to prevent progression of the disease and emergence of symptoms (Woolf et al., 2008). DNPs perform a variety of secondary prevention services and refer patients when necessary for advanced imaging modalities and evaluation by a medical specialist.

Tertiary prevention reduces the negative impact of an already established disease by restoring function and reducing disease-related complications (Woolf et al., 2008). This is accomplished in a rehabilitation setting, such as cardiac rehabilitation for the patient who has suffered from a myocardial infarction, or physical and cognitive rehabilitation for an individual who has suffered from a spinal cord injury or stroke. The DNP refers patients for care in these settings and maintains primary responsibility for the patients through communication with consultants to maximize the patients' function and independence, minimize complications, and prepare a plan for return to independent living in the community. For a C5 tetraplegic, this can include assessing the individual for independent driving and evaluating and taking measures to avoid skin breakdown, which allows for opportunistic infection and chronic pain.

THE DNP ROLE IN DISEASE MANAGEMENT

Patients present with a constellation of symptoms requiring critical evaluation by the DNP to determine what diagnostics are required to confirm or refute a suspected diagnosis and direct the plan of care for therapeutics and education. The DNP formulates differential diagnoses, diagnostic strategies, and therapeutic interventions with attention to scientific evidence, safety, cost, invasiveness, adherence, and efficacy. This is done for patients who present with new conditions and those with ambiguous or incomplete data, complex illnesses, comorbid conditions, and multiple diagnoses in all clinical settings. Additionally, DNPs appraise the acuity of the patient's condition, determine the need to transfer the patient to a higher acuity setting, and coordinate and manage transfer to optimize patient outcomes. DNPs utilize shared decision-making in developing a plan of care with the patient that addresses individual needs.

The delivery of high-quality, effective, and cost-efficient health care requires that the DNP understand the sociocultural background of patients, their families, and the environments in which they live (Like, Steiner, & Rubel, 1996). DNPs intervene with clients in culturally sensitive ways, incorporating cultural beliefs into the plan of care and involving the community in preventive health care programs. The DNP is aware of the impact of sociocultural factors on patients, practitioners, the clinical encounter, and interpersonal relationships. DNPs appreciate the heterogeneity that exists within cultural groups and the importance of providing culturally sensitive care to their patients. They work to recognize their own personal biases, to understand and explicate those values, assumptions, and beliefs, and to examine how these assumptions affect the care provided to patients that share or do not share a similar perspective.

THE DNP APPROACH TO COMPREHENISVE ADULT CARE

The challenge of providing comprehensive cross-site care of this magnitude and complexity requires a practitioner who is clinically knowledgeable and has the ability to communicate with patients and other health professionals accurately and with a focus on positive care outcomes. As a comprehensive provider, the DNP bases clinical decisions on the best evidence available and is able to determine if the evidence is applicable to the individual patient. In some cases, care decisions need to be made in the absence of evidence. The DNP in adult care uses critical thinking and clinical judgment at the highest level to integrate biophysical science, clinical evidence, assessment, and communication skills in the context of multiple health care settings.

References

Christmas, A.B., Reynolds, J., Hodges, S., Franklin, G.A., Miller, F.B., Richardson, J.D., & Rodriguez, J.L. (2005). Physician extenders impact trauma systems. *Journal of Trauma Injury Infection and Critical Care, 58,* 917–920.

Kaluski, E., Alfano, D., Randhawa, P., Palmaro, J., Jones, P., Romano, K., Dolny-Korasick, D., & Klapholz, M. (2008). Length of hospital stay after percutaneous coronary interventions. *Journal of Cardiovascular Nursing, 23,* 345–348.

Like, R.C., Steiner, R.P., & Rubel, A.J. (1996). *Recommended core curriculum guidelines on culturally sensitive and competent health care.* Retrieved August 11, 2009, from http://www.stfm .org/group/minority/guidelines.cfm

Naylor, M. (2004). Transitional care of older adults hospitalized with heart failure: A random-ized, controlled trial. *Journal of the American Geriatrics Society, 52,* 675–684.

Wood, C., & Hurley, C. (2007). Retrospective comparison of emergency department length of stay for procedural sedation and analgesia by nurse practitioners and physicians. *Pediatric Emergency Care, 23,* 709–712.

Woolf, S.H., Jonas, S., & Kaplan-Liss, E. (2008). *Health promotion and disease prevention in clinical practice* (2nd ed.). Baltimore: Lippincott Williams & Wilkins.

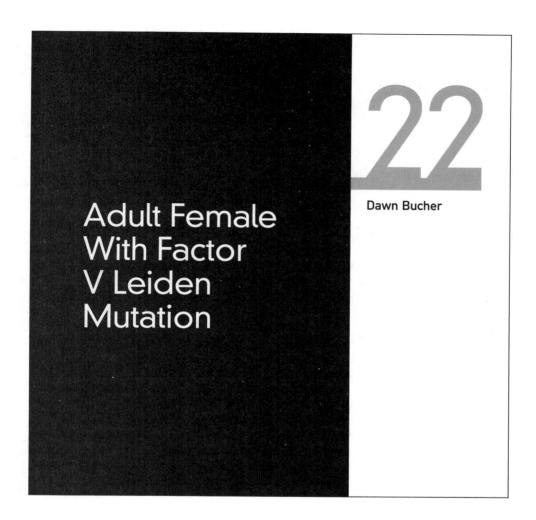

22

Dawn Bucher

Adult Female With Factor V Leiden Mutation

This case narrative describes the care I provided for a Medicaid-insured patient with a genetic condition, my intervention for risk reduction, and a collaborative consultation. The case narrative consists of three encounters and demonstrates my ability to meet the following Columbia University School of Nursing (CUSN) doctoral competencies for comprehensive direct patient care.

DOMAIN 1, COMPETENCY 1

Evaluate patient needs based on age, developmental stage, family history, ethnicity, and individual risk, including genetic profile, to formulate plans for health promotion, anticipatory guidance, counseling, and disease prevention services for healthy or sick patients and their families in any clinical setting.

PO A. Identify a potential genetic risk.
PO B. Diagnose a genetic condition.

PO C. Evaluate individual patient needs based on age, developmental stage, family history, ethnicity, and individual risk.

PO D. Formulate a plan that addresses health promotion, anticipatory guidance, and/or disease prevention for the individual.

PO E. Develop a plan that addresses health promotion, anticipatory guidance, and/or disease prevention for the family.

SUMMARY OF CARE (PROVIDED PRIOR TO THE CASE NARRATIVE)

Patient is a 51-year-old Caucasian female in good health who has received health care in this clinic for 25 years. She lives 30 miles away. My collaborating physician delivered all three of her children, years ago, when this small rural hospital offered delivery services.

ENCOUNTER CONTEXT

Encounter One (annual well-woman comprehensive examination)

DNP role: I am the doctor of nursing practice (DNP) student and certified nurse practitioner.

Identifying Information

Site: Rural health clinic.

Setting: Outpatient, ambulatory care.

Reason for encounter: Annual well-woman examination.

Informant: Patient and medical records. Patient is a 51-year-old female who appears to be a reliable historian.

Chief complaint: "I am here for my yearly gynecological well-woman exam and also have some questions about Factor V mutation."

History of Present Illness (HPI)

"My oldest daughter had her first baby three months ago and developed blood clots in her legs. She was given warfarin (Coumadin) for a short period of time, went off of it, and then developed some small clots in her lungs. She is back on warfarin (Coumadin) and tested positive for the Factor V mutation. She also had a miscarriage one year ago. I remember developing a blood clot after one of my pregnancies and was told it was not uncommon after a delivery. I wonder if I also have the Factor V mutation. Other than that I am feeling very well."

Woman's Health History

This patient is a 51-year-old woman, gravida 3, para 3, abortions 0. Her last menstrual period was 15 days ago. She reports menses every 28 to 30 days with three to four days of moderate flow. Her last Pap smear one year ago showed no dysplastic cells, and she has no history of an abnormal Pap smear. Her last mammogram one year ago showed benign calcifications of the left breast. She performs a self-breast exam monthly and does not note any abnormalities.

She has a history of menometrorrhagia treated with dilatation and curettage at age 35. She also had a tubal ligation at age 35. She reports sleeping well throughout the night, her appetite is normal, she has been exercising, and she has lost a few pounds over the past year. She denies vasomotor changes, night sweats, mood shift, change in self-concept, vaginal dryness, dysuria, or dyspareunia. She reports good sexual function and interest. Patient offers no complaints.

Past Medical History

- Rheumatic fever at age seven, treatment at that time unknown.
- Strep pharyngitis and erythema nodosum at age 35. Patient exhibited rash, fever, fatigue, and joint pains. She was treated symptomatically and with prednisone. She recovered within two months.
- Grade 1 systolic heart murmur with normal echocardiogram initially noted at age 35.
- Mild leukopenia at age 32. Patient asymptomatic, was seen by hematologist, and is monitored yearly, etiology unknown.
- History of iron deficiency anemia secondary to menometrorrhagia, treated with ferrous sulfate and dilation and curettage.
- Denies history of diabetes (DM), hypertension (HTN), myocardial infarction (MI), stroke (CVA), peptic ulcer disorder (PUD), asthma, emphysema, thyroid disease, liver disease, kidney disease, cancer, tuberculosis (TB), hepatitis, and sexually transmitted infection (STIs).

Erythema nodosum (EN) is red or violet subcutaneous nodules that develop on the anterior aspects of legs, but can also be present on the thighs, trunk, and upper extremities (Shojania, 2006).

The majorities of patients with EN have a streptococcal infection or have no identifiable etiology. Polyarthralgias, fever, and malaise are common finding with EN (Gonzalez-Gay, Garcia-Porrua, Pujol, & Salvarani, 2001).
Oxford Centre for Evidenced-Based Medicine (CEBM), level 5.

Past Surgical History

Tonsillectomy and adenoidectomy during childhood.
Tubal ligation at age 35.
Scalp laceration repaired with staples at age 38, due to a softball injury. No sequelae or other problems due to injury.

Current Health Status

Medications: None.

Dietary supplement: Multivitamin with iron by mouth daily.

Allergies: Penicillin allergy noted by rash. No known allergies to foods or environmental products.

Psychosocial History

Employment: She currently is working full-time in a grocery store.

Family: Patient has been married for 30 years. Husband is employed at local fertilizer plant.

Religious affiliation: Lutheran.

Alcohol: Socially consumes alcohol, approximately five times annually.

Tobacco and drugs: Never smoked cigarettes or used illegal drugs.

Caffeine: Occasional consumption of coffee. She does not drink tea.

Diet: Her appetite is good. She has lost three pounds over the last year by choice. She would like to lose more weight. She eats three meals per day and reports a variety selection of foods, including fruits, vegetables, meats, dairy products, and carbohydrates. She is not on a special diet.

Exercise: She has increased activity over the past year. She has been walking to and from work instead of driving.

Sleep patterns: Sleeps well, all night for at least eight hours.

Leisure: Enjoys spending time with family and friends, and loves to cook.

Safety measures: Uses seat belts all the time, smoke detectors installed in new home eight months ago. She knows to test smoke detectors every six months.

According to the United States Preventive Services Task Force (USPSTF) guidelines (2006), pelvic and Pap smear should be done every three years after having three normal (negative) Pap smear reports. Pap smears may be discontinued at age 65 unless high risk (frequent positive pap smears or previous cervical cancer). This patient has had a Pap/pelvic exam every year.

USPSTF also recommends yearly mammograms after age 50 and sexually transmitted infection (STI) screening if patient is at high risk (adolescent, prior STI, high prevalence, or multiple partners). Patient's last mammogram was last year and STI screening in 1985 (age 30), which predates the recommendations of the USPSTF.

Osteoporosis screening, based on USPSTF recommendations, should be done on all women over age 65 and in high-risk females at age 60 (smokers, weight <70 kg, family history, and/or alcohol use). This patient has never had an osteoporosis screening test, nor does she have a family history of osteoporosis or other risk factors.

Health Maintenance Review	Recommendation	Last Performed
Regular health exam	Annual	One year ago
Blood pressure	Annual	One year ago
Cholesterol	Every five years if in desired range	One year ago
Fasting glucose	Based on clinical judgment, recommended especially in adults with hypertension or hyperlipidemia	Three years ago
Mammography and clinical breast exam	Annual	One year ago
Pap smear	Every two to three years	One year ago
Pelvic examination	Annual	One year ago
Chlamydia screen	Under the age 24	Age 31
Colorectal cancer screening and fecal occult blood testing (FOBT)	Age 50 with average risk	Not done
Hearing screening	Periodic screening as indicated	Not indicated as she does not have hearing problems
Eye examination	Every two to four years between ages 40 and 54	One year ago
Bone mineral density	Age 65	Not indicated
PPD	Indicated in high-risk population or with occupational exposure	Never

USPSTF strongly recommends colorectal cancer screening for men and women 50 years of age or older. This patient has not had a colorectal cancer screen to date.

CEBM, level 5.

Immunization	Recommendation	Status
Tetanus	Td every 10 years, substitute one dose of Tdap	15 years ago
Measles-mumps-rubella	One dose recommended if another risk factor is present and lack evidence of immunity	Childhood illness
Varicella	Two doses recommended to all who lack evidence of immunity	Childhood illness
Influenza	Yearly greater than age 50	One year ago
Pneumococcal	One or two doses recommended if another risk factor is present	Never
Hepatitis B vaccine	Three doses recommended if another risk factor is present	Never

According to the CDC Adult Immunization Schedule (2006), Td booster is needed every 10 years; influenza every year, pneumococcal one dose after age 65 or younger in high-risk populations (chronic lung disease, CVD, DM, chronic liver disease, asplenia, etc.); Hep B vaccine series in patients with medical, behavioral, or occupational indications (asplenia, DM, chronic liver disease, COPD, heart disease, renal failure, HIV, malignancies); PPD to all patients at high risk (close contacts of persons with TB, HIV patients, illicit drug use, health care workers, foreign-born persons if immigrated within last 5 years from high prevalence country, medical underserved, low-income populations, nursing home residents, DM, renal disease, malignancies, silicosis, malabsorptive disease, GI cancers, immunosuppression).

CEBM, level 5.

Family History

Patient's parents, brother, sister, and youngest daughter have not been tested for Factor V Leiden deficiency. She denies family history of cancer, mental illness, diabetes, rheumatism, gout, goiter, obesity, nephritis, epilepsy, or drug addictions. No consanguinity.

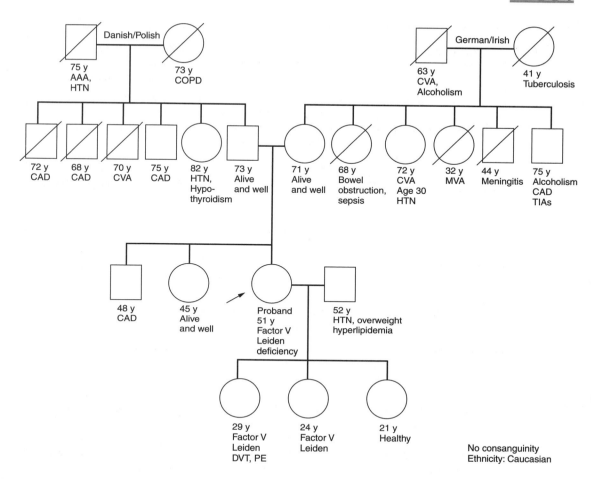

Danish/Polish	**German/Irish**

75 y
AAA,
HTN

73 y
COPD

63 y
CVA,
Alcoholism

41 y
Tuberculosis

72 y
CAD

68 y
CAD

70 y
CVA

75 y
CAD

82 y
HTN,
Hypo-
thyroidism

73 y
Alive
and well

71 y
Alive
and well

68 y
Bowel
obstruction,
sepsis

72 y
CVA
Age 30
HTN

32 y
MVA

44 y
Meningitis

75 y
Alcoholism
CAD
TIAs

48 y
CAD

45 y
Alive
and well

Proband
51 y
Factor V
Leiden
deficiency

52 y
HTN, overweight
hyperlipidemia

29 y
Factor V
Leiden
DVT, PE

24 y
Factor V
Leiden

21 y
Healthy

No consanguinity
Ethnicity: Caucasian

Review of Systems

General health: Denies fatigue, weakness, fever, chills, or night sweats.

Skin: Denies hair loss, nail changes, skin rash, itching, sores, lumps, or moles.

Head: Denies headache.

Eyes: Denies blurred vision, double vision. Last eye exam one year ago was normal without need for corrective lenses.

Ears: Denies ear pain, hearing loss, or neck pain.

Nose: Denies rhinorrhea or congestion.

Mouth and throat: Denies bleeding gums, hoarseness, sore throat, dysphagia. Last dental exam: one year ago with no cavities.

Neck: Denies lumps, swollen glands, goiter, pain, or stiffness.

Breast: Denies breast lumps, breast pain or discomfort, or nipple discharge. Self-breast exam monthly.

Respiratory: Denies shortness of breath, wheezing, cough, hemoptysis, asthma, or tuberculosis. Reports having "walking" pneumonia in her teens. Last chest x-ray 17 years ago was unremarkable.

Cardiovascular: History of rheumatic fever at age seven. It is not known if this was treated at time of diagnosis; history of Grade 1 systolic heart murmur; denies chest pains, palpitations, angina, dyspnea on exertion, orthopnea, edema, or hypertension. Last echocardiogram was within normal limits in 1990.

Gastrointestinal: Reports "good appetite"; denies nausea, vomiting, dysphagia, or indigestion. Reports bowel movement daily; denies diarrhea, hemorrhoids, melena, abdominal pain, jaundice, or hepatitis. Reports occasional constipation with iron supplements.

Gynecologic: See HPI.

Urinary: Denies urgency, frequency, or burning with urination. Denies polyuria, dysuria, hematuria, nocturia, incontinence, stones, or infections.

Endocrine: Denies polydipsia, polyphagia, temperature intolerance, hormone therapy, changes in hair and skin texture. Patient states she had thyroid-stimulating hormone (TSH) level evaluated one year ago with a normal result.

Musculoskeletal: Denies joint pain, stiffness, swelling, or redness. Denies muscle weakness, decreased range of motion, arthritis, or gout. Reports history of erythema nodosum at age 35, denies any residual effects.

Peripheral vascular: Reports history of blood clot in left leg after one of her pregnancies 28 years ago. Reports varicose veins bilaterally. Denies leg edema or claudication.

Hematologic: History of iron deficiency anemia secondary to menometrorrhagia. Denies transfusions, purpura, petechiae, or bruising.

Neurologic: Denies tremors, fainting, or blackouts. Denies numbness, tingling, or loss of sensation. Denies weakness or paralysis or history of seizures.

Psychiatric: Denies depression, anxiety, tension, or memory problems.

Physical Examination

General: Well-developed middle-aged white female in no acute distress, appears stated age.

Vital signs: 5'10," 166 ¾ lb, BMI = 24.0 = healthy, blood pressure 120/75, pulse 76, respiratory rate 20, SaO_2 98% room air.

Skin: Warm, dry, pink, intact without rashes.

HEENT:

Head: Normocephalic, no evidence of trauma.
Eyes: PERRLA, EOMI.
Ears: Symmetrical without bloody discharge.

Nose: Symmetrical, no deviation or inflammation. No bloody discharge.
Mouth and throat: No erythema or exudates. Teeth in good repair.

Neck: Supple, no thyromegaly or adenopathy, no masses or tracheal deviation.

Chest: Clear bilaterally without wheezing or rhonchi; respirations unlabored without use of accessory muscles.

Heart: Regular rate and rhythm, Grade 1/6 systolic murmur audible over pulmonary valve, right second intercostal space that goes away when she lies down in left lateral decubitus position.

Breast: No tenderness, masses, nipple discharge, or dimpling present.

Abdomen: Soft, nontender, no masses or hepatosplenomegaly; bowel sounds active in four quadrants; no costovertebral angle tenderness.

Pelvic: No vaginal lesions or discharge; no cervical motion tenderness; uterus retroflexed; no adnexal masses or tenderness; Pap smear obtained.

Rectal: Sphincter tone intact, no masses, occult stool blood negative.

Musculoskeletal: Moves all extremities without difficulty. No weakness or muscle atrophy. No swelling or redness of joints; gait stable; reflexes 2+ equal bilaterally.

Peripheral/vascular: No peripheral edema present. Mild varicose veins in lower mid-inner calves bilaterally; no carotid bruits audible bilaterally; peripheral pulses palpable, equal bilaterally.

Lymphatic: No cervical, intraclavicular, axillary, or inguinal adenopathy palpable.

Neurologic: Cranial nerves II–XII intact; gait steady; reflexes equal +2 bilaterally in upper and lower extremities.

Critical Appraisal

Although the USPSTF guidelines recommend Pap smears every three years after three consecutive normal Pap smears and this patient has had three normal Pap smears consecutively, our clinic continues to do yearly Pap smears on patients until age 65. I plan to begin discussion to establish protocol that adheres to guideline recommendations.

Impression

51-year-old Caucasian female in good health who presents to the clinic for a yearly comprehensive physical and gynecologic exam. Concern for Factor V Leiden mutation is raised due to daughter's recent diagnosis. Patient has a remote history of DVT, menometrorrhagia, and positive family history of Factor V Leiden mutation, and an aunt who had a stroke in her thirties. Genetic testing is indicated to determine if patient has an inherited thrombophilia.

Health Maintenance Needs

- Immunization for hepatitis B, influenza, and tetanus booster.
- Health screening.
  - Mammogram today because this patient is 51 years old and her last screening mammogram was last year.
  - Colonoscopy is scheduled for patient because she is 51 years old and she has not been screened.
  - Pap smear as per individual clinic guideline.
  - Influenza vaccine in one month is recommended because the flu vaccine is not available and it is not flu season yet.
  - Hepatitis B series is discussed with patient, and she will start series today because she resides in an underserved medical area and has a history of rheumatic heart disease.
  - Tetanus booster today because it has been more than 10 years since her last booster.

ICD-9 Codes

Well-woman gynecological exam (v72.3)
Perimenopause (9627.0)
History of rheumatic fever (398.90)
Family history of Factor V (Leiden) mutation (289.81)

Plan

Therapeutic Interventions
- Continue with current medication.
- Multivitamin with iron one table by mouth daily to prevent recurrence of iron deficiency anemia.

Health Care Maintenance
- Mammogram today.
- Colonoscopy screening scheduled next month at outside facility.
- Influenza immunization next month; recommended because the flu vaccine is not in yet and it is not flu season yet.
- Hepatitis B first immunization today; second immunization due in one to two months; third immunization due in six months.
- Pregenetic counseling for Factor V Leiden mutation performed to educate patient on possible positive test, what a positive test would mean, and to assess patient's perception and knowledge. The patient asked a few questions about Factor V Leiden mutation, but had done research prior to visit.

She was not anxious about the testing. She just wanted to know if her daughter inherited the mutation from her or her husband **(D1, C1, PO A, C, D).**

- Continue with diet and exercise wellness regimen.
- Adult tetanus today.
- Review results of CBC, ESR, Pipids, and BMP performed earlier today as per protocol.

Follow-up
- Will notify patient of test results.

> *According to the USPSTF Preventative Screening guidelines (2006), mammograms are recommended yearly at the age of 50.*
>
> *USPTF guidelines recommend begin screening for colorectal cancer at age 50.*
>
> *Adult Td was administered because the patient has not had a booster since 1989. According to the USPTF guidelines (2006), Td boosters are recommended every 10 years.*
>
> CEBM, level 5.

Encounter Two (telephone consultation one week after appointment)

I call the patient to notify her of her test results. Pap smear is negative for intraepithelial lesion or malignancy. Factor V mutation is positive for one copy of heterozygous R506Q (Factor V Leiden) mutation. I request patient to return to clinic to discuss the results.

> *Factor V Leiden is the most common cause of inherited thrombophilia. This hereditary blood coagulation disorder is found in 5% of Caucasians and 1.2% of African American population (De Stefano, Rossi, Za, & Leone, 2006; FVL, 2006). This disorder is associated with deep vein thrombosis, superficial thrombophlebitis, sinus vein thrombosis, mesenteric vein thrombosis, and Budd-Chiari syndrome (thrombosis in liver veins), pulmonary embolism, strokes, heart attacks, still birth or unexplained miscarriage, and/or preeclampsia/eclampsia (FVL, 2006). Risk of venous thromboembolism is increased 5–7 fold in patients with heterozygous form of factor V Leiden and 25 to 50 fold in patients with the homozygous form (Spencer, 2006). Screening in the general population is not recommended, but is recommended in patients with a family history of venous thromboembolism (De Stefano, 2006). Knowing that a patient has a factor V Leiden mutation is important for future care to prevent any thrombolytic events and to detect thrombolytic events early.*
>
> CEBM, level 5.

Laboratory Study	Result	Reference Range
WBC	4.8	4.1–10.9
Lym	1.4	0.6–4.1
Mid	0.8	0.0–1.8
Gran	4.6	2.0–7.8
HGB	12.8	12.0–18.0
HCT	36.4 Red cell indices and platelets normal	37.0–51.0
Urinalysis	Normal	Normal
ESR	18	0–30
Cholesterol	169	< 200
Triglycerides	49	< 150
HDL	68	> 45
LDL	91	< 130
Glucose	93	65–99
BUN	16	7–25
Creatinine	0.8	0.5–1.2
Sodium	136	135–145
Potassium	4.5	3.5–5.3
Calcium	9.5	8.5–10.4
Factor V mutation	Positive for one copy of heterozygous R506Q	Negative

Encounter Three (two weeks since comprehensive annual examination)

Patient presents to the clinic for discussion of laboratory results. This is a counseling visit. Patient reports feeling well and offers no complaints.

Impression

51-year-old Caucasian female in good health returns to discuss all laboratory results. We specifically focus our discussion on Factor V Leiden mutation. Testing is positive for one copy of the R506Q, Factor V Leiden mutation. The patient is not surprised to learn she has this disorder, nor is she upset. She wants to learn more about the disorder and ways to prevent venous thromboembolism (VTE) **(D1, C1, PO B)**.

Plan

Counseling
- We discuss positive Factor V Leiden results.

The literature reports that long-term therapy to prevent recurrence depends on the number of recurrences, the number of thrombophilic defects found, and patient preferences (Bauer, 2006).

Two large prospective studies found the incidence of venous thromboembolism in asymptomatic relatives with Factor V Leiden was low and in the European Prospective Cohort on Thrombophilia, the incidence among carriers were no different from that of controls (Middeldorp et al., 1998; Simioni et al., 2002; Vossen et al., 2005). According to the literature, studies have argued against long-term use of warfarin after a first thromboembolic event in patients with inherited thrombophilia. It was reported that the risk of death from hemorrhage would exceed the number of fatal pulmonary emboli with chronic warfarin therapy (Baglin et al., 1998). According to Christiansen et al. (2005), the risk of recurrent venous thrombosis in patients who developed their first deep vein thrombosis was similar to those without an inherited Factor V Leiden mutation.

CEBM, level 2b.

According to De Stefano et al. (2006), health care providers must balance risk and benefits of prophylactic treatment in patients with inherited thrombophilia, along with shared decision-making with the patient.

CEBM, level 5.

- I counsel the patient to avoid hormone replacement therapy (HRT) during menopause **(D1, C1, PO D).**

HRT is contraindicated in patients with a past history of venous thromboembolism. Women with a history of VTE who are receiving HRT have 8.5% per year risk of developing another VTE in comparison to placebo (1.1% risks) (Hoibraaten et al., 2000).

CEBM, level 1b.

- We discuss implications of this inherited disease for patient's daughters. Two of the three daughters have been tested for Factor V Leiden, and both of the daughters tested positive. These two daughters should never use oral contraceptives. The one daughter who has had two episodes of VTE should be on long-term warfarin therapy. For the daughter who has not been pregnant, I recommend she see her primary care provider and discuss the recommendation for clinical surveillance and the use of graduated compression stockings for prevention of VTE during pregnancy (De Stefano et al., 2006). I suggest that the youngest daughter, who is 21 years old and not taking oral contraceptives, see her primary care provider for Factor V Leiden testing **(D1, C1, PO E).**
- I recommend that any other relatives, brother, sister, and parents be tested for this genetic disorder **(D1, C1, PO E).**
- I discuss signs and symptoms of VTE and the need to call me immediately if any of the signs or symptoms are present.
- Factor V Leiden disorder handouts and written instructions are given **(D1, C1, PO D, E).**

Critical Appraisal

After discussing this case with my collaborating physician, we decide to recommend that this patient start on a baby acetylsalicylic acid (Aspirin) and clopidogrel (Plavix). Although the literature does not support or discuss the use of acetylsalicylic acid (Aspirin) and/or clopidogrel (Plavix), it is recommended by my collaborating physician because of the patient's history of rheumatic heart disease and increased risk of heart disease. This was discussed with the patient, and she agreed to treatment.

There is no evidence-based study in the literature regarding the use of Aspirin and clopidogrel prophylactically for inherited thrombophilia. The use of these two medications was based on the patient's history and shared decision-making.

Bauer, Leung, & Landaw (2009) recommend oral anticoagulants for a minimum of six to twelve months for patients with venous thromboembolism and an inherited thrombophilia. However, for patients who are at high risk for spontaneous thrombosis along with inherited thrombophilia, Bauer and colleagues recommend oral anticoagulation indefinitely. Scientific studies are lacking in the long-term management of patients with inherited thrombophilia who have had venous thrombosis and of patients exposed to the increased risk associated with pregnancy and surgery. There are only general guidelines for providers to use when treating such patients.

CEBM, level 5.

Medications (see Medications list at the end of chapter)

- Acetylsalicylic acid (Aspirin) 81 mg daily by mouth.
- Clopidogrel (Plavix) 75 mg daily by mouth.

Follow-up

- As needed.
- As scheduled for immunization series.
- Comprehensive health review in one year.
- Factor V Leiden: She is very comfortable calling the clinic with any questions. She is encouraged to do so at any time.

COMPETENCY DEFENSE

Domain 1, Competency 1. Evaluate patient needs based on age, developmental stage, family history, ethnicity, and individual risk, including genetic profile, to formulate plans for health promotion, anticipatory guidance, counseling, and disease prevention services for healthy or sick patients and their families in any clinical setting.

Defense. This competency is met by identifying a potential risk and confirming diagnosis of Factor V Leiden mutation. I develop a plan focusing on health promotion, anticipatory guidance, and disease prevention designed to meet the individual needs of this patient in the context of family and geographic location.

Medications

Drug: Acetylsalicylic Acid (Aspirin)

Dose: 81 mg daily.

Method of administration in this case: By mouth.

Mechanism of action: Inhibits prostaglandin synthesis, acts on the hypothalamus heat-regulating center to reduce fever, blocks prostaglandin synthetase action, which prevents formation of the platelet-aggregating substance thromboxane A2.

Clinical uses: Treatment of mild to moderate pain, inflammation, and fever; may be used as prophylaxis of myocardial infarction, stroke, and/or transient ischemic episodes; management of rheumatoid arthritis, rheumatic fever, osteoarthritis, and gout.

Side effects
Common: Tinnitus, hearing loss, nausea, GI distress, occult bleeding, dyspepsia, leucopenia, prolonged bleeding time, rash.
Serious: GI bleeding, thrombocytopenia, anaphylaxis, Reye's syndrome.

Drug: Clopidogrel (Plavix)

Dose: 75 mg daily.

Method of administration in this case: By mouth.

Mechanism of action: Platelet aggregation inhibitor.

Clinical uses: Reduction of atherosclerotic events in recent MI or stroke, peripheral arterial disease, non-ST-segment elevation acute coronary syndrome, or ST-segment elevation acute MI.

Side effects
Common: Bleeding, GI upset or ulcers, bruising, rash, pruritus, dizziness, headache.
Rare: Thrombotic thrombocytopenic purpura, neutropenia, agranulocytosis.

References

Baglin, C., Brown, K., Luddington, R., & Baglin, T. (1998). Risk of recurrent venous thromboembolism in patients with the factor V Leiden (FVR506Q) mutation: Effect of warfarin and prediction by precipitating factors. East Anglian Thrombophilia Study Group. *British Journal of Haematology, 100*(4), 764–768.

Bauer, K.A. (2006). *Management of inherited thrombophilia*. Retrieved November 18, 2006, from http://www.utdol.com/utd/content/topic.do?topicKey=coagulat/7802&view=print

Bauer, K.A., Leung, L.L.K., & Landaw, S.A. (2009). *Management of inherited thrombophilia*. Retrieved June 18, 2009, from http://12.130.132.45/online/content/topic.do?topicKey=coagulat/7820&voew=print

Centers for Disease Control and Prevention (CDC). (2006). *Recommended adult immunization schedule*. Retrieved October 21, 2006, from http://www.cdc.gov/nip/recs/adult.schedule.htm

Christiansen, S.C., Cannegieter, S.C., Koster, T., Van Der Broucke, J.P., & Rosendaal, F.R. (2005). Thrombophilia, clinical factors, and recurrent venous thrombotic events. *Journal of the American Medical Association, 293*(19), 2352–2361.

De Stefano, V., Rossi, E., Za, T., & Leone, G. (2006). Prophylaxis and treatment of venous thromboembolism in individuals with inherited thrombophilia. *Seminars in Thrombosis and Hemostasis, 32*(8), 767–780.

FVL. (2006). *Thrombophilia support page. Living with thrombophilia*. Retrieved December 16, 2006, from www.fvleiden.org

Gonzalez-Gay, M.A., Garcia-Porrua, C., Pujol, R.M., & Salvarani, C. (2001). Erythema nodosum: A clinical approach. *Clinical and Experimental Rheumatology, 19*(4), 365–368.

Hoibraaten, E., Qvigstad, E., & Arnesen, H. (2000). Increased risk of recurrent venous thromboembolism during hormone replacement therapy. Results of the randomized, double-blind, placebo controlled estrogen in venous thromboembolism trial (EVTET). *Thrombosis and Haemostasis, 84*(5), 961–969.

Middeldorp, S., Henkens, C.M., Koopman, M.M., van Pampus, E.C., Hamulyak, K., van de Meer, J., Prins, M.H., & Buller, H.R. (1998). The incidence of venous thromboembolism in family members of patients with factor V Leiden mutation and venous thrombosis. *Annals of Internal Medicine, 128*(1), 15–20.

Shojania, K.G. (2006). *Erythema nodosum*. Retrieved November 18, 2006, from http://utdol.com/utd/content/topic.do?topicKey=othrheum/6877&view=print

Simioni, P., Tormene, D., Prandoni, P., Zerbinati, P., Gavasso, S., Cefalo, P., & Girolami, A. (2002). Incidence of venous thromboembolism in asymptomatic family members who are carriers of factor V Leiden: A prospective cohort study. *Blood, 99*(6), 1938–1942.

Spencer, C. (2006). About factor V Leiden. *Nursing, 36*(12), 70.

USPSTF. (2006). *Guide to clinical preventative services*. Retrieved October 18, 2006, from http://www.ahrq.gov/clinic/pocketgd/gcps2.htm

Vossen, C.Y., Conard, J., Fontcuberta, J., Makris, M., van der Meer, F.J., Pabinger, I., Palareti, G., Preston, F.E., Scharrer, I., Souto, J.C., Svensson, P., Walker, I.D., & Rosendaal, F.R. (2005). Risk of first venous thrombotic event in carriers of a familial thrombophilic defect. The European Prospective Cohort on Thrombophilia (EPCOT). *Journal of Thrombosis and Haemostasis, 3*(3), 459–464.

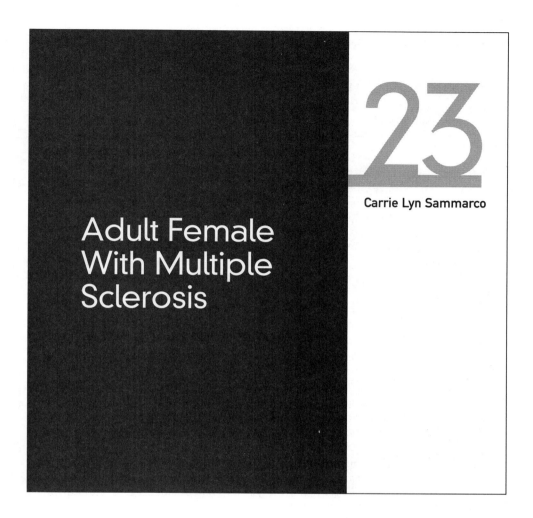

23

Carrie Lyn Sammarco

Adult Female With Multiple Sclerosis

This case describes the care I provided for a commercially insured 26-year-old woman with multiple sclerosis over an eight-month period in the ambulatory care setting. The case narrative demonstrates my ability to meet the following Columbia University School of Nursing (CUSN) doctoral competencies for comprehensive direct patient care.

DOMAIN 1, COMPETENCY 2

Evaluate population or geographically based health risk utilizing principles of epidemiology, clinical prevention, environmental health, and biostatistics.

PO A. Assess the patient or family *at risk* for a condition, incorporating epidemiologic principles and/or environmental factors that contribute to the risk or incidence of disease.

DOMAIN 2, COMPETENCY 1

Assemble a collaborative interdisciplinary network, and refer and consult appropriately while maintaining primary responsibility for comprehensive patient care.

PO A. Initiate referral to other health care professionals while maintaining primary responsibility for patient care.
PO D. Evaluate outcomes of interventions.
PO E. Provide ongoing patient follow-up, and monitor outcomes of collaborative network interventions.

SUMMARY OF CARE (PROVIDED PRIOR TO FOCUS OF THIS NARRATIVE)

The patient is a 26-year-old Caucasian female who has been seen in the Multiple Sclerosis Center for approximately 22 months. An ophthalmologist referred her for evaluation of optic neuritis (ON). Her past medical history is unremarkable. She does not have a history of surgery. She is single, lives with a female roommate, and denies cigarette smoking and alcohol intake. After a complete diagnostic evaluation, which included an MRI of the brain, cervical and thoracic cord, cerebrospinal fluid examination, serum review, and neurologic examination, she was diagnosed with multiple sclerosis (MS).

Since her last appointment, which was nearly eight weeks ago, she developed left foot numbness and her ankle "gave out." These symptoms resolved on their own within a "few hours." Four weeks ago she initiated interferon beta-1a, 30-mcg intramuscular injection (IFN-1a) (Avonex), weekly for long-term management of MS (see Medications list at the end of the chapter).

ENCOUNTER CONTEXT

Encounter One (one-month follow-up)

DNP role: Doctor of nursing practice resident and family nurse practitioner.

Identifying Information

Site: Urban academic medical center.

Setting: Neurology specialty practice.

Reason for encounter: Evaluation post initiation of IFN-1a (Avonex).

Informant: Patient and medical records. She appears to be a reliable historian.

History of Present Illness (HPI)

Patient arrives today with her mother. This is her one-month follow-up since initiating IFN-1a (Avonex). She has not yet titrated up to her full dose of medication. She does not like the idea of injecting herself, but she will if it is "good for her." She denies weakness, numbness or tingling in extremities, or problems with coordination.

Sometimes she is so tired she feels as though she could take a nap at work. She is not exercising as much as previously. She goes to the gym one to two times per week. She usually does 30 minutes of machine cardiovascular exercise. She feels "depressed" and anxious, especially regarding her diagnosis. She states that her friends and family have been very supportive.

She feels stressed about her work situation. Her boss is demanding, and she does not like her job. She admits to feeling depressed, anxious, and concerned about her future. She denies suicidal thoughts, homicidal thoughts, and changes in sleep at night or in appetite. She does not feel hopelessness, helplessness. She denies substance use.

When her mother leaves the room, she confides that she "does not want to worry" her parents by talking to them about MS. She is concerned that symptoms will return and be permanent.

Medications (see Medications list at the end of the chapter)

Interferon beta-1a (Avonex) 30-mcg intramuscular injection weekly. Ibuprofen (Motrin) 200 mg by mouth with weekly injection.

Allergies: No known allergies.

Review of Systems

General: Reports increased fatigue and hypersomnia. Denies fever, chills, weight loss.

Eyes: Denies visual change and eye pain.

ENT: Denies change in hearing, tinnitus, sore throat, dysphagia, dysarthria, epistaxis.

Cardiovascular: Denies chest pain or tightness, shortness of breath (SOB), palpitations, edema.

Respiratory: Denies cough, wheezing.

Gastrointestinal: Denies constipation, abdominal pain, diarrhea.

Urinary: Denies nocturia, increased frequency and urgency; recent urinary tract infection treated by her gynecologist with an antibiotic for one week, symptoms resolved without sequelae.

Gynecologic: Regular follow-up with gynecologist, last menstrual period 15 days ago, admits to being sexually active in the past with one partner and using condoms for contraception. Denies dyspareunia, history of sexually transmitted infections, violence, or abuse.

Musculoskeletal: Denies muscle aches or joint pain.

Neurologic: See HPI.

Endocrine: Denies intolerance to temperature change, change in skin or hair.

Psychiatric: See HPI.

Physical Examination

Vital signs: Respiratory rate 16, pulse 70, blood pressure 118/68, height 5'7", weight 148 lb, BMI 23.31.

General: Alert and oriented × 3, well groomed, in no acute distress (NAD), maintains good eye contact, good historian.

Skin: Warm; dry, intact, no rashes or lesions, no tattoos; examination of injection site areas (thighs) unremarkable.

HEENT:

Head: Normocephalic.
Eyes: PERRLA, EOMs intact, visual acuity using near card both eyes 20/20 with brisk constriction.
Ears: Hearing equal bilaterally.
Nose: Straight without deviation, no discharge.
Oropharynx: Without redness or exudates.

Neck: Supple, no adenopathy, thyromegaly.

Respiratory: Without adventitious sounds bilaterally.

Heart: Regular rate, rhythm with S1, S2 heard, no murmurs, gallops, rubs.

Abdomen: Soft, without tenderness.

Genitourinary: Deferred.

Rectal: Deferred.

Neurologic:

Mental status: Alert and cooperative.
Cranial nerves: CN II–XII intact.
Motor system: Muscle tone and bulk are equal bilaterally to upper and lower extremities, motor strength 5/5 equal bilaterally to upper and lower extremities.
Coordination: Finger-nose-finger and Heel-to-shin intact, rapid alternating movements without decrement.
Sensory: Light touch, pin sensation equal and intact bilaterally, vibration slight decrease distal lower left extremity, proprioception intact.
Reflexes: deep tendon reflexes (DTRs) 2 in bilateral upper extremities and 2+ in bilateral lower extremities, toes down-going bilaterally.
Gait: Regular stance, cadence, heel-to-toe walk intact, balances on one foot and hops five times bilaterally, Romberg negative.

Impression

26-year-old Caucasian female with a history of MS who began treatment with IFN-1a (Avonex) one month ago returns for follow-up evaluation. MS symptoms and physical examination are without change since last appointment. Patient reports depressed mood, hypersomnia, concentration difficulties at work, decreased energy, impaired capacity to work or study, and fatigue. These symptoms are consistent with depression, which occurs in persons with MS. The onset of these symptoms in relation to initiation of IFN therapy is considered. The patient also complains of fatigue, which may be secondary to MS, exacerbated by depression or a medication side effect. This patient does not have suicidal or homicidal ideation and has a strong informal support network. Frequent outpatient monitoring may be indicated due to IFN-1a (Avonex) and depression symptoms in this patient with MS **(D1, C2, PO A)**.

The nine symptoms of depression are divided into two subgroups: psychologic (four symptoms) and physical (five symptoms). The diagnosis of depression requires the presence of depressed mood or the inability to experience pleasure, plus four other symptoms. Thus, five of nine symptoms must be present. Inclusion, exclusion and duration criteria must also be met. The symptoms are not accounted for by bereavement, general medical conditions, medications, or drug or alcohol abuse. The symptoms must result in significant impairment of social, occupational or school functioning (American Psychiatric Association, 1994).
                    Oxford Centre for Evidence-Based Medicine (CEBM), level 5.

ICD-9 Codes

MS (340.0)
Fatigue (780.7)
Depression (300.4)

Plan

Medications
- Continue to titrate IFN-1a (Avonex) 30-mcg intramuscular weekly to full dose; premedicate with ibuprofen (Motrin) 400 mg orally as needed.
- Start modafinil (Provigil) 200 mg, one-half tablet orally in morning as needed for fatigue.

Data from a study to assess the efficacy and safety of modafinil for the treatment of fatigue in multiple sclerosis (MS) suggest that 200 mg/day modafinil (Provigil) significantly improves fatigue and is well tolerated in patients with MS (Rammohan, et al., 2002).
                                        CEBM, level 1b.

Up to one-half of depressed patients have partial or no response to anti-depressant monotherapy. A multicenter, placebo-controlled study evaluated the efficacy of modafinil (Provigil) augmentation in major depressive disorder (MDD) patients with fatigue and excessive sleepiness despite selective serotonin reuptake inhibitor (SSRI) monotherapy. Findings suggest that modafinil (Provigil) is a well-tolerated and potentially effective augmenting agent for SSRI partial responders with fatigue and sleepiness (Fava, Thase, & DeBattista, 2005).

CEBM, level 1b.

- Start escitalopram (Lexapro) 10 g, one-half tablet, orally in morning for one week; titrate to 10 mg as tolerated for depression; may also benefit fatigue. Use as-needed dose of modafinil (Provigil) until escitalopram (Lexapro) is titrated to a therapeutic level. Monitor use to determine if fatigue is neurogenic or related to depression.

Diagnostics
Complete blood count (CBC) and liver function tests (LFTs) one month (V58.9).

Referrals
Social work to assess for possible benefit of talk therapy regarding mood and coping skills regarding new diagnosis **(D2, C1, PO A).**

Counseling and Education
- Extensive discussion of medication use, dosing schedule, and adverse reactions.
- Discussion of disease management and symptom management.
- Review why an improvement in her fatigue may help with her work concerns.
- I encourage her to continue her exercise regimen.
- I also encourage her to call me to discuss issues she may not feel comfortable talking about with her parents or friends.

Follow–up
Return one month for follow-up regarding mood and fatigue; sooner for new or worsening symptoms **(D2, C1, PO A).**

Interim Summary of Care

Patient's fatigue improved immediately after initiating modafinil (Provigil). She titrated up to escitalopram (Lexapro) 10 mg orally every day after one week and started seeing a social worker outside of the MS center for weekly therapy. Within one month she reported significant improvement in her depression. She also began looking for a new job.

Five months later she had an exacerbation of MS. She developed "numbness and tingling" in her legs with mild exertion of walking three blocks.

Trace weakness was noted on her exam. She was treated with methylpred-nisolone sodium succinate (Solu-medrol) 1 g intravenously for one day, fol-lowed by an oral prednisone taper. Her symptoms resolved completely for approximately one month. She then reported transient, mild numbness in her knees and shins, especially with exercise or exertion. She denied weak-ness or altered gait. These symptoms would resolve with rest.

Encounter Two (six months after initial narrative encounter)

Patient presents for a routine follow-up visit. Her mother accompanies her. She reports she has been "feeling well" with a decrease in her lower extremity "tingling." She is exercising three to four times per week. Her fatigue contin-ues to benefit from modafinil (Provigil) 200 mg orally on workdays. Her mood has been stable on escitalopram (Lexapro) 10 mg orally, and she is seeing her therapist weekly.

Social

She states that her alcohol consumption is "two glasses of wine or margaritas three times during the week" and five vodka drinks on Friday and Saturday evenings. This pattern has been going on for the past three months. She denies any impact on work. She describes herself as "social." She enjoys going out with her friends to meet guys. She always goes home with her girlfriends, though she does not always remember leaving establishments or how she arrives home. Further discussion reveals "blacking out" during drinking. This has occurred two times in the last eight weeks. She describes these events as having no recollection of leaving one bar and heading to the second. She remembers later events from the evening. She describes waking up at home in her previous night's clothes the next morning. This has occurred "a few times." She states that most of her friends drink alcohol frequently and it would be hard to stop. She states that she wants to "cut back" and thinks she "might have a problem." She is frank regarding her concerns and answers questions without hesitation.

> As alcohol consumption increases, the magnitude of the memory impairments increases. Large amounts of alcohol, rapidly consumed, can produce partial or complete blackouts. Blackouts are much more common among social drink-ers than was previously assumed. Mechanisms underlying alcohol-induced memory impairments include disruption of activity in the hippocampus (White, 2004).
>
> CEBM, level 5.

Medications

IFN-1a (Avonex) 30-mcg intramuscular injection weekly.
Ibuprofen (Motrin) 400 mg orally with injections.

Escitalopram oxalate (Lexapro) 10 g, one-half tablet orally in morning for one week; titrate to 10 mg thereafter.
Modafinil (Provigil) 200 mg orally daily.

Allergies: No known allergies.

Review of Systems

General: Decreased daytime fatigue, denies altered sleep, denies fever, chills, weight loss.

Eyes: Denies visual change and eye pain.

ENT: Denies change in hearing, tinnitus, sore throat, dysphagia, dysarthria, epistaxis.

Pulmonary: Denies cough, wheezing.

Cardiovascular: Denies chest pain or tightness, SOB, palpitations, edema.

Gastrointestinal: Denies constipation, abdominal pain, diarrhea.

Urinary: Denies nocturia, increased frequency, urgency, and incontinence.

Gynecologic: Regular follow-up with gynecologist, LMP two days ago, denies sexual dysfunction or abuse.

Musculoskeletal: Denies muscle aches or joint pain.

Neurologic: Episodic "tingling" in legs with exertion; see HPI.

Endocrine: Denies intolerance to temperature change, change in skin or hair, increased fatigue.

Psychiatric: Mood stable; see HPI.

Physical Examination

Vital signs: Respiratory rate 16, pulse 70, blood pressure 118/68, height 5'7", weight 148 lb, BMI 23.31.

General: Alert and oriented × 3, well groomed, in NAD, maintains good eye contact, good historian.

Skin: Warm, dry, intact, no rashes or lesions, no tattoos; examination of injection site areas, thighs, unremarkable.

HEENT:

Head: Normocephalic.
Eyes: PERRLA, EOMs intact; visual acuity using near card OU 20/20; OU brisk constriction.
Ears: Hearing equal bilaterally.
Nose: Straight without deviation, no discharge.
Oropharynx: Without redness or exudates.

Neck: Supple, no adenopathy, thyromegaly.

Respiratory: No wheezing, rhonchi.

Heart: Regular rate, rhythm, S1, S2 present without murmurs, gallops, rubs.

Abdomen: Soft, without tenderness.

Genitourinary: Deferred.

Rectal: Deferred.

Neurologic:

Mental status: Alert and cooperative.
Cranial nerves: CN II–XII intact.
Motor system: Muscle tone and bulk symmetric without atrophy. Motor strength: 5/5 bilateral upper and lower extremities.
Coordination: Finger-nose-finger, heel-to-shin: intact; rapid alternating movements without decrement.
Sensory: Light touch sensation intact, pin sensation intact throughout, vibration slight decrease distal lower extremities, proprioception intact.
Reflexes: DTRs 2 bilateral in upper extremities and 2+ bilateral in lower extremities, toes down-going bilaterally.
Gait: Regular stance, cadence, tandem intact, balances on one foot and hops five times bilaterally, negative Romberg.

Diagnostics Review: Last laboratory studies, performed three months ago, included CBC with differential, LFTs, and TSH, all within normal range.

Impression

26-year-old Caucasian female with a history of MS treated with IFN-1a for seven months. She is tolerating therapy well by history and laboratory results. Resolving sensory symptoms, and stable physical examination compared with last examination. Fatigue improved on modafinil (Provigil). Depression improved on escitalopram (Lexapro) and weekly talk therapy with social worker.

Patient presents with possible alcohol abuse for approximately three months associated with blackouts.

American Psychiatric Association, 1994.

A maladaptive pattern of substance use leading to clinically significant impairment or distress [is] manifested by three (or more) of the following, occurring at any time in the same 12-month period:
- *Substance is often taken in larger amounts or over longer period than intended*
- *Persistent desire or unsuccessful efforts to cut down or control substance use*
- *A great deal of time is spent in activities necessary to obtain the substance (e.g., visiting multiple doctors or driving long distances), use the substance (e.g., chain smoking), or recover from its effects*

- *Important social, occupational, or recreational activities given up or reduced because of substance abuse*
- *Continued substance use despite knowledge of having a persistent or recurrent psychological or physical problem that is caused or exacerbated by use of the substance*
- *Tolerance, as defined by either:*
  1. *need for increasing amounts of the substance in order to achieve intoxication or desired effect; or*
  2. *markedly diminished effect with continued use of the same amount*
- *Withdrawal, as manifested by either:*
  1. *characteristic withdrawal syndrome for the substance; or*
  2. *the same (or closely related) substance is taken to relieve or avoid withdrawal symptoms (NIH, 2004).*

CEBM, level 5.

ICD-9 Codes

MS (340.0)
Fatigue (780.7)
Depression (300.4)
Substance abuse (305.0) (v65.4) (v58.69)

Plan

Medications

- Continue on IFN-1a (Avonex) 30 mcg intramuscularly weekly for MS, and continue premedication with ibuprofen (Motrin) 400 mg by mouth to decrease flu-like side effects.
- Continue modafinil (Provigil) 200 mg orally as needed for fatigue.
- Continue escitalopram (Lexapro) 20 mg by mouth daily for depression.

CNS Drugs—Given the primary CNS effects of escitalopram, caution should be used when it is taken in combination with other centrally acting drugs. Alcohol—Although Lexapro did not potentiate the cognitive and motor effects of alcohol in a clinical trial, as with other psychotropic medications, the use of alcohol by patients taking Lexapro is not recommended.

http://www.lexapro.com/about-lexapro/lexapro-side-effects.aspx

Diagnostics
CBC with differential, comprehensive metabolic panel with LFTs.

Referrals
Continue weekly follow-up with therapist; discuss Alcoholics Anonymous (AA) for alcohol abuse if therapist and patient agree that counseling with therapist alone is not adequate. I also refer her to the social worker at the MS

Center. She agrees that I may discuss her case with the social worker **(D2, C1, PO D, E)**.

Counseling and Education

In the presence of patient's mother, we discuss concerns regarding patient's alcohol consumption, such as health implications, both physical and emotional, along with safety concerns. The patient agrees that her alcohol consumption is concerning and a possible problem and states that she wishes to address it. We discuss potential options, including one-on-one therapy and group therapy, such as Alcoholics Anonymous (AA). I encourage her to discuss this with her therapist. She feels comfortable doing so and agrees that her therapist would support her. I advise her that she can contact me, the other nurse practitioner, or the social worker at the MS Center with any questions or concerns, via either e-mail or telephone. At the end of this extensive discussion regarding substance abuse, potential complications, and counseling options, she reports that she is going to think about her options and talk to her therapist.

Follow-up

- Patient will contact either me or other nurse practitioner in one week with progress report **(D2, C1, PO D, E)**.
- I encourage her to schedule a follow-up office visit for one month.
- We will see her in the office sooner if symptoms worsen or if there is an increased concern regarding her alcohol abuse. We will maintain e-mail contact if she is in counseling and improving until her next visit.
- In the interim, I will discuss her case with the social worker on staff at the MS Center. I will request updates from the social worker when she has contact with the patient **(D2, C1, PO E)**.

Alcoholics Anonymous (AA) is a voluntary program for people with problem drinking, based on fellowship and a belief in a spiritual basis for recovery. Abstinence is encouraged on a "one day at a time" basis. The Twelve-Step program entails acknowledgment that alcohol has led to loss of control, that recovery is a spiritual journey through belief in a higher power, and through personal exploration and acceptance. More information about AA can be found on their website: www.alcoholics-anonymous.org.

CEBM, level 5.

Telephone Encounter (14 days after last visit)

The patient informs me that, after meeting with her therapist and with the encouragement and support of her family, she joined AA and is 13 days sober. She has also established a telephone relationship with the social worker at the MS Center. I encourage her sobriety.

COMPETENCY DEFENSE

Domain 1, Competency 2. Evaluate population or geographically based health risk utilizing principles of epidemiology, clinical prevention, environmental health, and biostatistics.

Defense. I formulated a diagnosis of depression using the *DSM-IV* criteria. Given her current symptoms of depressed mood, hypersomnia, concentration difficulties at work, decreased energy, and fatigue, I devised a treatment regimen that included pharmacologic and nonpharmacologic interventions. Psychiatric disorders, especially depression, are frequent in patients with MS. Depression can be reactive (related to the psychosocial impact of a chronic, often progressive, and potentially disabling illness) and/or organic in nature (related to cerebral demyelination). Complicating this matter, the medication used to manage MS and its symptoms, such as corticosteroids and possibly interferon (IFN), may also have depressogenic effects, though there is little evidence to support the latter. Similarly, symptoms of depression may be confused with or confounded by MS fatigue and cognitive impairment. Depression in MS, as in other conditions, is most effectively treated with psychotherapy and medication. Because major depressive disorders and incidents of suicidal ideation are increased in MS patients, it is especially important to do a careful assessment of mood.

Domain 2, Competency 1. Assemble a collaborative interdisciplinary network, and refer and consult appropriately while maintaining primary responsibility for comprehensive patient care.

Defense. Multiple sclerosis has a highly variable disease course. Although it is unpredictable, many patients eventually have a progressive disease course resulting in an accumulation of wide-ranging disabilities, including physical, psychological, and cognitive changes. These disabilities can have a significant impact on the individual with MS, affecting mood, role and relationships, schooling, employment, and socialization. To adequately address these complex needs, a detailed assessment of physical, psychological, and social functioning by a multidisciplinary team is needed. Collaboration among members of the health care team is essential to ensure that all the patient's needs are addressed. Specific team members may be better equipped to address certain issues based on their training and experience. As part of my treatment plan for management of the patient's depression and alcohol use problem, I referred her to the MS social worker for evaluation.

Medications

Drug: Interferon Beta-1a (Avonex)

Dose range: 30-mcg intramuscular injection weekly.

Method of administration in this case: Intramuscular injection.

Mechanism of action: Mechanism in MS is unknown. However, it is thought to interfere with the actions of interferon gamma, which appears to provoke exacerbations of the disease. Interferons are a family of proteins and glycoproteins that are potent cytokines with antiviral, immunomodulating, and antiproliferative actions.

(continued)

Clinical uses: MS, relapsing forms.

Side effects
Common: *Neurologic:* Headache. *Other:* Influenza-like illness, fever, chills, myalgia.
Serious: *Hematologic:* Anemia, leukopenia, thrombocytopenia. *Hepatic:* Increased liver enzymes, injury of liver, liver failure (rare). *Immunologic:* Anaphylaxis (rare). *Neurologic:* Seizure. *Psychiatric:* Mental disorder.

Drug: Ibuprofen (Motrin)

Dose range: 200 mg, two tablets.

Method of administration in this case: By mouth, taken with Avonex injection.

Mechanism of action: Nonsteroidal anti-inflammatory drug (NSAID) that exhibits analgesic and antipyretic activities by inhibiting prostaglandin synthesis.

Clinical uses: Decrease side effects of Avonex.

Side effects
Common: *Cardiovascular:* Hypotension. *Dermatologic:* Rash. *Endocrine metabolic:* Hypernatremia, hypoalbuminemia, hypoproteinemia, elevated serum lactate dehydrogenase level. *Gastrointestinal:* Flatulence, heartburn, nausea, vomiting. *Hematologic:* Thrombocytosis. *Immunologic:* Bacteremia. *Neurologic:* Dizziness, headache. *Renal:* Serum blood urea nitrogen raised, urinary retention. *Respiratory:* Bacterial pneumonia.
Serious: *Cardiovascular:* Congestive heart failure, hypertension, myocardial infarction, thrombotic tendency observations. *Dermatologic:* Erythema multiforme, erythroderma, Stevens-Johnson syndrome, toxic epidermal necrolysis. *Gastrointestinal:* Gastrointestinal hemorrhage, gastrointestinal perforation, gastrointestinal ulcer, inflammatory disorder of digestive tract, melena, pancreatitis. *Hematologic:* Agranulocytosis, anemia, aplastic anemia, bleeding, hemolytic anemia, neutropenia, thrombocytopenia, wound hemorrhage. *Hepatic:* Fulminant hepatitis (rare), hepatic necrosis (rare), hepatitis, hepatotoxicity (rare), jaundice, liver failure, vanishing bile duct syndrome. *Immunologic:* Anaphylactoid reaction, immune hypersensitivity reaction. *Neurologic:* Aseptic meningitis, cerebrovascular accident. *Ophthalmic:* Amblyopia. *Otic:* Hearing loss. *Psychiatric:* Depression. *Renal:* Acute renal failure, hematuria, renal azotemia. *Other:* Reye's syndrome.

Drug: Escitalopram Oxalate (Lexapro)

Dose range: 10 mg daily.

Method of administration in this case: By mouth.

Mechanism of action: A selective serotonin reuptake inhibitor (SSRI) and S-enantiomer of racemic citalopram, this drug enhances serotonergic activity in the central nervous system (CNS) as a result of its inhibition of serotonin (5-HT) reuptake in CNS neurons.

(continued)

Clinical uses: Major depressive disorder.

Side effects
Common: *Cardiovascular:* Palpitations. *Dermatologic:* Diaphoresis. *Endocrine metabolic:* Weight increase. *Gastrointestinal:* Constipation, diarrhea, indigestion, nausea, xerostomia. *Hematologic:* Anemia, contusion, epistaxis, hematoma. *Neurologic:* Agitation, dizziness, feeling nervous, headache, insomnia, lightheadedness, somnolence, tremor. *Reproductive:* Disorder of ejaculation, impotence. *Other:* Fatigue.
Serious: *Cardiovascular:* Heart failure, myocardial infarction, prolonged QT interval, torsades de pointes. *Endocrine metabolic:* Diabetes mellitus, syndrome of inappropriate antidiuretic hormone secretion. *Gastrointestinal:* Pancreatitis, rectal hemorrhage. *Neurologic:* Grand mal seizure, neuroleptic malignant syndrome. *Psychiatric:* Depression, worsening (rare), suicidal thoughts (rare), suicide (rare). *Other:* Serotonin syndrome.

Drug: Modafinil (Provigil)

Dose range: 200 mg orally once daily in the morning.

Method of administration in this case: By mouth.

Mechanism of action: Uncertain.

Clinical uses: Improve wakefulness in patients with excessive daytime sleepiness.

Side effects
Common: *Dermatologic:* Rash. *Gastrointestinal:* Nausea. *Neurologic:* Dizziness, headache, insomnia. *Psychiatric:* Anxiety, feeling nervous.
Serious: *Cardiovascular:* Hypertension. *Dermatologic:* Drug hypersensitivity syndrome, Stevens-Johnson syndrome, toxic epidermal necrolysis due to drug. *Immunologic:* Hypersensitivity reaction, multiorgan. *Psychiatric:* Mania.

Source: http://www.thompsonhc.com

References

American Psychiatric Association. (1994). *Diagnostic and statistical manual of mental disorders* (4th ed.). Washington, DC: Author.
Clanet, M.G., & Brassat, D. (2000). The management of multiple sclerosis patients. *Current Opinion in Neurology, 13,* 263–270.
Fava, M., Thase, M.E., & DeBattista, C. (2005). A multicenter, placebo-controlled study of modafinil augmentation in partial responders to selective serotonin reuptake inhibitors with persistent fatigue and sleepiness. *Journal of Clinical Psychiatry, 66*(1), 85–93.
Francis, G.S., Rice, G.P., & Alsop J.C. (2005). Interferon beta-1a in MS: Results following development of neutralizing antibodies in PRISMS. *Neurology, 65*(1), 48–55.
Goeb, J.L., Even, C., Nicholas, G., Gohier, B., Dubas, F., & Garre, J.B. (2006). Psychiatric side effects of interferon-beta in multiple sclerosis. *European Psychiatry, 21*(3), 186–193.

Hauser, S.L., & Goodin, D.S. (2006). Multiple sclerosis and other demyelinating diseases. Chapter 359 in *Diseases of the central nervous system*. Retrieved from Harrison's Internal Medicine, http://www.accessmedicine.com

Hoogervorst, E.L.J., de Jonge, P., Jelles, B., Huyse, F.J., Heere, I., et al. (2003). The INTERMED: A screening instrument to identify multiple sclerosis patients in need of multidisciplinary treatment. *Neurology, Neurosurgery and Psychiatry, 74,* 20–24.

Kappos, L., Clanet, M., Sandberg-Wollheim, M., Radue, E.W., Hartung, H.P., Hohlfeld, R., Xu, J., Bennett, D., Sandrock, A., & Goelz, S. (2005). Neutralizing antibodies and efficacy of interferon beta-1a: A 4-year controlled study. *Neurology, 65*(1), 40–47.

Kaufman, M. (2006). *Treatment of multiple sclerosis symptoms.* Retrieved October 2006 from http://www.medlink.com/MedLinkContent.asp

National Institute of Health (NIH), National Institute on Alcohol Abuse and Alcoholism. (2004). *Alcohol alert.* Retrieved October 2006 from http://www.niaaa.nih.gov

Panitch, H., Goodin, D.S., Francis, G., Chang, P., Coyle, P.K., O'Connor, P., Monaghan, E., Li, D., & Weinshenker, B. (2002). Randomized, comparative study of interferon beta-1a treatment regimens in MS: The EVIDENCE Trial. *Neurology, 59*(10), 1496–1506.

Rammohan, K.W., Rosenberg, J.H., Lynn, D.J., Blumenfeld, A.M., Pollak, C.P., & Nagaraja, H.N. (2002). Efficacy and safety of modafinil (Provigil) for the treatment of fatigue in multiple sclerosis: A two centre phase 2 study. *Journal of Neurology, Neurosurgery and Psychiatry, 72*(2), 179–183.

White, A.M. (2004). *What happened? Alcohol, memory blackouts, and the brain.* Retrieved May 15, 2009, from http://pubs.niaaa.nih.gov/publications/arh27–2/186–196.htm

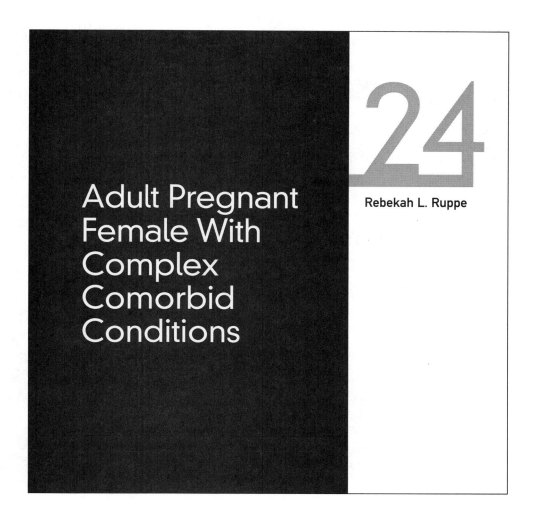

Adult Pregnant Female With Complex Comorbid Conditions

Rebekah L. Ruppe

24

This case describes the care I provided for a commercially insured patient during pregnancy with complex comorbidities. The narrative describes eight encounters that occurred over a period of seven months and demonstrates my ability to meet the following Columbia University School of Nursing (CUSN) doctoral competencies for comprehensive direct patient care.

DOMAIN 1, COMPETENCY 4

Appraise acuity of patient condition, determine need to transfer patient to higher acuity setting, coordinate, and manage transfer to optimize patient outcomes.

PO A. Assess the acuity of patient status.
PO B. Determine the most appropriate treatment setting based on level of acuity.
PO C. Formulate a transfer plan.

PO D. Implement plan to transfer the patient to a higher level of care utilizing written and oral communication.
PO E. Coordinate care during transition to the higher acuity setting
PO F. Co-manage care in person.
PO G. Co-manage care though written and verbal instructions.
PO H. Make recommendations for patient disposition from the higher acuity location.
PO I. Coordinate post-discharge care.

DOMAIN 2, COMPETENCY 1

Assemble a collaborative interdisciplinary network, and refer and consult appropriately while maintaining primary responsibility for comprehensive patient care.

PO A. Initiate referral to other health care professionals while maintaining primary responsibility for patient care.
PO B. Accept referrals from other health care professions, and communicate consultation findings and recommendations to the referring provider and collaborative network.
PO C. Utilize consultation recommendations for decision-making while maintaining primary responsibility for care.
PO D. Evaluate outcomes of interventions.
PO E. Provide ongoing patient follow-up, and monitor outcomes of collaborative network interventions.

ENCOUNTER CONTEXT

Encounter one (initial prenatal visit)

DNP role: I am the attending nurse midwife and DNP student providing prenatal care.

Identifying Information

Site: Private midwifery practice, urban setting.

Setting: Private midwifery practice that is affiliated with a university tertiary care and community hospital.

Reason for encounter: Initial prenatal visit, 6 weeks 3 days gestation.

Informant: Julia is a 30-year-old gravida 2 para 1 (G2P1001) who presents as a new patient for an initial prenatal visit. She appears to be a reliable historian.

Chief complaint: Patient states, "I'm pregnant. I'm here for my first prenatal visit."

History of present illness (HPI): Julia's last menstrual period (LMP) was six weeks and three days ago. She reports regular periods with 28-day cycles. Her first positive urine pregnancy test was two weeks ago. She denies febrile illnesses, uterine cramping, vaginal bleeding, vomiting, constipation, or diarrhea since her last menstrual period. She reports occasional nausea approximately four to five times per week, which is relieved with snacking.

Comprehensive Health History

Medical History

- Asthma, diagnosed as teen, currently controlled with montelukast sodium (Singulair). Patient denies history of hospitalization or intubation. Last exacerbation was two years ago before she began current therapy. She reports minimal symptoms with montelukast sodium (Singulair). In the past, symptoms have been exacerbated by cold weather and occasionally exercise. Julia states that she has a peak flow meter and knows how to use it. Since initiating montelukast sodium (Singulair) therapy two years ago, she has had minimal asthma-related symptoms and has not had to use her short-acting inhaler in over 18 months. She has not had any change in symptom presentation, frequency, or severity since her LMP.
- Graves' disease, diagnosed four years ago; thyroid was ablated with radioactive iodine. Patient is now hypothyroid and takes levothyroxine (Synthroid) daily. Her dose was recently increased by her endocrinologist.
- Pre-pregnancy weight is reported as 192 pounds. Patient reports no significant weight gain or loss in the past year.

Past surgical history
Patient has not had prior surgeries.

Prior obstetric history
Normal spontaneous vaginal birth of live female infant weighing nine pounds two years ago. Labor was induced after a sonogram at 39 weeks supported the clinically suspected diagnosis of large-for-gestational-age status of fetus (> 90th percentile). There were no perinatal or peripartum complications.

Gynecologic history
Denies history of abnormal Pap smears, sexually transmitted infections, or infertility. Her last Pap smear was over one year ago. Last menstrual period was six weeks and three days ago. Prior to conception she had regular periods every 28 days, with five to six days of moderate bleeding. Dysmenorrhea on days one and two, relieved with ibuprofen (Motrin).

Sexual history
Husband is sexual partner for nine years. She reports two lifetime partners, denies difficulties or pain with sexual intercourse, and reports sexual satisfaction.

Contraceptive history

History of combined contraceptive pill use before birth of daughter, approximately four years. She denies associated complications or adverse events. She used condoms prior to present pregnancy.

Family history

Patient denies family history of thyroid disease, kidney disease, stroke, or seizure disorder. No consanguinity in this pedigree.

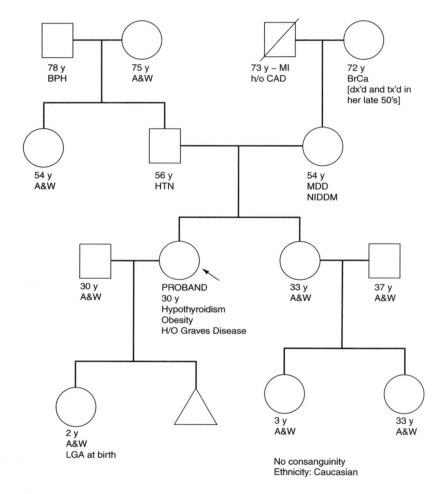

Genetic history

Patient denies known genetic disorders in her own family and in her partner's family.

Psychosocial history

Denies history of depression, anxiety, or partner violence. She is happy in current relationship with husband of six years. She lives with husband and two-year-old daughter in two-bedroom urban apartment in an elevator building. She denies history of or current tobacco or substance use. Prior to conception, she consumed two to three servings of caffeine daily and two to three alcoholic beverages per week. She currently does not consume caffeine or alcohol.

Nutrition and exercise history
Review of typical breakfast, lunch, dinner, and snacks reveals generally well-balanced diet of lean proteins, occasional red meat, fruits, vegetables, and grains daily. She reports eating "too much sugar" as she has candy, pastry, or other desert item daily. Although she does not have a regular exercise routine, she walks to work daily.

Medications (see Medications list at end of chapter)
- Montelukast sodium (Singulair) 10 mg by mouth, daily.
- Levothyroxine (Synthroid) 0.137 mg by mouth, daily (recently increased, preconceptively, from 0.125 mg).
- Prenatal vitamin by mouth daily.

Allergies
Denies known drug, food, or environmental allergies.

Review of Systems

Constitutional: Denies weight loss, fatigue, weakness, fever, chills, or night sweats. No change in appetite or general activity level. She reports a pre-pregnancy weight of 192 pounds and a recent gain of approximately 5 pounds, most of which she attributes to snacking to avoid nausea.

Skin and hair: Denies rashes or lesions. No change in hair amount, texture, or consistency.

Head, ears, eyes, nose, and throat: Denies headache. No changes in visual, auditory, olfactory acuity. No problems eating, swallowing.

Neck: Denies masses, tenderness, stiffness, or limitations in movement.

Breast: Denies breast lumps, pain or tenderness, or discharge.

Chest: Denies cough, chest pain, shortness of breath, wheezing. Reports asthma, well controlled.

Cardiovascular: Denies chest pain, palpitations, dyspnea on exertion, edema.

Gastrointestinal: Denies appetite changes, nausea, vomiting, diarrhea, constipation, changes in stool or stooling pattern.

Urinary: Reports frequency and dysuria for the past week, which she describes as "mild." Denies urgency, nocturia, or incontinence of urine.

Genitalia: Denies vaginal irritation, discharge, malodor, lesions, or abnormal vaginal bleeding or spotting.

Musculoskeletal: Denies myalgia and arthralgia. No redness, swelling, or tenderness of joints. No limitations in movement or range of motion.

Neurologic: Denies dizziness, weakness, numbness, coordination problems, loss of consciousness, or alteration in mood, sleep, and memory.

Psychologic: Denies depression, anxiety, and loss of energy or ability to concentrate.

Focused Physical Examination

Vital signs: Blood pressure 100/64, heart rate 72, respiratory rate 16, temp 36.5°C, weight 196 lb, height 5'7", BMI (pre-pregnancy) 30.

General: Appropriate affect, good hygiene, appears well nourished.

Neck: Supple, lymph nodes not enlarged; thyroid smooth, not enlarged.

Heart: Regular rate and rhythm (RRR), no murmur, no rub, no gallop.

Lungs: Clear to auscultation (CTA), anterior, posterior, bilaterally. No adventitious sounds.

External Genitalia: Appropriate hair distribution. No lesions, masses, erythema, edema. No abrasions or excoriations.

Vagina: Pink mucosa, rugae present. Smooth, homogenous, white secretions noted. No malodor, lesions, or discharge noted. Good vaginal tone.

Cervix: Approximately 3.5 centimeters long. Parous os. No lesions or discharge noted. No cervical motion tenderness.

Uterus: Retroverted, nontender, no masses. Difficult to fully evaluate due to uterine position and maternal habitus.

Adnexa: Nontender, no masses bilaterally. Right and left ovaries approximately 2 × 3 centimeters.

Rectal: No visible hemorrhoids or lesions; internal exam deferred.

Impression

Julia is a 30-year-old gravida 2 para 1 (G2P1001) at 6 weeks 3 days gestation based on certain last menstrual period. Her history is significant for mild persistent asthma controlled with montelukast sodium (Singulair) and Graves' disease with post-ablative hypothyroidism, which is treated with levothyroxine (Synthroid). Her physical exam is significant for obesity (BMI = 30). Total weight gain this pregnancy is four pounds. Uterine size was difficult to assess due to the retroverted position of her uterus and her habitus.

Uterine size should be assessed at the initial prenatal visit to make a clinical estimation of gestational age and confirm gestational age based on menstrual dating. Obesity and other factors affecting the ability to palpate the uterus (i.e., retroverted position) interfere with accurate clinical assessment of gestational age (MacKenzie, Stephenson, & Funai, 2007).
Oxford Centre for Evidence-Based Medicine (CEBM), level 5.

The review of symptoms reveals mild nausea, relieved with snacking and urinary frequency and dysuria. Given that her nausea is not accompanied by vomiting or acute abdominal pain and is relieved with snacking, it is most likely a common discomfort of early pregnancy due to hormonal changes.

Most women develop nausea between six and 12 weeks gestation. If nausea (with or without vomiting) is accompanied by pain, abdominal distention, fever, vertigo, diarrhea or headache, then other diagnoses should be considered (Bastian & Brown, 2007).
CEBM, level 5.

The differential diagnoses for her urinary symptoms of dysuria and frequency are urinary tract infection and urinary frequency of early pregnancy. In the absence of dysuria, pyuria, and hematuria, urinary frequency of early pregnancy is most likely.

Urinary frequency is a common early pregnancy complaint. Urinary tract infection should be considered if dysuria, pyuria or hematuria is present (Bastian & Brown, 2007).
CEBM, level 5.

ICD-9 Codes

V22.2 Supervision of normal pregnancy with non-obstetric complication (active)
278.00 Obesity (active)
244.1 Hypothyroidism, acquired, due to ablation (active)
493.10 Asthma, intrinsic, unspecified (active)
597.80 Urethritis, unspecified (active)
787.02 Nausea (active)
376.21 Thyrotoxic exophthalmos (Graves' disease) (inactive)

Plan

Laboratory and Diagnostic Studies
- I perform phlebotomy and order initial prenatal laboratory studies that include an obstetric panel composed of blood type, Rh factor, antibody screen, CBC, HBsAg, rubella titer, varicella titer, hemoglobin electrophoresis, VDRL, and HIV.

- HIV counseling and consent obtain prior to phlebotomy.
- Pap smear and gonorrhea and chlamydia screening (Lockwood & Magriples, 2008).

  CEBM, level 5.

- Urine culture to rule out urinary tract infection.

  In addition to history and physical examination, urine culture should be used in the evaluation of pregnant patients with dysuria (Komaroff, 2007).

  CEBM, level 5.

- TSH and free T4 to evaluate thyroid function. Given this patient's history of Graves' disease and her current treatment for hypothyroidism, it is important to evaluate thyroid hormones TSH and free T4.

  Serum TSH should be measured four to six weeks after conception, four to six weeks after any change in the dose of T4, and at least once each trimester. Increased estrogen in pregnancy results in decreased clearance of serum thyroxine-binding globulin (TBG) concentrations. TBG excess leads to an increase in both serum total thyroxine (T4) and triiodothyronine (T3) concentrations, but not serum free T4 and T3 concentrations; therefore, free T3/T4 is a better indicator of thyroid function during pregnancy (Ross, 2007).

  CEBM, level 5.

- I refer patient for a pelvic ultrasound to confirm gestational age of pregnancy.

  Ultrasound is often used to establish gestational age when the uterine size estimated on physical examination differs from menstrual dating. Generally this difference may be due to uterine fibroids, retroverted uterus, multiple gestation or inaccurate menstrual dates (MacKenzie et al., 2007).

  CEBM, level 5.

Patient Education and Counseling

- I explain initial prenatal lab studies and discuss the need for further evaluation to diagnose urinary tract infection. I encourage adequate daily fluid intake and frequent voiding for comfort and to prevent urinary stasis.
- I discuss asthma management issues, including the importance of recognizing signs and symptoms of asthma, avoiding triggers, taking medications as directed, and receiving prompt care for acute exacerbations. I explain that continuing asthma medication during pregnancy is considered safer than having symptoms or exacerbations during pregnancy. I also discuss the common pregnancy discomfort of "shortness of breath" and encourage the patient to report any changes in her breathing or breathing effort. I share with her that shortness of breath with cough or wheeze is not likely a discomfort, but more likely a sign of worsening asthma. I encourage her to monitor peak expiratory flow rates (PEFR) at home. Julia states her

understanding of the importance of continued therapy, monitoring PEFRs, and reporting increased symptoms.

Asthma may improve, worsen, or remain unchanged in severity during pregnancy. Prevention of acute episodes and optimizing pulmonary function continue to be the primary goals of asthma care in pregnancy. When a pregnant asthmatic woman experiences dyspnea, it is important to determine whether this symptom is an exacerbation of asthma or physiologic dyspnea of pregnancy. The presence of cough and wheezing suggests asthma. Using PEFR or FEV1 can provide additional objective information—reductions in either suggest asthma exacerbation. It is important to monitor pulmonary function as decreased function during pregnancy is associated with adverse perinatal outcomes (Schatz & Weinberger, 2008).

CEBM, level 5.

- I counsel Julia on the guidelines for a recommended weight gain of 11 to 20 pounds in pregnancy with a pre-pregnancy BMI of 30 (Institute of Medicine, 2009).

CEBM, level 5.

- I explain the basis for these guidelines and the importance of having adequate intake and nutrition for fetal growth and development. I recommend a cautious balance between snacking to relieve nausea and snacking that introduces excessive or "empty" calories to her daily intake. For additional resources, I refer her to the pregnancy food pyramid online.

The interactive site http://www.mypyramid.gov/mypyramidmoms/ provides food suggestions and recommends daily and weekly intake amounts to meet the expected demands of pregnancy for specific parameters entered by the pregnant woman (age, BMI, activity level and weeks gestation) (United States Department of Agriculture Center for Nutrition Policy and Promotion, n.d.).

CEBM, level 5.

- Julia understands that with a BMI of 30 she just meets the criteria for "obese." Although this information is difficult to hear, she acknowledges that she is above her ideal "healthy" weight. She was only able to lose about half of the weight that she gained with her previous pregnancy. Her first pre-pregnancy weight was 165 pounds, and she gained 55 pounds. She lost approximately 30 pounds in the first six months after her son was born.

One of the strongest reasons for staying within the upper limit of IOM's recommendation comes from studies showing postpartum maternal weight retention and future risk of obesity, which is consistent with Julia's history. The IOM recommends that obese women gain between 11 and 20 pounds during pregnancy (Tse & Macones, 2008; Institute of Medicine, 2009).

CEBM, level 5.

- With a current total weight gain of four pounds, Julia is already at the target gain for the first trimester. I explain to her that some women gain more in the first trimester when they have significant nausea, as she has had. We agree to focus more on the coming months and to make a plan to monitor intake and weight gain together. Julia understands that "dieting" in pregnancy is not recommended, but we do discuss keeping a food diary to better evaluate specific nutritional intake and portion sizes. She agrees to develop a weekly eating plan but declines a nutritional consult at this time.

Anticipatory Guidance

- I discuss common discomforts of early pregnancy, including mild headache, mild nausea with or without vomiting, and urinary frequency or urgency (Bastian & Brown, 2007).

CEBM, level 5.

- I recommend vitamin B_6 (pyridoxine) supplementation, 25 mg by mouth three times a day, to help control nausea; I also recommend healthy snacks throughout the day.

Vitamin B_6 (pyridoxine) supplementation has been shown to reduce pregnancy related nausea (Jewell & Young, 2003).

CEBM, level 1a.

- I review signs of early pregnancy complication, including abdominal or uterine cramping, vaginal bleeding, severe nausea, and vomiting, and encourage patient to report these symptoms promptly (Lockwood & Magriples, 2008).

CEBM, level 5.

- I discuss prenatal genetic screening tests for aneuploidy and open neural tube defects (ONTD) and offer the following options:
  - Decline screening
  - Screen with ultrasound alone
  - Screen with combined first-trimester screening only
  - First- and second-trimester screening (integrated, sequential, or contingent)
  - Second-trimester screening alone

Julia elects to proceed with contingent screening. She will have first-trimester screening for aneuploidy, and if these results are reassuring and show low risk, she will have a second trimester screen for ONTDs with maternal serum alpha fetoprotein (msAFP). If these results are not reassuring, showing intermediate or high risk, she will continue with the sequential screen, msAFP, inhibin A, estradiol, and human chorionic gonadotropin. She will not undergo amniocentesis regardless of the results.

"Combined first trimester screening" is prenatal genetic screening of the fetus via nuchal translucency thickness measures and maternal serum biochemical

markers to detect elevated risk of aneuploidy (American College of Obstetricians and Gynecologists, 2007).

CEBM, level 5.

Detection rates for trisomy 21 using combined first trimester screening alone are 82–87%. When performed step-wise (sequential) with second trimester maternal serum testing the detection rate for trisomy 21 increases to 95%. When performed as an integrated screen (no results are given until after the second phase of testing) the detection rate improves to 96% (Malone et al., 2005).

CEBM, level 1b.

Contingent screening is a more cost effective approach to first and second trimester screening and is performed as follows: first trimester results are classified as low-risk, intermediate risk and high-risk. Low-risk results do not require follow-up. Intermediate risk results are an indication to proceed with second trimester screening for aneuploidy. High-risk results are an indication for amniocentesis, which the woman may accept or decline (Ball et al., 2007).

CEBM, level 2b.

Second trimester maternal serum screening can also detect elevated risk of open neural tube defects. This can be performed in various combinations with combined first trimester screening (as described above) or alone. Fetal chromosomal screening should be offered to all pregnant women regardless of age (American College of Obstetricians and Gynecologists, 2007).

CEBM, level 5.

Referral for perinatology consultation

Perinatology consult to be made after lab results are received and reviewed **(D2, C1, PO A).**

When a woman is pregnant and has multiple pre-existing comorbidities it is appropriate to obtain a perinatology consult during the course of prenatal care (Varney, Kriebs, & Gegor, 2004).

CEBM, level 5.

Prescriptions

None given.

Critical Appraisal

According to our facility's birthing center guidelines, a perinatal consult is required for patients with certain comorbid conditions who wish to give birth in the birth center. The perinatology group will decide whether it is appropriate for the patient to labor and birth in the birthing center.

Follow-up

- I will call patient with results of urine culture, thyroid function tests, and initial prenatal laboratory testing.
- After confirmation of gestational age, I will refer Julia for combined first trimester screening.

It is important to have accurate dates before scheduling combined first trimester screening. Screening is performed between 10 weeks three days and 13 weeks six days gestation (Malone et al., 2005).

CEBM, level 1b.

- Julia will have an early glucose challenge test (GCT) screen at 16 weeks gestation. Julia's history of giving birth to an infant weighing over 4,000 g increases her risk of gestation diabetes for this pregnancy. It is recommended that she have an early GCT screening test. There are no specific guidelines for when to perform the early screening test. We decide to perform the test at 16 weeks, when she will be having second trimester blood drawn for either contingent screen or msAFP.

All pregnant women should be screened for gestation diabetes between 24 and 28 weeks gestation unless they have risk factors (i.e., personal history of GDM, having a previous infant with birth weight > 4,000 grams, strong family history of diabetes mellitus) that warrant earlier testing (American College of Obstetricians and Gynecologists, 2001).

CEBM, level 5.

- Julia will return to office in four weeks for routine follow-up, or sooner as needed.

Encounter Two

Laboratory results from initial prenatal visit at 7 weeks 3 days gestation: CBC with differential, hemoglobin electrophoresis are within normal range. Hepatitis B surface antigen, VDRL, HIV, gonorrhea, chlamydia, urine culture, and Pap smear are negative. Blood type is O+ with negative antibody screen. Varicella and rubella antibody detected.

Telephone consult to endocrinologist after laboratory review: I fax the thyroid function test results to Julia's endocrinologist and follow up with a phone call to discuss her results and possible changes to her levothyroxine (Synthroid) dose. Since her levothyroxine (Synthroid) dose was increased six weeks ago and she is taking her medication as prescribed, the laboratory results are likely an accurate measurement of her thyroid function on 0.137 mg/day. The endocrinologist recommends an increase in levothyroxine (Synthroid) to 0.175 mg/day and reevaluation of TSH and FT4 in four to six weeks **(D2, C1, PO A).**

TSH and FT4 should be checked four to six weeks after any dose adjustment (Ross, 2007).

CEBM, level 5.

Test	Result	Reference Range	Interpretation
TSH	5.35 mIU/L	0.40–4.50 mIU/L Pregnant: 1st trimester 0.20–4.70 mIU/L 2nd trimester 0.30–4.10 mIU/L 3rd trimester 0.40–2.70 mIU/L	Elevated
Free T4	0.9 ng/dL	0.8–1.8 ng/dL	Within normal range

Encounter Three (telephone consult with patient one week after initial visit, 7 weeks 4 days gestation)

I call Julia after reviewing her initial laboratory results and discussing her thyroid management with her endocrinologist. I explain that all values were within normal range except for her TSH, which was elevated. Julia confirmed that she had increased her dose from 0.125 mg to 0.137 mg over six weeks ago and reported taking the prescribed amount daily. Her TSH and FT4 levels had not been reevaluated since her therapy change. She denies any symptoms of hypothyroidism. I explain the endocrinologist's recommendation to increase her daily dose to 0.175 mg/day and to reassess her thyroid function in four to six weeks **(D2, C1, PO C).**

Women with pre-pregnancy diagnosed hypothyroidism have increased requirements of thyroid hormone in pregnancy. Many women who are taking synthetic thyroid hormone for hypothyroidism need to increase doses during the preconception period or the first trimester (Ross, 2007). Mandel and colleagues found an increase of nearly 50% in mean thyroxine dosage (0.1 mg/d to 0.148 mg/d)(Mandel, Larsen, Seely, & Brent, 1990).

CEBM, level 2b.

Encounter Four (follow-up prenatal visit at 27 weeks 0 days gestation)

Interval History (between 8 and 27 weeks gestation)

Julia continued to receive prenatal care with our practice and attended visits at routine intervals. The results of her prenatal genetic screening in the first trimester were reassuring, as was her screening for ONTDs, both demonstrating low risk for the respective fetal anomalies. The early GCT performed at 16 weeks was within normal range. Her second trimester TSH and FT4 were also within normal range. Her ultrasound at 20 weeks revealed normal fetal anatomy, size consistent with dates, normal amniotic fluid volume, and a posterior implanted placenta. Blood pressure readings were 100–110/60–76. Fetal growth, as assessed by fundal height measurements at each visit, was adequate throughout the second trimester. Julia has followed an eating plan modified from the mypyramid.gov site and has gained weight at a rate of approximately 0.5 pound per week. She has not had any signs of pregnancy complications, asthma exacerbation, or hypothyroidism.

Review of Perinatal Consult

Julia was seen by our consulting perinatologist at 19 weeks gestation to receive recommendations regarding her care during this pregnancy with comorbid conditions **(D2, C1, PO E).**

The perinatologist supported continued midwifery care and recommended thyroid function tests each trimester to evaluate thyroid function and adequacy of control, serial ultrasounds to assess fetal growth, and weekly fetal surveillance via non-stress test and biophysical profile starting at 34 weeks to assess fetal well-being. There were no recommendations made to alter management of weight gain or asthma. There were no recommendations to alter prenatal care or fetal monitoring based on these stable conditions.

The perinatal consultant was not willing to make a decision on Julia's eligibility for the birth center at this time. He was concerned about her thyroid control given elevated TSH despite recent increases of levothyroxine (Synthroid) daily dosage. He requested a return consult in two months to reevaluate her thyroid control and to consider birth center eligibility based on her status at that time. He did state that he was fairly certain she would not be a suitable candidate for the birth center, but he was willing to reevaluate her situation at the end of the second trimester.

Chief complaint: Julia continues to feel well and is happy about the pregnancy. She presents for a routine follow-up at 27 weeks gestation and to rescreen for gestational diabetes and thyroid function.

History of Previous Illness: Julia reports daily fetal movement. She denies vaginal bleeding or spotting, abdominal pain or cramping, fever, fatigue, changes in vaginal discharge, leaking of fluid from the vagina, severe headache, or visual changes.

Julia continues taking montelukast sodium (Singulair) and levothyroxine (Synthroid) daily and denies any adverse effects or symptoms of asthma or hypothyroidism.

Review of Systems

Constitutional: Denies weight loss, fatigue, weakness, fever, chills, or night sweats. No change in appetite or general activity level. No excessive weight gain. No difficulty falling asleep or staying asleep.

Skin and hair: Denies rashes or lesions. No change in hair amount, texture, or consistency.

Head, ears, eyes, nose, and throat: Denies headache. No changes in visual, auditory, olfactory acuity. No problems eating, swallowing. No voice changes.

Neck: Denies masses, tenderness, stiffness, or limitations in movement.

Breast: Denies breast lumps, pain or tenderness, or discharge.

Chest: Denies cough, chest pain, shortness of breath, wheezing.

Cardiovascular: Denies chest pain, palpitations, dyspnea on exertion, edema.

Gastrointestinal: Denies appetite changes, nausea, vomiting, diarrhea, constipation, changes in stool or stooling pattern.

Urinary: Denies frequency, urgency, dysuria, nocturia, or incontinence of urine.

Genitalia: Denies vaginal bleeding, malodorous discharge, lesions, or pain.

Musculoskeletal: Denies pain or tenderness. No limitation in movement or range of motion.

Neurologic: Denies dizziness, weakness, numbness, coordination problems, loss of consciousness, or alteration in mood, sleep, and memory.

Psychologic: Denies depression, anxiety, and loss of energy or ability to concentrate.

Focused Prenatal Physical Exam

BP: 104/66.

Weight: 208 lb (16 lb total weight gain).

Uterus: Soft, nontender, fundal height 27 cm.

FHR: 150s.

Urine: Protein: negative; glucose: negative.

Impression

30-year-old G2P1001 at 27 weeks 4 days gestation. Current fetal status is reassuring, as evidenced by fetal heart rate of 150s and subjective observation of daily fetal movement. Fundal height is appropriate for estimated gestational age.

Her prenatal course is complicated by a history of Graves' disease with postablative hypothyroidism treated with levothyroxine (Synthroid), which has been increased during this pregnancy in response to elevated TSH levels. She has not demonstrated signs or symptoms of hypothyroidism, but monitored lab values show that her thyroid function has not been well controlled **(D2, C1, PO D)**.

The goal of synthetic hormone therapy during pregnancy is to normalize maternal TSH concentration (Ross, 2007).

CEBM, level 5.

Total weight gain of 16 pounds is within normal limits.

An obese-weight woman (pre-pregnancy BMI ≥ 30) should gain at least 11 pounds, with an expected/target weight gain of one half pound per week in the third trimester and a total weight gain of less than 20 pounds (Institute of Medicine, 2009).

CEBM, level 5.

Fetal growth remains adequate as evidenced by fundal height measurements that are within expected range for estimated gestational age.

Fundal height in centimeters should be consistent with number of weeks gestation after the 22nd week. Overall trend of growth should also be evaluated. Further investigation and possible sonographic evaluation are indicated if fundal height and weeks gestation differ by more than 2 (Varney et al., 2004).

CEBM, level 5.

ICD-9 Codes

V22.2 Supervision of normal pregnancy with non-obstetric complication (active)
278.00 Obesity (active)
244.1 Hypothyroidism, acquired, due to ablation (active)
493.10 Asthma, intrinsic, unspecified (active)
376.21 Thyrotoxic exophthalmos (Graves disease) (inactive)

Plan

Laboratory diagnostics
I perform phlebotomy and order a GCT, TSH, and FT4.

Education and Counseling
I explain the laboratory studies to Julia and review the importance of monitoring her TSH levels at routine intervals and after levothyroxine (Synthroid) dose changes. I also review the reason for rescreening for GDM with another GCT at this point in the pregnancy.

Serum TSH should be measured four to six weeks after conception, four to six weeks after any change in the dose of thyroid hormone, and at least once each trimester. Since increased estrogen levels in pregnancy result in elevations of total T3 and T4, FT4 is a better indicator of thyroid function in pregnancy (Ross, 2007).

CEBM, level 5.

For women with risk factors and negative early GCT screening it is appropriate to rescreen at 24–28 weeks gestation, as in routine care. Insulin resistance increases as pregnancy progresses (American College of Obstetricians and Gynecologists, 2001).

CEBM, level 5.

I congratulate Julia on her excellent weight management and share that her weight gain is appropriate for this point in pregnancy. I ask how she is coping with dietary changes and meal planning. Julia reports feeling very satisfied with her weight management so far this pregnancy. I discuss and reinforce the need to have adequate nutritional intake and to avoid large portions and foods with high fats, sugars, and calories that do not provide significant nutrition. I ask if she feels stress or frustration when keeping to her daily eating guidelines. She admits that she does have difficulty—logistically and emotionally—adjusting to the routine of food planning but is happy that the health of her pregnancy and new baby are motivating her to change her eating habits. I encourage her to continue her new eating habits through to term. I discuss typical fetal growth patterns and explain that the majority of fetal mass is gained in the third trimester and that this fetal growth can be affected by excessive maternal intake and weight gain. She states that she will continue this lifestyle change for herself and her family even after giving birth.

Success in weight management begins with self-motivation and willingness to make lifestyle changes. Overweight and obese individuals need active support in planning and achieving weight loss and optimal weight maintenance (Costain & Croker, 2005).

CEBM, level 5.

In a recent study, overweight and obese women who did have excessive gestational weight gain tended to increase total caloric intake and carbohydrates and sugars during the third trimester of pregnancy. Those who consumed a stable number of calories throughout pregnancy were less likely to have excessive gestational weight gain and perinatal complications (Olafsdottir, Skuladottir, Thorsdottir, Hauksson, & Steingrimsdottir, 2006).

CEBM, level 2c.

I discuss fetal movement awareness and encourage the patient to contact the office or the midwife on call if she feels a decrease fetal movement.

Fetal death may be preceded by subjective observation of decreased movement (American College of Obstetricians and Gynecologists, 2000). Movement awareness and counting is considered a low-tech, non-invasive method of fetal assessment. Formal movement counting is not indicated in low-risk pregnancies until 34–36 weeks, but awareness of fetal movement and perception of decreased movement is reviewed at each prenatal encounter (Varney et al., 2004).

CEBM, level 5.

I review signs and symptoms of preeclampsia and preterm labor and encourage the patient to contact the office or the midwife on call if she experiences any symptoms.

Pre-eclampsia is defined as gestational hypertension (onset after 20 weeks gestation) with proteinuria. Symptoms may include: severe headache, visual changes, right upper quadrant or epigastric pain, excessive swelling (generalized or periorbital). A woman with symptoms of pre-eclampsia should be evaluated promptly as symptoms generally present as the conditions worsens (Varney et al., 2004).

CEBM, level 5.

Symptoms of preterm labor include: menstrual-like cramps, dull lower backache, suprapubic pain or pressure, pelvic pressure, change in vaginal secretions, uterine contractions > six per hour not relieved by rest. Screening for preterm labor in low-risk women includes reviewing signs and symptoms at each visit and encouraging the woman to be aware and report any symptoms. Preterm labor leads to preterm birth in approximately 12% of all U.S. births and is associated with 75% of perinatal deaths and 50% of neurological deficits of infancy (Varney et al., 2004).

CEBM, level 5.

Anticipatory Guidance
- I review routine late second trimester anticipatory guidance.
- I review the perinatal recommendations for fetal testing in the third trimester and explain to Julia the purpose of the planned surveillance to evaluate fetal growth and identify signs of fetal compromise.
- Julia accepts the plan made in consult with the perinatologist. She understands that her current pregnancy will be managed differently than her first due to her current hypothyroid state. She understands that the proposed fetal testing is to ensure that the fetus is developing well and being supported adequately by the intrauterine environment **(D2, C1, PO C, E).**

Consult
I confirm the perinatology follow-up consult with the patient. She has an appointment with the perinatologist in one week.

Prescriptions
None given.

Follow-up
I will call patient with the results of today's laboratory tests and fax a copy of the reports to the perinatal associates' office. The patient will return to this office in two weeks for routine prenatal follow-up visit.

Laboratory results from encounter at 27 weeks
Glucose challenge test results in the normal range, and thyroid-stimulating hormone continues to be elevated at 4.53 mIU/L.

Encounter Five (telephone consult with patient at 28 weeks 3 days gestation)

Since the last encounter, Julia's lab results have been received, reviewed, and sent to the perinatology associates' office. Her GCT is within normal range,

TSH is elevated, and FT4 is within normal range. She has been notified of these results. She had her perinatal consult two days ago.

I call Julia after receiving a faxed report from her perinatology consult. During the consultation, the perinatologist discussed Julia's prenatal course and focused primarily on her thyroid function. He was concerned about the apparent poor control during pregnancy and recommended another increase in levothyroxine (Synthroid) (from 0.175 to 0.200 mg/day). He restated his recommendations for weekly fetal surveillance after 34 weeks. He recommended that she give birth on the labor and delivery unit instead of at the birth center.

I review all these points with Julia. She states that the perinatologist has thoroughly explained the recommendations for care and she understands the basis for these recommendations. She remains happy about the course of pregnancy to date. She expresses disappointment regarding the recommendation to birth on the labor and delivery unit but is grateful that she can continue with midwifery care **(D2, C1, PO C, E)**.

Encounter Six (telephone consult with patient at 29 weeks 5 days gestation)

I receive a call from Julia at the practice office.

Chief complaint: "I was working, and my right eye went cloudy and dim, and I had some tingling in my right hand."

HPI: While at work today Julia experienced a sudden vision loss in the periphery of her right eye that she describes as "cloudy and dim." There was no change in vision of the left eye. Shortly after, she felt tingling of the right arm and hand. She denies eye pain, headache, nausea, palpitations, weakness in the extremities, slurred speech, muscle or joint pain, gait disturbances, dizziness, or vertigo. The symptoms resolved after one hour. She denies any change in activity level. She denies any new medications or use of recreational drugs.

She reports active fetal movement and denies vaginal bleeding or spotting, abdominal pain or cramping, fever, fatigue, changes in vaginal discharge, leaking of fluid from the vagina, or severe epigastric or right upper quadrant pain.

Pertinent Review of Systems

Head, ears, eyes, nose, and throat: Denies headache. No changes in visual, auditory, olfactory acuity. No problems eating, swallowing. No voice changes or slurred speech.

Neck: Denies masses, tenderness, stiffness, or limitations in movement.

Cardiovascular: Denies chest pain, palpitations, dyspnea on exertion, edema.

Musculoskeletal: Denies pain or tenderness. No limitation in movement or range of motion.

Neurologic: See HPI.

Psychologic: Denies depression, anxiety, and loss of energy or ability to concentrate.

Impression

30-year-old G2P1001 at 29 weeks 5 days with acute onset and rapid resolution of visual disturbance accompanied by ipsilateral arm tingling and numbness in the absence of pain, weakness, and palpitations. The event began two to three hours ago and resolved approximately one hour ago. She is now asymptomatic.

Cerebrovascular and cardiovascular causes of symptoms require immediate evaluation and physical examination. Possible etiologies for symptoms include migraine, which is unlikely because she does not report headache. Optic neuritis is unlikely because it generally develops over days to weeks and resolves slowly. Preeclampsia is an unlikely diagnosis but an important pregnancy complication to consider when a pregnant women presents with visual changes. Transient ischemic attack or stroke must be considered and requires immediate evaluation.

Plan

I explain to Julia that these are not typical symptoms of pregnancy. I explain my concern about the possibility of neurologic or cardiovascular problems that need to be evaluated. I refer her to the emergency department at our affiliated institution, which is 15 city blocks from her office. She is very willing to present for evaluation. She plans to arrive by cab and have her husband meet her in the hospital. I call the hospital and alert the staff that she is en route for evaluation of a transient visual loss and sensory disturbance. Her initial evaluation will be in the obstetrical triage area. I will follow up with the chief resident after her initial evaluation **(D1, C4, PO A, B, C, D, E)**.

Encounter Seven (telephone consult with chief obstetric resident, 120 minutes later the same day)

I call the obstetrical triage area and receive the following verbal report.

The patient presented for evaluation to obstetrical triage approximately two hours prior. She was accompanied by her husband. Her symptoms were completely resolved and she denied any recurrent symptoms. She denied new visual, neurologic, focal, or peripheral symptoms since her initial reported episode. The resident reported vital signs within normal limits. Fetal heart rate was being monitored continuously, and the baseline ranged from 140 to 150. She was not experiencing uterine contractions. Her oxygen saturation was 100 percent on room air. A bedside neurologic exam was performed and all parameters were within normal limits. They planned to admit her for 24-hour observation. In that time they would arrange for an MRI of the brain, an MRI angiogram of the head, a neurologic consult, and possibly a cardiac consult to exclude structural abnormalities, cardiac masses, or atherosclerotic disease. I will coordinate as midwifery service consultant.

Summary of Hospital Course and Discharge Plan

Julia was discharged from the hospital after 24 hours of observation. All diagnostic testing was unremarkable.

In collaboration with the hospital staff, we schedule a transesophageal echocardiogram and a follow-up neurology consult with a neurologist in our facility's stroke prevention program. Julia will continue to present at routine intervals for prenatal care managed by the midwifery group practice provided she does not have continued or recurrent symptoms. She will call to report recurrent or new-onset symptoms, including weakness, pain, palpitations, dizziness, or changes in vision, movement, sensation, or speech (**D1, C4, PO G, H, I**).

Encounter Eight (follow-up prenatal visit at 34 weeks 2 days gestation)

Interval History (29–34 Weeks Gestation) by Chart Review

Julia has continued to receive prenatal care with our practice and has attended visits at routine intervals. Blood pressure readings have been 104–110/64–70. Fetal growth, as assessed by fundal height measurements at each visit, has been adequate throughout the third trimester. Julia continues her modified eating plan and has gained weight at a rate of approximately 0.5 pound per week for the second and third trimesters. She has not had any signs of preterm labor, preeclampsia, asthma exacerbation, or hypothyroidism.

The results of her inpatient evaluation for transient visual and sensory disturbance at 29 weeks suggest a probable transient ischemic attack. Since she is pregnant and may have had an associated hypercoagulable state, the neurology team decided to perform a complete stroke evaluation that included MRI, MRI angiography of head and neck, and transesophageal echocardiogram. The results of the MRI and MRI angiogram performed during her hospitalization were unremarkable. She was released after 24 hours of observation with no recurrent symptoms and unremarkable studies. At discharge from the hospital a transesophageal echocardiogram was arranged to evaluate for cardiac mass, structural abnormality, patent foramen ovale, or significant atherosclerotic disease. The results of that study were also unremarkable. She had a follow-up evaluation by the neurologist in an ambulatory setting.

Review of Neurology Consult

Julia was seen by the neurologist at 30 weeks 3 days gestation. She was accompanied by her husband. At the consult the patient reported compliance with her low-dose anti-platelet therapy, aspirin (Ecotrin) 81 mg/day, and she denied any change in status or any recurrent symptoms. The neurologist reviewed the presumed diagnosis of transient ischemic attack and the results of the evaluation to date. There was no evidence of a recent CNS injury, intra- or extracranial vascular stenosis, or structural cardiac abnormality. No specific abnormalities were found to explain the apparent interruption in blood flow to the brain. The event was categorized as "cryptogenic stroke." Testing for hypercoagulopathy was performed at this consult. The neurologist recommended continued anti-platelet therapy with aspirin (Ecotrin) 81 mg/day and repeat hypercoagulopathy testing before future pregnancies.

It is unclear why hypercoagulopathy studies were not initiated during Julia's hospitalization. Since they were not performed previously, the neurologist ordered testing at her consult. Julia's workup included testing to evaluate all possible mechanisms for cryptogenic stroke.

> *Ischemic strokes without well-defined etiologies are labeled cryptogenic and account for 30–40% of all ischemic strokes. Various mechanisms have been associated with cryptogenic stroke (CS): paradoxical embolism secondary to patent foramen ovale, thrombophilia, occult cardiac embolism secondary to aortic atherosclerotic disease, preclinical or subclinical cerebrovascular disease, and inflammatory processes. Ultimately cryptogenic stroke is a diagnosis of exclusion that follows a thorough investigation of possible causes (Prabhakaran & Elkind, 2008).*
>
> CEBM, level 5.

Chief complaint: "I'm here for a follow-up visit, and I feel pretty good. I just had my first non-stress test and biophysical today. They said the fluid was 'low' and the report would be faxed over."

HPI

- Julia reports daily fetal movement. She denies vaginal bleeding or spotting, abdominal pain or cramping, fever, fatigue, changes in vaginal discharge, leaking of fluid from the vagina, severe headache, or visual changes.
- Episode of visual loss and transient ipsilateral arm numbness five weeks ago: Julia denies repeat episodes of visual changes, loss of vision, blurred vision, or any other sensory changes since her initial episode at 29 weeks. She continues to work at her office job but plans to begin her maternity leave at 36 weeks. She generally feels well but is concerned about the possible diagnosis of a "transient ischemic attack" and what it could mean to the pregnancy. She is taking a baby aspirin (Ecotrin) daily as recommended by the neurologist. She denies any abnormal bleeding or bruising.
- Asthma: Continues taking montelukast sodium (Singulair) daily. She denies cough, chest pain, shortness of breath, wheezing. She continues to monitor PEFRs at home.
- Hypothyroidism: Continues taking levothyroxine (Synthroid) daily and denies any adverse effects of medication or symptoms of hyperthyroidism

or hypothyroidism, including weight loss or significant gain, fatigue, weakness, palpitations, fever, chills or night sweats, change in appetite or general activity level, slow movement or speech, cold or heat intolerance, constipation, change in hair amount, texture, or consistency, or voice changes.

Review of Systems

Constitutional: See HPI. No difficulty falling to sleep or staying asleep.

Skin and hair: Denies rashes or lesions.

Head, ears, eyes, nose, and throat: Denies headache. No changes in visual, auditory, olfactory acuity. No problems eating, swallowing.

Neck: Denies masses, tenderness, stiffness, or limitations in movement.

Breast: Denies breast lumps, pain or tenderness, or discharge.

Chest: See HPI.

Cardiovascular: See HPI. Denies chest pain, dyspnea on exertion, edema.

Gastrointestinal: Denies appetite changes, nausea, vomiting, diarrhea, constipation, changes in stool or stooling pattern.

Urinary: Denies frequency, urgency, dysuria, nocturia, or incontinence of urine.

Genitalia: Denies vaginal bleeding, malodorous discharge, lesions, or pain.

Musculoskeletal: Denies pain or tenderness. No limitation in movement or range of motion.

Neurologic: See HPI. Denies loss of consciousness or alteration in mood, sleep, or memory.

Psychologic: Denies depression, anxiety, and loss of energy or ability to concentrate.

Ultrasound and Fetal Testing Report (performed today prior to office visit)

One fetus in vertex presentation.
Fetal cardiac activity observed.
Placenta anterior.
Amniotic fluid volume decreased (4 cm).
Fetal size consistent with gestational age (86th percentile).
Fetal kidney, bladder, stomach, ventricles are within normal limits.
Non-stress test (NST): reactive.
Biophysical profile (BPP): 8/10.
Recommendation: Follow-up in two days to reevaluate amniotic fluid volume.
    Increase fluid intake, perform kick counts daily.

Focused Prenatal Physical Exam

BP: 110/70.

Weight: 213 lb (21 lb total weight gain).

Uterus: Soft, nontender, fundal height 34 cm.

FHR: 140s.

Urine: Protein: negative; glucose: negative.

Impression

Julia is a 30-year-old G2P1001 at 34 weeks 2 days gestation. Current fetal status is reassuring as evidenced by fetal heart rate of 140s and subjective observation of daily fetal movement as well as recent fetal testing showing a reactive NST and a BPP score of 8/10.

Oligohydramnios is present based on sonogram evaluation today showing an AFI of 4 centimeters.

> *Oligohydramnios is defined at AFI < 5 (Beloosesky & Ross, 2007).*
>
> CEBM, level 5.

Her prenatal course is complicated by a recent episode of right-sided visual and sensory disturbance that was evaluated acutely as an inpatient and followed up with an outpatient neurology consult. The results of all tests have been unremarkable. She has been diagnosed with a probable transient ischemic attack (TIA) or cryptogenic stroke (CS). She takes 81 mg of aspirin (Ecotrin) daily for stroke prevention.

Her course is further complicated by a history of Graves' disease with post-ablative hypothyroidism, treated with levothyroxine (Synthroid), which has been increased during this pregnancy in response to elevated TSH levels. She has not demonstrated signs or symptoms of hypothyroidism, but based on monitored lab values her thyroid function has not been well controlled.

> *The goal of synthetic hormone therapy during pregnancy is to normalize maternal TSH concentration (Ross, 2007).*
>
> CEBM, level 5.

Total weight gain of 21 pounds is above recommended range.

> *An obese-weight woman (pre-pregnancy BMI ≥ 30) should gain at least 11 pounds, with an expected/target weight gain of one half pound per week in the third trimester and a total weight gain of less than 20 pounds (Institute of Medicine, 2009).*
>
> CEBM, level 5.

Fetal growth remains adequate as evidenced by fundal height measurements within expected range for estimated gestational age and by sonogram biometrics performed today. Fetus size is in the 86th percentile for this gestational age.

ICD-9 Codes

V22.2 Supervision of normal pregnancy with non-obstetric complication (active)
674.0 Cerebrovascular disorder (active)
278.00 Obesity (active)
244.1 Hypothyroidism, acquired, due to ablation (active)
493.10 Asthma, intrinsic, unspecified (active)
376.21 Thyrotoxic exophthalmos (Graves' disease) (inactive)

Plan

Laboratory studies
None ordered today.

Follow-up
Patient has a scheduled AFI follow-up in two days.

Education and Counseling
- I discuss the finding of oligohydramnios on ultrasound today. I explain to Julia that this finding can be transient or persistent and that is why follow-up testing in needed. If persistent, oligohydramnios can be a sign that the fetus is not receiving adequate blood flow and therefore adequate oxygenation in the uterus.

In the third trimester AFI is inversely related to adverse pregnancy outcomes secondary to umbilical cord compression, uteroplacental insufficiency and meconium aspiration (Beloosesky & Ross, 2007).

CEBM, level 5.

- I review the neurology consult report with Julia and explain the diagnosis of cryptogenic stroke. I explain the recommendation for continued aspirin (Ecotrin) therapy given that pregnancy is a hypercoagulable state and she had experienced a probable TIA/CS. She was shocked by the idea of having a stroke at age 30 and during pregnancy. I explain again that this is a diagnosis of exclusion and we are managing the situation conservatively. We are awaiting the results of hypercoagulable testing to determine whether aspirin (Ecotrin) therapy is necessary and if so whether it is sufficient **(D2, C1, PO C, E).**

The short-term risk of recurrent stroke after CS is intermediate. Long-term prognosis is good. Risk reduction includes antiplatelet therapy and risk factor modification (weight loss; smoking cessation; control of diabetes, hypertension, hyperlipidemia; moderate alcohol intake; and adequate physical activity) (Prabhakaran & Elkind, 2008).

CEBM, level 5.

- I follow up on Julia's eating plan. She continues with success—daily intake, emotional satisfaction, and appropriate weight gain. I encourage her to maintain motivation for healthy eating and to continue after the prenatal period, particularly in light of her probable diagnosis with TIA/CS.
- I discuss fetal movement awareness and encourage the patient to contact the office or the midwife on call if she feels decreased fetal movement.
- I review signs and symptoms of preeclampsia and preterm labor and encourage the patient to contact the office or the midwife on call if she experiences any symptoms.
- I encourage rest and increased fluid intake over the next week in hopes to increase amniotic fluid volume. She has a follow-up sonogram scheduled in one week.

Rest and increased oral hydration have been shown to increase amniotic fluid volume (Hofmeyr & Gulmezoglu, 2002).

CEBM, level 5.

- During our visit, Julia expresses concern that she may no longer be eligible for midwifery care. I explain to her that although she has multiple conditions being monitored and treated during this gestation, her pregnancy is progressing well and the fetal status is reassuring. Provided that her conditions remain stable and there are no signs of serious fetal compromise, she can remain in our care. It is appropriate to request another perinatology consult at this time to evaluate Julia, the fetus, and our current plan of care **(D2, C1, PO A, E).**

Anticipatory Guidance
- I review routine third-trimester anticipatory guidance.
- I review the perinatal recommendations for fetal testing in the third trimester and explain to Julia the purpose of the planned surveillance. I also discuss the various outcomes from her follow-up testing: normal amniotic fluid volume on the next evaluation would be an indication to return to weekly testing, as planned previously due to her hypothyroid condition; continued biweekly testing until she gives birth if oligohydramnios persists; and possible labor induction if oligohydramnios worsens or if other signs of fetal compromise are identified in follow-up evaluations.
- I remind Julia that we will be sending another TSH and FT4 to evaluate her thyroid control at her next visit.

Serum TSH should be measured four to six weeks after conception, four to six weeks after any change in the dose of thyroid hormone, and at least once each trimester. Since increased estrogen levels in pregnancy result in elevations of total T3 and T4, FT4 is a better indicator of thyroid function in pregnancy (Ross, 2007).

CEBM, level 5.

Consultation request: I request a perinatology consult to review the findings and recommendations of the neurologist and the appropriateness of continued midwifery care.

Prescriptions: None given.

Follow-up: I will follow up with the neurologist regarding the coagulopathy testing performed.

Return to office in two weeks for routine prenatal follow-up visit and TSH/FT4 testing.

ADDENDUM AND SUMMARY OF CONTINUED CARE

Julia continued to be seen weekly at our midwifery practice. Blood pressures, weight gain, and fetal growth and activity were all within expected ranges. She had no symptoms of pregnancy complications. The perinatologist recommended continued antiplatelet therapy with aspirin (Ecotrin) 81 mg/day until delivery based on her clinical diagnosis of probable TIA/CS. Results from the hypercoagulopathy studies were unremarkable. She had no continued or recurrent symptoms of TIA/CS. She continued biweekly fetal evaluation and amniotic fluid monitoring for oligohydramnios. AFI measurements ranged from four to eight centimeters, and fetal status was reassuring. At 36 weeks 4 days gestation, the AFI was 2.2 and the decision to induce labor was made in consult with the perinatologist. She continued under midwifery care and had a spontaneous vaginal birth of a 3,375-g live male infant at 36 weeks 5 days. One- and five-minute Apgars were nine and nine.

COMPETENCY DEFENSE

Domain 1, Competency 4. Appraise acuity of patient condition, and determine need to transfer patient to higher acuity setting, coordinate, and manage transfer to optimize patient outcomes.

Defense. Competency 4 was met when Julia called with a new onset of visual disturbance and I coordinated her emergency department evaluation and neurology follow-up care post hospitalization.

Domain 2, Competency 1. Assemble a collaborative interdisciplinary network, and refer and consult appropriately while maintaining primary responsibility for comprehensive patient care.

Defense. Julia presented with multiple chronic illnesses that required assembling an interdisciplinary network including consultants from neurology, perinatology, and emergency services to ensure an optimal outcome for both mother and baby.

Medications

Aspirin (Ecotrin)

Indication: Stroke prevention.

Class: Salicylate.

Mechanism: Inhibits prostaglandin synthesis and platelet aggregation by inactivates cyclooxygenase via acetylation.

Dose: 81 mg tablet, daily.

(continued)

Side effects
Common: Indigestion, nausea, vomiting.
Serious: Gastrointestinal ulcer, bleeding, tinnitus, bronchospasm, angioedema.
Pregnancy class: Category D (avoid in the third trimester).

Drug: Levothyroxine Sodium (Synthroid)

Indication: Hypothyroidism.

Class: Synthetic thyroid hormone.

Mechanism: Mimics thyroid hormone activity, thought to act by binding to thyroid receptor proteins attached to DNA and activating gene transcription and protein synthesis.

Dose: Titrated depending on comorbid conditions, age, and severity of hypothyroidism.

Side effects: Tachycardia, hyperactivity, fever, vomiting, diarrhea, diaphoresis, flushing.
Adverse effects: Seizure, osteopenia, myocardial infarction.
Pregnancy class: Category A.

Drug: Montelukast Sodium (Singulair)

Indication: Asthma.

Class: Leukotriene receptor antagonist.

Mechanism: Binds to cysteinyl leukotriene receptor 1 in the upper and lower airways to prevent leukotriene-mediated effects associated with asthma and allergic rhinitis (airway edema, smooth muscle contraction, and other respiratory inflammation).

Dose: 10-mg tablet, daily.

Side effects: Fatigue, fever, dyspepsia, gastroenteritis, dizziness, headache, nasal congestion, cough, rash.
Adverse effects (rare): Allergic granulomatosis angiitis, cholestatic hepatitis, aggressive behavior, agitation, dream disorder, hallucinations, altered behavior, suicidal thoughts.
Pregnancy class: Category B.

Drug: Vitamin B$_6$ (Pyridoxine)

Dose: 50 mg three times daily.

Indications: To alleviate pregnancy-related nausea.

Adverse effects (common): Paresthesias, numbness, unsteady gait.

Serious effects: May occur, none reported.

Source: American Society of Health-System Pharmacists, 2008; Thomson Micromedex Healthcare, 2008.

References

American College of Obstetricians and Gynecologists. (2000). Antepartum fetal surveillance (ACOG Practice Bulletin No. 9; replaces Technical Bulletin No. 188, January 1994). *Int J Gynaecol Obstet, 68*(2), 175–185.

American College of Obstetricians and Gynecologists. (2001). Gestational diabetes (ACOG Practice Bulletin No. 30; Replaces Technical Bulletin No. 200, December 1994, reaffirmed 2008). *Obstet Gynecol, 98*(3), 525–538.

American College of Obstetricians and Gynecologists. (2007). Screening for fetal chromosomal abnormalities (ACOG Practice Bulletin No. 77). *Obstet Gynecol, 109*(1), 217–227.

American Society of Health-System Pharmacists. (2008). *AHFS drug information.* Retrieved October 24, 2008, from http://online.statref.com

Ball, R.H., Caughey, A.B., Malone, F.D., Nyberg, D.A., Comstock, C.H., Saade, G.R., et al. (2007). First- and second-trimester evaluation of risk for Down syndrome. *Obstet Gynecol, 110*(1), 10–17.

Bastian, L.A., & Brown, H.L. (2007). *Diagnosis and clinical manifestations of early pregnancy.* Retrieved November 10, 2008, from http://www.uptodateonline.com

Beloosesky, R., & Ross, M.G. (2007). *Oligohydramnios.* Retrieved November 20, 2008, from http://www.uptodateonline.com

Costain, L., & Croker, H. (2005). Helping individuals to help themselves. *Proc Nutr Soc, 64*(1), 89–96.

Hofmeyr, G.J., & Gulmezoglu, A.M. (2002). Maternal hydration for increasing amniotic fluid volume in oligohydramnios and normal amniotic fluid volume. *Cochrane Database Syst Rev, 1,* CD000134.

Institute of Medicine (U.S.), Committee to reexamine IOM Pregnancy Weight Guidelines; Food and Nutrition Board; Board on Children, Youth, and Families. (2009). *Weight gain during pregnancy: reexamining the guidelines.* Washington, DC: National Academy Press.

Jewell, D., & Young, G. (2003). Interventions for nausea and vomiting in early pregnancy. *Cochrane Database Syst Rev, 4,* CD000145.

Komaroff, A.L. (2007). *Dysuria in adult women.* Retrieved November 10, 2008, from http://www.uptodateonline.com

Lockwood, C.J., & Magriples, U. (2008). *The initial prenatal assessment and routine prenatal care.* Retrieved November 10, 2008, from http://www.uptodateonline.com

MacKenzie, A.P., Stephenson, C.D., & Funai, E.F. (2007). *Prenatal assessment of gestational age.* Retrieved November 10, 2008, from http://www.uptodateonline.com

Malone, F.D., Canick, J.A., Ball, R.H., Nyberg, D.A., Comstock, C.H., Bukowski, R., et al. (2005). First-trimester or second-trimester screening, or both, for Down's syndrome. *N Engl J Med, 353*(19), 2001–2011.

Mandel, S.J., Larsen, P.R., Seely, E.W., & Brent, G.A. (1990). Increased need for thyroxine during pregnancy in women with primary hypothyroidism. *N Engl J Med, 323*(2), 91–96.

Olafsdottir, A.S., Skuladottir, G.V., Thorsdottir, I., Hauksson, A., & Steingrimsdottir, L. (2006). Maternal diet in early and late pregnancy in relation to weight gain. *Int J Obes (Lond), 30*(3), 492–499.

Prabhakaran, S., & Elkind, M.S. (2008). *Cryptogenic stroke.* Retrieved November 20, 2008, from http://www.uptodateonline.com

Ross, D.S. (2007). *Overview of thyroid disease in pregnancy.* Retrieved November 10, 2008, from http://www.uptodateonline.com

Schatz, M., & Weinberger, S.E. (2008). *Management of asthma during pregnancy.* Retrieved November 10, 2008, from http://www.uptodateonline.com

Thomson Micromedex Healthcare. (2008). *DrugPoint system.* Retrieved October 24, 2008, from http://online.statref.com

Tse, G., & Macones, G. (2008). *Weight gain in pregnancy.* Retrieved November 10, 2008, from http://www.uptodateonline.com

United States Department of Agriculture Center for Nutrition Policy and Promotion. (n.d.). *MyPyramid for pregnancy and breastfeeding.* Retrieved November 10, 2008, from http://www.mypyramid.gov/mypyramidmoms/

Varney, H., Kriebs, J.M., & Gegor, C.L. (2004). *Varney's midwifery* (4th ed.). Sudbury, MA: Jones and Bartlett.

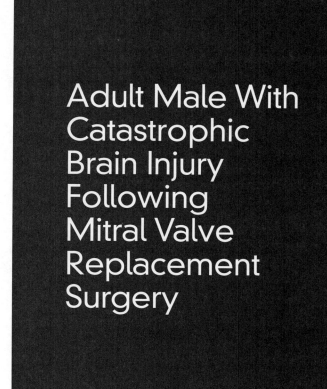

25

Adult Male With Catastrophic Brain Injury Following Mitral Valve Replacement Surgery

Dallas D. Regan

This case narrative focuses on the care I provided for a 60-year-old man with commercial medical insurance who suffered catastrophic brain injury following mitral valve replacement surgery. The case narrative focuses on care provided in the intensive care unit over eight hours in the immediate postoperative period. This case narrative demonstrates my ability to meet the following Columbia University School of Nursing (CUSN) doctoral competencies for comprehensive direct patient care.

DOMAIN 1, COMPETENCY 3

Formulate differential diagnoses and diagnostic strategies and therapeutic interventions with attention to scientific evidence, safety, cost, invasiveness, simplicity, acceptability, adherence, and efficacy for patients who present with new conditions and those with ambiguous or incomplete data, complex illnesses, comorbid conditions, and multiple diagnoses in all clinical settings.

PO A. Formulate a differential diagnosis for a patient who presents with new undifferentiated signs and symptoms.

PO B. Formulate a differential diagnosis for a patient who presents with ambiguous or incomplete data, complex illnesses, comorbid conditions, and potential multiple diagnoses.

PO C. Discuss the rationale for the differential diagnosis.

PO D. Discuss the rationale for the diagnostic evaluation with attention to scientific evidence, safety, cost, invasiveness, simplicity, acceptability, adherence, and efficacy.

PO E. Discuss the rationale for the therapeutic intervention with attention to scientific evidence, safety, cost, invasiveness, simplicity, acceptability, adherence, and efficacy.

DOMAIN 2, COMPETENCY 1

Assemble a collaborative interdisciplinary network, and refer and consult appropriately while maintaining primary responsibility for comprehensive patient care.

PO A. Initiate referral to other health care professionals while maintaining primary responsibility for patient care.

PO C. Utilize consultation recommendations for decision-making while maintaining primary responsibility for care.

PO D. Evaluate outcomes of interventions.

DOMAIN 1, COMPETENCY 7

Facilitate and guide the process of palliative care and/or planning end-of-life care by discussing diagnoses and prognosis, clarifying and validating patient desires and priorities, and promoting informed choices and shared decision-making by patient, family, and members of the health care team.

PO A. Facilitate and guide the palliative care process by discussing diagnoses and prognosis, clarifying and validating patient desires and priorities, and promoting informed choices and shared decision-making by patient, family, and members of the health care team.

PO B. Facilitate and guide planning end-of-life care by discussing diagnoses and prognosis, clarifying and validating patient desires and priorities, and promoting informed choices and shared decision-making by patient, family, and members of the health care team.

ENCOUNTER CONTEXT

Encounter Number One (post-operative day zero)

DNP role: I am the attending nurse practitioner as well as a DNP resident. I am assuming responsibility of care for this patient.

Identifying Information

Site: Urban academic medical center.

Setting: Adult cardiothoracic intensive care unit (CTICU).

Reason for encounter: Postoperative recovery and stabilization.

Informant: Chart review, surgical team report, and anesthesia report. The patient is mechanically ventilated and sedated following mitral valve replacement.

Summary of Care Previously Provided

Mr. P is a 60-year-old man with a complicated medical history including Hodgkin's lymphoma, coronary artery disease, and aortic stenosis diagnosed in 1994, for which he underwent coronary artery bypass grafting (CABG) and aortic valve replacement with a mechanical valve that same year.

One year prior to this admission, he experienced shortness of breath and dyspnea on exertion. He was taken to another hospital and was diagnosed with a non-ST elevation myocardial infarction (NSTEMI). He underwent cardiac catheterization, and a drug-eluting stent was placed in the vein graft of his prior CABG. Mild mitral valve regurgitation was noted at that time.

Four months prior to this admission, he complained of shortness of breath and dyspnea on exertion again. He was seen by his cardiologist, who performed a cardiac catheterization.

Mr. P was placed on medical therapy, but after several months with no relief, he was referred to this medical center for evaluation and possible surgical intervention.

Coronary Arteries	
Left main (LM)	No luminal irregularities
Left anterior descending (LAD)	100% proximal stenosis
Left circumflex (LCx)	Minor luminal irregularities with no flow limitation
Right coronary artery (RCA)	80% ostial lesion
Bypass grafts	Saphenous vein graft from aorta to mid-LAD with minor luminal irregularities
Valves	
Aortic	Mechanical prosthesis with normal function and no regurgitation or stenosis
Mitral	Mitral valve prolapse with 3+ mitral regurgitation
Other Data	
Left ventriculogram	EF 50% with no wall motion abnormalities

Mitral valve prolapse accounts for the vast majority of mitral valve regurgitation in developed countries. Other primary causes include rheumatic disease, trauma, and infective endocarditis. Mitral annular calcification is a common occurrence in older patients with an incidence of 20% in those aged 60 to 70, and increases with age. Some studies have shown that patients with severe mitral annular calcification have better outcomes with mitral repair versus replacement; however, the limited access to the surgical field by minimally invasive approaches makes repair more difficult (Aronow & Kronzon, 1987; Feindel, Tufail, David, Ivanov, & Armstrong, 2003; Otto, 2008).

Centre for Evidence-Based Medicine (CEBM), level 5.

Because of his history of lymphoma with radiation therapy to the thorax as well as his history of sternotomy for previous cardiac surgery, there was concern that a repeat sternotomy would be difficult from a technical standpoint and increase Mr. P's risk of poor wound healing. As a result, the surgical approach chosen was a "mini" thoracotomy to avoid the mediastinum.

Therapeutic radiation therapy is associated with histologic changes in the affected tissue, which can disrupt the normal healing process and make surgical dissection more difficult. Alterations in healing have been attributed to the changes in cutaneous blood vessels, fibroblasts, collagen, and keratinocytes of the affected tissues (Tokarek, Bernstein, Sullivan, Uitto, & Mitchell, 1994).

CEBM, level 5.

Minimally invasive mitral valve replacement is most commonly performed via a limited right thoracotomy. The mitral valve is exposed either directly through the left atrium or through the right atrium and an atrial septal incision. Benefits of the minimally invasive approach include avoidance of a sternotomy, decreased risk of sternal wound infections, and faster healing. Disadvantages of this approach include a higher degree of technical skill required of the surgeon, limited views of the surgical field, and difficult or inadequate emptying of air from the left ventricle (Aldea, 2006).

CEBM, level 5.

Medical History

- Hodgkin's lymphoma, diagnosed in 1992 and treated with radiation therapy and chemotherapy. No history of recurrence.
- Retroperitoneal sarcoma, diagnosed in 1994 and treated with surgical resection.
- Hypertension, diagnosed in 1994 and controlled with medication.
- Aortic stenosis and coronary artery disease, diagnosed in 1994 and treated medically and surgically.
- Thyroid goiter, diagnosed in 1997 and treated with iodine, resulting in hypothyroidism. Hypothyroidism is stable and treated medically with levothyroxine (Synthroid).
- Hemorrhagic cerebrovascular accident (CVA) due to supratherapeutic anticoagulation in 2001 with residual left upper extremity paralysis and left lower extremity weakness.

- Fibromyalgia, diagnosed in 2004 and treated medically.
- Myocardial infarction in 2007, treated with percutaneous coronary intervention and medication.
- Mitral valve prolapse with severe mitral regurgitation, diagnosed in 2007 and treated medically.
- Ulcerative colitis for unknown period of time with unknown treatment.
- Asthma for unknown period of time, treated medically and well controlled on a leukotriene inhibitor. He has never been hospitalized or intubated for asthma.
- Severe gastroesophageal reflux disease for unknown period of time, treated medically.
- Benign prostatic hyperplasia for unknown period of time, with no medical or surgical treatment documented.

Surgical History

- Splenectomy in 1972 for unknown reason.
- Mechanical aortic valve replacement and coronary artery bypass grafting performed in 1994.
- Surgical resection of sarcoma from unknown location in 1994.
- Percutaneous coronary intervention in 2007.

Medications

Medication	Dose	Unit	Route	Frequency
Warfarin (Coumadin)	7	mg	Orally	Daily
KCl (Klor-con)	10	mEq	Orally	Twice a day
Esomeprazole (Nexium)	40	mg	Orally	Three times daily
Furosemide (Lasix)	80	mg	Orally	Daily
Clopidogrel (Plavix)	75	mg	Orally	Daily
Diltiazem CD (Cardizem CD)	360	mg	Orally	Daily
Levothyroxine (Synthroid)	188	mcg	Orally	Daily
Montelukast (Singulair)	10	mg	Orally	Daily
Fluvastatin XL (Lescol XL)	80	mg	Orally	Daily
Buproprion SR (Wellbutrin SR)	200	mg	Orally	Three times daily
Domperidone (Motillium)	10	mg	Orally	Two times daily
Tizanidine (Zanaflex)	4	mg	Orally	As needed
Nizatidine (Axid)	300	mg	Orally	Daily
Ezetimibe (Zetia)	10	mg	Orally	Daily

Allergies: No known drug allergies. No known food or environmental allergies.

Social and family history: Mr. P has been on permanent disability since the time of his CVA in 2001 as a result of his paralysis and weakness. He previously worked as an investment banker for 28 years, prior to his stroke. He has been married for 31 years and has two sons ages 24 and 26. He lives with his wife and youngest son in a single-level home.

Operative Course

The patient underwent mitral valve replacement via limited right thoracotomy. The aortic arch was noted to be heavily calcified. After failed attempts to use the femoral artery as the arterial cannulation site, the decision was made to use a noncalcified spot on the aorta. The mitral valve leaflets and the mitral annulus were heavily calcified, making the dissection and sewing of the new valve very difficult. Due to excess bleeding, the surgeon requested circulatory arrest to allow for better visualization. The patient was cooled to 20°C for organ protection. Toward the end of the procedure, a large bubble of air was noted traveling down the aorta on transesophageal echocardiogram (TEE).

The total bypass time for this procedure was 4 hours and 26 minutes. There was no aortic cross-clamping, and the total circulatory arrest time was 1 hour and 13 minutes. Mr. P received 3 units of packed red blood cells, 1 unit of Cell Saver blood, 4 units of fresh-frozen plasma, and 12 packs of platelets. His anesthetic agents included midazolam (Versed) 23 mg, fentanyl citrate (Fentanyl) 2,100 mcg, rocuronium bromide (Zemuron) 100 mg, and vecuronium bromide (Norcuron) 30 mg. Of note, he received vecuronium bromide (Norcuron) just prior to leaving the operating room. He was admitted to the CTICU on the following infusions: nitroglycerin 30 mcg/min and propofol (Diprivan) 30 mcg/kg/min; no vasopressors or inotropes.

Postoperative TEE showed a normal left ventricular size with left ventricular ejection fraction > 55 percent, no regional wall motion abnormalities, normal right ventricular size and function, left atrial enlargement, trace aortic regurgitation, properly functioning mechanical mitral valve with trace mitral regurgitation but no paravalvular leak, and no aortic dissection.

The surgeon spoke with the family and explained that the operation was very difficult and that he was extremely concerned about a possible stroke given the air and calcification encountered during the operation. Per the surgeon, the wife told him that they did not want Mr. P to suffer and that he had a living will stating that he did not wish to be kept alive should he suffer a catastrophic event. The patient and his family had all discussed his wishes concerning continuation or withdrawal of care.

Time: 0 minutes

On admission to the CTICU, the patient is observed to be hemodynamically stable, overbreathing the ventilator, with minimal drainage from his chest tubes. He is maintained on a propofol (Diprivan) infusion.

At this time, Mr. P's wife and children are allowed to come into the CTICU to visit. I introduce myself and explain that I will be with him overnight. I explain that we will not be able to wake him immediately, but that as soon as it is safe, we will decrease his propofol (Diprivan) infusion and allow him to emerge from sedation to assess his neurologic status. I assure the family that I will vigilantly monitor him throughout the night and will contact Mrs. P at home to update her on his status later in the evening.

The ED$_{95}$ for vecuronium (Norcuron) is 0.05 mg/kg, meaning that this drug performs its therapeutic intent in 95% of patients with that dose. The intubating dose of vecuronium (Norcuron) is 0.12 mg/kg and has a half-life of 45–90 minutes (Morgan, Mikhail, & Murray, 2006).

CEBM, level 5.

Vitals: BP 106/58, HR 76, RR 13, SpO$_2$ 100%, temp 36.4°C.

Ventilator settings: Assist/Control, rate 10, tidal volume 600 mL, PEEP 5, FiO$_2$ 100%.

Parameter	Patient Value	Normal Values	Unit of Measure
Central venous pressure	8	1–6	mmHg
Pulmonary artery pressure	39/16	15–30/8	mmHg
Pulmonary artery wedge pressure	Not obtained	6–12	mmHg
Cardiac index	2.4	2.4–4	L/min/m^2
Systemic vascular resistance	1,185	1,200–1,500	dynes•s•cm^{-5}

I/O: UOP 500 mL from operating room, current UOP approximately 40 mL/hr, right chest tube draining approximately 20–30 mL/hr.

Medications: Esomeprazole (Nexium) 40 mg IV three times daily, acetylsalicylic acid (Aspirin) 300 mg PR daily, chlorhexidine gluconate (Peridex) mouthwash 0.12% 15 mL orally every 8 hours, levothyroxine (Synthroid) 95 mcg IV daily.

Infusions: Nitroglycerin 30 mcg/min, propofol (Diprivan) 35 mcg/kg/min, insulin 1 U/hr.

Physical Examination

General: Sedated and intubated.

Neurovascular: Ramsay score 6, PERRL, pupil size 3 mm equal bilaterally.

Cardiovascular: Regular rate and rhythm, no rub, murmur, or gallop appreciated.

Respiratory: Left-sided lung fields are clear throughout; however, the right lung demonstrates diminished breath sounds and scattered crackles in the base. No wheezes or rhonchi are appreciated. Right-side chest tube to low wall suction with no air leak.

Gastrointestinal: Abdomen soft, nondistended, absent bowel sounds.

Extremities: 2+ palpable pulses in all four extremities; extremities warm and well perfused.

Wounds: Right femoral cannulation site dressing clean, dry, and intact; right thoracotomy dressing clean, dry, and intact; sanguinous chest tube drainage.

Diagnostics

EKG on admission: HR 80s, normal sinus rhythm, left atrial enlargement.

Chest x-ray on admission: Left lung parenchyma clear, right lower lobe atelectasis, right internal jugular introducer sheath with pulmonary artery catheter in good position, endotracheal tube with tip approximately 2 cm above the carina.

Laboratory findings:

Parameter	Patient Value	Normal Values	Unit of Measure
	Arterial Blood Gas		
pH	7.46	7.35–7.45	
$PaCO_2$	34	32–43	mmHg
PaO_2	392	72–104	mmHg
BE	1	–2 to +2	mM/l
HCO_3	24	22–30	mM/l
O_2 saturation	99.9	95–99	%
	Basic Metabolic Profile		
Na^+	140	136–146	mM/l
K^+	3.8	3.6–5.0	mM/l
Cl^-	104	102–109	mM/l
CO_2	22	25–33	mM/l
BUN	23	7–20	mg/dL
Cr	1.0	0.5–0.9	mg/dL
Glu	192	70–105	mg/dL
Mg^{2+}	1.9	1.5–2.3	mg/dL
PO_4^{-2}	3.8	2.5–4.3	mg/dL
Ca^{2+}	9.1	8.4–9.8	mg/dL
	Complete Blood Count		
WBC	12.0	3.54–9.06	10*9/l
Hb	8.9	12.0–15.8	g/dL
Hct	27.1	35.4–44.4	%
Plt	225	165–415	10*9/l

(continued)

Parameter	Patient Value	Normal Values	Unit of Measure
Coagulation Studies			
INR	1.48	0.88–1.12	units
PTT	35.9	23.3–32.3	sec
Mixed Venous Oxygen Saturation			
SvO_2	79.8%	>70%	%

Impression

This is a 60-year-old man with a complicated medical history who has undergone a mitral valve replacement. He is at high risk for embolic stroke and/or anoxic brain injury given the air embolism seen on TEE, the prolonged bypass, the circulatory arrest times, and the calcification of his aorta and mitral valve. His pupillary, gag, and corneal reflexes are intact. His respiratory center is intact, as evidenced by his overbreathing the ventilator. I am unable to wake him up immediately given recent administration of neuromuscular blockade and residual effects of cardiac anesthesia. It is imperative that his neurologic status be assessed as soon as possible in order to initiate any treatment as indicated. At this time he cannot be anticoagulated, as he is at risk for hemorrhagic stroke given his operative course and current coagulopathy. Because intravenous nitroglycerin can cause hypotension, potentially negating the body's stress response to stroke, elevation of the blood pressure by pharmacologic means may be necessary to maintain cerebral perfusion pressure.

> *The incidence of peri-operative stroke during cardiac surgery involving valve replacement is 1.8 percent. It is most commonly caused by cerebral hypoperfusion or emboli. Embolic sources include gas, thrombus, and atheroma. Atheroemboli and thromboemboli may occur during aortic cross clamping, during excision of a valve, or by turbulent flow in the aorta during the operation. Gas emboli most commonly occur when air enters the cardiac chambers during the operation or from the cannulation sites for cardio-pulmonary bypass (Anyanwu, Filsoufi, Salzberg, Bronster, & Adams, 2007; McGarvey, Cheung, & Stecker, 2008).*

CEBM, level 5.

He is hemodynamically stable and is not requiring vasopressor or inotropic agents. He remains on nitroglycerin infusion, which was started in the operating room, for moderate pulmonary hypertension and he has been very responsive to this therapy. His current pulmonary artery pressures are still elevated despite valve replacement. The chronic cardiopulmonary changes observed in pulmonary hypertension do not immediately reverse after correction of a valvulopathy. His pulmonary arterial hypertension could also be a result of primary pulmonary hypertension; however, this cannot be elucidated at this time. Our treatment in either case will be the same, and he is tolerating these pulmonary pressures, as evidenced by the absence of pulmonary edema or right ventricular failure.

> *Pulmonary hypertension is a condition in which the arterial pressure of the pulmonary vasculature is elevated. As in this case, mitral disease can result in the transmission of high left-sided intracardiac pressures to the pulmonary circulation and subsequently to the right heart. Intravenous nitroglycerin can be used in the operative setting to alleviate pulmonary hypertension. Nitroglycerin dilates peripheral arteries and veins with a more pronounced effect on venous vessels. This is believed to benefit pulmonary hypertension by decreasing left ventricular afterload and decreasing cardiac preload. Small studies have demonstrated a 19% reduction in mean pulmonary artery pressures, a 43% reduction in pulmonary vascular resistance, and a 50% increase in cardiac index (Pearl, Rosenthal, Schroeder, & Ashton, 1983; Rubin & Hopkins, 2008).*
>
> CEBM, levels 4 (Pearl et al., 1983), 5 (Rubin & Hopkins, 2008).

He is currently ventilator dependent given recent administration of general anesthesia with high doses of benzodiazepines and opioids. His respiratory rate is higher than the rate set on the ventilator, indicating that his respiratory center in the brain stem is intact. His arterial blood gas shows a mild alkalosis, which is not concerning at this time. His arterial partial pressure of oxygen is high as a result of his high fraction of inspired oxygen delivered via the ventilator. The right lower lobe atelectasis observed on the chest x-ray is a normal finding after single lung ventilation and compression of the right lung during the operation.

His hemoglobin and hematocrit are low. Nonetheless, he is hemodynamically stable off vasopressors, has adequate arterial oxygenation, and normal mixed venous blood oxygen saturation. Based on these findings, he is tolerating this level of anemia without consequence. He has no evidence of active bleeding from his chest tubes and does not display signs of cardiac tamponade. His platelet count is normal; however, given his long bypass time, he is likely to have a qualitative platelet defect. His bleeding times are mildly prolonged and are consistent with the high levels of anticoagulation received during cardiac surgery as well as the dilution of clotting factors commonly observed after cardiac surgery. A less likely explanation of his prolonged bleeding times is impaired hepatic coagulation factor synthesis as a result of hepatic injury. His white blood cell count is mildly elevated, which is most likely an inflammatory response to his prolonged bypass time; however, postoperative infection cannot be ruled out at this time.

> *Mixed venous oxygen saturation (SvO_2) is an indirect indicator of systemic oxygen consumption, and can be used to evaluate the effectiveness of perfusion and oxygenation of tissues and thus cardiac output. Mixed venous blood samples are taken from the distal port of the pulmonary artery catheter, which sits in the pulmonary artery. An SvO_2 of 70% is considered normal (Bojar, 2005).*
>
> CEBM, level 5.

Large amounts of intravenous fluids, and often times blood products, are administered to the patient during cardiopulmonary bypass. Due to bleeding and hemodilution, post-cardiopulmonary bypass patients are commonly anemic. Hematocrit levels as low as 22–24% are often tolerated in post-cardiopulmonary bypass patients without serious consequence (Bojar, 2005).

CEBM, level 5.

Leukocytosis not related to infection can be seen in the perioperative period and may be related to the release of pro-inflammatory cytokines or other unknown etiology (Jakobsen, Pedersen, & Egeberg, 1986).

CEBM, level 2b.

Although his creatinine and blood urea nitrogen are slightly elevated, his urine output is adequate at this time. Given his operative course, however, he is at high risk for postoperative renal failure as a result of embolism or acute tubular necrosis.

Renal dysfunction is a common complication following cardiac surgery. In fact, up to 30% of patients undergoing cardiac surgery develop acute renal failure in the post-operative period, and 1–5% of those patients will require hemodialysis. Risk factors for renal failure following cardiac surgery include hypotension, hypothermia, loss of pulsatile flow and embolism (Corwin, Sprague, DeLaria, & Norusis, 1989; Silvestry, 2008).

CEBM, levels 4 (Corwin et al., 1989), 5 (Silvestry, 2008).

His blood glucose level is elevated despite the fact that he does not have diabetes. His hyperglycemia is most likely a result of the normal stress response during surgery; however, he could have undiagnosed underlying type 2 diabetes. He is currently on an insulin infusion for glucose control.

Problem List

1) High risk of embolic stroke and/or anoxic brain injury
2) Pulmonary artery hypertension
3) Postoperative pulmonary insufficiency
4) Atelectasis
5) Postoperative anemia
6) Coagulopathy, mild
7) Hyperglycemia
8) Hypothyroidism
9) Severe GERD

Plan

1) Continue sedation for now given potential residual neuromuscular blockade. In one hour, begin wean of sedation to allow for assessment of neurologic status. If he does not awaken two to three hours after discontinuation of sedation, he should be taken for STAT computed tomography (CT) scan of the head, and an acute stroke consult should be obtained, if appropriate, based on the radiologic findings. Start norepinephrine (Levophed) infusion

as needed to maintain mean arterial pressure (MAP) > 70 mmHg to maintain adequate cerebral perfusion pressure.

2) Slowly wean nitroglycerin off as tolerated by pulmonary pressures. Keep pulmonary artery systolic pressure less than 40 mmHg.

3) Continue mechanical ventilatory support until the patient is alert and meets extubation criteria. Wean FiO_2 to 0.4 as tolerated based on serial arterial blood gases. Start albuterol (Proventil) nebulizers via ventilator every 6 hours for bronchodilation. Continue chlorhexidine gluconate (Peridex) mouthwash per ventilator-associated pneumonia prevention protocol.

4) Maintain positive end-expiratory pressure at 5 cm H_2O. Maintain chest tube to wall suction. Perform percussion and vibration as tolerated to promote alveolar recruitment. Initiate chest physical therapy and early mobilization as soon as possible.

5) Monitor complete blood count every six hours. Monitor chest tube output closely. Transfuse packed red blood cells as needed for increased blood loss associated with clinical deterioration or hematocrit less than 25 percent with decreased mixed venous oxygen saturation.

6) Monitor prothrombin time and partial thromboplastin time. Transfuse fresh-frozen plasma and/or cryoprecipitate as needed if there is significant bleeding.

7) Continue intensive insulin therapy per hospital protocol to maintain blood glucose levels of 80–110 mg/dL.

8) Begin levothyroxine (Synthroid) 95 mcg IV daily tomorrow and convert to oral dose once he is extubated.

9) Resume esomeprazole (Nexium) 40 mg IV every 8 hours per home medication regimen. Initiate aspiration precautions: head of bed > 30 degrees, NPO status.

(D1, C3, PO A, B, C.)

ICD-9 Codes

348.1   Anoxic brain damage
416.9   Chronic pulmonary heart disease unspecified
518.5   Pulmonary insufficiency following trauma and surgery
518.0   Pulmonary collapse
285.9   Anemia unspecified
790.92 Abnormal coagulation profile
251.3   Postsurgical hypoinsulinemia
244.2   Iodine hypothyroidism
530.81 Esophageal reflux

The risk of pharmacologically increasing MAP at this time would be increased bleeding should he have a hemorrhagic stroke or conversion of an embolic stroke to hemorrhagic **(D1, C3, PO E).**

Hypotension during acute stroke is associated with poor outcomes. Cerebral perfusion pressure (CPP) is calculated by subtracting intracranial pressure (ICP) from the MAP (CPP = MAP–ICP). Therefore, if ICP is constant, then an increase in MAP should result in increased CPP (Bongard & Sue, 2002; Oliveira-Filho & Koroshetz, 2008).

CEBM, level 5.

Perioperative hyperglycemia is observed in non-diabetic patients undergoing cardiac surgery and is a result of the physiologic stress response to surgery. This retrospective, observational study concluded that patients with a 20 mg/dL increase in mean intraoperative glucose levels were 30% more likely to reach one of the study endpoints. The most commonly observed endpoints were atrial fibrillation, prolonged mechanical ventilation, delirium, and urinary tract infections (Gandhi et al., 2005).

CEBM, level 2b.

Encounter Time: 4 hours after admission

Four hours after discontinuation of sedation and narcotic infusions, the patient has not emerged from anesthesia. He is non-responsive to painful stimuli and his respiratory rate is no longer higher than the rate set on the ventilator. At this point, I order and accompany the patient for a non-contrast CT scan.

Magnetic Resonance Imaging (MRI) is more sensitive for identifying acute stroke and acute or chronic hemorrhage. This prospective blind comparison study enrolled a series of patients presenting with acute stroke. Both MRI (with diffusion weighted images and susceptibility weighted images) and CT were obtained. The images were evaluated by four experts who were blinded to clinical information. MRI showed a sensitivity of 83% while CT showed a 26% sensitivity for the detection of any stroke. Despite the superior detection with MRI, the acquisition times are significantly longer which keeps a critically ill patient away from the ICU for a prolonged period of time. Additionally, cardiac surgical patients have temporary epicardial pacing wires containing metal, which would preclude MRI (Chalela et al., 2007).

CEBM, level 5.

(D1, C3, PO D.)

Telephone Consult with Patient's Wife

While the staff are preparing for transport to the radiology suite, I call the patient's wife at her home. I explain that Mr. P has not woken up and that we are taking him for an emergent CT scan of his head. I tell her I will notify her of the findings as soon as the test is performed. Mrs. P begins to cry. She explains that her husband has been sick for many years and has suffered tremendously over the last 5 to 10 years. Mr. P and his family have talked about his quality of life and what he would want should something unforeseeable happen to him during the operation. She expresses concern that the medical staff will think she is a bad person for wanting her husband to die rather than survive a devastating stroke. I explain to Mrs. P that we are completely understanding of her family's feelings. I explain that not wanting her husband to suffer is not something she should feel guilty for; rather, it is a very compassionate and selfless response. I tell her that without the CT scan, we still do not know if he has definitely suffered a stroke, and the test will be quick. I promise to call as soon as the test is done and I have additional information.

The need for information is one of the most important needs that family members have when a loved one is in the intensive care unit. Families want "timely, clear, and honest" information from providers who are familiar with the patient's status, and they want providers to listen to their concerns (Treece, 2007).

CEBM, level 5.

Encounter Time: 4 hours 10 minutes after admission

CT Scan of the Head without Contrast

Multiple large hypodensities are seen throughout both cerebral hemispheres. A large hypodensity is seen in the right temporal lobe and right occipital lobe, extending into the right parietal lobe in the right posterior cerebral artery distribution. Additionally, a large hypodensity is seen involving most of the right frontal lobe. Left frontal and left posterior temporal hypodensities are seen. Medial superior left frontoparietal hypodensity is also noted. In addition, multiple hypodensities are seen within the cerebelli. Mass effect is noted upon the right lateral ventricle. There is mild right-to-left midline shift. Mild mass effect is noted upon the right basal cisterns. There is presently no evidence of hemorrhage. An old right basal ganglia infarct is seen.

Encounter Time: 4 hours 30 minutes after admission

Upon returning to the CTICU from radiology, I call and activate the hospital acute stroke team **(D2, C1, PO A).**

Neurology/Stroke Resident Consult

The stroke resident comes to the ICU immediately. We review the CT scan and identify the multiple large infarcts involving both hemispheres of the brain. Additionally, the mass effect and midline shift are very worrisome for cerebral edema and increased intracranial pressure. The neurology consultant examines the patient and feels that Mr. P's exam reveals severe neurologic deficits and is consistent with the radiographic findings. He recommends institution of mannitol (Osmitrol) therapy and obtaining a neurosurgery consult. He notes, however, that these measures are unlikely to have any significant effect on the clinical course of the stroke and that Mr. P's prognosis is dismal given the severity of the findings.

Vitals: BP 123/72, HR 72, RR 10, SpO$_2$ 100%, temp 37.1°C.

Ventilator settings: Assist/Control, rate 10, tidal volume 600 mL, PEEP 5, FiO$_2$ 40%.

Parameter	Patient Value	Normal Values	Unit of Measure
Central venous pressure	7	1–6	mmHg
Pulmonary artery pressure	34/13	15–30/8	mmHg
Pulmonary artery wedge pressure	Not obtained	6–12	mmHg
Cardiac index	Not obtained	2.4–4	L/min/m^2
Systemic vascular resistance	Not obtained	1,200–1,500	dynes•s•cm^{-5}

I/O: UOP 40–50 mL/hr, right chest tube draining approximately 20 mL/hr.

Medications: Esomeprazole (Nexium) 40 mg IV three times daily, acetyl-salicylic acid (Aspirin) 300 mg PR daily, chlorhexidine gluconate (Peridex) mouthwash 0.12 percent 15 mL orally every 8 hours, levothyroxine (Synthroid) 95 mcg IV daily.

Infusions: Nitroglycerin 30 mcg/min, propofol (Diprivan) 0 mcg/kg/min, and insulin 2 U/hr.

Physical Examination

General: Sedated and intubated, motionless.

Neurovascular: Eyes closed with no spontaneous movement and no response to deep nailbed pressure in any extremity. No blink to threat, pupils 2 mm and reactive to light bilaterally. Both eyes deviated to the left with positive dolls eyes but do not cross midline. Corneal reflexes intact bilaterally. No facial asymmetry. No gag reflex. Not overbreathing the ventilator. 2+ deep tendon reflexes throughout. Positive Babinski sign bilaterally.

Cardiovascular: Regular rate and rhythm, no rub, murmur, or gallop appreciated.

Respiratory: Left-sided lung fields are clear throughout, right lung demonstrates diminished breath sounds and scattered crackles in the base. No wheezes or rhonchi are appreciated. Right-sided chest tube to low wall suction with no air leak.

Gastrointestinal: Abdomen soft, nondistended, absent bowel sounds.

Extremities: 2+ palpable pulses in all four extremities; extremities warm and well perfused.

Wounds: Right femoral cannulation site dressing clean, dry, and intact; right thoracotomy dressing clean, dry, and intact; minimal sanguinous chest tube drainage.

Laboratory findings:

Parameter	Patient Value	Normal Values	Unit of Measure
Arterial Blood Gas			
pH	7.59	7.35–7.45	
$PaCO_2$	24	32–43	mmHg
PaO_2	151	72–104	mmHg
BE	3	–2 to +2	mM/l
HCO_3	23	22–30	mM/l
O_2 saturation	99.9	95–99	%
Basic Metabolic Profile			
Na^+	143	136–146	mM/l
K^+	3.5	3.6–5.0	mM/l
Cl^-	107	102–109	mM/l
CO_2	25	25–33	mM/l
BUN	24	7–20	mg/dL
Cr	1.1	0.5–0.9	mg/dL
Glu	175	70–105	mg/dL
Mg^{2+}	1.6	1.5–2.3	mg/dL
PO_4^{-2}	2.0	2.5–4.3	mg/dL
Ca^{2+}	8.5	8.4–9.8	mg/dL
Complete Blood Count			
WBC	16.1	3.54–9.06	10*9/l
Hb	9.0	12.0–15.8	g/dL
Hct	27.1	35.4–44.4	%
Plt	279	165–415	10*9/l
Coagulation Studies			
INR	1.25	0.88–1.12	units
PTT	28.8	23.3–32.3	sec
Mixed Venous Oxygen Saturation			
SvO_2	64.3%	>70%	%

Impression

Mr. P has suffered a catastrophic stroke involving both cerebral hemispheres with diffuse cerebral edema. His physical exam reveals loss of multiple cranial nerve responses. The etiology of his stroke is not clear based on the CT scan; however, it can be presumed that it was caused by air embolus. He is not eligible for systemic or intracranial administration of recombinant tissue-type plasminogen activator (tPA) given his recent surgery. Due to the size and extent of the infarcts, he is experiencing cerebral edema and shows signs of brain stem herniation evidenced on CT scan. We cannot place the patient on systemic anticoagulation for further potential embolic prevention. Furthermore, this would be unlikely to provide any benefit given that the embolic source is most likely air. Efforts to minimize intracranial edema should be instituted immediately. It is possible that craniotomy or another surgical procedure may be of benefit. Neurology consultant feels that treatment, medical or otherwise, is unlikely to have any significant effect on his clinical outcome and that his prognosis is extremely poor.

The administration of systemic tPA is contraindicated in patients who have undergone surgery in the 14 days following up to proposed thrombolytic therapy. Furthermore, brain edema or mass effect imposes an increased risk of intracerebral hemorrhage (Oliveira-Filho, Koroshetz, & Samuels, 2008).

CEBM, level 5.

The most common causes of death in the first few days following stroke are cerebral edema and stroke. Mannitol (Osmitrol) can be used in this setting in order to produce an osmotic diuresis with the goal of decreasing swelling in the brain, hopefully preventing herniation of the brain. It is possible to perform a craniectomy or strokectomy in some cases in order to prevent swelling (Fink, 2005).

CEBM, level 5.

Mr. P remains hemodynamically stable and does not require vasopressor or inotropic agents. He continues on nitroglycerin infusion for moderate pulmonary hypertension. His pulmonary artery pressures remain mildly elevated, and no further intervention is necessary at this time. His right-sided filling pressures are adequate following cardiac surgery. His mixed venous oxygen saturation is somewhat lower; however, it is still acceptable. Given that he remains off vasopressors, is maintaining an adequate blood pressure, and has an acceptable hematocrit, this is most likely of little consequence.

He continues to require mechanical ventilation, and in fact his intrinsic respiratory rate has fallen below the settings on the ventilator. His arterial blood gas shows partially compensated respiratory alkalosis. Therapeutic hypocapnia may actually be beneficial in the setting of cerebral edema with resultant elevated intracranial pressure. His oxygenation is adequate on the current ventilator settings. At this time, it is unlikely that he will regain an adequate ventilatory drive and will most likely be ineligible for extubation.

Hyperventilation causes cerebral vasoconstriction, which results in decreased cerebral blood flow to the brain. Therapeutic hyperventilation to a $PaCO_2$ of

26–30 mmHg has been show to quickly reduce intracranial pressure. Further-more, the respiratory alkalosis which is produced by these means is felt to buffer the acid produced from tissue damage. Unfortunately, this treatment is only temporary and may only last several hours (Smith & Amin-Hanjani, 2008).

CEBM, level 5.

His hemoglobin and hematocrit remain low, but are stable. For reasons previously stated, we will not transfuse exogenous blood products at this time. Should his mixed venous oxygen saturation continue to drop, transfusion of packed red blood cells may be beneficial. His chest tube output is acceptable after this procedure. His platelet count remains at an acceptable level, and his bleeding times are trending toward normal levels. The etiology of his increased leukocytosis is still unclear, but may possibly be a result of an inflammatory process related to his massive strokes and cerebral edema. Infection should also be considered, but without fever or other microbiologic data to support this, antibiotics are not warranted.

His serum creatinine and blood urea nitrogen levels are slightly elevated. This most likely represents normal intra-laboratory variation. Although less likely, early acute renal failure as a result of renal hypoperfusion or renal artery air embolus are potential complications as well.

Problem List

1) Extensive bilateral brain infarcts with diffuse cerebral edema and herniation
2) Pulmonary artery hypertension, stable
3) Postoperative pulmonary insufficiency, worsening
4) Atelectasis
5) Postoperative anemia, stable
6) Coagulopathy, improved
7) Hyperglycemia, stable
8) Hypothyroidism
9) Severe gastroesophageal reflux disease (GERD)

Plan

1) Hold sedation or other medications that might alter neurologic exam. Elevate head of bed to 30 degrees. Start mannitol (Osmitrol) 1 g/kg IV every six hours in an effort to minimize cerebral edema and further herniation. Check serum osmoles and basic metabolic profile every six hours to guide hyperosmolar therapy. Discontinue mannitol (Osmitrol) for serum sodium > 150, serum osmolality > 320 mOsm, or evidence of worsening renal function. Despite the impression of a poor prognosis by the neurology consultant, I will obtain neurosurgery consult to assess whether craniectomy or other surgical intervention might be beneficial.
2) Maintain nitroglycerin infusion at current rate. Keep pulmonary artery systolic pressure less than 40 mmHg.
3) Continue mechanical ventilatory support. Continue therapeutic hyperventilation to decrease ICP with goal $PaCO_2$ 25–30 mmHg. Continue albuterol

(Proventil) nebulizers via ventilator every six hours for bronchodilation. Continue chlorhexidine gluconate (Peridex) mouthwash per ventilator-associated pneumonia prevention protocol. Currently, there are no plans for extubation.

4) Continue positive end-expiratory pressure at 5cm H_2O. Maintain chest tube to wall suction. Perform percussion and vibration as tolerated to encourage alveolar recruitment. Continue chest physical therapy.

5) Continue to monitor complete blood count every eight hours. Monitor chest tube output closely. Will consider transfusion of packed cells only if mixed venous oxygen saturation continues to decrease or if neurology consult feels that increasing serum hemoglobin will benefit in terms of meeting cerebral metabolic requirements for oxygen.

6) Continue to monitor prothrombin time and partial thromboplastin time. No need for transfusion of coagulation factors at this time.

7) Continue intensive insulin therapy per hospital protocol to maintain blood glucose levels of 80–110 mg/dL.

8) Continue levothyroxine (Synthroid) 95 mcg IV daily.

9) Continue esomeprazole (Nexium) 40 mg IV every eight hours, as per home medication regimen. Continue aspiration precautions: head of bed > 30 degrees, NPO status.

(D1, C3, PO A, B, C, D; D2, C1, PO A, C.)

ICD-9 Codes

997.02 Iatrogenic cerebrovascular infarction or hemorrhage
416.9   Chronic pulmonary heart disease unspecified
518.5   Pulmonary insufficiency following trauma and surgery
518.0   Pulmonary collapse
285.9   Anemia unspecified
790.92 Abnormal coagulation profile
251.3   Postsurgical hypoinsulinemia
244.2   Iodine hypothyroidism
530.81 Esophageal reflux

Aggressive diuresis with mannitol (Osmitrol) results in a loss of free water potentially resulting in severe hypernatremia. Likewise, massive volume losses can result in renal failure. Subsequently, renal failure can result in accumulation of mannitol (Osmitrol) within the circulation and possibly result in volume expansion, hyponatremia, hyperkalemia, and metabolic acidosis (Rose, 2008).

CEBM, level 5.

Encounter Time: 5 hours 15 minutes after admission

Attending physician consult: The CTICU fellow, the covering CTICU attending, and the cardiothoracic surgeon are all notified of the findings and agree with the treatment plan as outlined above.

Encounter Time: 5 hours 20 minutes after admission

Telephone conversation with Mrs. P: I call Mrs. P as promised. I explain that the CT scan shows that Mr. P has suffered massive bilateral strokes. Mrs. P says, "Oh my God," and begins to cry. I wait until she is able to speak. She asks what this means for Mr. P. She says, "You can tell me. I can handle this and need to hear the truth." I explain that, based on the CT scan, his physical examination, and the neurologist's assessment, Mr. P has little hope of any meaningful recovery. He is not breathing adequately on his own and his brain is herniating due to swelling. She expresses concern that her children will be upset if he has to suffer. She asks what is needed to withdraw ventilator support. Mrs. P is extremely worried about "this getting dragged out," translating into a prolonged and painful death for Mr. P. We agree that she and her family will come to the hospital and meet with myself, the CTICU attending physician, and the surgeon.

Encounter Time: 5 hours 30 minutes after admission

Neurosurgery consult: Mr. P is seen by neurosurgery, and the information is discussed with the neurosurgery chief and the neurosurgery attending on call. Given the situation, they feel there would be no benefit from any surgical intervention. They recommend continuation of the current medical management and discussion of withdrawal of care with the family.

The patient has now been off all sedation for four and a half hours, and the patient is reexamined with the neurology resident.

Vitals: BP 116/68, HR 68, RR 10, SpO$_2$ 100%, temp 37.1°C.

Ventilator settings: Assist/Control, rate 10, tidal volume 600 mL, PEEP 5, FiO$_2$ 40%.

Parameter	Patient Value	Normal Values	Unit of Measure
Central venous pressure	9	1–6	mmHg
Pulmonary artery pressure	38/16	15–30/8	mmHg
Pulmonary artery wedge pressure	Not obtained	6–12	mmHg
Cardiac index	Not obtained	2.4–4	L/min/m^2
Systemic vascular resistance	Not obtained	1,200–1,500	dynes•s•cm^{-5}

I/O: UOP 150–200 mL/hr, right chest tube draining approximately 10 mL/hr.

Medications: Esomeprazole (Nexium) 40 mg IV three times daily, acetylsalicylic acid (Aspirin) 300 mg PR daily, chlorhexidine gluconate (Peridex) mouthwash 0.12 percent 15 mL orally every 8 hours, levothyroxine (Synthroid) 95 mcg IV daily, mannitol (Osmitrol) 1 g/kg IV every 6 hours.

Infusions: Nitroglycerin 30 mcg/min, propofol (Diprivan) 0 mcg/kg/min, insulin 4 U/hr.

Focused Physical Examination

General: Sedated and intubated, motionless.

Neurovascular: Eyes closed, no spontaneous movement and no response to deep nailbed pressure in any extremity. No grimace to pain. No blink to threat, pupils 4 mm and nonreactive to light bilaterally. Both eyes deviated to the left. Corneal reflexes absent bilaterally. Cold caloric test negative, dolls eyes negative. No facial asymmetry. No gag reflex. Not overbreathing the ventilator.

Most recent laboratory findings:

Parameter	Patient Value	Normal Values	Unit of Measure
Arterial Blood Gas			
pH	7.66	7.35–7.45	
$PaCO_2$	25	32–43	mmHg
PaO_2	247	72–104	mmHg
BE	8	–2 to +2	mM/l
HCO_3	28	22–30	mM/l
O_2 saturation	100	95–99	%
iSTAT Point of Care Test Results			
Na^+	145	136–146	mM/l
K^+	2.9	3.6–5.0	mM/l
Hgb	10.2	12.0–15.8	g/dl
Hct	30	35.4–44.4	%
Glucose	160	70–105	mg/dL
Calculated serum osmolality	313	285–295	mOsm/L
iCa^{2+}	1.18	1.12–1.32	mM/L
Mixed Venous Oxygen Saturation			
SvO_2	72%	>70%	%

Impression

Mr. P's massive infarcts have caused significant cerebral swelling as evidenced by radiographic imaging. His physical exam is deteriorating, and he now has fixed pupils that are unresponsive to light. We have been successful with hyperventilation therapy and osmotic diuresis with mannitol (Osmitrol), but this has had little to no effect on his clinical status. In fact, his clinical exam has dramatically deteriorated. All involved agree that Mr. P's prognosis is very poor and are in favor of the family's wishes to withdraw care. The CTICU attending and the cardiothoracic surgeon have examined the patient and are also in agreement with this course of action.

Mr. P remains hemodynamically stable and continues on the nitroglycerin infusion for pulmonary hypertension. At this point, attempts to wean these infusions are unnecessary given his imminent demise and we do not want to do anything to cause instability before his family arrives. He may require volume if he becomes hypotensive due to the hyperosmolar diuresis.

He continues to be ventilator-dependent, and his partial pressure of carbon dioxide has been purposefully decreased by hyperventilation in order to decrease cerebral blood flow with the hope of lowering intracranial pressure. His arterial blood gas shows an uncompensated respiratory alkalosis. His oxygenation remains adequate.

His hemoglobin and hematocrit are stable. His mixed venous oxygen saturation reflects adequate systemic oxygenation. His chest tube output is acceptable.

His urine output has increased as a result of treatment with mannitol (Osmitrol). This will likely cause his intravascular space to become depleted, and we may have to replace his fluid losses at some point. His calculated serum osmolality is elevated as called for. This could potentially increase his risk of renal failure; however, even the slight chance of neurologic benefit from hyperosmolar diuresis outweighs the risk of renal failure at this point.

His family has been notified of these catastrophic events. Fortunately, Mr. P and his family have discussed his wishes in the event that these circumstances were to arise. Mr. P has a living will that states the following: "If at any time I should have an incurable and irreversible injury, disease, or illness judged to be a terminal condition by my attending physician who has personally examined me and has determined that my death is imminent except for death delaying procedures, I direct that such procedures which would only prolong the dying process be withheld or withdrawn, and that I be permitted to die naturally with only the administration of medication, sustenance, or the performance of any medical procedure deemed necessary by my attending physician to provide me with comfort care." Mrs. P had also been designated, in writing, by Mr. P as his health care proxy.

Problem List

1) Extensive bilateral brain infarcts with diffuse cerebral edema and herniation, worsening
2) Pulmonary artery hypertension, stable
3) Central respiratory failure
4) Atelectasis
5) Postoperative anemia, stable
6) Coagulopathy, improved
7) Hyperglycemia, stable
8) Hypothyroidism
9) Severe GERD

Plan

1) Continue hyperosmolar diuresis, keeping serum osmolality at 310–320 mOsm/L. Discontinue therapeutic hyperventilation. At this point, we will await the arrival of the family in order to have a discussion about their wishes for withdrawal of support and allow them time with the patient. We will start midazolam (Versed) 1 mg/hr and fentanyl citrate (Fentanyl) 25 mcg/hr for comfort and prevention of possible seizures. Maintain elevation of head of bed above 30 degrees.

2) Maintain nitroglycerin infusion at current rate. Keep pulmonary artery systolic pressure less than 40 mmHg.

3) Continue mechanical ventilatory support. Discontinue therapeutic hyperventilation. Adjust ventilator settings to maintain pCO_2 35–45 mmHg. Continue albuterol (Proventil) nebulizers via ventilator every 6 hours for bronchodilation. Continue chlorhexidine gluconate (Peridex) mouthwash per ventilator-associated pneumonia prevention protocol. Currently, there are no plans for extubation.

4) Continue positive end-expiratory pressure at 5 cm H_2O. Maintain chest tube to wall suction.

5) No transfusions at this time. Continue to monitor complete blood count every eight hours. Monitor chest tube output closely.

6) Continue to monitor prothrombin time and partial thromboplastin time. No need for transfusion of coagulation factors at this time.

7) Continue intensive insulin therapy per hospital protocol to maintain blood glucose levels of 80–110 mg/dL.

8) Continue levothyroxine (Synthroid) 95 mcg IV daily.

9) Continue esomeprazole (Nexium) 40 mg IV every 8 hours per home medication regimen. Continue aspiration precautions: head of bed > 30 degrees, NPO status.

(D1, C3, PO A, B, C, D; D2, C1, PO D; D1, C7, PO A.)

ICD-9 Codes

997.02 Iatrogenic cerebrovascular infarction or hemorrhage
348.4 Compression of the brain
416.9 Chronic pulmonary heart disease unspecified
799.1 Respiratory arrest
518.0 Pulmonary collapse
285.9 Anemia unspecified
790.92 Abnormal coagulation profile
251.3 Postsurgical hypoinsulinemia
244.2 Iodine hypothyroidism
530.81 Esophageal reflux

The attending surgeon and the CTICU attending arrive and evaluate the patient and radiographic data. They agree with the assessment of the neurologist and neurosurgeon. The surgeon, CTICU attending, myself, and the bedside nurse meet with the family upon their arrival to the unit. The wife and her sons are crying and clearly distraught. They again express Mr. P's wishes, as well as their own. They wish to avoid any further pain or suffering for Mr. P. The surgeon explains the difficulties incurred in the operating room and conveys his regret of the outcome. The family states they understand and do not express any anger. At the conclusion of the meeting, it is decided that the family will have as much time as they need with the patient. When they are ready, we will terminally extubate Mr. P, allowing him to die. I emphasize to the family that I am available and will ensure adequate sedation and analgesia so that Mr. P will not suffer unnecessarily.

The family spends approximately 30 minutes alone with their loved one. They notify me when they are ready. They want to be present for his death. The nurse and I enter the room and ask the family whether there is anything we can do for them before we extubate Mr. P. They say no, and we extubate Mr. P in a calm and caring manner. All alarms are deactivated, and we leave the room to allow for privacy. Mr. P makes no effort to breathe, and within five minutes he becomes bradycardic and then asystolic. As the family leaves, I hug Mrs. P and tell her I am sorry for her loss. The family thanks us for the care we provided **(D1, C7, PO B).**

The provider is left with a heavy burden . . . to determine whether to honor patient autonomy and possibly withdraw care, or continue treatment with the hope of not causing harm to the patient (Fink, 2005).

CEBM, level 5.

COMPETENCY DEFENSE

Domain 1, Competency 3. Formulate differential diagnoses and diagnostic strategies and therapeutic interventions with attention to scientific evidence, safety, cost, invasiveness, simplicity, acceptability, adherence, and efficacy for patients who present with new conditions and those with ambiguous or incomplete data, complex illnesses, comorbid conditions, and multiple diagnoses in all clinical settings.

Defense. I was able to formulate several differential diagnoses in this case. It was clear that Mr. P had suffered a severe stroke, but it was unclear whether this was a hemorrhagic stroke or embolic stroke. Despite the superior sensitivity of MRI, I ordered a CT scan of the head and outlined my reasoning for this diagnostic strategy. It was then determined that this was not a hemorrhagic stroke, but was most likely an air embolus. Unfortunately, this did not allow for many therapeutic options. Even had this been a blood clot that had embolized, we were unable to provide tPA because of recent surgery. Furthermore, tPA would have been useless had this been a calcium or air embolus. Despite a lack of definitive etiology, our treatment would be the same: supportive care.

Domain 2, Competency 1. Assemble a collaborative interdisciplinary network, and refer and consult appropriately while maintaining primary responsibility for comprehensive patient care.

Defense. Upon radiographic confirmation of stroke, I made the decision to initiate an emergent consultation with the acute stroke team. Based upon their recommendations, we instituted mannitol therapy and therapeutic hyperventilation. I assessed the patient on multiple occasions and determined that therapeutic goals had been met. Subsequently, I initiated a second consult from the neurosurgical team. Additionally, I consulted with the attending CTICU surgeon and cardiothoracic surgeon. While using these consults, I maintained primary care of both the patient and the family.

Domain 1, Competency 7. Facilitate and guide the process of palliative care and/or planning end-of-life care by discussing diagnoses and prognosis, clarifying and validating patient desires and priorities, and promoting informed choices and shared decision-making by patient, family, and members of the health care team.

Defense. This case allowed me to demonstrate my ability to care for patients and families at the end of life. I made myself a contact person for this family and maintained consistent communication with them. When information about the patient's status was available, I called Mrs. P to inform her right away. I did my best to portray an honest and caring dialogue during this difficult time and expressed understanding and respect for the wishes of both the patient and the family about end-of-life care. I presented information to them and facilitated a meeting with the surgeon, attending CTICU physician, the bedside nurse, and myself. Furthermore, when it was clear that there would be no heroic measures, I instituted sedatives and opioids to maintain patient comfort. I promoted a calm and caring environment during the dying process and made time for the family to be alone with their loved one.

Medications

Drug: Albuterol (Proventil)

Dose range: 2–4 mg PO tid-qid.

Method of administration in this case: Inhaled.

Mechanism of action: Stimulates beta 2-adrenergic receptors, relaxing airway smooth muscle.

Clinical uses: Bronchospasm.

Side effects
Common: Tremor, nervousness, headache, nausea, tachycardia, muscle cramps, palpitations, insomnia, dizziness.
Serious: Hypersensitivity reactions, paradoxical bronchospasm, HTN, angina, MI, hypokalemia, arrhythmias.

Drug: Bupropion (Wellbutrin SR)

Dose range: 150 mg bid.

Method of administration in this case: Orally.

(continued)

Mechanism of action: Mechanism for smoking cessation unknown; exact mechanism of action for depression unknown, inhibits neuronal uptake of norepinephrine and dopamine (aminoketone).

Clinical uses: Major depressive disorder, smoking cessation, attention deficit disorder.

Side effects
Common: Dry mouth, headache, agitation, nausea, dizziness, constipation, tremor, sweating, abnormal dreams, insomnia, tinnitus, pharyngitis, anorexia, weight loss, infection, abdominal pain, diarrhea, anxiety, flatulence, rash, palpitations, myalgia/arthralgia, chest pain, blurred vision, urinary frequency.
Serious: Seizures, arrhythmias, tachycardia, Stevens-Johnson syndrome, erythema multiforme, anaphylactic/anaphylactoid rxns, hallucinations, mania, psychosis, suicidality, depression, worsening, hepatotoxicity, HTN, severe, elevated IOP, migraine.

Drug: Chlorhexidine Gluconate Mouthwash (Peridex)

Dose range: 15 mL swish/spit bid.

Method of administration in this case: Orally.

Mechanism of action: Active against various bacteria.

Clinical uses: Gingivitis, ventilator-associated pneumonia prevention (non-FDA approved use).

Side effects
Common: Dental deposits, staining of teeth, taste changes, parotiditis.
Serious: May occur but none reported.

Drug: Clopidogrel (Plavix)

Dose range: 75 mg daily.

Method of administration in this case: Orally.

Mechanism of action: Inhibits adenosine diphosphate binding to platelet receptors.

Clinical uses: Acute coronary syndrome, thrombotic event prevention.

Side effects
Common: Nausea, dyspepsia, diarrhea, abdominal pain, hemorrhage, purpura, rash, pruritus, influenza-like symptoms, cough, bronchitis, dizziness, headache, fatigue, arthralgia, chest pain, palpitations, epistaxis, urinary tract infection.
Serious: Bleeding, hemorrhage, thrombocytopenic purpura (rare), neutropenia (rare), anaphylactoid reactions, serum sickness, angioedema, hypersensitivity reaction, Stevens-Johnson syndrome, toxic epidermal necrolysis, erythema multiforme, hepatitis, liver failure, pancreatitis.

(continued)

Drug: Diltiazem (Cardizem CD)

Dose range: 120–480 mg daily.

Method of administration in this case: Orally.

Mechanism of action: Inhibits calcium ion influx into vascular smooth muscle and myocardium, relaxing smooth muscle, decreasing peripheral vascular resistance, dilating coronary arteries, and prolonging atrioventricular (AV) node refractory period.

Clinical uses: Chronic, stable angina, vasospastic angina, hypertension.

Side effects
Common: Peripheral edema, headache, dizziness, asthenia, orthostatic hypotension, dyspepsia, constipation, rash, bradycardia, first-degree AV block, elevated liver transaminases.
Serious: Bradycardia, AV block, arrhythmias, severe hypotension, syncope, cardiac failure, CHF, acute hepatic injury, erythema multiforme, exfoliative dermatitis.

Drug: Domperidone (Motilium)

Dose range: 10–20 mg up to three times daily, before meals and at night, symptomatically.

Method of administration in this case: Orally.

Mechanism of action: Facilitates gastrointestinal smooth muscle activity by inhibiting dopamine at the D1 receptors and inhibiting the release of neural acetylcholine by blocking D2 receptors.

Clinical uses: Gastroparesis.

Side effects (serious): Ventricular fibrillation, cardiac arrest, injection site pain, galactorrhea, gynecomastia, extrapyramidal side effects, neuroleptic malignant syndrome, seizure.

Drug: Esomeprazole (Nexium)

Dose range: 20–40 mg daily.

Method of administration in this case: Orally.

Mechanism of action: Inhibits gastric parietal cell hydrogen-potassium ATPase (proton pump inhibitor).

Clinical uses: GERD, erosive esophagitis, *H. pylori* infection, hypersecretory conditions, NSAID-associated gastric ulcer risk reduction.

Side effects
Common: Headache, diarrhea, abdominal pain, nausea.
Serious: Blood dyscrasias (rare), hepatic dysfunction (rare), Stevens-Johnson syndrome (rare), toxic epidermal necrolysis (rare), erythema multiforme (rare), pancreatitis (rare), interstitial nephritis (rare), hip fracture (long-term, > 50 years old).

(continued)

Drug: Ezetimibe (Zetia)

Dose range: 10 mg daily.

Method of administration in this case: Orally.

Mechanism of action: Inhibits cholesterol absorption at small intestinal brush border.

Clinical uses: Hypercholesterolemia, mixed dyslipidemia, homozygous familial hypercholesterolemia, homozygous familial sitosterolemia.

Side effects
Common: Upper respiratory infection, diarrhea, nasopharyngitis, arthralgia, sinusitis, myalgia, extremity pain, fatigue, back pain, influenza.
Serious: Hypersensitivity reaction, anaphylaxis, angioedema, pancreatitis, hepatitis, cholecystitis, cholelithiasis, thrombocytopenia, rhabdomyolysis (rare), depression.

Drug: Fentanyl Citrate (Fentanyl)

Dose range: 2–50 mcg/kg.

Method of administration in this case: Intravenous.

Mechanism of action: Binds to various opioid receptors, producing analgesia and sedation.

Clinical uses: Analgesia, anesthetic adjunct, postoperative pain.

Side effects
Common: Somnolence, nausea, vomiting, confusion, asthenia, constipation, dry mouth, sweating, dizziness, urinary retention, nervousness, euphoria, hallucinations, dyspnea, pruritus, hypotension, bradycardia, muscle rigidity, biliary spasm, incoordination.

(continued)

Serious: Respiratory depression, respiratory arrest, dependency, abuse, bradycardia, severe, hypotension, severe, anaphylaxis, laryngospasm, bronchoconstriction, severe muscle rigidity, cardiac arrest, circulatory collapse, arrhythmias, intracranial pressure, delirium, seizures, paralytic ileus.

Drug: Fluvastatin (Lescol XL)

Dose range: 80 mg daily.

Method of administration in this case: Orally.

Mechanism of action: Inhibits 3-hydroxy-3-methylglutaryl-coenzyme A (HMG-CoA) reductase.

Clinical uses: Hypercholesterolemia, cardiovascular event risk reduction, atherosclerosis.

(continued)

Side effects
Common: Headache, dyspepsia, abdominal pain, diarrhea, nausea, insomnia, fatigue, flatulence, sinusitis, myalgia, elevated creatinine kinase, elevated liver transaminases.
Serious: Myopathy, rhabdomyolysis (rare), renal failure, acute (rare), hepatotoxicity, pancreatitis, hypersensitivity reactions (rare), anaphylaxis (rare), angioedema (rare), lupus-like syndrome (rare), polymyalgia rheumatica (rare), dermatomyositis (rare), vasculitis (rare), thrombocytopenia (rare), leukopenia (rare), hemolytic anemia (rare), photosensitivity (rare), toxic epidermal necrolysis (rare), erythema multiforme (rare), Stevens-Johnson syndrome (rare).

Drug: Furosemide (Lasix)

Dose range: 10–120 mg.

Method of administration in this case: Intravenous.

Mechanism of action: Inhibits loop of Henle and proximal and distal convoluted tubule sodium and chloride resorption.

Clinical uses: Edema, acute pulmonary edema, hypertension, hypercalcemia.

Side effects
Common: Urinary frequency, dizziness, nausea or vomiting, weakness, muscle cramps, hypokalemia, hypomagnesemia, orthostatic hypotension, blurred vision, anorexia, abdominal cramps, diarrhea, pruritus, rash, hyperuricemia, hyperglycemia, hypocalcemia, tinnitus, paresthesias, photosensitivity.
Serious: Hypokalemia, electrolyte imbalance, metabolic alkalosis, hypovolemia or dehydration, ototoxicity, thrombocytopenia, anemia, aplastic anemia (rare), leucopenia, agranulocytosis (rare), anaphylaxis (rare), vasculitis, interstitial nephritis, necrotizing angiitis, erythema multiforme, exfoliative dermatitis, pancreatitis, cholestatic jaundice, systemic lupus erythematous exacerbation, thrombosis.

Drug: Levothyroxine (Synthroid)

Dose range: 50–200 mcg daily.

Method of administration in this case: Orally.

Mechanism of action: Produces various physiologic effects, including increasing metabolism (synthetic T4).

Clinical uses: Hypothyroidism, myxedema coma.

(continued)

Side effects
Common: Palpitations, appetite increase, tachycardia, nervousness, tremor, weight loss, diaphoresis, diarrhea, abdominal cramps, insomnia, fever, headache, alopecia, heat intolerance, menstrual irregularities, nausea, anxiety.
Serious: Arrhythmias, CHF, HTN, angina, pseudotumor cerebri (peds), craniosynostosis (infants), premature epiphyseal closure, seizures (rare).

Drug: Mannitol (Osmitrol)

Dose range: 0.25–2.00 g/kg.

Method of administration in this case: Intravenous.

Mechanism of action: Elevates glomerular filtrate osmolarity (osmotic diuretic).

Clinical uses: Oliguria prevention, oliguria treatment, cerebral edema, elevated intraocular pressure/intracranial pressure.

Side effects
Common: Headache, nausea, vomiting, polyuria, dizziness, rash, blurred vision, thrombophlebitis, fluid imbalance, electrolyte disorders, acidosis, dehydration, thirst, urticaria, hypotension, tachycardia.
Serious: Seizures, CHF, cardiovascular collapse, pulmonary edema, osmotic nephrosis, renal failure, CNS depression, coma, extravasation necrosis.

Drug: Midazolam (Versed)

Dose range: 0.30–0.35 mg/kg once.

Method of administration in this case: Intravenous.

Mechanism of action: Binds to benzodiazepine receptors; enhances GABA effects.

Clinical uses: Sedation, anesthesia.

Side effects
Common: Nausea, vomiting, sedation, headache, hypotension, agitation, involuntary movements, retrograde amnesia, euphoria, hallucinations, confusion, ataxia, dizziness, metallic taste, dry mouth, constipation, urticaria, rash, local burning or discomfort.
Serious: Respiratory arrest, cardiac arrest, withdrawal symptoms (prolonged use).

Drug: Milrinone (Primacor)

Dose range: 0.375–0.750 mcg/kg/min.

Method of administration in this case: Intravenous.

(continued)

Mechanism of action: Inhibits cAMP phosphodiesterase.

Clinical uses: Congestive heart failure, cardiac output maintenance.

Side effects
Common: Ventricular arrhythmias, ventricular ectopy, ventricular tachycardia, supraventricular arrhythmias, hypotension, headache.
Serious: Ventricular arrhythmia, torsades de pointes (rare), anaphylactic shock, bronchospasm, infusion site reaction.

Drug: Montelukast (Singulair)

Dose range: 10 mg daily.

Method of administration in this case: Orally.

Mechanism of action: Selectively binds to cysteinyl leukotriene receptors.

Clinical uses: Asthma maintenance, allergic rhinitis, exercise-induced bronchospasm.

Side effects
Common: Headache, influenza-like symptoms, abdominal pain, cough, dizziness, fatigue, asthenia, rash, fever, gastroenteritis, elevated ALT, AST, bilirubin, pruritus, urticaria, otitis media (peds), URI (peds), sleep disorders, anxiety or irritability, restlessness, tremor.
Serious: Angioedema, anaphylaxis, erythema nodosum, Churg-Strauss syndrome (rare), hepatic eosinophilic infiltration (rare), hepatotoxicity (rare).

Drug: Nitroglycerin (Generic)

Dose range: 5–200 mcg/min.

Method of administration in this case: Intravenous.

Mechanism of action: Stimulates cGMP production, resulting in vascular smooth muscle relaxation.

Clinical uses: Acute angina, angina prophylaxis, HTN, CHF.

Side effects
Common: Headache, light-headedness, dizziness, flushing, orthostatic hypotension, reflex tachycardia, burning oral sensation, tingling oral sensation, edema.
Serious: Hypotension, severe, tolerance or dependence (continued use), bradycardia, paradoxical (rare), anaphylactoid reactions (rare), methemoglobinemia (rare).

(continued)

Drug: Nizatidine (Axid)

Dose range: 150–300 mg daily.

Method of administration in this case: Orally.

Mechanism of action: Selectively antagonizes histamine H2 receptors (H2 blocker).

Clinical uses: GERD, active duodenal ulcer, duodenal ulcer prophylaxis, active gastric ulcer.

Side effects
Common: Headache, rhinitis, abdominal pain, nausea, dizziness, vomiting, dyspepsia, confusion, depression, agitation, anemia, elevated LFTs, constipation, sinusitis, insomnia, somnolence.
Serious: Hepatitis, thrombocytopenic purpura, exfoliative dermatitis, leucopenia, pneumonia.

Drug: Norepinephrine (Levophed)

Dose range: 2–12 mcg/min.

Method of administration in this case: Intravenous.

Mechanism of action: Stimulates alpha and beta 1-adrenergic receptors.

Clinical uses: Acute hypotension, cardiac arrest adjunct.

Side effects
Common: Headache, anxiety, bradycardia, dyspnea.
Serious: Severe HTN, anaphylaxis, asthma exacerbation, arrhythmias.

Drug: Potassium Chloride (Klor-con)

Dose range: 20–100 mEq daily.

Method of administration in this case: Orally.

Mechanism of action: Replaces potassium, a major intracellular cation involved in physiologic processes such as nerve impulse conduction, cardiac, skeletal, and smooth muscle contraction, and in maintaining normal renal function.

Clinical uses: Hypokalemia.

Side effects
Common: Nausea, vomiting, flatulence, abdominal pain or discomfort, diarrhea, hyperkalemia.
Serious: Hyperkalemia, arrhythmias, GI obstruction, GI bleed, GI ulceration or perforation.

(continued)

Drug: Propofol (Diprivan)

Dose range: 5–50 mcg/kg/min.

Method of administration in this case: Intravenous.

Mechanism of action: Induces GABA receptor-mediated hypnosis.

Clinical uses: Anesthesia induction and maintenance, procedural sedation, ICU sedation.

Side effects
Common: Injection site reaction, hypotension, involuntary muscle movements, respiratory acidosis during weaning, hyperlipidemia, rash, pruritus.
Serious: Anaphylactic or anaphylactoid reactions, including fatal, propofol infusion syndrome, including fatal, bradycardia, asystole, cardiac arrest (rare), seizures (rare), opisthotonus (rare), pancreatitis (rare), pulmonary edema (rare), phlebitis (rare), thrombosis (rare), renal tubular toxicity (rare), unconsciousness (rare).

Drug: Rocuronium (Zemuron)

Dose range: 600–1,200 mcg/kg.

Method of administration in this case: Intravenous.

Mechanism of action: Antagonizes motor endplate acetylcholine receptors.

Clinical uses: Endotracheal intubation, neuromuscular blockade induction and maintenance.

Side effects
Common: Transient hypotension, hypertension.
Serious: Prolonged paralysis (long-term use), respiratory depression, apnea, anaphylactic reaction (rare), bronchospasm, arrhythmias.

Drug: Tizanidine (Zanaflex)

Dose range: 8 mg every 6 to 8 hours.

Method of administration in this case: Orally.

Mechanism of action: Exact mechanism of action unknown; binds to central alpha 2-adrenergic receptors, increasing presynaptic motor neuron inhibition and reducing spasticity (centrally acting muscle relaxant).

Clinical uses: Spasticity.

Side effects
Common: Dry mouth, somnolence, asthenia, dizziness, hypotension, orthostatic hypotension, bradycardia, UTI, infection, constipation, elevated liver transaminases, vomiting, speech disturbance, urinary frequency,

(continued)

blurred vision, flu syndrome, dyskinesia, nervousness, pharyngitis, rhinitis, hallucinations, spasticity/tone increase.
Serious: Hepatotoxicity, severe bradycardia, severe hypotension, HTN, rebound, tachycardia, hallucinations, retinal degeneration (animal studies), corneal defects (animal studies), QT prolongation (animal studies).

Drug: Vecuronium (Norcuron)

Dose range: 80–100 mcg/kg.

Method of administration in this case: Intravenous.

Mechanism of action: Antagonizes motor endplate acetylcholine receptors.

Clinical uses: Neuromuscular blockade induction and maintenance.

Side effects
Common: Muscle weakness.
Serious: Prolonged paralysis (long-term use), respiratory depression, apnea, hypersensitivity reaction (rare), bronchospasm (rare).

Drug: Warfarin (Coumadin)

Dose range: 2–10 mg daily.

Method of administration in this case: Orally.

Mechanism of action: Inhibits vitamin K-dependent coagulation factor synthesis (II, VII, IX, X, proteins C and S).

Clinical uses: Anticoagulation.

Side effects
Common: Bleeding, bruising easily, abdominal cramps or pain, nausea or vomiting, diarrhea, flatulence or bloating, fatigue or malaise, lethargy, asthenia, headache, dizziness, taste changes, pruritus, edema, dermatitis, rash or urticaria, fever, cold intolerance, paresthesias, alopecia.
Serious: Hemorrhage, skin or tissue necrosis, gangrene, cholesterol embolism, purple toes syndrome, fetal or neonatal harm or death (in utero exposure), hypersensitivity reaction, anaphylactic reaction, cholestatic jaundice, hepatitis, vasculitis, tracheobronchial calcification, anemia, syncope.

Source: Epocrates Online, 2009

References

Aldea, G. (2006). *Minimally invasive aortic and mitral valve surgery.* Retrieved January 2, 2008, from http://www.uptodateonline.com/online/content/topic.do?topicKey=valve_hd/15179

Anyanwu, A.C., Filsoufi, F., Salzberg, S.P., Bronster, D.J., & Adams, D.H. (2007). Epidemiology of stroke after cardiac surgery in the current era. *J Thorac Cardiovasc Surg, 134*(5), 1121–1127.

Aronow, W.S., & Kronzon, I. (1987). Correlation of prevalence and severity of mitral regurgitation and mitral stenosis determined by Doppler echocardiography with physical signs of mitral regurgitation and mitral stenosis in 100 patients aged 62 to 100 years with mitral anular calcium. *Am J Cardiol, 60*(14), 1189–1190.

Bojar, R.M. (2005). *Manual of perioperative care in adult cardiac surgery* (4th ed.). Malden, MA: Blackwell.

Bongard, F.S., & Sue, D.Y. (2002). *Current critical care diagnosis and treatment* (2nd ed.). New York,: Lange Medical Books/McGraw-Hill.

Chalela, J.A., Kidwell, C.S., Nentwich, L.M., Luby, M., Butman, J.A., Demchuk, A.M., et al. (2007). Magnetic resonance imaging and computed tomography in emergency assessment of patients with suspected acute stroke: A prospective comparison. *Lancet, 369*(9558), 293–298.

Corwin, H.L., Sprague, S.M., DeLaria, G.A., & Norusis, M.J. (1989). Acute renal failure associated with cardiac operations. A case-control study. *J Thorac Cardiovasc Surg, 98*(6), 1107–1112.

Epocrates Online. (2009). *Epocrates online.* Retrieved February 12, 2009, from https://online.epocrates.com/home

Feindel, C.M., Tufail, Z., David, T.E., Ivanov, J., & Armstrong, S. (2003). Mitral valve surgery in patients with extensive calcification of the mitral annulus. *Journal of Thoracic and Cardiovascular Surgery, 126*(3), 777–781.

Fink, M.P. (2005). *Textbook of critical care* (5th ed.). Philadelphia: Elsevier Saunders.

Gandhi, G.Y., Nuttall, G.A., Abel, M.D., Mullany, C.J., Schaff, H.V., Williams, B.A., et al. (2005). Intraoperative hyperglycemia and perioperative outcomes in cardiac surgery patients. *Mayo Clinic Proceedings, 80*(7), 862–866.

Jakobsen, B.W., Pedersen, J., & Egeberg, B.B. (1986). Postoperative lymphocytopenia and leucocytosis after epidural and general anaesthesia. *Acta Anaesthesiol Scand, 30*(8), 668–671.

Malawer, M.H., & Sullivan, B.L. (2005). Sarcomas of the bone. In V.H. DeVita & S. Rosenberg (Eds.), *Cancer: Principles and practice of oncology* (7th ed., pp. 1673–1676). Philadelphia: Lippincott, Williams, and Wilkin.

McGarvey, M., Cheung, A., & Stecker, M. (2008). *Neurologic complications of cardiac surgery.* Retrieved January 18, 2009, from http://www.uptodateonline.com/online/content/topic .do?topicKey=cc_neuro/4752&linkTitle=STROKE&source=preview&selectedTitle=3~150 &anchor=3#3

Morgan, G.E., Mikhail, M.S., & Murray, M.J. (2006). *Clinical anesthesiology* (4th ed.). New York: Lange Medical Books/McGraw Hill Medical.

Oliveira-Filho, J., & Koroshetz, W. (2008). *Initial assessment and management of acute stroke.* Retrieved January 19, 2009, from http://www.uptodateonline.com/online/content/topic .do?topicKey=cva_dise/6754&selectedTitle=4~35&source=search_result

Oliveira-Filho, J., Koroshetz, W., & Samuels, O. (2008). *Fibrinolytic (thrombolytic) therapy for acute ischemic stroke.* Retrieved February 1, 2008, from http://www.uptodateonline. com/online/content/topic.do?topicKey=cva_dise/6308&selectedTitle=5~150&source=sea rch_result

Otto, C. (2008). *Etiology, clinical features, and evaluation of chronic mitral regurgitation.* Retrieved January 2, 2008, from http://www.uptodateonline.com/online/content/topic .do?topicKey=valve_hd/11034

Pearl, R.G., Rosenthal, M.H., Schroeder, J.S., & Ashton, J.P. (1983). Acute hemodynamic effects of nitroglycerin in pulmonary hypertension. *Ann Intern Med, 99*(1), 9–13.

Rose, B.D. (2008). *Complications of mannitol therapy.* Retrieved February 2, 2009, from http:// www.uptodateonline.com/online/content/topic.do?topicKey=fldlytes/24396&selectedTitl e=13~150&source=search_result

Rubin, L., & Hopkins, W. (2008). *Overview of pulmonary hypertension.* Retrieved January 18, 2009, from http://www.uptodateonline.com/online/content/topic.do?topicKey=ven_pulm /5112&selectedTitle=1~150&source=search_result

Silvestry, F. (2008). *Overview of postoperative management of patients undergoing cardiac surgery.* Retrieved January 18, 2009, from http://www.uptodateonline.com/online/content/ topic.do?topicKey=cc_medi/22438&selectedTitle=1~150&source=search_result#20

Smith, E.R., & Amin-Hanjani, S. (2008). *Evaluation and management of elevated intrcranial pressure in adults.* Retrieved February 2, 2009, from http://www.uptodateonline.com/

online/content/topic.do?topicKey=cc_neuro/4543&selectedTitle=2~150&source=searc h_result#33

Tietze, K., & Fuchs, B. (2008). *Use of sedative medications in critically ill patients.* Retrieved March 9, 2009, from http://www.uptodateonline.com/online/content/topic.do?topicKey=cc_medi/ 14409&selectedTitle=1~150&source=search_result

Tokarek, R., Bernstein, E.F., Sullivan, F., Uitto, J., & Mitchell, J.B. (1994). Effect of therapeutic radiation on wound healing. *Clinics in Dermatology, 12*(1), 57–70.

Treece, P. D. (2007). Communication in the intensive care unit about the end of life. *AACN Adv Crit Care, 18*(4), 406–414.

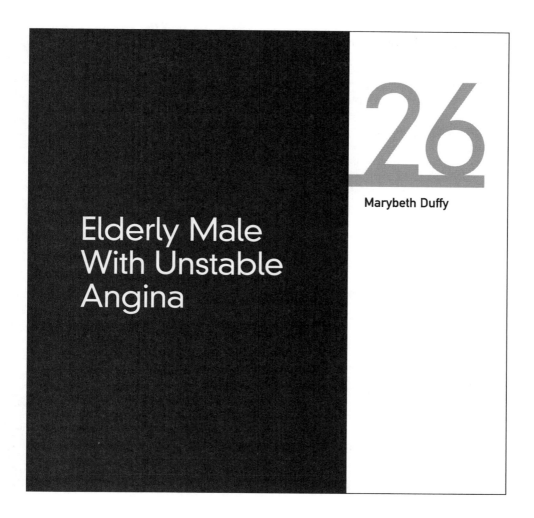

26

Marybeth Duffy

Elderly Male With Unstable Angina

I have selected this case narrative to document the comprehensive management of a commercially insured 68-year-old Caucasian male who presented for evaluation of new increasing fatigue, shortness of breath, and occasional chest pressure upon minimal exertion. The case narrative focuses on six encounters that occurred over two weeks. The encounters consist of one initial ambulatory outpatient evaluation, four in-hospital encounters, and one outpatient follow-up visit with this patient. This case addresses the following CUSN Comprehensive Direct Care patient-specific elements of doctoral competency.

DOMAIN 1, COMPETENCY 3

Formulate differential diagnoses, and diagnostic strategies and therapeutic interventions with attention to scientific evidence, safety, cost, invasiveness, simplicity, acceptability, adherence, and efficacy for patients who present with new conditions and those with ambiguous or incomplete data, complex illnesses, co-morbid conditions, and multiple diagnoses in all clinical settings.

PO A. Formulate a differential diagnosis for a patient who presents with new undifferentiated signs and symptoms.

PO B. Formulate a differential diagnosis for a patient who presents with ambiguous or incomplete data, complex illnesses, comorbid conditions and potential multiple diagnoses.

PO C. Discuss the rationale for the differential diagnosis.

PO D. Discuss the rationale for the diagnostic evaluation with attention to scientific evidence, safety, cost, invasiveness, simplicity, acceptability, adherence, and efficacy.

PO E. Discuss the rationale for the therapeutic intervention with attention to scientific evidence, safety, cost, invasiveness, simplicity, acceptability, adherence, and efficacy.

DOMAIN 3, COMPETENCY 1

Construct and evaluate outcomes of a culturally sensitive, individualized intervention that addresses the specific needs of a patient in context of family and community.

PO A. Assess culturally specific needs of patient in context of family, and community.

PO B. Construct a culturally sensitive intervention to address needs of patient in context of family, and community.

PO C. Evaluate outcomes of the intervention.

DOMAIN 2, COMPETENCY 1

Assemble a collaborative interdisciplinary network; refer and consult appropriately while maintaining primary responsibility for comprehensive patient care.

PO A. Initiate referral to other healthcare professionals while maintaining primary responsibility for patient care.

PO B. Accept referrals from other health care professions and communicate consultation findings and recommendations to the referring provider and collaborative network.

PO C. Utilize consultation recommendations for decision making while maintaining primary responsibility for care.

PO D. Evaluate outcomes of interventions.

PO E. Provide ongoing patient follow-up and monitor outcomes of collaborative network interventions.

DOMAIN 3, COMPETENCY 2

Evaluate gaps in health care access that compromise optimal patient outcomes, and apply current knowledge of the organization and financing of health care systems to ameliorate negative impact.

PO A. Identify gaps in access that compromise patient's optimum care.

PO B. Identify gaps in reimbursement that compromise patient's optimum care.

PO C. Demonstrate patient advocacy in the provision of continuous and comprehensive care.

PO D. Apply current knowledge of the organization to ameliorate negative impact.

PO E. Apply current knowledge of health care systems to ameliorate negative impact.

ENCOUNTER CONTEXT

Encounter One (initial assessment, cardiac clinic ambulatory setting)

Doctor of nursing practice (DNP) role: I am the DNP student and nurse practitioner seeing this patient, with an attending cardiologist, for the first time in an outpatient cardiology clinic.

Identifying Information

Site: Urban academic medical center.

Setting: Cardiology outpatient clinic.

Reason for encounter: This patient is referred for a cardiology consult by the patient's primary care provider (PCP). The patient's prior medical care had been provided at another medical center; however, the patient was dissatisfied with the care and requested a cardiology referral to this private office.

Informant: Patient medical records, brought by patient, who is a reliable historian.

Chief complaint: When walking less than one block at a fast pace, or upon walking uphill, the patient states that he will immediately experience "burning" or "pressure" in the chest and occasional radiating "aching or numbness" in the left shoulder, left forearm, and neck, accompanied by shortness of breath and increasing fatigue. Patient reports, "I gained 20 pounds over the last four years. My lifestyle has become very sedentary the last few months because of this chest pain."

History of Present Illness (HPI)

This is a 68-year-old male who had progressive chronic lymphocytic leukemia (CLL) with large nodes in his neck and abdomen. He was treated in 2008 with Fludara (fludarabine phosphate) and Cytoxan (cyclophosphamide) with Rituxan (rituximab), which is a monoclonal antibody chemotherapy. He had some significant shrinkage of all his adenopathy, but also had pancytopenia with lowest platelet count of 45,000 during chemotherapy treatment and a most recent platelet count of 70,000. He has been classified as Stage IV CLL by his oncologist.

The patient reports that his first episode of chest "burning," "aching," and/or "numbness" radiating to left arm, shoulder, and neck, associated with shortness of breath, occurred after his first chemotherapy treatment, in 2008. Patient also complains of decreased exercise tolerance since chemotherapy treatments began in 2008.

Over the last few weeks, his exercise tolerance has progressively decreased. Patient can walk one block at a slow to moderate pace. However, if he quickens the pace or walks uphill, he will immediately experience "burning" or "pressure" in the chest and occasional radiating "aching or numbness" in the left shoulder, left forearm, and neck. He has orthopnea, dyspnea, and shortness of breath on minimal exertion. Symptoms have progressively worsened over the last four to six months. Symptoms are quickly relieved with rest. Patient has never taken nor been prescribed sublingual nitroglycerine (NitroStat) tablets. He has intermittent swelling in the lower extremities, which is relieved with elevation. The edema has decreased since he began taking hydrochlorothiazide (HydroDiuril) a few months ago.

He reports that he has become much more sedentary over the last few years, especially over the last few months. He has experienced a weight gain of 20 pounds over the last four years that he attributes to his present sedentary lifestyle and activity level that is limited by chest pain.

He states that he was diagnosed with hypercholesterolemia and hypertension (HTN) more than twenty years ago. Over the last several years, his cholesterol levels have been and continue to be fairly well controlled on atorvastatin (Lipitor) 40 milligrams, which he continues to take daily. His total cholesterol (TC) remains less than 120, high-density lipoprotein (HDL) is low at 40, triglycerides 130, and low-density lipoproteins (LDL) 110. Although his most recent LDL is 110, the patient says it is normally 100 or less.

According to the Third Report of the National Cholesterol Education Program (NCEP) Expert Panel on Detection, Evaluation, and Treatment of High Blood Cholesterol in Adults Treatment Panel (2002), if he does have CAD, the optimal LDL target is < 70 mg.DL (Grundy et al., 2004).
        Oxford Centre for Evidence-Based Medicine (CEBM), level 5.

His HTN is well controlled with losartan (Cozaar) 30 milligrams by mouth every hour of sleep, and hydrochlorothiazide (HydroDiuril) 12.5 milligrams by mouth daily, as his average systolic blood pressure (SBP) ranges from 110 to120 mmHg, and his average diastolic blood pressure (DBP) ranges from 70 to 80 mmHg. He maintains a low-salt, low-cholesterol diet and reports compliance with medications, which has likely contributed to these outcomes. However, as he mentioned, he is very sedentary and does not exercise.

Medical Record Review

Previous stress sestamibi test 16 years ago showed moderately positive anterior ischemia; however, patient was without symptoms at that time and was unaware of his test results. Now, patient presents with Class III angina with a markedly positive stress test, performed two weeks ago, that demonstrates severe anterior ischemia.

Medical History

- CLL was diagnosed in 2003 with marker studies done on peripheral blood smear that reported cluster of differentiation (CD) 38 negative, which is indicative of a longer survival outcome. CD 5, 23, 52, and CD 31 were positive, and therefore CLL was diagnosed.
- Paroxysmal atrial arrhythmia, with first episode 20 years ago. Most recent episode five years ago, with spontaneous resolution to normal sinus rhythm that is well controlled on diltiazem (Cardizem) and with avoidance of caffeine.
- Sleep apnea diagnosed eight years ago. Sleep apnea treated with continuous positive airway pressure (CPAP). Patient wakes up feeling more rested and energized since using CPAP.
- Gastroesophageal reflux (GERD), effectively treated with lansoprazole (Prevacid).
- Chronic sinusitis, treated with antihistamines and antibiotics when necessary.

Allergies: No known allergies (drugs, food, or environmental).

Surgical procedures: Cataracts removed several years ago.

Hospitalizations: None.

Trauma: None.

Transfusions: None prior to this admission.

Routine health maintenance: Pneumococcal vaccination (2004, 2009); influenza vaccination (2009); colonoscopy (2008).

Family History

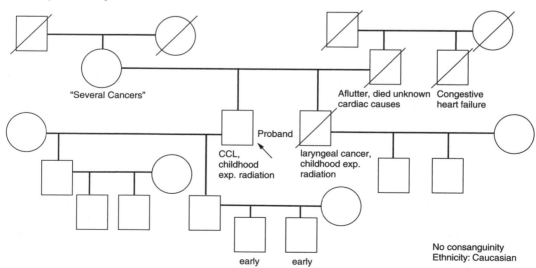

Psychosocial History

Patient denies smoking, and reports that he drinks a glass of wine once a month but has had none in the last year during chemotherapy treatment. Denies illicit drug use. Patient lives with wife of 40 years and works as a computer analyst. Patient observes an orthodox religion and requests that plan of care be scheduled congruent with his beliefs. Expresses concern for his children and grandchildren's risks for cancer and heart disease, and with regard to burdening his wife.

Education

Graduate school.

Present Medications (prescribed by patient's PCP)

- Acetylsalicylic acid (ASA) 81 mg by mouth daily, started three weeks prior to this encounter by PCP.
- Losartan (Cozaar) 30 milligrams by mouth every hour of sleep.
- Diltiazem (Cardizem) 30 milligrams by mouth daily.
- Hydrochlorothiazide (HydroDiuril) 12.5 milligrams by mouth daily.
- Metoprolol succinate (Toprol XL) XL 25 milligrams by mouth daily.
- Atorvastatin (Lipitor) 40 milligrams by mouth daily.
- Fexofenadine (Seldane) 60 milligrams by mouth daily.
- Zolpidem (Ambien) 5 mg milligrams by mouth every hour of sleep as needed.
- Montelukast (Singulair) 10 milligrams by mouth daily as needed.
- Lansoprazole (Prevacid) 30 milligrams by mouth daily as needed.
- Guaifenesin (Robitussin) 600 mg by mouth as needed.
- Docusate (Colace) 100 milligrams up to three times daily as needed for constipation.
- Dextroamphetamine (Dexedrine) 10 milligrams by mouth daily as needed for daytime somnolence.

Review of Systems

General: Reports a twenty-pound weight gain over the last four years. Denies fevers, chills, night sweats, malaise, lethargy.

Neurologic: Denies CVA, seizures, paresthesia, tremors, headaches. Complains of numbness to left shoulder and left arm on exertion after initial "twinge" of pain in chest upon minimal exertion.

Psychiatric: No clinical depression or other psychiatric disorders.

Integumentary: No rashes, petechiae, or lesions.

Ears: No tinnitus/vertigo, or hearing deficit.

Eyes: Wears glasses for presbyopia and nearsightedness. No glaucoma. Cataracts surgically removed several years ago.

Nose: No sinus pain, drainage, or pressure.

Throat/Mouth: No dentures, has own teeth in good repair.

Pulmonary: See HPI. No history of asthma, bronchitis, tuberculosis, cough, and hemoptysis.

Cardiovascular: See HPI.

Gastrointestinal: No nausea/vomiting; no black, tarry, or bloody stools. Reports bowel movements every one to two days; denies change in appetite.

Genitourinary: No incontinence, urgency, frequency, or pain on urination; no bloody or discolored urine; reports occasional hesitancy.

Endocrine: No diabetes; no thyroid abnormalities; no cold or heat intolerance; no polydypsia, polyphagia, or polyuria.

Immune: See HPI.

Musculoskeletal: Fully independent in activities of daily living (ADL). Denies joint pain, swelling, stiffness, back, or neck pain.

Hematology: See HPI.

Health Maintenance: Up-to-date with all recommended screening exams and tests, including pneumonia and influenza vaccine, colonoscopy, electrocardiogram (EKG), and stress test. Recent colonoscopy without abnormal findings.

Physical Examination

General: Patient is ambulatory. He is obese, well groomed, appropriate, and appears to be his stated age. He is an excellent historian.

Vital Signs: Blood pressure 130/80, heart rate 73, respiratory rate 20, tympanic temp 98.2°F. Height 69 inches; weight 250 pounds; basal metabolic index (BMI) 36.9.

Skin: No rashes or petechiae. Warm, no mottling or discoloration.

Nodes: Palpable 2-cm left supraclavicular node and 1-cm submental node; no palpable periauricular, axillary, cervical, inguinal, abdominal or right supraclavicular nodes.

Head: Atraumatic, round.

Neck: Short, supple. No trachea deviation noted.

Eyes: Pupils equal and reactive to light and accommodation. No cataracts noted.

Neuropsychologic: Awake, alert, and oriented to person, place, and time. Affect is flat. Patient denies depressed feelings and is willing to discuss condition and plan of care collaboratively and proactively.

Cardiac: S1, S2 regular rate and rhythm (RRR), no murmurs, gallops, rubs, heaves, or lifts. Plus two to three radial, femoral, and dorsalis pedis pulses bilaterally; trace dependent bilateral pedal edema; no jugular venous distention; negative hepatojugular reflux.

Pulmonary: Auscultation bilaterally reveals no crackles, rhonchi, or wheezing.

Gastrointestinal: Abdomen soft, round, obese, non-tender; normoactive bowel sounds in all four quadrants. No palpable hepatomegaly or splenomegaly noted.

Genitourinary: Deferred.

Musculoskeletal: Ambulatory, normal gait. No myopathies, tremors, or dyskinetic movements noted. Strength is equal in both upper and lower extremities, five out of five.

Diagnostic Test Review

Colonoscopy (2008): Negative.

Endoscopy (2008): Benign tubular adenoma.

Baseline EKG: Normal sinus rhythm 73 beats per minute; no q waves or ST or t wave abnormalities; normal axis.

Stress sestamibi (1993): Abnormal; consistent with moderate apical, mild inferior, and minimal anterior ischemia. No follow-up because patient was unaware of results and was asymptomatic.

Stress thallium (2009): Ischemic ST segment response with one-millimeter ST depression in inferior and lateral leads. Large area of severe ischemia involving the left anterior descending (LAD) and diagonal areas with stress-induced stunning of the apex suggesting a greater than 90 percent occlusion.

Laboratory Values (outside laboratory; one week prior to initial visit)

Laboratory	Patient's Value	Reference Range
White Blood Cells	3.7	4,300–10,800 cells/_L/cu mm
Hemoglobin (Hgb)	11.9	Male: 13–18 gm/dL
Hematocrit (Hct)	35	Male: 45–62%
Platelets	70	150,000–350,000/mL
Sodium (Na)	140	136–146 mM/L
Potassium (K)	4.0	3.6–5.0 mM/L
Chloride (Cl)	104	102–109 mM/L
HCO3	27	25–33 mM/L
Blood urea nitrogen (BUN)	31	7–20 mg/dL
Creatinine	1.1	0.5–1.4 mg/dL
Glucose	128	70–110 mg/dL

(continued)

Laboratory	Patient's Value	Reference Range
Aspartate aminotransferase	27	12–38 U/l
Alanine aminotransferase	19	7–41 U/l
Alkaline phosphatase	81	33–96 U/l
Total bilirubin	0.2	0.30–1.20 mg/dL
Direct bilirubin	0.6	0.04–0.4 mg/dL
Total protein	6.2	6.0–8.6 g/dL
Albumin	3.4	3.5–5.0 g/dL
Magnesium	1.9	1.5–2.0 mEq/L
Partial thromboplastin (PT)/International normalized ratio (INR)	13.04/1.0	12.0–15.0 seconds/0.8–1.2
Activated partial thromboplastin time (APTT)	29	24.0–40.0 seconds
Triglycerides	130	80–150 mg/dL
Total cholesterol	120	120–200 mg/dL
High-density lipoproteins	40	50–110 mg/dL
Low-density lipoproteins	110	60–100 mg/dL

Impression and Plan

Patient is a 68-year-old obese Caucasian male who presents to this cardiology center for second opinion regarding recent escalation of symptoms, which include exertional chest pain relieved with rest, and decreased exercise tolerance. A stress thallium test performed three weeks ago demonstrates a large area of severe ischemia involving the LAD and diagonal areas with stress-induced stunning of the apex suggesting a greater than 90 percent occlusion.

The patient's past medical history is significant for CLL diagnosed in 2003, treated in 2008 with FCR chemotherapy. This resulted in significant shrinkage of all his adenopathy, currently classified as Stage IV due to subsequent pancytopenia.

Although the patient's symptoms may be related to CLL and a side effect of chemotherapy treatments, in light of his recent escalation in symptoms despite cessation of chemotherapy, it is reasonable to consider that the patient is more likely presenting with Canadian Class (CCS) III angina due to ischemic heart disease caused by underlying CAD, as demonstrated by his most recent markedly positive stress test.

Printzmetal's angina is considered, though unlikely because chest pain does not occur intermittently at rest. Anemia may also be considered as a contributing factor; however, the patient's hemoglobin and hematocrit have remained stable over the last several months.

It is not clear what his atrial irregular rhythm is, although the patient is certain it is not atrial fibrillation. More likely, he experiences atrial tachycardia, and this may cause worsening of his symptomatology in times of exertion and stress. However, even if this is the case, the rapid rate would likely cause near-syncope, dizziness, and perhaps headache (which the patient denies). If in fact he does have an underlying arrhythmia that provokes his symptoms, he should also initially be evaluated for CAD. Therefore, I recommended the following **(D1, C3, PO A, B, C)**:

- Transthoracic echocardiography to assess left ventricular (LV) size and function and to evaluate valvular function. LV function to be assessed prior to cardiac catheterization in order to avoid excess dye given during left ventriculogram. Although patient's creatinine is normal at this time, even small risk of injury to kidneys should be avoided **(D1, C3, PO C, D)**.
- Cardiac catheterization scheduled in two days to evaluate for CAD. Scheduled on a day that would not impact patient's observance of the Sabbath **(D 3, C1, PO B)**.

Critical Appraisal

It may be argued that the patient is not on an optimal medical regimen, as he is not taking any anti-ischemic medications or nitrates such as NitroStat (nitroglycerin), Imdur, or Ranexa, and therefore he should be started on a nitrate prior to ordering an invasive cardiac catheterization/PCI procedure. However, given the abrupt recent onset and escalation of his symptoms and the history of mild to moderate ischemia in the anterior (LAD) territory diagnosed 15 years ago by stress sestamibi, which has now progressed to severe ischemia, I am compelled to take a more invasive approach.

- Continue present medications (as listed).
- Stop taking lanzopezole (Prevacid) while on clopidogrel (Plavix). Instruct patient to report any stomach discomfort or pain. Will resume if aggravating abdominal symptoms develop, and/or after clopidogrel (Plavix) cessation.
- Started on clopidogrel (Plavix) 75 milligrams by mouth daily to initiate that day in the event patient warrants a percutaneous coronary intervention (PCI) or stent to his coronary arteries.
- Clinic appointment scheduled for one week after cardiac catheterization.
- He is not yet confirmed to have CAD; therefore an LDL of 110 is acceptable. However, if he does have CAD, optimal LDL is 70, and to reach this target we can increase Lipitor to 80 mg orally daily or add Zetia (as recommended by the American Heart Association [AHA] and NCEP/ATP III).
- Copy of medical records given to patient and faxed to primary care provider **(D2, C1, PO B)**.

ICD-9 Codes

Canadian Class III Unstable Angina 411.1
Ischemic Heart Disease 414.9
Printzmetal's Angina 413.1
Anemia 281
Atrial Arrythmia 427.0

(D1, C3, PO A.)

Diagnostic Test Review

Echocardiogram is performed on the day of initial encounter.
Results: Normal LV size and function. Ejection fraction = 60 percent. No mitral, aortic, tricuspid, or pulmonic valvular stenosis or regurgitation seen.

Encounter Two (two days after initial evaluation; cardiac catheterization)

Laboratory Ambulatory Intake Area

Hematology consult requested prior to possible PCI with anticoagulant and clopidogrel (Plavix). Patient seen by hematologist, who agrees with plan to give bivalirudin (Angiomax) and the implant of a bare metal stent, with clopidogrel (Plavix) for only one month in the event the patient requires a stent **(D2, C1, PO A)**.

History and Physical Examination (performed by me)

General: Patient is ambulatory. He is obese, well groomed, and appropriate.

Vital signs: Blood pressure 136/84, heart rate 76 beats per minute (bpm), respiratory rate 20, temp 98.0°F.
Ht. 69 inches, wt. 250 pounds, BMI 36.9.

Skin: No rashes or petechiae. Warm, no mottling or discoloration.

Nodes: Palpable 2-cm left supraclavicular node and 1-cm submental node; no palpable periauricular, axillary, cervical, inguinal, abdominal, or right supraclavicular nodes.

Head: Atraumatic, round.

Neck: Short, supple. No trachea deviation noted.

Eyes: Pupils equal and reactive to light and accommodation. No cataracts noted.

Neuropsychologic: Awake, alert, and oriented to person, place, and time. Appears anxious, talking fast and asking numerous—though relevant—questions regarding the procedure. Denies anxiety and refuses oral anti-anxiety agent offered prior to procedure.

Cardiac: S1, S2 RRR; no murmurs, gallops, rubs, heaves, or lifts. Plus two to three radial, femoral and dorsalis pedis pulses bilaterally, trace-dependent bilateral pedal edema, no jugular venous distention, negative hepatojugular reflux.

Pulmonary: Clear to auscultation bilaterally; no crackles, rhonchi, or wheezing.

Gastrointestinal: Abdomen soft, round, obese; non-tender, normoactive bowel sounds in all four quadrants. No palpable hepatomegaly or splenomegaly noted.

Genitourinary: Deferred.

Musculoskeletal: Ambulatory, normal gait. No myopathies, tremors, or dyskinetic movements noted. Strength is equal in both upper and lower extremities, five out of five.

Laboratory findings and electrocardiogram were performed within the past month and can be accepted for an elective procedure as per institutional protocol.

Informed Consent

Discussion and consent for diagnostic and possible coronary intervention. I explain risk factors, including but not limited to a three percent risk of bleeding, infection, myocardial infarction (MI), stroke, neurovascular injury, hematoma, pseudoaneurysm, and death. It is explained that the patient's preexisting CLL and thrombocytopenia predispose him to a greater risk of infection and bleeding that may warrant the transfusion of blood products and/or antibiotics. In the event of any emergency such as cardiac arrest or lethal arrhythmia, cardiopulmonary resuscitation and emergent insertion of an intra-aortic balloon pump (IABP), urgent CABG, or vascular surgery may be warranted. Benefits include relief of anginal pain, allowing for increased activity without chest pain and, therefore, enhancement of quality of life.

The patient informs us that he has researched options, risks, and benefits of each procedure, and if at all possible PCI would be his choice because it is least invasive. If PCI does not alleviate his symptoms, he will opt for CABG at a later date. Consent is signed according to protocol.

Encounter Three (catheterization laboratory procedure room; two days after initial consult; one hour after obtaining consent in the ambulatory intake area)

I am present and assist the attending interventional cardiologist during the entire diagnostic and interventional procedure. I am responsible for obtaining femoral artery access and assisting in all aspects of the diagnostic and interventional procedure.

The diagnostic left heart catheterization demonstrates two vessel CAD, 95% proximal left anterior descending (LAD), mild irregularities to the proximal and distal left circumflex, and 70% occlusion to the mid right coronary artery (RCA) segment.

To avoid additional dye being given to the patient, a left ventriculogram is not performed, because the left ventricle (LV) was normal in appearance and function on a transthoracic echocardiogram (TTE) performed within the past month.

An appropriateness (A) criteria set forth by Patel (2009) for coronary revascularization states the appropriateness level of revascularization for a patient with

2-vessel CAD involving the proximal LAD with

- *High-risk findings on noninvasive testing and*
- *Receiving no or minimal anti-ischemic medical therapy is (A)(8) and for a patient with*

2-vessel CAD involving the proximal LAD A (9)

- *High-risk findings on noninvasive testing*
- *Receiving a course maximal anti-ischemic medical therapy A (9)*

Appropriateness for 2-vessel CAD with proximal LAD stenosis for PCI is A (8)* and for CABG A (8)* as well, on a scale from one to ten, for this patient (Patel, 2009).

CEBM, level 5.

Although this patient was not on adequate anti-ischemic medications, his appropriateness score for revascularization is eight out of ten, given that he has two-vessel CAD involving the proximal LAD and presents with Class III unstable angina symptoms.

At this time during the procedure, the patient has received conscious sedation, midazolam (Versed) given intravenously; however, he is conscious. Immediately after the diagnostic catheterization, the attending physician and I reiterate the risks and benefits of revascularization treatment options with the patient, including PCI stenting of the LAD as opposed to coronary artery bypass grafting (CABG). I again discuss with the patient the risks and benefits of all possibilities. The patient wants a PCI if at all possible, instead of optimal medical management or CABG. The patient remains consistent in his decision.

Critical Appraisal

The attending interventional cardiologist and I also decided upon PCI for numerous factors.

Although there is evidence to support either CABG or PCI to treat this patient's unstable angina pain caused by CAD, he is at increased risk for bleeding with either procedure, due to his thrombocytopenia, and he is at increased risk for infection due to his immunocomprised state from the CLL.

CABG remains the standard of care for patients with three-vessel or left main coronary artery disease, since the use of CABG, as compared with PCI, resulted in lower rates of the combined end point of major adverse cardiac or cerebrovascular events at 1 year (Serruys et al., 2009).

CEBM, level 1b.

As an initial management strategy in patients with stable coronary artery disease, PCI did not reduce the risk of death, myocardial infarction, or other major cardiovascular events when added to optimal medical therapy (Boden et al., 2007).

CEBM, level 1b.

CABG would predispose him to potential sternal wound and leg-bypass graft wound infections, and the majority of patients receive blood products (Samuels, Kaufman, Morris, Styler, & Brockman, 1999). He may also be prone to subsequent infections, as they would most likely harvest his left internal mammary artery (LIMA), as the patency rate is superior to that of a vein graft—leaving his chest wall with collateral circulation only, after the LIMA is dissected and rerouted to provide blood flow to the LAD artery.

> *The report by Samuels et al. (2009) is not CEBM-rated because it is a report of twelve patients diagnosed with CLL that had CABG (nine patients), CABG and valve repair (one patient), and valve repair alone (two patients). Hospital mortality occurred in two (17%) patients. Both patients died of sepsis. Hospital morbidity occurred in seven (58%) patients. The most common complications were infections. Transfusion of blood products was required in eight (67%) patients. The average length of stay was 15. Follow-up was complete. Late mortality occurred in four patients at a mean of seven months, all non-cardiac related (Samuels et al., 2009).*

Heparin is used to anticoagulate the blood to decrease the risk of thromboembolism and stroke during cardiopulmonary bypass. The use of heparin predisposes the patient to possible heparin-induced thrombocytopenia (HIT) and further decreased platelet count.

Although PCI performed with the administration of bivalirudin (Angiomax) as an anti-thrombin agent and clopidogrel (Plavix) use for one month also predispose the patient to worsening thrombocytopenia, it is much less invasive than CABG and can be performed without the use of heparin.

The Acute Catheterization and Urgent Intervention Triage strategy (ACUITY) trial consisted of 13,819 moderate and high-risk NSTE/Acute Coronary Syndrome (ACS) patients randomized to either bivalirudin (Angiomax) monotherapy, bivalirudin (Angiomax) plus provisional use of a IIb/IIIa inhibitor or unfractionated heparin (UFH)/enoxaparin (Lovenox) plus a IIb/IIa inhibitor. Bivalirudin (Angiomax) monotherapy demonstrated significantly fewer bleeding complications in comparison to the UFH/enoxaparin (Lovenox) plus IIb/IIIa inhibitors and the bivalirudin (Angiomax) plus provisional IIb/IIIa inhibitor groups. It should also be noted that patients with thrombocytopenia were excluded from entry into this trial (White et al., 2008).

> *In the ACUITY trial, 13,819 patients with moderate- and high-risk Non ST Elevation Acute Coronary Syndrome (NSTE-ACS) were randomized to one of three groups: unfractionated heparin or Enoxaparin (Lovenox) plus Glyco Protein (GP) IIb/IIIa inhibitors; bivalirudin (Angiomax) plus IIb/IIIa inhibitors; or bivalirudin (Angiomax) monotherapy with provisional use of GP IIb/IIIa inhibitors for ischemic complications. Results of*

the overall study showed the best outcomes in the bivalirudin (Angiomax) monotherapy group, which had a similar rate of ischemic complications but a reduced rate of bleeding 2.5% bivalirudin (Angiomax) versus 4.9% unfractionated heparin/Enoxaparin (Lovenox) or bivalirudin (Angiomax) given concomitantly with a IIb/IIa inhibitor in the naïve anticoagulant and antithrombin patients demonstrating a statistically significant p value < 0.01 (White et al., 2008).

CEBM, level 1b.

The attending physician and I order bivalirudin (Angiomax) (Krolich, 2006), which I administer intra-arterially via the right femoral artery, prior to the intervention. When the patient's activated clotting time (ACT) reaches 322, the LAD lesion is stented with a bare metal stent rather than a drug-eluting stent. A bare metal stent (BMS) is chosen over a drug-eluting stent (DES) because a BMS requires only one month of clopidogrel (Plavix) after the PCI, as opposed to the one year required after a DES stent, to prevent the life-threatening complication of acute in-stent thrombosis.

Krolich (2006), a single case study that demonstrated safety in administering bivalirudin (Angiomax®) to a single patient diagnosed with CLL and thrombocytopenia (platelet count circa 40,000)during PCI [. . .], suggests that bivalirudin (Angiomax) may be safely used in patients who are at an increased risk of bleeding undergoing PCI.

Krolich, 2006.

Studies have shown that DES stents have less risk of reocclusion or in-stent restenosis, but the necessity for clopidogrel (Plavix) over an entire year, combined with daily baby aspirin (Ecotrin), would put this patient at risk for bleeding. If it became necessary to stop the clopidogrel (Plavix), this patient would be at great risk for acute stent thrombosis and possible death.

The lesion is crossed with a wire, and a BMS stent is deployed at the ostial and proximal LAD lesion without complication. The patient experiences chest pain that he describes as "usual" during balloon inflation to expand the stent. The pain is immediately relieved with balloon deflation, which is less than twelve seconds. The RCA vessel is not intervened upon because it is considered the non-culprit vessel, given that there is no ischemia in this area on the stress sestamibi. We will consider revascularization in the future, if after discharge home the patient continues with the same or worsening symptoms (Boden et al., 2007) **(D1, C3, PO E).**

After the procedure is completed, I deploy a ProGlide 5–8F Suture-Mediated Closure System (Perclose) closure device to the patient's right femoral artery, which is occlusive without hematoma, oozing, or complications.

The ProGlide(tm) 5–8F Suture-Mediated Closure System (Perclose®) device was safe and effective for closing arteriotomy sites in patients undergoing neurointerventional procedures, including those receiving anticoagulation/ anti-platelet therapy or those previously treated with the device one or two times (Khaghany, Al-Ali, Spigelmoyer, Pimentel, & Wharton, 2005).

CEBM, level 1b.

Encounter Four (telemetry unit, two days after initial consult, four hours after the PCI procedure)

I admit the patient to a telemetry-monitored bed for overnight observation, due to patient's preexisting comorbid conditions. Although the patient is stable and had no intraprocedural or post-procedural complications, and the femoral insertion site has no inadvertent venous or multiple arterial punctures, his medical history is significant for CLL and thrombocytopenia. He is at greater risk for possible late bleeding complications at the femoral insertion site. His platelets were 70,000, and he received an anti-thrombin agent, bivalirudin (Angiomax), which has been shown to reduce bleeding risk in PCI patients; however, the trials were done on patients with baseline platelet counts above 150,000.

One documented case narrative by Krolick (2006) demonstrated safety of the use of bivalirudin (Angiomax) in a patient with CLL and a platelet count of less than 50,000; however, this is not sufficient evidence to suggest that this patient is not still at risk (Krolich, 2006). The lack of sufficient evidence-based clinical trials and data regarding bivalirudin (Angiomax) use in CLL patients with thrombocytopenia prompts me to admit the patient overnight for further observation and laboratory monitoring of platelet count **(D3, C2, PO B, C, D, E).**

New Medicare guidelines require same-day discharge for PCI patients less than 75 years old unless adequate documentation explicitly states reasonable need for overnight admission. If not documented properly or to Medicare's satisfaction, the hospital will be denied reimbursement for the overnight stay. Under Medicare, the Quality Improvement Organization (QIO), for each hospital is responsible for deciding, during review of inpatient admissions on a case-by-case basis, whether the admission was medically necessary. Medicare law authorizes the QIO to make these judgments and the judgments are binding for purposes of Medicare coverage. The physician or other practitioner responsible for a patient's care at the hospital is also responsible for deciding whether the patient should be admitted as an inpatient.

Resnic, 2007.

Encounter Five (eight hours post-PCI follow-up)

Patient reports feeling well, no chest pain, no shortness of breath, groin pain, or discomfort, and no abdominal discomfort. Wife is visiting with patient.

Physical Examination

General: Patient feels well, no complaints of chest discomfort or groin discomfort.

Vital signs: Blood pressure 120/75, heart rate 70, normal sinus rhythm, respiratory rate 18, temp 98.7°F.

Cardiac: S1, S2 regular rate and rhythm.

Pulmonary: Clear to auscultation bilaterally.

Gastrointestinal: Normoactive bowel sounds; obese; nontender.

Extremities: Right groin site with dressing clean, dry, dressing intact; no hematoma, ecchymosis, bruit, oozing. Mild tenderness to palpation.

Vascular: Plus two to three femoral and dorsalis pedis pulses, which is unchanged prior to PCI.

Laboratory Values

Laboratory	Patient's Value 8 Hours After PCI	Reference range
White blood cells	4.3	4,300–10,800 cells/µL/cu mm
Hemoglobin (Hgb)	11.4	Male: 13–18 gm/dL
Hematocrit (Hct)	32.4	Male: 45–62%
Platelets	95	150,000–350,000/mL
Sodium (Na)	140	136–146 mM/L
Potassium (K)	4.2	3.6–5.0 mM/L
Chloride (Cl)	106	102–109 mM/L
HCO3	27	25–33 mM/L
Blood urea nitrogen (BUN)	33	7–20 mg/dL
Creatinine	1.2	0.5–1.4 mg/dL
Glucose	102	70–110 mg/dL
Aspartate aminotransferase (AST)	13	12–38 U/l
Alanine aminotransferase (ALT)	18	7–41 U/l
Alkaline phosphatase	79	33–96 U/l
Partial thromboplastin (PT)/International normalized ratio (INR)	12.2/1.0	12.0–15.0 seconds/0.8–1.2
Triglycerides	87	80–150 mg/dL
Total cholesterol	113	120–200 mg/dL
High-density lipoproteins	31	50–110 mg/dL
Low-density lipoproteins	65	60–100 mg/dL
Troponin	0	
Creatinine kinase myocardial band (CKMB)	5	

Impression

68-year-old male with history of CLL, three-vessel CAD with unstable angina status post-successful PCI with bare metal stent to ostial and proximal LAD, chosen in lieu of CABG is clinically stable eight hours post procedure.

Plan

Teaching and post-PCI follow-up, all CAD ramifications, blood pressure, and cholesterol parameters, risk factors, and dietary and exercise recommendations discussed in detail.

Encounter Six (post-PCI day one)

Discharge Note: Patient reports feeling well, with no chest pain, shortness of breath, groin pain, or discomfort, and no abdominal discomfort. Patient reports that he is ready to go home.

Physical Examination

General: Patient feels well; no complaints of chest discomfort or groin discomfort.

Vital signs: Blood pressure 115/75, heart rate 70s, normal sinus rhythm, respiratory rate 20, temp 98.5°F.

Cardiac: S1, S2 regular rate and rhythm.

Pulmonary: Clear to auscultation bilaterally.

Gastrointestinal: Normoactive bowel sounds; obese, nontender.

Extremities: Right groin site with dressing clean, dry, and intact; no hematoma; no ecchymosis; no bruit, no oozing, no tenderness to palpation.

Vascular: Plus two to three femoral and dorsalis pedis pulses (no change from prior to PCI).

EKG: NSR 68; no ST/T wave ischemic changes or q waves.

Impression

68-year-old male with history of CLL, three-vessel CAD with unstable angina now one day post-PCI, bare metal stent to ostial and proximal LAD, no intra- or post-procedural complications, stable, symptom-free, and ready for discharge home.

Plan

Counseling and Education

Laboratory results reviewed with patient, and discharge teaching and follow-up instructions reiterated with patient and patient's wife.

Medications

Continue medications as prescribed in past medical history.

- Continue atorvastatin (Lipitor) 40 milligrams by mouth daily because patient's fasting LDL 65 is within target range of < 70.
- Clopidogrel (Plavix) 75 milligrams by mouth daily for one month.
- Hold lansoprazole (Prevacid) until clopidogrel (Plavix) has been stopped.

Discharge

Patient discharged home with wife.

> *Concomitant use of clopidogrel (Plavix®) and PPI after hospital discharge for Acute Coronary Syndrome (ACS) was associated with an increased risk of adverse outcomes than use of clopidogrel (Plavix®) without PPI, suggesting that use of PPI may be associated with attenuation of benefits of clopidogrel (Plavix®) after ACS (Ho, 2009).*
>
> CEBM, level 2b.

Encounter Seven (post-initial consult 13 Days; post-PCI day 11)

Follow-Up Visit (Cardiac outpatient center)

Patient states, "I felt much better the first three days after the stent. I was able to exercise on the treadmill for thirty minutes, and I lost five pounds. But the fourth day after the procedure, I was feeling tired after I exercised for only fifteen minutes." Patient requests to restart dextroamphetamine (Dexedrine) for his daytime sleepiness. He had stopped taking it after his positive stress test over a month ago. Although the CPAP helps him to awaken less sleepy, he still suffers from daytime somnolence due to the sleep apnea.

Physical Examination

Vital signs: Blood pressure 110/60; heart rate 76, regular rate and rhythm; respiratory rate 20; temp 98.5°F; weight 245 pounds (five pounds less than eleven days prior).

Skin: Warm, intact. No petechiae, ecchymosis, rashes.

Neurologic: Alert and oriented ($\times$ 3).

Cardiac: S1, S2 regular rate and rhythm.

Pulmonary: No wheezing or rhonchi noted bilaterally.

Extremities: No pedal edema; plus two dorsalis pedal pulses; right groin no swelling, hematoma, ecchymosis, or tenderness.

EKG: NSR 68, no ST/T wave ischemic changes or q waves.

Laboratory results from 11 days ago reviewed. Platelets are drawn today and are 92,000.

Impression

This is a 68-year-old male with a past medical history of CLL diagnosed in 2003 and treated with radiation and chemotherapy in 2008 with subsequent pancytopenia, which categorizes him as Stage IV CLL. Several months ago, he had a positive stress test that revealed markedly severe ischemia in the anterior territory, and patient exhibited signs of CCS III angina. An echocardiogram shows that he has normal left ventricular size and function. He is now eleven days s/p cardiac catheterization, which showed two-vessel CAD, 95% proximal LAD and 70% mid RCA stenosis. Bivalirudin (Angiomax) was used during the procedure, and patient was given and is still continued on clopidogrel (Plavix) with no side effects. Last platelet count is 92,000. He had a bare metal stent implanted in the proximal LAD lesion, and the RCA was not revascularized because the stress test did not reveal ischemia to this area.

It appears that the patient is angina-free and able to exercise without chest pain. His fatigue is likely due to overexertion after months of inactivity rather than ischemia, given that his EKG and physical examination are unremarkable at this time. I discuss this with the patient, and advise him to attend cardiac rehabilitation. Monitored supervision will give him confidence to engage in an active progression of activity, exercise, and lifestyle changes.

Plan

Therapeutics
- Continue medications as prescribed in medical history.
- Continue atorvastatin (Lipitor) 40 milligrams by mouth daily, as patient lower-density lipoprotein (LDL) 65 is within target range of < 70.
- Clopidogrel (Plavix) 75 milligrams by mouth daily for one month; continue for 19 more days.
- Continue to hold lansoprazole (Prevacid) until clopidogrel (Plavix) has been stopped.
- Discontinue hydrochlorothiazide (HydoDiuril) and losartan (Cozaar), and change to hydrochlorothiazide/losartan (Hyzaar) 50/12.5 mg by mouth daily.
- In regard to dexoamphetamine (Dexedrine), per patient request, I assure him it is safe to use for combating daytime sleepiness; however, I advise

him to stop taking it immediately if he experiences palpitations or dizziness, and to call me or the cardiologist or go to the emergency department if symptoms are severe.

Referral
- Refer to cardiac rehabilitation program located in hospital.
- Medical history and insurance forms forwarded to the rehabilitation facility. Patient says he is a "workaholic" and fears he will not have time to go. The rehabilitation facility is in close proximity to his work, and together we plan for at least two days during the week when it would be possible for him to attend.

Education and counseling
- Recommend low-fat, low-cholesterol, heart-healthy diet, exercise and weight loss regimen.

Diagnostic tests
- Will not revascularize right coronary artery at this time because patient's exercise tolerance has improved.
- If patient continues to complain of fatigue after active participation in rehabilitation program, we will consider a repeat thallium stress test and possible cardiac catheterization to evaluate LAD stent patency and possible revascularization of the RCA.
- Repeat stress thallium in six months unless symptomatic, warranting the test or revascularization earlier.
- Repeat platelet count in three weeks. Patient appears to be doing well on clopidogrel (Plavix) and aspirin (Ecotrin).

Follow-up appointment in three weeks to check complete blood count and platelets, and to reevaluate cardiac rehabilitation and exercise, as well as diet and weight loss regimen.

CASE SUMMATION

The patient is stable post-PCI (BMS) to proximal LAD and exhibits increasing exercise tolerance and weight loss. He is to start cardiac rehabilitation to assist in transitioning to mandatory lifestyle changes in order to counteract CAD progression. He will return to the clinic in three weeks to have his CBC and platelet count checked after his clopidogrel (Plavix) has been stopped. He will be monitored closely while on lifelong aspirin (Ecotrin).

COMPETENCY DEFENSE

Domain 1, Competency 3. Formulate differential diagnoses, and diagnostic strategies and therapeutic interventions with attention to scientific evidence, safety, cost, invasiveness, simplicity, acceptability, adherence, and efficacy for patients who present with new conditions and those with ambiguous or incomplete data, complex illnesses, comorbid conditions, and multiple diagnoses in all clinical settings.

Defense. I formulated several differential diagnoses (Class III angina, Printzmetal's angina, anemia, atrial arrythmia) for this patient who presented with new, undifferentiated signs and symptoms of shortness of breath, fatigue, and increasing lack of exercise tolerance. Evidence was cited for the echocardiogram, cardiac catheterization diagnostic tools, and for the therapeutic intervention of stent implantation to his LAD artery. I also cited evidence for not intervening on the RCA.

Domain 3, Competency 1. Construct and evaluate outcomes of a culturally sensitive, individualized intervention that addresses the specific needs of a patient in context of family and community.

Defense. The patient and his wife adhere to a strict observance of the Sabbath. At his request, I arranged for the echocardiogram and cardiac catheterization to be performed on a day that would not interfere with their family gathering and ceremony. He was discharged home the day after his PCI and was home in time to spend the Sabbath with his family.

Domain 2, Competency 1. Assemble a collaborative interdisciplinary network, refer and consult appropriately while maintaining primary responsibility for comprehensive patient care.

Defense. I initiated referral to other health care professionals, including a hematologist and cardiac rehabilitation specialists, while maintaining primary responsibility for this patient's care.

I, with the attending cardiologist, accepted the referral of this patient from his primary care provider and interpreted his stress test, ordered an echocardiogram and diagnostic cardiac catheterization, and assisted in his PCI. I evaluated outcomes of this patient's LAD intervention and did not intervene on his RCA because this was not the area of ischemia noted on the stress test. I will continue to follow up with this patient and will only intervene on the RCA if patient's chief complaints and symptoms persist after discharge. The COURAGE trial results reveal that optimal medical management has better outcomes for patients with stable angina than for those that have a PCI.

I provided ongoing patient follow-up and monitored outcomes of collaborative network interventions. The hematologist followed the patient throughout his hospital stay and documented the patient's agreement with a bivilarudin (Angiomax), aspirin (Ecotrin), and clopidogrel (Plavix) regimen. I scheduled a follow-up appointment for this patient within one to two weeks of his PCI and enrolled him in a cardiac rehabilitation program. I will follow up on his progress in rehabilitation at the next follow-up visit.

I was responsible for the patient's care in the hospital and collaborated with the telemetry nurse practitioner and the attending cardiologist, and consulted with a hematologist regarding optimal care. The hematologist agreed with a bivilarudin (Angiomax), aspirin (Ecotrin), and clopidogrel (Plavix) regimen and close monitoring of the patient to observe for any adverse effects.

I coordinated post-discharge care and scheduled a cardiology clinic appointment for one week after PCI. Patient already had scheduled follow-up appointments with his oncologist.

Domain 3, Competency 2. Evaluate gaps in health care access that compromise optimal patient outcomes, and apply current knowledge of the organization and financing of health care systems to ameliorate negative impact.

Defense. The patient's history of CLL and pancytopenia predisposed him to infection, bleeding, and complications post-PCI, such as thrombocytopenia exacerbated by anticoagulant therapy of bivilarudin (Angiomax) and antiplatelet therapies clopidogrel (Plavix) and aspirin (Ecotrin). In the last month or so, Medicare changed the policy regarding reimbursement for PCI. According to the revised policy, a patient less than 75 years old who has a stent placement with no complications should be discharged home the same day. If the patient remains overnight, the hospital will only be reimbursed for the procedure and not the overnight stay, unless the provider documents acceptable reasons for keeping the patient in the hospital. The attending cardiologist and I admitted this patient to the telemetry unit overnight for observation because his history of CLL warranted close follow-up and documented these reasons in the chart.

As discussed above, I admitted this patient despite Medicare's policy that makes it cumbersome to do so and therefore may easily lead to improper reimbursement if the proper documentation is not strictly adhered to. I demonstrated patient advocacy in the provision of continuous and comprehensive care.

Medications

Drug: Acetylsalicylic acid (ASA)

Dose range: 81 mg to 325 mg per day.

Method of administration in this case: Oral.

Mechanism of action: Inhibitor of both prostaglandin synthesis and platelet aggregation producing analgesic, anti-inflammatory, antipyretic effects; irreversibly inhibits platelet aggregation.

Clinical uses in this case: Acute coronary syndrome, myocardial infarction, stroke, and thrombotic event prevention; PCI, angina.

Side effects: Indigestion, nausea, vomiting, gastrointestinal ulcer, bleeding, tinnitus, bronchospasm, angioedema, Reye's syndrome.

Drug: Losartan (Cozaar)

Dose range: 25 mg to 100 mg per day.

Method of administration in this case: Oral.

Mechanism of action: Selectively antagonizes angiotensin II AT1 receptors.

Clinical uses in this case: HTN.

(continued)

Side effects: Hypotension, hyperkalemia, renal impairment, leukopenia, neutropenia, agranulocytosis, rhabdomyolysis, hepatitis, dizziness, headache, fatigue, musculoskeletal pain, dyspepsia, edema, diarrhea, cough, pruritis, rash, elevated liver enzymes, BUN and/or creatinine.

Drug: Diltiazem (Cardizem)

Dose range: 180 mg to 360 mg per day.

Method of administration in this case: Oral.

Mechanism of action: Inhibits calcium ion influx into vascular smooth muscle and myocardium, relaxing smooth muscle, decreasing peripheral vascular resistance, dilating coronary arteries, and prolonging AV node refractory.

Clinical uses: Angina, HTN.

Side effects: Bradycardia, atrioventricular (AV) node block, arrhythmias, hypotension, syncope, cardiac failure, hepatic injury, peripheral edema, headache, dizziness, hypotension, dyspepsia, constipation, rash, elevated liver transaminases.

Drug: Hydochlorothiazide (Hydrodiuril)

Dose range: 12.5 mg to 25 mg per day.

Method of administration in this case: Oral.

Mechanism of action: Enhances excretion of sodium, chloride, and water by interfering with transport of sodium ions across renal tubular epithelium.

Clinical uses in this case: HTN.

Side effects: Hypokalemia, electrolyte imbalance, arrhythmias, pancreatitis, hypotension, dizziness, diarrhea, abdominal pain, headache, weakness, muscle cramps, photosensitivity, rash.

Drug: Atorvastatin (Lipitor)

Dose range: 10 mg to 80 mg per day.

Method of administration in this case: Oral.

Mechanism of action: Inhibits 3-hydroxy-3-methylglutaryl-coenzyme A (HMG-CoA) reductase.

Clinical uses in this case: Hypercholesterolemia, hypertriglyceridemia, cardiovascular event risk reduction.

(continued)

Side effects: Myopathy, rhabdomyolysis, renal failure, hepatotoxicity, pancreatitis, myalgia, diarrhea, dyspepsia, constipation, flatulence, elevated CPK.

Drug: Clopidogrel (Plavix)

Dose range: 5 mg to 150 mg per day, preloading dose 300 mg to 60 mg.

Method of administration in this case: Oral.

Mechanism of action: Inhibits adenosine diphosphate binding to platelet receptors (platelet aggregation inhibitor).

Clinical uses in this case: Thrombotic event prevention, peripheral arterial disease (PAD), PCI, angina.

Side effects: Bleeding, hemorrhage, TTP, neutropenia, anaphylactoid reaction, angioedema, hepatic failure, pancreatitis, nausea, dyspepsia, diarrhea, abdominal pain, purpura, rash, pruritis.

Drug: Metoprolol succinate (ToprolXL)

Dose range: 12.5 mg to 100 mg in a single dose, no greater than 400 mg in a day.

Method of administration in this case: Oral.

Mechanism of action: Beta-adrenergic blocker with selective activity on beta (one) adrenoreceptors located mainly in cardiac muscles. At higher doses, it also inhibits beta (two) adrenoreceptors of bronchial and vascular smooth muscles.

Clinical uses in this case: HTN, unstable angina.

Side effects: Bradyarrhythmia, cold extremities, heart failure, hypotension, pruritus, rash, constipation, diarrhea, indigestion, nausea, dizziness, fatigue, headache, depression, dyspnea, wheezing.

Source: Epocrates, https://online.epocrates.com. All drug information from Micromediex Health Series is available through institutional or personal license at www.micromedex.com.

References

Anti-Anginal Therapeutic Strategy. CCS Angina. Retrieved August 25, 2009 from http://www.cvtoolbox.com/downloads/cpe/Therapeutic_Strategy.pdf

Boden, W.E., et al. (2007). Optimal medical therapy with or without PCI for stable coronary disease. *N Engl J Med, 356*(15), 1503–1516.

Grundy, S.M., Cleeman, J.I., Merz, C.N., Brewer, H.B., Jr., Clark, L.T., Hunninghake, D.B., et al. (2004). Implications of recent clinical trials for the National Cholesterol Education Program Adult Treatment Panel III Guidelines. *J Am Coll Cardiol, 44*(3), 720–732.

Harper S.A., Fukuda K., Uyeki T.M., Cox N.J., Bridges C.B., Singleton, J.A. (2005). Prevention and control of influenza: Recommendations of the advisory committee on immunization practices (ACIP). *MMWR Recomm Rep, 54*(RR-8),1–40; Erratum in *Morb Mortal Wkly Rep, 2005, 54*(30),750.

Ho, P.M., Maddox, T.M., Wang, L., Fihn, S.D., Jesse, R.L., Peterson, E.D., & Rumsfeld, J.S. (2009). Risk of adverse outcomes associated with concomitant use of clopidogrel and proton pump inhibitors following acute coronary syndrome. *Journal of the American Medical Association, 301*(9), 937–944.

Jackson, G. (2007). Stable and also unstable coronary disease—COURAGE and the importance of optimal medical therapy. *Int J Clin Pract, 61*(6), 883.

Khaghany, K., Al-Ali, F., Spigelmoyer, T., Pimentel, R., & Wharton, K. (2005). Efficacy and safety of the perclose closer s device after neurointerventional procedures: Prospective study and literature review. *Am J Neuroradiol, 26*(6), 1420–1424.

King, S.B., et al. (2008). 2007 focused update of the ACC/AHA/SCAI 2005 guideline update for percutaneous coronary intervention: A report of the American College of Cardiology/American Heart Association Task Force on Practice guidelines. *J Am Coll Cardiol, 51*(2), 172–209.

Krolick, M.A. (2006). Successful percutaneous coronary intervention using bivalirudinin a patient with chronic lymphocytic leukemia and thrombocytopenia. *European Journal of Haematology, 77*(4), pp. 355–357.

Lopes, R.D., et al. (2009). Advanced age, antithrombotic strategy, and bleeding in non-ST-segment elevation acute coronary syndromes: Results from the ACUITY (Acute Catheterization and Urgent Intervention Triage Strategy) trial. *J Am Coll Cardiol, 53*(12), 1021–1030.

Patel, M.R., Dehemer, G.J., Hirsfield, J.W., Smith, P.K., & Spertus, J.A. (2009). ACCF/SCAI/STS/AATS/AHA/ASNC 2009 Appropriateness Criteria for Coronary Revascculariszation: A report by the American College of Cardiology Foundation Appropriateness Criteria Task Force, Society for Cardiovascular Angiography and Interventions Society of Thoracic Surgeons, American Association for Thoracic Surgery, American Heart Association, and American Society of Nuclear Cardiology, Endorsed by the American Society of Echocardiography, the Heart Failure Society of America and the Society of Cardiovascular Computer Tomography. *J Am Coll Cardiol, 53*(6), 530–553.

Pitt, B. (2007). Percutaneous coronary intervention plus optimal medical therapy was not more effective than medical therapy alone in stable CAD. *Evid-Based Med, 12*(4), 107.

Resnic, F.S. (2007). The case for outpatient coronary intervention: Balancing charges and discharges. *Circulation, 115*(17), 2248–2250.

Samuels, L.E., Kaufman, M.S., Morris, R.J., Styler, M., & Brockman, S.K. (1999). Open heart surgery in patients with chronic lymphocytic leukemia. *Leuk Res, 23*(1), 71–75.

Serruys, P.W., et al. (2009). Percutaneous coronary intervention versus coronary-artery bypass grafting for severe coronary artery disease. *N Engl J Med, 360*(10), 961–972.

Sever, P.S., Dahlof, B., Poulter, N.R., Wedel, H., Beevers, G., Caulfield, M., Ostergren, J. (2003). Prevention of coronary and stroke events with atorvastatin in hypertensive patients who have average or lower-than-average cholesterol concentrations, in the Anglo-Scandinavian Cardiac Outcomes Trial—Lipid Lowering Arm (ASCOT-LLA): A multicentre randomized controlled trial. *Lancet, 361*(9364), 1149–1158.

Smith, S.C., Jr., et al. (2006). AHA/ACC guidelines for secondary prevention for patients with coronary and other atherosclerotic vascular disease: 2006 update endorsed by the National Heart, Lung, and Blood Institute. *J Am Coll Cardiol, 47*(10), 2130–2139.

Third Report of the National Cholesterol Education Program (NCEP) Expert Panel on Detection, Evaluation, and Treatment of High Blood Cholesterol in Adults (Adult Treatment Panel III) Final Report. (2002). *Circulation, 106*(25), 3143–3421.

White, H.D., et al. (2008). Safety and efficacy of bivalirudin with and without glycoprotein IIb/IIIa inhibitors in patients with acute coronary syndromes undergoing percutaneous coronary intervention: 1-year results from the ACUITY (Acute Catheterization and Urgent Intervention Triage strategY) trial. *J Am Coll Cardiol, 52*(10), 807–814.

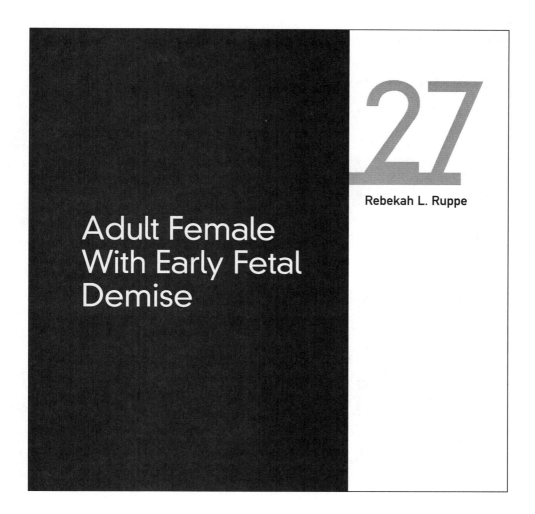

27

Rebekah L. Ruppe

Adult Female With Early Fetal Demise

The following case narrative addresses the initial comprehensive management of an unexplained early fetal death. This case narrative describes care provided during four encounters for this commercially insured patient in an urban academic medical center. The case narrative addresses the following Columbia University School of Nursing (CUSN) doctoral competencies for comprehensive direct patient care.

DOMAIN 1, COMPETENCY 3

Formulate differential diagnoses and diagnostic strategies and therapeutic interventions with attention to scientific evidence, safety, cost, invasiveness, simplicity, acceptability, adherence, and efficacy for patients who present with new conditions and those with ambiguous or incomplete data, complex illnesses, comorbid conditions, and multiple diagnoses in all clinical settings.

PO A. Formulate a differential diagnosis for a patient who presents with new undifferentiated signs and symptoms.

PO B. Formulate a differential diagnosis for a patient who presents with ambiguous or incomplete data, complex illnesses, comorbid conditions, and potential multiple diagnoses.

PO C. Discuss the rationale for the differential diagnosis.

PO D. Discuss the rationale for the diagnostic evaluation with attention to scientific evidence, safety, cost, invasiveness, simplicity, acceptability, adherence, and efficacy.

PO E. Discuss the rationale for the therapeutic intervention with attention to scientific evidence, safety, cost, invasiveness, simplicity, acceptability, adherence, and efficacy.

DOMAIN 1, COMPETENCY 4

Appraise acuity of patient condition, determine the need to transfer patient to higher acuity setting, coordinate, and manage transfer to optimize patient outcomes.

PO A. Assess the acuity of patient status.

PO B. Determine the most appropriate treatment setting based on level of acuity.

PO C. Formulate a transfer plan.

PO D. Implement plan to transfer the patient to a higher level of care utilizing written and oral communication.

PO E. Coordinate care during transition to the higher acuity setting

PO F. Co-manage care in person.

PO G. Co-manage care though written and verbal instructions.

PO H. Make recommendations for patient disposition from the higher acuity location.

PO I. Coordinate post-discharge care.

DOMAIN 1, COMPETENCY 5

Evaluate and direct care during hospitalization, and design a comprehensive discharge plan for patients from an acute care setting.

PO A. Assess the acuity of the patient's condition and determine the most appropriate inpatient treatment setting based on level of acuity.

PO B. Actively participate in the admission process to the appropriate inpatient treatment setting.

PO C. Actively co-manage patient care during hospitalization.

PO D. Formulate plan for ongoing care to be provided in a subacute setting, such as a long-term care facility, rehabilitation facility, or home or community setting.

PO D. Coordinate ongoing comprehensive care to be provided in a subacute setting, such as a long-term care facility, rehabilitation facility, or home or community setting.

DOMAIN 3, COMPETENCY 1

Construct and evaluate outcomes of a culturally sensitive, individualized intervention that addresses the specific needs of a patient in the context of family and community.

PO A. Assess culturally specific needs of the patient in the context of family and community.
PO B. Construct a culturally sensitive intervention to address the needs of patient in the context of family and community.
PO C. Evaluate outcomes of the intervention.

DOMAIN 3, COMPETENCY 2

Evaluate gaps in health care access that compromise optimal patient outcomes, and apply current knowledge of the organization and financing of health care systems to ameliorate negative impact.

PO A. Identify gaps in access that compromise the patient's optimum care.
PO B. Identify gaps in reimbursement that compromise the patient's optimum care.
PO C. Demonstrate patient advocacy in the provision of continuous and comprehensive care.
PO D. Apply current knowledge of the organization to ameliorate negative impact.
PO E. Apply current knowledge of health care systems to ameliorate negative impact.

DOMAIN 1, COMPETENCY 7

Facilitate and guide the process of palliative care and/or planning end-of-life care by discussing diagnoses and prognosis, clarifying and validating patient desires and priorities, and promoting informed choices and shared decision-making by patient, family, and members of the health care team.

PO A. Facilitate and guide the palliative care process by discussing diagnoses and prognosis, clarifying and validating patient desires and priorities, and promoting informed choices and shared decision-making by patient, family, and members of the health care team.
PO B. Facilitate and guide planning end-of-life care by discussing diagnoses and prognosis, clarifying and validating patient desires and priorities, and promoting informed choices and shared decision-making by patient, family, and members of the health care team.

DOMAIN 3, COMPETENCY 2

Synthesize the principles of legal and ethical decision-making, and analyze dilemmas that arise in patient care, interprofessional relationships, research, or practice management to improve outcomes.

PO A. Synthesize ethical principles to address a complex practice dilemma.
PO B. Apply ethical principles to resolve the dilemma.
PO C. Synthesize legal principles to address a complex practice dilemma.
PO D. Apply legal principles to resolve the dilemma.

ENCOUNTER CONTEXT

Initial Encounter (call to pager from patient)

DNP role: I am a DNP resident and the attending midwife on call for the midwifery service.

Identifying Information

Site: Urban academic medical center.

Setting: Telephone triage.

Reason for encounter: Telephone call from patient.

Informant: Patient.

Danielle is a 38-year-old Caucasian/Ashkenazi Jewish gravida 4 para 3 (G4P3) at 24 weeks 2 days gestation who paged me, the on-call midwife, to report decreased fetal movement.

Chief complaint: "I'm not feeling much movement from the baby. I haven't really noticed much during this pregnancy at all, but I'm 24 weeks and I thought I should really be noticing it. I don't know if I should be concerned."

History of Present Illness

This is Danielle's fourth pregnancy. She has not noted vigorous or frequent movement during this pregnancy. At her last visit she reported sensing occasional movement. She had attributed her low sensitivity to fetal movement to her busy days taking care of three children and preparing for a move to Canada next week. Fetal heart tones were auscultated by a midwife colleague at her last visit at 22 weeks.

She denies vaginal bleeding or spotting, abdominal pain or cramping, changes in vaginal discharge, leaking of fluid from the vagina, severe headache, or visual changes. She denies any recent toxic exposures; denies medication, drug, or alcohol ingestion; and denies any injury, fall, or blow to the abdomen.

Impression

Danielle is a 38-year-old G4P3 at 24 weeks 2 days gestation by last menstrual period with essentially uncomplicated prenatal course. She describes decreased fetal movement (DFM) as evidenced by subjective maternal assessment. The differential diagnosis for this subjective finding is perceived DFM, fetal compromise due to fetal hypoxia, hypoxemia, impaired fetal growth, and fetal death that requires urgent obstetrical evaluation **(D1, C3, PO A, C; D1 C4, PO A, B, C, D).**

Perceived DFM does not mean the fetus is compromised. A mother may sense decreases or alterations in fetal movement due to early gestational age, decreased amniotic fluid, maternal drug ingestion, fetal position, or fetal sleep state. DFM in the third trimester is associated with poor pregnancy outcome. It is not known how prevalent DFM is in the second trimester or whether it is of any clinical significance. When DFM is reported, fetal viability should be confirmed (Froen, 2008). Fetal death may be preceded by subjective observation of decreased movement (American College of Obstetricians and Gynecologists, 2000).
Oxford Centre for Evidence-Based Medicine (CEBM), level 5

Plan

Patient will present to the obstetric emergency department for evaluation **(D1, C4, PO A, B, C, D).**

Patient education and counseling

I explain to Danielle that her sense of decreased fetal movement could be a misperception due to fetal or placenta position. I also explain that it can be a "warning sign" from the fetus and that it is important to evaluate fetal status promptly. She is appropriately concerned and agrees to present right away for evaluation. We plan to meet at the obstetric (OB) emergency department (ED) for evaluation.

Follow-up Encounter: Obstetric Emergency Triage (1 hour after first encounter)

I meet Danielle in OB triage for evaluation of decreased fetal movement **(D1, C4, PO F).** Her status had not changed since our earlier telephone conversation. She has not sensed fetal movements. She has not experienced vaginal bleeding, uterine cramping, or loss of fluid per vagina.

Comprehensive Health History

Past medical history: Patient denies history of diabetes, hypertension, heart disease, kidney disease, liver disease, seizure disorder, thyroid dysfunction, asthma, tuberculosis, major accident, or blood transfusion.

Past surgical history: No prior surgeries.

Prior Obstetric History: Patient reports three prior vaginal births. She denies history of termination of pregnancy, miscarriage, or ectopic.

- 2003: Spontaneous vaginal birth at 36 weeks gestation of live male infant weighing 2,778 g. Preterm premature rupture of membranes preceded spontaneous preterm labor. Length of labor was 12 hours. There were no perinatal or peripartum complications.

- 2004: Spontaneous vaginal birth at 37 weeks 3 days gestation of live male infant weighing 3,175 g. Length of labor was 8 hours. There were no perinatal or peripartum complications.
- 2006: Spontaneous vaginal birth at 39 weeks 5 days gestation of live male infant weighing 3,487 g. Length of labor was less than 6 hours. There were no perinatal or peripartum complications.

Gynecologic and contraceptive history: Denies history of sexually transmitted infections or recurrent vaginitis. No history of abnormal Pap smears. Reports using condoms and fertility awareness for pregnancy planning and spacing. Menarche at age 11. Reports regular menses every 28 to 30 days with four to five days of moderate flow without dysmenorrhea. Her last menstrual period began 24 weeks two days ago.

Family history: Denies family history of diabetes, heart disease, stroke, thyroid disorder, seizure disorder, dyslipidemia, or hypertension.

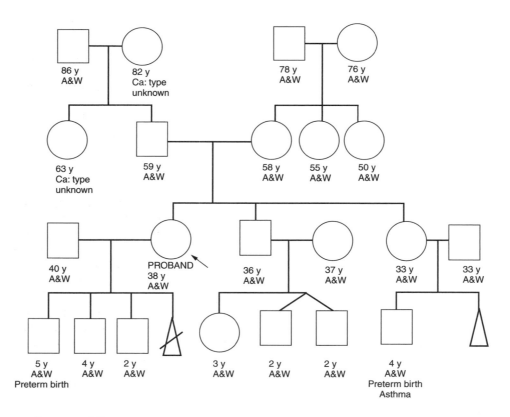

No consanguinity
Ethnicity: Caucasian

Genetic history: Danielle will be 38 years old when her child is born. She is Ashkenazi Jewish and had negative carrier screening during a previous pregnancy. Both her parents and grandparents are also Ashkenazi Jewish, and her family was originally from Eastern Europe.

Individuals of Ashkenazi Jewish descent commonly carry genetic mutations for one of many "Jewish genetic disorders" (Bloom syndrome, cystic fibrosis, Riley-Day syndrome, Fanconi's anemia, Gaucher disease, Mucolipidosis type IV [MLIV], Niemann-Pick disease type A [NPDA], Tay-Sachs disease). Carrier testing is recommended for any individual who has at least one grandparent of Ashkenazi Jewish ancestry or has one relative affected with any of the above disorders (Roman, 2008).

CEBM, level 5

There is no known history of genetic anomalies or illnesses in Danielle's family or in her husband's family. She denies known history of Jewish genetic disorders, hemophilia, Huntington chorea, neural tube defects, limb deformities, congenital abnormalities, birth defects, hemophilia, sickle cell, thalassemia, muscular dystrophy, polycystic kidney disease, or congenital adrenal hyperplasia. Denies history of Downs, Turner, and Kleinfelter syndromes or other chromosomal abnormalities. She has no history of multiple miscarriages, fetal demise, or still birth.

Psychosocial history: Denies history of anxiety or depression. Denies alcohol or substance use or abuse. She has sex with men and reports three lifetime sexual partners. She is monogamous with her husband of 12 years. She denies history of physical or sexual abuse or violence and feels safe and happy in her current relationship. She lives with husband and three children, ages five, four, and two, in a three-bedroom house. She practices Modern Orthodox Judaism. She is a homemaker, and her husband is a teacher. Her family is planning a move to the west coast at 25 weeks gestation.

Nutrition and exercise history: Reports eating a Kosher diet that includes a variety vegetables, dairy, fruits, and whole grains. She reports a "mostly vegetarian diet" but eats some fish and poultry. Primary protein sources include dairy, eggs, beans, legumes, nuts, and occasionally tofu. Typical daily intake includes: breakfast of cereal with 2 percent milk and fruit or bagel and fruit; snack of yogurt, cheese toast, or peanut butter toast; lunch of sandwich with protein and vegetables or salad greens and mix of vegetables with chickpeas, cottage cheese, or nuts and seeds; dinner varies but generally includes a protein, usually fish, poultry, or beans or legumes with cooked vegetables and rice or potato. She does not drink caffeinated coffee but does drink one to two cups of black or green tea daily. She practices yoga daily.

Medications: Does not take prescription or over-the-counter medications. Takes prenatal vitamins one tablet daily by mouth. Does not take other nutritional supplements. (See Medications list at the end of the chapter.)

Allergies: Denies known medication, environmental, or seasonal allergies..

Current Prenatal History

Danielle initiated prenatal care at this practice at 10 weeks gestation by certain last menstrual period. Dating was confirmed with early clinical exam. Initial prenatal labs were collected and sent. All values were within expected ranges or negative for pathology and required no additional follow-up. Ashkenazi genetic carrier testing from previous pregnancy was negative and was not repeated.

She has been seen at approximately four-week intervals with a total of five visits. Her prenatal course has been uncomplicated to date. She declined prenatal genetic screening. The fetal anatomy scan at 20 weeks and three days revealed a fetus in vertex presentation with normal cardiac activity, anterior attached placenta, appropriate levels of amniotic fluid, and normal anatomy.

Her last routine prenatal visit was two weeks ago. At that time, fetal movement was noted and the fetal heart rate was 140 bpm. Sonogram results were reviewed with the patient by a midwife colleague.

Review of Systems

Constitutional: Denies weight gain or loss, fatigue, weakness, fever, chills, or night sweats. No change in appetite or general activity level.

Skin and hair: Denies rashes or lesions. No change in hair amount, texture, or consistency.

Head, ears, eyes, nose, and throat: Denies headache. No changes in visual, auditory, olfactory acuity. No problems eating or swallowing.

Neck: Denies masses, tenderness, stiffness, or limitations in movement.

Breast: Denies breast lumps, pain or tenderness, or discharge.

Chest: Denies cough, chest pain, shortness of breath, wheezing.

Cardiovascular: Denies chest pain, palpitations, dyspnea on exertion, edema.

Gastrointestinal: Denies appetite changes, nausea, vomiting, diarrhea, constipation, changes in stool or stooling pattern.

Urinary: Denies frequency, urgency, dysuria, nocturia, or incontinence of urine.

Genitalia: Denies vaginal irritation, discharge, malodor, lesions, or abnormal vaginal bleeding or spotting.

Musculoskeletal: Denies myalgia and arthralgia. No redness, swelling, or tenderness of joints. No limitations in movement or range of motion.

Neurologic: Denies dizziness, weakness, numbness, coordination problems, loss of consciousness, or alteration in mood, sleep, and memory.

Psychologic: Denies depression, anxiety, or loss of energy or ability to concentrate.

Focused Physical Examination

Vital signs: Blood pressure 94/62, heart rate 80, respiratory rate 18, temp 98.8°F.

General: Appropriate affect, appears concerned. Well groomed, appears well nourished.

Heart: RRR, no murmur, no rub, no gallop.

Lungs: Clear to auscultation anterior, posterior, bilaterally. No adventitious sounds.

Abdomen: Gravid, nontender, no masses; uterine fundus is three finger-breadths above umbilicus.

Fetal heart tones: Not heard with Doppler device on external fetal-monitoring system.

Cervix: Deferred at this time.

Impression

38-year-old gravida 4 para 3 (G4P3003) at 24 weeks and 2 days gestation by last menstrual period with essentially normal prenatal course presents with subjective assessment of decreased fetal movement. Fetal heart tones not appreciated with Doppler. Fetal demise is strongly suspected; however, need ultrasound for diagnostic confirmation **(D1, C3, PO A, B, C, D)**.

Plan

Diagnostic ultrasound: I call the chief resident to perform a sonogram to locate fetal heart tones.

Patient education and counseling: I explain to Danielle that it is unusual to not hear the heart tones with the Doppler device but that we sometimes have technical difficulties. I explain that we will find the fetal heart with the sonogram. At this point I do share with Danielle that I am very concerned for the baby's well-being but won't know any specifics about the baby until the sonogram is performed. While we wait for the sonogram, my focus is to keep her calm without giving her false reassurances.

> Women who report decreased fetal movement have greater risk of adverse pregnancy outcome, including fetal demise. When suspected, diagnosis must be confirmed by sonogram showing the absence of fetal cardiac activity (Fretts, 2008).
>
> CEBM, level 5.

Bedside sonogram (performed by chief resident within minutes of request): Fetal cardiac activity not observed. Estimated fetal weight: 468 g.

Impression

38-year-old gravida 4 para 3 (G4P3003) at 24 weeks and 2 days gestation by last menstrual period with essentially normal prenatal course presents with subjective assessment of decreased fetal movement. Fetal heart tones not heard with Doppler. Sonographic findings show no fetal cardiac activity consistent with fetal demise **(D1, C3, PO A, C).**

> *Fetal death may be preceded by subjective observation of decreased movement (American College of Obstetricians and Gynecologists, 2000).*
>
> CEBM, level 5.

ICD-9 Codes

659.63 Other advanced maternal age antepartum condition or complication (active).
656.43 Intrauterine death, antepartum (active).

Plan

Patient Education and Counseling

I explain the diagnosis of intrauterine fetal demise to the patient and her husband. I review maternal risks associated with fetal demise and discuss management options, which include awaiting onset of spontaneous labor or intervening with dilation and evacuation or medication induction **(D1, C4, PO F; D1, C7, PO A).**

> *Most women will have spontaneous labor within two weeks of fetal demise. Intrauterine fetal demise without birth or expulsion ("retained fetus") is associated with consumptive coagulation related to placental release of thromboplastin into maternal circulation. This is more prevalent if the fetus is retained for more than two to four weeks (Fretts, 2008).*
>
> CEBM, level 5.

Risk/Benefits Discussion

I explain to Danielle that her baby has died in the womb. After giving a few moments of quiet for her and her husband to process what has happened, I explain that we do not know when the baby passed or why. I let them know that there are a variety of tests we can do after the baby is born to try to determine a cause, but many times the testing is inconclusive. I also share with them that most women will have spontaneous labor within two weeks of fetal death. I explain the potential risks to her health, which include infection and consumptive coagulation if the baby is not birthed within two to four weeks of the fetus's death. I offer expected management or active management and briefly explain the two methods of active management, dilation and evacuation (D&E) and induction **(D1, C3, PO D, E).**

Danielle and her husband share they would not feel comfortable waiting for spontaneous labor onset knowing that the baby has died. They elect for active management to reduce maternal risks and to get back to their three children more quickly. The process of D&E is not an option for Danielle and her husband because of their religious beliefs. Danielle prefers to "give birth" to her child and to remain under midwifery care, so she elects to be induced with misoprostol (Cytotec) ("DrugPoints System," 2008). I then explain what she can expect with misoprostol (Cytotec) induction. She and her husband are grief-stricken. They understand the management plan and agree to admission and induction with misoprostol.

Admitting Orders
Admit to labor and delivery unit for management of early intrauterine fetal death with patient in stable condition **(D1, C5, PO A, B, C).**

Vital signs: every four hours.
No known drug, food, or environmental allergies.
Activity: Bedrest with bathroom privileges.
Notify attending midwife if temperature greater than 101°F, heart rate > 100 or < 60, systolic blood pressure > 160 or < 90; diastolic blood pressure > 100 or < 60; respiratory rate > 30 or < 10.
Diet: clear liquids.
IV fluid: 1,000 mL D5LR at 125 cc/hr.
Medication: Misoprostol (Cytotec) 100 mcg per vagina every four hours until birth of fetus.

There is no consistently recommended dose, route or frequency of administration for misoprostol use in the management of intrauterine fetal demise. Doses range from 100–400 mcg given every three to 12 hours given orally, sublingually or vaginally (Fretts, 2008).

CEBM, level 5.

Critical Appraisal

It is our routine practice to administer 100 mcg vaginally every four hours until the fetus is expelled.

Diagnostic studies: blood type, antibody screen, complete blood cell count, prothrombin time, partial thromboplastin time, fibrinogen and Kleihauer-Betke test.

Blood type, antibody screen and complete blood cell count are routine admission labs for obstetrical patients. Coagulation studies are indicated in the event of fetal demise as retention of a dead fetus is associated with coagulopathy (Fretts, 2008).

CEBM, level 5.

Kleihauer-Betke test to detect fetal-maternal hemorrhage may be performed in cases of unexplained stillbirth as a large hemorrhage may result in fetal death (Roberts, 2008a).

CEBM, level 5.

Patient advocacy: I speak with the charge nurse and request a room as far from the central staff station as possible to minimize traffic and noise. There is a room on the far end of the unit available for Danielle **(D3, C1, PO C).**

Inpatient Management: Labor Induction (0 hours)

Subjective

Danielle is admitted to a labor and delivery room, and I begin labor induction for intrauterine fetal demise. At this time she reports no pain (0/10). Danielle's husband is at the bedside and supportive. The couple are tearful but open to discussing their loss.

Objective

Vital signs: Blood pressure 90/60, heart rate 84, respiratory rate,18, temp 98.8°F.

General: Tearful and grieving, responsive.

Cervix: Long, closed, posterior. I place misoprostol 100 mcg in the posterior vaginal fornix.

Admission laboratory results: Pending.

Assessment

Patient is a 38-year-old gravida 4 para 3 with an intrauterine fetal demise at 24 weeks 2 days gestation by LMP admitted to the labor and delivery unit for medical induction and vaginal delivery of her deceased fetus according to religious custom. Her vital signs are stable. She is in no apparent distress; however, she is grieving the loss of this baby.

Plan

Monitor vital signs, maternal pain, coping, and induction progress.
Continue misoprostol (Cytotec) 100 mcg per vagina every four hours until
    birth of fetus.
Provide emotional support to the couple.

Discuss bereavement consult.
Review laboratory results when available.
Anticipate vaginal stillbirth.
(D1, C5, PO C.)

Patient Counseling
I express my sympathy and offer to answer any questions they might have about the loss or the process of induction. They have no specific questions and request to have time alone with interruptions only for medically necessary interventions. I explain the need for vital sign monitoring and misoprostol (Cytotec) placement every four hours and agree to return to the room at their request or in four hours to reevaluate and place the second dose of misoprostol (Cytotec). I discuss the bereavement counseling group and their services and offer to call them with the couple's permission. They are interested in speaking to a grief counselor but want to wait until after the birth process is complete. I share this plan with the support staff, who also agree to give the couple privacy and keep interactions to the minimum necessary **(D1, C5, PO C; D3, C2, PO C; D1, C7, PO B).**

Critical Appraisal

At our facility, the bereavement team is lead by psychiatric nurse practitioners who specialize in bereavement care for families. With patient permission, they are contacted by phone to set up a consultation. After the initial evaluation they may be referred to the Parent Support Group, a grief counselor for further therapy, or both. They may also continue to make and receive contact from the bereavement psychiatric nurse practitioner for as long as it is beneficial and desired.

Inpatient Management: Labor Induction (4 hours)

Subjective

I return to the patient's room to place the second misoprostol (Cytotec) dose. Danielle is in the patient bed, and her husband is sitting in a chair beside her. They are both quiet but responsive. Danielle reports some uterine cramping, which she rates as 2/10. I offer pharmacologic pain management, which she declines.

Objective

Vital signs: Blood pressure 90/60, heart rate 74, respiratory rate 16, temp 98.6°F.

General: Quiet with sad affect.

Cervix: Very soft and posterior. 1-cm dilation/50% effacement /–3 station. I place the second dose of misoprostol 100 mcg in the posterior vaginal fornix.

Admission laboratory results reviewed:

Test	Result	Reference Range	Interpretation
Blood type	A	A, B, AB, or O	Within normal range
Rh factor	Positive	Positive or negative	Within normal range
Antibody screen	Negative	Negative	Within normal range
White blood cells	9.3	3.8–10.8 × 1,000/mcL	Within normal range
Hemoglobin	12.5	11.7–15.5 g/dL	Within normal range
Hematocrit	38.1%	35–45%	Within normal range
Platelets	281	140–400 × 1,000/mcL	Within normal range
Prothrombin time	13.2	10–14 seconds	Within normal range
Partial thromboplastin time	32	32–45 seconds	Within normal range
Fibrinogen	310	160–450 mg/dL	Within normal range
Kleihauer-Betke	Negative	Negative	Within normal range

Assessment

Patient is a 38-year-old gravida 4 para 3 with an intrauterine fetal demise at 24 weeks 2 days gestation by LMP undergoing induction with misoprostol (Cytotec). Her vital signs are stable. Her cervical exam reveals response to misoprostol administration as evidenced by dilation to 1 cm with 50 percent effacement. She is in no apparent distress but is appropriately emotional and grieving the loss of this baby. She is coping well with uterine pain and declines medication for pain.

Plan

Review admission laboratory results with patient.

Monitor vital signs, induction progress, maternal pain, and coping.

Continue misoprostol (Cytotec) 100 mcg per vagina every four hours until birth of fetus.

Provide emotional support to the couple.

Discuss pain management options available.

I review the possible pain management options with Danielle and her husband. She had not used analgesia or anesthesia in previous labor and declines using it now.

Anticipate vaginal stillbirth.

(D1, C5, PO C.)

Inpatient Management: Labor Induction (6 hours 47 minutes)

Subjective

I return to the patient's room per Danielle's request. She reports increased painful uterine cramping, which she rates as a 7/10. She also reports increased pelvic pressure.

Objective

Vital signs: Blood pressure 90/60, heart rate 70, respiratory rate 16, temp 98.6°F.

Vaginal exam: 8-cm dilation/90% effacement/0 station; bulging amniotic sac palpated in vaginal vault at +2 to +3 station; cervix very soft and pliable.

Assessment

Patient is a 38-year-old gravida 4 para 3 with an intrauterine fetal demise at 24 weeks 2 days gestation by LMP undergoing induction with misoprostol. Her vital signs are stable. Her cervical exam reveals adequate response to misoprostol administration as evidenced by 8-cm dilation with 90% effacement and fetus at 0 station. She is in no apparent distress but is grieving the loss of this baby. She is coping well with uterine pain and declines medication for pain.

Plan

Provide emotional support to the couple.
Encourage pushing efforts as desired or tolerated by the patient.
Anticipate vaginal stillbirth.
(D1, C5, PO C.)

Patient education: I explain to Danielle and her husband that she is eight centimeters dilated and the pressure she is feeling is from the full amniotic sac descending into the vagina. I share that she can push the baby out whenever she is ready or she can wait for her body to push it out completely. She asks for time with her husband to discuss the options. There are no studies to evaluate the benefit or effectiveness of active or passive management of second stage in cases of fetal demise. Since the fetus can be expelled with or without maternal pushing efforts, I explain this to Danielle and offer the choice. She and her husband decide she will push and "give birth" to the baby. They also state that they want to complete the process, see the baby, and begin the recovery **(D1, C3, PO E).**

Inpatient Management: Vaginal Stillbirth (7 hours 35 minutes)

Delivery Note

38-year-old gravida 4 now para 3103 at 24 weeks and 2 days from LMP was induced with misoprostol (Cytotec) 100 mcg two doses indicated by intrauterine fetal demise. She began pushing at time 6h58m and vaginally expelled the 423-g male fetus along with the membranes and placenta over an intact perineum at time 7h06m. Apgars were zero and zero at one and five minutes. The fetus was mildly macerated with peeling skin noted approximately three centimeters around the umbilical insertion and skin slippage around the scrotal area and groin. There were no signs of compression, fetal hydrops, or gross anomalies or malformations. The umbilical cord had two arteries and one vein, was shiny, white, and covered uniformly with Wharton's jelly, had no knots, and was centrally inserted into the placenta. The placenta was complete and intact, and there were no signs of vasa previa or placental infarct. The fundus was firm and estimated maternal blood loss was 200 cc. The placenta will be sent to pathology for evaluation. Danielle is stable in the labor and delivery room with her husband at her side **(D1, C3, PO D; D1, C5, PO C).**

> *Gross examination of the placenta can reveal signs of placental infarct, abruption, vessel rupture or cord anomalies including true knots or nodules which may be associated with fetal compromise or death (Roberts, 2008b). Placental pathology is recommended in the evaluation of intrauterine fetal demise to rule out infection or placental infarct as a cause of fetal death. Placental studies may be particularly helpful when complete autopsy is declined (Roberts, 2008a).*
>
> CEBM, level 5.

After examining the fetus, placenta, and membranes, I explain to Danielle that her son had some signs of skin breakdown from being in the amniotic fluid for a while after passing in the uterus, but no obvious signs of abnormalities. I ask Danielle and her husband if they would like to see or hold the baby. They both accept, so I wrap him in a receiving blanket and I offer Danielle her baby. I ask Danielle if she would like me to contact the bereavement counselor. I also tell her that we have a keepsake box that we will put together with footprints and a photograph. She agrees to the photographs, footprints, and consultation with the bereavement counselor. She and her husband request that we give them some time alone with the baby and return in about an hour **(D1, C7, PO B).**

> *When considering the psychosocial management of a stillbirth, health care providers focus care on the parents and family in order to facilitate the grief process and help with recovery (Hughes & Riches, 2003). There are few studies that evaluate the benefit or risk to the parents and their grief process when they have contact with the stillborn. Trends in management have gone from a beneficent, protective approach of 'no contact' to 'encouraged contact.'*

Contact with the stillborn is thought to facilitate attachment and prevent dysfunctional attachment that can complicate the grieving process (Hughes & Riches, 2003).

CEBM, level 5.

A large retrospective study in which most parents viewed the stillborn found no association between length of time spent with the stillborn or delay of delivery after diagnosis and anxiety levels after three years (Radestad, Nordin, Steineck, & Sjogren, 1998).

CEBM, level 3b.

Another study found higher levels of depression in women who had contact with their stillborn compared to those who did not (Hughes, Turton, Hopper, & Evans, 2002).

CEBM, level 3b.

There is evidence, however, that parents who choose to view the infant's body value the experience and the memory (Cuisinier, Kuijpers, Hoogduin, de Graauw, & Janssen, 1993; Rand, Kellner, Revak-Lutz, & Massey, 1998).

CEBM, levels 3b, 2b.

In these studies the parents elected to view or not view the body. It is very likely that the psychological state of the parents that informs this decision is related to the psychological state that persists after this experience. Most professionals and bereaved parents agree that parental autonomy should guide decisions about stillborn viewing and physical contact (Hughes & Riches, 2003).

CEBM, level 5.

Inpatient Management: Immediate Postpartum Care (8 hours 30 minutes)

Subjective

Danielle is one hour 24 minutes postpartum. She has spent the past hour with her husband and stillborn son and now requests that he is taken for footprinting and photographing. She is no longer tearful but expresses sadness over the loss of her son. She reports moderate vaginal bleeding and mild uterine cramping.

Objective

Vital signs: Blood pressure 90/60, heart rate 78, respiratory rate 16, temp 98.8°F.

General: Saddened affect; grieving, but responsive.

Heart: RRR, no murmur, no rub, no gallop.

Lungs: Clear to auscultation anterior, posterior, bilaterally. No adventitious sounds.

Abdomen: Nontender, no masses, bowel sounds present; diastasis rectii is one fingerbreadth.

Fundus: Firm, nontender; one fingerbreadth below umbilicus.

Perineum: Intact, no edema or ecchymoses present.

Lochia: Scant rubra, no odor present.

Extremities: No edema, no varices.

Assessment

38-year-old G4P3103 is 1 hour 24 minutes status post vaginal birth of stillborn son with unremarkable postpartum exam. She is grieving the loss of her son and appears to be coping well with the support of her husband.

Plan

Transfer to medical unit **(D1, C5, PO C).**
Vital signs: Every shift.
Diet: Regular Kosher diet.
Activity: Ambulate as tolerated.
Notify attending midwife if temperature > 101°F, heart rate < 100 or > 60, systolic blood pressure > 160 or < 90, diastolic blood pressure > 100 or < 60, respiratory rate > 30 or < 10.
IV fluids: Discontinue IV fluids and saline lock.
Medications: Ibuprofen (Motrin) 400 mg by mouth every four to six hours as need for pain ("AHFS Drug Information," 2008; "DrugPoints System," 2008).
Labs: Complete blood cell count with differential.

Patient Education and Counseling
I explain to Danielle and her husband about the hospital's bereavement counseling services and offer to call the bereavement counseling group, which they accept. I encourage the couple to utilize the services of the bereavement counselor **(D1, C7, PO B).**

I discuss the increased risk of postpartum depression among women who have pregnancy losses and review signs and symptoms of postpartum grief versus postpartum depression. I encourage Danielle and her husband to utilize their support system and to avoid social isolation during this difficult time.

Danielle and her husband are still planning a move later in the week. They have movers coming to pack the house. I am concerned that this additional stress will make her grieving process more difficult, but they are not able or interested in postponing the move. Danielle is originally from the west coast, and she will be closer to her family. She states that in spite of the stress of the actual move, she is looking forward to relocating and will feel more at ease with her family nearby.

I discuss postnatal testing—chromosome analysis, pathology studies, and autopsy—to try to determine the cause of fetal death. I also explain that many times the cause of death is not found.

> *When studies are performed after fetal demise approximately 35 percent have major structural anomalies, 20 percent have dysmorphic features or skeletal abnormalities and eight percent have chromosomal abnormalities (Cunningham & Williams, 2005). In 25 to 60 percent of cases no cause of death is found (Fretts, 2008).*
>
> CEBM, level 5.

Although Danielle and her husband practice Modern Orthodox Judaism, I offer postnatal testing and explain what each form of testing would entail to allow them to make an informed decision. They decline all testing, citing their belief in the sacredness of the body. I further explain that there are tests that could be performed without disrupting the baby's body. They still decline. They are "intellectually" accepting of the outcome, and they state that no testing could alter the outcome or their experience. They explain that they do not want to "drag out" the process, but rather grieve their loss and try to move on. I document this decision in the hospital record and share it with the staff **(D1, C5, PO C; D3, C1, PO A, B, C; D3, C2, PO C).**

> *While observant Jewish families may typically decline autopsy studies after perinatal losses, some may elect to do so if information found may prevent a future loss. If autopsy is performed, all body parts must be returned for burial (Shuzman, 2003). If a couple declines autopsy they should be informed of other less invasive testing that is available to evaluate the stillborn for possible causes of death ("Obstetric and Medical Complications," 2007).*
>
> CEBM, level 5.

Referrals
Bereavement counseling.

Anticipatory guidance
I tell Danielle and her husband that they can expect discharge home tomorrow. After transfer to the medical unit, her husband will have to follow visiting hours and cannot stay overnight. Danielle prefers to stay overnight and have some "quiet time." Her husband offers to bring food and her journal.

Follow-up plan
Postpartum day 1 evaluation tomorrow. Discharge home if stable.

Encounter 3: Inpatient Management (postpartum day 1)

Subjective

Patient encountered resting in bed in a private room on the medical floor. She feels upset and confused about the pregnancy loss and is anxious about going home. She is eager to see her three children and to have the burial ceremony, which she and her husband have already planned for tomorrow.

She reports light vaginal bleeding and mild afterbirth pains (3/10), which are relieved with ibuprofen. She denies breast fullness or tenderness. She has no difficulty ambulating, eating, voiding, or stooling. She reports some difficulty sleeping through the night, which she attributes to the "uncomfortable hospital bed," but also states that she had difficulty "quieting her mind" and was thinking about the pregnancy and the baby "that isn't there anymore." She denies feelings of hopelessness or depression, but does feel sadness. She and her husband spoke with the bereavement counselor yesterday and they received the keepsake box. She hasn't yet told her children about the baby's death, but she has informed her family and her husband's family.

Objective

Vital signs: Blood pressure 112/68, heart rate 68, respiratory rate 16, temp 98.6°F.

General: Saddened affect, grieving, but responsive.

Heart: RRR, no murmur, no rub, no gallop.

Lungs: Clear to auscultation, anterior, posterior, bilaterally. No adventitious sounds.

Breast: Soft, nontender, no masses, nipples intact.

Abdomen: Nontender, no masses, bowel sounds present; diastasis rectii is one fingerbreadth.

Fundus: Firm, nontender; three fingerbreadths below umbilicus.

Perineum: Intact, no edema or ecchymoses present.

Lochia: Scant rubra, no odor present.

Extremities: No edema, no varices.

Postpartum laboratory results

Test	Result	Reference Range	Interpretation
White blood cells	10.6	3.8–10.8 × 1,000/mcL	Within normal range
Hemoglobin	11.7	11.7–15.5 g/dL	Within normal range
Hematocrit	35.3%	35–45%	Within normal range
MCV	89.6	80–100 fL	Within normal range
MCH	31.2	27–33 pg	Within normal range
MCHC	34.8	32–36 g/dL	Within normal range
RDW	13	11–15%	Within normal range
Platelets	298	140–400 × 1,000/mcL	Within normal range
MPV	8.9	7.5–11.5 fL	Within normal range
Total neutrophils	56.9	38–80%	Within normal range
Total lymphocytes	35.2	15–49%	Within normal range
Monocytes	4.7	0–13%	Within normal range
Eosinophils	2.1	0–8%	Within normal range
Basophils	1.1	0–2%	Within normal range
Neutrophils, absolute	4,154	1,500–7,800 cells/mcL	Within normal range
Lymphocytes, absolute	2,570	850–3,900 cells/mcL	Within normal range
Monocytes, absolute	343	200–950 cells/mcL	Within normal range
Eosinophils, absolute	153	15–550 cells/mcL	Within normal range
Basophils, absolute	80	0–200 cells/mcL	Within normal range

Assessment

38-year-old G4P3103 on postpartum day 1 after induction for unexplained fetal demise at 24 weeks and two days gestation with an unremarkable postpartum physical exam. She is experiencing grief over the loss of her son.

Plan

Patient Education and Counseling

I review signs and symptoms of postpartum complication and morbidity, including increased uterine pain, increased vaginal bleeding, elevated temperature over 100.4°F, pain or redness in breasts, feelings of helplessness, uselessness, or hopelessness, thoughts of hurting self or children (Varney, Kriebs, & Gegor, 2004).

I review perinatal grief and bereavement, postpartum blues, and postpartum depression and encourage Danielle to contact her midwifery care providers if she experiences any feelings of hopelessness, helplessness, or inability to cope (Varney et al., 2004).

I review perineal care, breast care, and postpartum exercise, including Kegel's and abdominal exercises. I advise her to begin any exercise routine slowly and recommend she wait until after the postpartum lochial discharge is gone (Varney et al., 2004).

I encourage her to continue with her prenatal vitamins until her postpartum visit. I also encourage foods rich in iron, vitamin C, calcium, and protein to aid in postpartum recovery and healing (Varney et al., 2004).

I share with Danielle that everyone's experience of grief is very personal. Although there is no way I could truly understand her experience, I could share my experiences of supporting women through this process. I share that the loss of a child is one of the most difficult losses a person can face, and when that loss happens during pregnancy it can be especially difficult because the hopes and dreams for the child are lost as well. I share with her that parents cope with grief in very individualized ways and her husband's grief experience may be different from her own, but not less. In my experience, women have coped better when they can communicate with their partners and support people about the loss and avoid being isolated in the experience. I also share with Danielle that the grief process is a way to remember and honor her baby.

Danielle will be in her new home by the end of this week. I encourage her to keep in contact with the bereavement counselor. I explain the need for evaluation at four to six weeks postpartum and for contact with a health care professional in the interim should she have symptoms of postpartum complications or depression. She has already contacted a midwifery group for a transfer of care. She plans to meet with them after the move and will see them for her routine postpartum visit and any interval concerns **(D3, C3, PO B)**.

Patient will be discharged home today.

Postpartum visit in four to six weeks.

Discharge Summary Note

Patient was admitted yesterday for induction of labor due to intrauterine fetal demise diagnosed at 24 weeks and two days gestation. She is discharged today on postpartum day 1 with the diagnoses of intrauterine fetal demise, delivered. Rebekah L. Ruppe, MS, CNM, DNP(c), is the attending of record.

Procedures: Induction of labor, spontaneous vaginal birth.

Brief history, pertinent physical findings, and lab data: Patient presented to OB triage with reports of decreased fetal movement. She had a previously uncomplicated prenatal course. This was her fourth pregnancy.

Hospital course: Fetal demise was confirmed by ultrasound. She was admitted and induced with misoprostol (Cytotec) per vagina. She delivered a slightly macerated stillborn male with no gross anomalies. The family declined autopsy or chromosomal testing of the fetus. At the time of discharge, placental pathology is pending. The patient's postpartum course was uncomplicated. She was seen by the bereavement counselor.

Condition at discharge: Stable.

Disposition: Patient is discharged to home.

Discharge medications: Ibuprofen (Motrin) 400 mg by mouth every four to six hours as needed for pain.

Discharge instructions and follow-up: Call midwife with increased pain or vaginal bleeding, temperature elevated greater than 100.4°F, pain or redness in breasts, feelings of helplessness, uselessness, or hopelessness, thoughts of hurting self or children. Patient should avoid inserting anything into the vagina, avoid vaginal intercourse, and avoid heavy lifting. Follow-up in four to six weeks for routine postpartum visit or earlier as needed.

Encounter 4: Telephone Call to Midwifery Practice Office from Hospital (one day following discharge)

I am in the office the day after Danielle's discharge when we receive a call from the hospital requesting completion of a death certificate.

I am informed there was an error in the processing of the death certificate, and the family's funeral director is requesting a copy to proceed with the funeral arrangements. Since I was the "attending of record," the office called our midwifery practice to complete the certificate perhaps, not knowing that midwives are not permitted to "certify death." I call the labor and delivery floor to speak with a resident or attending physician to ask if they could complete and sign the form based on information provided. This is acceptable procedure because a physician "in attendance or one acting on his behalf can certify the cause of death" (New York State, 2005). Although this was a case of unexplained ambulatory fetal death, no one was "comfortable" signing a death certificate.

> In New York State midwives can certify the birth of a dead infant but cannot certify the death.
>
> "In each case where a physician was in attendance at, or after, a fetal death it shall be the duty of such physician to certify to the birth and to the cause of death on the fetal death certificate. Where a nurse-midwife was in attendance at a fetal death it shall be the duty of such nurse-midwife to certify to the birth but she shall not certify to the cause of death on the fetal death certificate." (New York State, 2005)
>
> "When a fetal death occurs in a hospital, except in those cases where certificates are issued by coroners or medical examiners, the person in charge of such hospital or his designated representative shall promptly present the certificate to the physician in attendance or a physician acting in his behalf who shall promptly certify to the facts of birth and of fetal death, provide the medical information required by the certificate, sign the medical certificate of birth and death and thereupon return such certificate to such person, so that the seventy-two hour registration time limit prescribed in section four thousand one hundred sixty of this chapter can be met." (New York State, 2005)

CEBM, level 5.

Response to phone call: I rearrange the afternoon schedule to permit an hour break to go to the hospital and fill out the death certificate. I then physically take it to the labor and delivery unit, explain the situation to the attending physician on call, and ask if she could sign the certificate so the family can have the funeral proceedings. The attending then agrees and signs the form, which I deliver to the hospital administrator **(D3, C2, PO C; D3, C3, PO C, D).**

Addendum

When last contacted by phone, Danielle was settled in her new home with her family, had met with the local midwifery group, and was still grieving. She stated she was coping as well as could be expected. She was busy with her three children and was in close contact with her family. She was no longer in contact with the bereavement counselor and had declined grief therapy.

Medications

Drug: Misoprostol (Cytotec)

Indication: Cervical ripening and labor induction (unlabeled use).

Class: Prostaglandin (synthetic analog of prostaglandin E_1).

Mechanism: Synthetic prostaglandin that has been shown to induce uterine contractions.

Dose: 100 mcg intravaginally.

Adverse effects: Diarrhea, abdominal pain, headache, constipation, flatulence, nausea, dyspepsia, vomiting.

Contraindications: Hypersensitivity to misoprostol, prostaglandins, or any component of the formulation; pregnancy (when used to reduce NSAID-induced ulcers).

Cautions: Cardiovascular disease or renal impairment.

Metabolism: Hepatic; rapidly de-esterified to active metabolite, misoprostol acid.

Drug interactions: May enhance therapeutic effects of oxytocin.

Drug: Ibuprofen (Motrin)

Indication: Pain.

Class: Nonsteroidal anti-inflammatory drug (NSAID).

Mechanism: Inhibits prostaglandin synthesis, resulting in antipyretic and analgesic effects.

Dose: 400 mg orally every four to six hours as needed.

Adverse effects
Common: Body fluid retention, rash, abdominal pain, constipation, diarrhea, heartburn, indigestion, nausea, stomatitis, vomiting, increased liver function test, dizziness, headache, somnolence, tinnitus.
Serious: Congestive heart failure, hypertension, myocardial infarction, thrombotic tendency observations, erythema multiforme, scaling eczema, Stevens-Johnson syndrome, toxic epidermal necrolysis, gastrointestinal hemorrhage, perforation, or ulcer, inflammatory disorder of digestive tract, melena, pancreatitis, agranulocytosis, anemia, hemolytic anemia,

(continued)

neutropenia, thrombocytopenia, hepatitis, jaundice, anaphylactoid reaction, aseptic meningitis (rare), cerebrovascular accident, confusion, amblyopia, hearing loss, depression, acute renal failure, hematuria, renal azotemia.

Contraindications: Treatment of perioperative pain in the setting of coronary artery bypass graft (CABG) surgery, active intracranial hemorrhage or gastrointestinal bleeding, coagulation defects, congenital heart disease, renal function impairment, thrombocytopenia, or necrotizing enterocolitis.

Cautions: History of coagulation defects, gastrointestinal ulceration, bleeding, or perforation, liver dysfunction or renal disease; hypertension, fluid retention, congestive heart failure; avoid in late pregnancy—may cause premature closure of patent foramen ovale.

Metabolism: Primarily renal; rapidly metabolized.

Drug interactions: Anticoagulants, thrombolytics, other NSAIDs, lithium, angiotensin-converting enzyme inhibitors and angiotensin II receptor antagonists, diuretics, methotrexate.

Supplement: Prenatal Multivitamin

Vitamin A (palmitate and beta-carotene) 400 IU
Vitamin C ascorbic acid 100 mg
Vitamin D cholecalciferol 400 IU
Vitamin E d-alpha tocopheryl succinate 100 IU
Vitamin K phytonadione 65 mcg
Thiamin (B_1) 10 mg
Riboflavin (B_2) 10 mg
Niacin (B_3) 20 mg
Vitamin B_6 pyridoxine 15 mg
Folate, folic acid 800 mcg
Vitamin B_{12} cyanocobalamin 25 mcg
Biotin 300 mcg
Pantothenic acid vitamin B-5 15 mg
Calcium carbonate, citrate-malate 200 mg
Iron amino acid chelate 30 mg
Iodine from kelp 150 mcg
Magnesium oxide 100 mg
Zinc citrate 15 mg
Selenium selenomethionine 100 mcg
Copper amino acid chelate 2 mg
Manganese citrate 2 mg
Chromium amino nicotinate 120 mg
Molybdenum amino acid chelate 75 mcg
Potassium citrate 10 mg
Boron glycinate 1 mg
Choline bitartrate 10 mg
Inositol 10 mg
PABA 10 mg
Protease 660 HUT

(continued)

Lipase 226 DU
Amylase 2 LU
Cellulase 3 CU
Spirulina 20 mg
Ginger 20 mg
Red raspberry leaf (2:1 extract) 50 mg

Source: "Prenatal One Vitamin," n.d.

References

AHFS Drug Information. (2008). American Society of Health-System Pharmacists, Inc. Retrieved October 24, 2008, from http://online.statref.com

American College of Obstetricians and Gynecologists. (2000). Antepartum fetal surveillance (ACOG Practice Bulletin No. 9; replaces Technical Bulletin No. 188, January 1994). *Int J Gynaecol Obstet, 68*(2), 175–185.

Cuisinier, M.C., Kuijpers, J.C., Hoogduin, C.A., de Graauw, C.P., & Janssen, H.J. (1993). Miscarriage and stillbirth: Time since the loss, grief intensity and satisfaction with care. *Eur J Obstet Gynecol Reprod Biol, 52*(3), 163–168.

Cunningham, F.G., & Williams, J.W. (2005). *Williams obstetrics* (22nd ed.). New York: McGraw-Hill Professional.

DrugPoints System. (2008). Thomson Micromedex Healthcare. Retrieved December 24, 2008, from http://online.statref.com

Fretts, R.C. (2008). *Etiology and management of antepartum fetal death.* Retrieved December 11, 2008, from http://www.uptodateonline.com

Froen, J.F. (2008). *Evaluation of decreased fetal movements.* Retrieved December 8, 2008, from http://www.uptodateonline.com

Hughes, P., & Riches, S. (2003). Psychological aspects of perinatal loss. *Curr Opin Obstet Gynecol, 15*(2), 107–111.

Hughes, P., Turton, P., Hopper, E., & Evans, C.D. (2002). Assessment of guidelines for good practice in psychosocial care of mothers after stillbirth: A cohort study. *Lancet, 360*(9327), 114–118.

New York State. (2005). Public health law, article 41 title 5 §4161, *Fetal death certificates; form and content; physicians, midwives and hospital administrators.* Retrieved January 5, 2009, from http://law.onecle.com/new-york/public-health/PBH04161_4161.html

Obstetric and medical complications. (2007). In *Guidelines for perinatal care* (6th ed.). Washington, DC: American College of Obstetricians and Gynecologists.

Prenatal One Multivitamin. (n.d.). Rainbow Light Nutritional Systems. Santa Cruz, CA. Retrieved December 11, 2008, from http://www.rainbowlight.com

Radestad, I., Nordin, C., Steineck, G., & Sjogren, B. (1998). A comparison of women's memories of care during pregnancy, labour and delivery after stillbirth or live birth. *Midwifery, 14*(2), 111–117.

Rand, C.S., Kellner, K.R., Revak-Lutz, R., & Massey, J.K. (1998). Parental behavior after perinatal death: Twelve years of observations. *J Psychosom Obstet Gynaecol, 19*(1), 44–48.

Roberts, D.J. (2008a). *Evaluation of stillbirth.* Retrieved December 22, 2008, from http://www.uptodateonline.com

Roberts, D.J. (2008b). *Gross examination of the placenta.* Retrieved January 1, 2009, from http://www.uptodateonline.com

Roman, A.S. (2008). *Prenatal screening for genetic disease in the Ashkenazi Jewish population.* Retrieved December 8, 2008, from http://www.uptodateonline.com

Shuzman, E. (2003). Facing stillbirth or neonatal death. Providing culturally appropriate care for Jewish families. *AWHONN Lifelines, 7*(6), 537–543.

Varney, H., Kriebs, J.M., & Gegor, C.L. (2004). *Varney's midwifery* (4th ed.). Sudbury, MA: Jones and Bartlett.

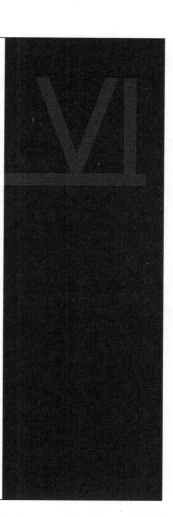

DNP Approach and Clinical Case Management in Anesthesia Care

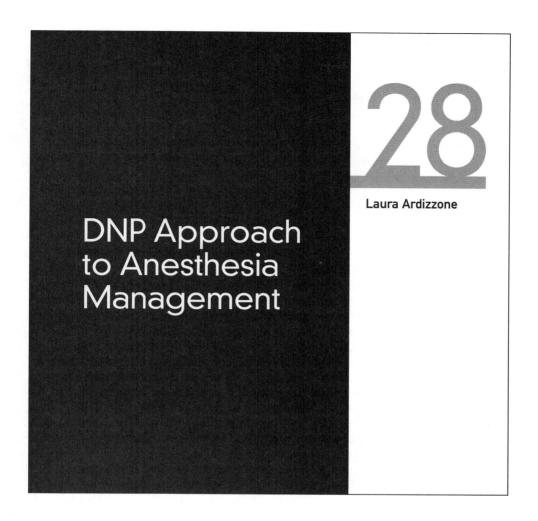

28

Laura Ardizzone

DNP Approach to Anesthesia Management

Established in the late 1800s, the specialty of nurse anesthesia is now recognized as a key component of health care delivery. Nurses were the first professional group to provide anesthesia services in the United States. Nurse anesthesia developed in response to the request of surgeons who sought a solution to the high morbidity and mortality attributed to anesthesia during this period. Surgeons viewed nurses as professionals who would give their complete attention to the patient during surgical procedures. Nurse anesthetists are now involved in the full range of specialty surgical procedures, as well as in the refinement of anesthesia techniques and the development of anesthesia equipment.

Certified registered nurse anesthetists (CRNAs) administer approximately 30 million anesthetics in the United States each year (AANA, 2009). CRNAs practice in every setting where anesthesia is delivered and are the sole anesthesia providers in more than two-thirds of all rural hospitals. They administer every type of anesthetic and provide anesthesia for every type of surgery and procedure.

The American Association of Nurse Anesthetists (AANA), founded in 1931, is the umbrella organization responsible for certification and recertification of nurse anesthesia professionals and is the professional organization for more than 90 percent of the nation's 39,000 CRNAs (AANA, 2009). The AANA's mission is to promote patient safety and provide excellence in anesthesia (AANA, 2009). The mission is guided by four core values: integrity, professionalism, advocacy, and quality. In 1975, the AANA became a leader among professional organizations in the United States because of its formation of autonomous multidisciplinary councils. These councils currently have public representation and perform the profession's certification, accreditation, and public interest functions.

As of February 2008, there were 109 nurse anesthesia programs in the United States, all affiliated with academic institutions. These master's or doctoral degree programs range in length from 24 to 36 months. This educational system provides more than 4,200 students with a graduate-level science foundation and with clinical anesthesia experiences (AANA, 2009).

In 2007, after a two-year task force study, the AANA board of directors endorsed doctoral education as the minimal requirement for entry into practice. All CRNA programs must convert to doctoral level by 2025. This new level of education must encompass technological and pharmaceutical advances, informatics, evidence-based practice, and a systems approach to quality improvement. This conversion echoes that of the American Association of Colleges of Nursing (AACN) regarding advanced practice nurses and the AACN's recommendation that all programs have doctoral-level education by 2015 (AACN, 2009; Martin-Sheridan, Ouellette, & Horton, 2006).

The vision and practice of a CRNA who has a doctor of nursing practice (DNP) degree is controversial. At last count, 8 schools out of 109 offer doctoral degrees as an option in nurse anesthesia programs, with other schools in the process of developing programs. A barrier to the development of doctoral education in nurse anesthesia is that more than half of the accredited programs are not housed within a school or division of nursing. They are contained within schools of allied health sciences or medical schools, which do not necessarily recognize the AACN doctoral recommendation. This results in some variability in degrees being offered and developed. For example, a doctor of practice management (DPMA) is being offered at Charleston Area Medical Center School of Nurse Anesthesia, and a doctor of nurse anesthesia practice (DNAP) degree is currently being offered at Virginia Commonwealth University and Texas Wesleyan University. These additional degree types add to nursing's continual problem of degree dilution and public and payer confusion.

DNP nurse anesthesia providers have expanded practice roles and the advanced clinical education to support them. These clinicians have advanced clinical skills and the tools and expertise needed to transform their practices. DNP nurse anesthetists are able to provide care to patients across health care settings in a comprehensive manner and not solely in the peri-anesthetic period. DNP clinicians are able to critically appraise and evaluate their current practice of anesthesia. DNPs also use their practices to develop and successfully address clinical questions, having acquired the skills to conduct practice-based research, either alone or with their research colleagues. DNP nurse anesthetists use their knowledge of informatics to change and influence health care systems and policy.

The role of a doctorally educated CRNA is in its infancy, and change is inevitable. CRNAs should be energized for the future and embrace this new and exciting opportunity.

CASE NARRATIVE

A scholarly case narrative by a nurse anesthetist must demonstrate evidence behind the practice of anesthesia. Case narratives described in the following section use the Columbia University School of Nursing direct patient care competencies.

The first step is to choose a potential case by examining one's clinical practice to find interesting cases that allow the DNP student to demonstrate the ability to meet the performance objectives of a clinical competency. Examples include a patient who has had an intraoperative event or a rare comorbid condition, a patient seen on multiple occasions, or a case in which the clinician uses a new technique or performs a novel procedure.

Once the case is chosen, the DNP resident systematically evaluates the care provided, the evidence to support the clinical decisions, and the interventions. In the CUSN case narrative format, objective data are written in Times New Roman 12-point font. Evidence supporting clinical practice is written in italics. Graphics, charts, and tables are included as appropriate. An important aspect of this process is the evaluation of the supporting evidence. The source used in the CUSN model to evaluate the evidence is the Center for Evidence-Based Medicine (CEBM), which provides a process and system for leveling the evidence (CEBM, 2009). A pre-anesthesia airway assessment may be written as follows:

Airway: Poor dentition and gingiva noted. Loose tooth #9, #10. Chip noted #6 and missing several lower teeth. Mallampati Class III airway, thyromental distance > 7 cm, full neck range of motion and good mouth opening.

Evidence suggests that there is a correlation between poor oral health, specifically tooth loss, and coronary heart disease (Joshipura et al., 1996).

CEBM, level 2b.

Recent data indicates that using the Mallampati score alone has a poor sensitivity and specificity of predicting a difficult intubation. The use of this measurement along with thyromental distance [measure from upper edge of thyroid cartilage to chin with the head fully extended—should be > 7 cm], mouth opening, patient height, neck mobility and dentition increases the sensitivity and specificity of predicting a difficult intubation (Lee, Fan, Gin, Karmakar, & Ngan Kee, 2006; Naguib et al., 2006).

CEBM, level 2a.

Another example would be the use of standard monitoring equipment during the operative procedure. The objective data are in Times New Roman 12-point font, the evidence is in italics, and the strength of the evidence presented is noted:

Patient was transported to operating room. A five-lead electrocardiogram (EKG) with automatic ST segment monitoring in Leads II and V, pulse oximeter, and blood pressure cuff were all applied.

Vital signs: Blood pressure 150/85, normal sinus rhythm with a rate of 86, respirations 20.

> *Leads II and V have been the suggested optimal leads to detect intra-operative ischemia based on prior exercise treadmill data. This was later validated through correlations with 12-lead EKG monitoring. In this study, sensitivity to ischemia using a single lead was greatest in V5 (75%) and V4 (61%). The remaining leads demonstrated either moderate to very low sensitivity or exhibited no ischemic changes (I and a VL). When leads V4 and V5 were combined sensitivity to ischemia increased to 90% [the standard clinical combination, II and V5, is only 80% sensitive]. Sensitivity to ischemia also increased to 96% by combining II, V4, and V5. This study confirms previous recommendations for the routine use of a V5 lead (either uni or bipolar) in all patients at risk for ischemia. V4 is more sensitive than lead II, and should be considered as a second choice. However, lead II, superior for detection of atrial dysrhythmias, is more easily obtained with conventional monitors. The use of all three would appear to be the optimal arrangement for most clinical needs, and is recommended if the clinician has the capability (London et al., 1988).*
>
> CEBM, level 1b.

An additional example includes physical examination, evidence supporting the practice, strength of the evidence, and the clinician's reflective thinking, which is included in a free text box.

The patient was pre-oxygenated for 3 minutes, cricoid pressure was applied, and rapid sequence intubation was performed with 150 mcg of fentanyl (Sublimaze), 200 mg of propofol (Diprivan), and 140 mg of succinylcholine (Anectine). Subsequent laryngoscopy was atraumatic, and a size 8.0 endotracheal tube was placed and confirmed. Patient was a grade III airway.

> *Three minutes of pre-oxygenation with a tight fitting mask seal and normal patient respiration has been found to be the appropriate amount of time for effective de-nitrogenation of exhaled patient air (Berthoud, Read, & Norman, 1983; Gambee, Hertzka, & Fisher, 1987).*
>
> CEBM, level 2b.

> *Rapid sequence intubation is a technique used to secure a patent airway while minimizing the risk of aspiration pneumonitis in patients who are at high risk. Reasons for high risk include body habitus, co-morbid conditions and/or disease state. The use of cricoid pressure was originally documented in 1961 and was based on a single small prospective study of 26 patients who were at risk for aspiration pneumonia (Sellick, 1961). Since then there has been limited evidence to substantiate its widespread use; however, it has become the gold standard in the prevention of the aspiration of stomach contents.*
>
> CEBM, level 2b.

Critical Appraisal

Although the evidence is weak regarding the utility of rapid sequence intubation and there is debate among clinicians as to what classifies patients as at risk for aspiration, I chose to treat this patient as a "full stomach." She had a history of non-insulin dependent diabetes, which can decrease gastric motility, she had some significant adiposity in the central region of her trunk, and she reported occasional gastroesophageal reflux disease (GERD). In this case, rapid sequence intubation was as follows: pre-oxygenation, application of cricoid pressure by an assistant, administration of induction agents, followed by immediate intubation ~ 60 seconds post drug administration, confirmation of tube position and removal of cricoid pressure.

Another step in this process is to note any education and patient follow-up that is provided. Once again, the care delivered to the patient is indicated in Times New Roman 12-point font, reflective thinking is in a text box, evidence is italicized, and levels of evidence are indicated. Note the addition of documentation of an achieved performance objective (PO).

Education

I discussed with the patient the anesthesia plan, risks and benefits, and potential complications associated with general anesthesia. I explained that all forms of anesthesia involve some risks, and no guarantees or promises can be made concerning the results of the procedure. Although rare, unexpected severe complications with anesthesia can occur and include the possibility of infection, bleeding, drug reactions, blood clots, loss of sensation, loss of limb function, paralysis, stroke, brain damage, heart attack, or death.

At this time, the patient was also instructed about what to expect in the postoperative period in terms of pain management, use of incentive spirometer, and early ambulation.

Evidence supports preoperative instruction and patient teaching as an intervention that has a positive effect on operative outcomes when it occurs at multiple intervals (Hathaway, 1986).

CEBM, level 1a.

Critical Appraisal

There is no requirement for written informed consent that is specific to my anesthesia department. Our services are bundled in to the general surgical consent form, which also includes blood transfusion consent. I always have a robust conversation with patients about the risks of anesthesia and document this in the medical record. I follow the practice guidelines on informed consent from my professional association, and I use my clinical knowledge about patient care to individualize the discussion (AANA, 2009) **(D4, C3, PO C, D)**.

Finally, the case study narrative author should briefly defend how each CUSN direct care patient competency was fulfilled. In the following example, a specific competency is described along with a discussion of how this competency was met in a case narrative that involved providing care for a surgical patient who was a Jehovah's Witness.

Domain 4, Competency 1. Construct and evaluate outcomes of a culturally sensitive, individualized intervention that addresses the specific needs of a patient in the context of family and community.

Defense. This competency was met by evaluation and assessment of the patient's needs in light of his religious beliefs. An immediate perioperative plan was discussed and implemented with the patient. This included the avoidance of blood products and the use of alternate methods of fluid resuscitation that included hetastarch and an intraoperative cell salvage device with use of a leukocyte reduction filter. The plan was evaluated postoperatively, and the patient was found to be stable. Long-term follow-up shows the patient alive and in rehabilitation therapy.

A case narrative is written in chronological order to ensure logical progression for the reader. Clinical data must be differentiated from evidence, and the strength of the evidence must be cited. Illustrations should be used as appropriate. Performance objectives are identified within the narrative. The performance objectives provide the basis for a cogent defense of the fulfilled competencies at the conclusion of the narrative.

The appendix includes several formats that CRNA DNP residents can use to structure their case narrative documentation in different settings.

References

AACN. (2009). *American Association of Colleges of Nursing.* Retrieved June 2009 from www .aacn.nche.edu

AANA. (2009). *American Association of Nurse Anesthetists.* Retrieved June 2009 from www .aana.com

Berthoud, M., Read, D.H., & Norman, J. (1983). Pre-oxygenation—how long? *Anaesthesia, 38*(2), 96–102.

CEBM. (2009, June). *Centre for Evidence-Based Medicine—Levels of evidence.* Retrieved June 1, 2009, from http://www.cebm.net/index.aspx?o=1025

Gambee, A.M., Hertzka, R.E., & Fisher, D.M. (1987). Preoxygenation techniques: Comparison of three minutes and four breaths. *Anesthesia and Analgesia, 66*(5), 468–470.

Hathaway, D. (1986). Effect of preoperative instruction on postoperative outcomes: A meta-analysis. *Nursing Research, 35*(5), 269–275.

Joshipura, K.J., Rimm, E.B., Douglass, C.W., Trichopoulos, D., Ascherio, A., & Willett, W.C. (1996). Poor oral health and coronary heart disease. *Journal of Dental Research, 75*(9), 1631–1636.

Lee, A., Fan, L.T., Gin, T., Karmakar, M.K., & Ngan Kee, W.D. (2006). A systematic review (meta-analysis) of the accuracy of the Mallampati tests to predict the difficult airway. *Anesthesia and Analgesia, 102*(6), 1867–1878.

London, M.J., Hollenberg, M., Wong, M.G., Levenson, L., Tubau, J.F., Browner, W., et al. (1988). Intraoperative myocardial ischemia: Localization by continuous 12-lead electrocardiography. *Anesthesiology, 69*(2), 232–241.

Martin-Sheridan, D., Ouellette, S.M., & Horton, B.J. (2006). Is doctoral education in our future? *AANA Journal 74*(2), 101–104.

Naguib, M., Scamman, F.L., O'Sullivan, C., Aker, J., Ross, A.F., Kosmach, S., et al. (2006). Predictive performance of three multivariate difficult tracheal intubation models: A double-blind, case-controlled study. *Anesthesia and Analgesia, 102*(3), 818–824.

Sellick, B.A. (1961). Cricoid pressure to control regurgitation of stomach contents during induction of anaesthesia. *Lancet, 2*(7199), 404–406.

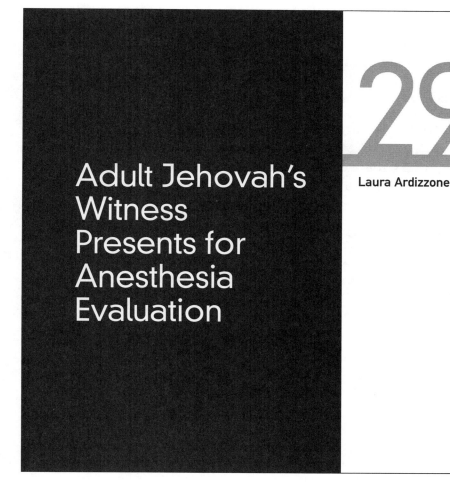

29

Adult Jehovah's Witness Presents for Anesthesia Evaluation

Laura Ardizzone

I have selected this case to illustrate the care of a patient who required an alternate plan of anesthesia care due to religious beliefs. I had two encounters with this commercially insured patient over a two-day period in an acute care inpatient setting in an academic medical center. The case narrative demonstrates my ability to meet the following Columbia University School of Nursing comprehensive doctoral competencies for direct patient care.

DOMAIN 3, COMPETENCY 1

Construct and evaluate outcomes of a culturally sensitive, individualized intervention that addresses the specific needs of a patient in the context of family and community.

PO A. Assess culturally specific needs of the patient in the context of family and community.
PO B. Construct a culturally sensitive intervention to address needs of the patient in the context of family and community.
PO C. Evaluate outcomes of the intervention.

DOMAIN 3, COMPETENCY 3

Synthesize the principles of legal and ethical decision-making and analyze dilemmas that arise in patient care, interprofessional relationships, research, or practice management to improve outcomes.

PO A. Synthesize ethical principles to address a complex practice dilemma.
PO B. Apply ethical principles to resolve the dilemma.
PO D. Apply legal principles to resolve the dilemma.

SUMMARY OF CARE PREVIOUSLY PROVIDED

The patient is a 54-year-old African American (AA) male who was seen in the orthopedic clinic because of a soft tissue mass on the right thigh that was causing pain and was protruding from the skin. The patient was seen and examined by the orthopedic surgeon. During the initial interview, the patient explained that he was a practicing Jehovah's Witness who would not accept blood or blood product transfusions. As definitive surgery was indicated, surgery and preoperative evaluation were deferred until the patient could be seen and examined by the hematology service.

The hematology service placed the patient on a three-week course of epoetin alfa (Epogen) and a four-week course of ferrous sulfate (Feosol) supplementation. The patient was scheduled for surgical resection approximately one month later.

There have been several anecdotal and case reports of the use of epoetin alfa and ferrous sulfate as an adjunct to the perioperative management and preparation for Jehovah's Witnesses undergoing major surgeries. Of the most notable have been case studies of patients who underwent a major liver resection, pancreatic resection, cardiac surgery and large gynecologic surgery (Barakat et al., 2007; Gyamfi & Yasin, 2000; Magner et al., 2006). Researchers have tried to extrapolate the use of epoetin alfa in these single case reports to other populations in the hopes to standardize dosing for surgical anemia prophylaxis as well as expand the potential use of this agent. In 1996 a randomized placebo controlled study of 185 patients undergoing orthopedic surgery demonstrated those who had epoetin alfa preoperatively had a 50% reduction in transfusion rates (Faris, Ritter, & Abels, 1996).

Centre for Evidence-Based Medicine (CEBM), levels 5 (Barakat et al., 2007; Gyamfi & Yasin, 2000; Magner et al., 2006), 1b (Faris, Ritter, & Abels, 1996).

A recent black box warning has been issued on epoetin alfa by the US Food and Drug Administration (FDA) with regard to cardiac risk and the judicious use of epoetin alfa for routine surgical prophylaxis to prevent transfusions is indicated. Specifically the FDA recommends that due to the risk of serious heart problems such as heart attack, stroke, heart failure, and a higher chance of death patients treated with an Erythropoiesis-Stimulating Agent (ESA) the target hemoglobin level should not be above 12 g/dL (FDA, 2009).

CEBM, level 5.

ENCOUNTER CONTEXT

Encounter one (initial evaluation for anesthesia)

DNP role: I am the nurse anesthetist seeing this patient prior to the administration of anesthesia.

Identifying Information

Setting: Academic medical center.

Reason for encounter: Immediate preoperative evaluation for anesthesia.

Informant: Information was obtained from chart review and patient.

Minute: Zero.

Chief complaint: "Mass on thigh."

History of Present Illness

Reason for anesthesia care: 54-year-old African American male presents for wide surgical resection of a soft tissue sarcoma on right midthigh.

> *Soft tissue sarcomas are uncommon tumors that are usually managed by wide excision surgery and radiotherapy and represent about 1% of all cancers. They can arise anywhere in the body but are most commonly found in the limb, pelvis or retroperitoneal area. Half of patients with soft tissue sarcomas will die from their disease (Clark, Fisher, Judson, & Thomas, 2005).*
>
> *There are four methods of surgical excision with varying rates of local recurrence post surgical excision. While the method of radical resection has the lowest recurrence rate it has the most detrimental effect on the patient's quality of life especially when performed on a limb.*
>
> CEBM, level 2a.

Anesthesia history: General anesthesia (GA) without complications for previous bunionectomy and laparoscopic cholecystectomy. Family history is unremarkable for problems with anesthesia.

NPO status: 10 hours, including medications.

Relevant History for Anesthesia Risk

Cardiovascular
Hypertension (HTN). Patient has been treated for HTN by his primary care provider for over 10 years with good control of blood pressure. He is medically managed with metoprolol (Toprol) and has a moderately active lifestyle. Patient reports he eats a balanced diet and avoids table salt when possible.

> *Hypertension is one of the most common diagnoses in the United States adult population and has a prevalence in excess of 50% of individuals older than*

65 years. Mild to moderate hypertension (stage 1 or stage 2 hypertension) affects patients with systolic blood pressure (BP) below 180 mm Hg and diastolic BP below 110 mm Hg. Evidence suggests that these patients do not appear to be at increased operative risk for cardiovascular adverse outcomes. For patients with severe hypertension (stage 3, systolic BP >180 mm Hg and diastolic BP >110 mm Hg), many investigators believe that BP should be controlled prior to proceeding to elective non-cardiac surgery. However, these recommendations have been based upon studies with small sample sizes with various study outcomes. The strongest evidence suggests that the patient with stage 1 or 2 hypertension and no evidence of end-organ damage or other comorbid cardiovascular diseases may safely proceed to surgery without escalation of therapy. For those patients with stage 3 hypertension (diastolic pressure >110 mm Hg), there is insufficient evidence to determine the approach leading to the best outcome, though some authors have suggested that postponement of elective surgery for 6 to 8 weeks with aggressive antihypertensive therapy may allow amelioration of the vascular changes associated with hypertension. This practice should be balanced against the urgency of the surgery and acknowledgment of the lack of data to determine if such practices will improve outcome. Minimally, medications should be initiated or titrated preoperatively to achieve a more normal BP prior to undergoing surgery (Fleischer, 2002).

CEBM, level 2a.

Endocrine

Type 2 diabetes mellitus (type 2 DM). Patient reports that he was diagnosed with type 2 DM about three years ago and started on metformin (Glucophage) about two years ago, having failed conservative therapy of diet and exercise modification. He does not routinely monitor his blood sugar levels but states he is sure they are checked when he sees his primary care provider. Preoperative glucose is 139.

Patients with diabetes are at increased risk of myocardial ischemia, cerebrovascular infarction and renal ischemia because of an increased incidence of coronary artery disease, arterial atherosclerosis and renal parenchyma disease. Increased mortality is found in all diabetics undergoing surgery as compared to non-diabetic patients. Although insulin dependent diabetes patients are particularly at risk for post-operative complications, non-insulin dependent diabetes patients should have their condition appropriately managed prior to surgery. Increased wound complications are associated with diabetes and anastomotic healing is severely impaired when glycemic control is sub-optimal during the peri-operative period (McAnulty, Robertshaw, & Hall, 2000).

CEBM, level 2a.

Current Medications (see Medications list at the end of the chapter)

Metoprolol (Toprol)—75 mg by mouth twice daily
Metformin (Glucophage)—500 mg by mouth twice daily
Cetirizine hydrochloride (Zyrtec)—5 mg by mouth once daily

Epoetin alfa (Epogen)—20,000 U subcutaneously weekly (last dose morning of surgery)

Ferrous sulfate (Feosol)—5 mg by mouth three times daily (discontinued day prior to surgery)

Allergies

Penicillin (rash) and seasonal allergies.

Hospitalizations

No recent hospitalizations.

Past medical history

HTN, type 2 DM.

Surgical history

2006: bilateral bunionectomies; 2005: laparoscopic cholecystectomy.

Social history

Denies cigarette smoking and recreational drug use. Occasional social drinking. Married with two children. Self-employed and able to independently care for self as well as elderly mother. Good social support system with large family in the immediate area who are able and willing to support patient during his recovery period. Practicing Jehovah's Witness.

Jehovah's Witnesses believe that blood transfusion is forbidden for them by select biblical passages. While these passages in the bible are not stated in medical terms, Witnesses interpret them as ruling out the possibility of transfusions of whole blood, packed red blood cells, plasma and platelets. However, their religious understanding does not absolutely prohibit the use of components such as albumin or immunoglobulins. Each patient must decide individually if they can accept these.

Jehovah's Witnesses believe that blood removed from the body should be disposed of, so they do not accept autologous blood. Techniques for intraoperative blood collection or hemodilution that involve blood storage may be objectionable to them. However, many patients permit the use of dialysis and bypass equipment (non-blood-prime) as well as intraoperative salvage if the extracorporeal circulation is uninterrupted; the provider should consult with the individual patient to assess their wishes.

These patients do not feel that the Bible comments directly on organ transplants; therefore decisions regarding cornea, kidney, or other tissue transplants must be made by the individual Witness (Dixon & Smalley, 1981; Singelenberg, 1990).

CEBM, level 5.

Critical Appraisal

I was specifically told about this patient the day before the case was scheduled so that I could review the chart and formulate a plan of care in consultation with the attending anesthesiologist and the surgeon. The patient had been well managed preoperatively and had been seen by the hematology service. The patient was started on epoetin alfa and ferrous sulfate supplements and was scheduled to arrive a half-hour earlier than usual so there would be ample time for discussion with the patient (D3, C1, PO A, B).

Family history

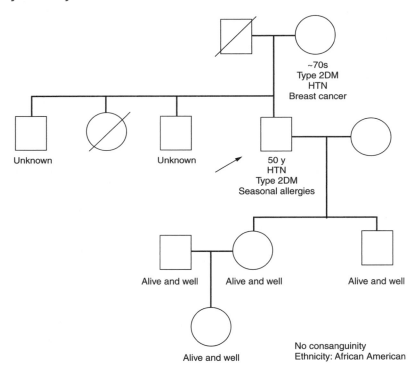

Review of Systems

General: Denies recent changes in weight, appetite, or energy level.

Skin: Denies recent rashes, pruritus, or skin lesions.

Head: Denies recent head trauma, syncopy, or tenderness.

Eyes: No changes in vision, wears reading glasses. Recent eye exam by provider.

Ears: No changes in hearing and denies tinnitus, ear pain, or current ear infection.

Nose: No changes in sense of smell. Patient reports no current sinus infection but seasonal allergies have been "acting up."

Mouth and throat: No lesions or ulcerations reported in mouth. Recent dental exam by dentist.

Neck: Denies pain, stiffness, or swollen glands.

Breast: Denies lumps or pain.

Respiratory: Denies current or recent infection, shortness of breath, or dyspnea on exertion.

Cardiovascular: Denies murmurs, edema, palpitations, or dyspnea on exertion.

Gastrointestinal: Denies changes in bowel habits or stool, nausea or vomiting, or food habits. Occasional reflux (GERD) after a large meal. Patient denies having had an esophagogastroduodenoscopy or colonoscopy.

Urinary: Denies changes in bladder habits, incontinence, or urinary tract infections.

Endocrine: Type 2 DM managed by primary care provider and treated with medications, diet, and exercise. Denies thyroid problems.

Musculoskeletal: Denies arthritis, recent trauma, joint swelling, or tenderness. Full range of motion. Moderately active lifestyle.

Peripheral vascular: Denies blood clots or intermittent claudication. Denies parasthesias.

Hematologic: Denies bruising or bleeding tendencies or swollen lymph nodes.

Neurologic: Denies syncopy, seizures, or alterations in sensation, memory, mood, or sleep pattern.

Psychiatric: Patient reports feeling depressed about possible loss of limb function and his role as the provider for the family.

Physical Examination

General: African American man appears stated age. Pleasant and answers questions easily.

Vital signs: 98.7°F (oral); pulse 64; respirations regular, 20; blood pressure 143/78 (left arm); height 73 inches (185.4 cm); weight 97 kg; BMI 28.2.

Airway: Teeth intact, partial upper dentures removed, Mallampati class II airway, full range of motion of neck.

Skin: No rashes, eruptions, scars, or wounds noted.

Lymph nodes: No swollen or tender lymph nodes.

HEENT:

Head: Normocephalic.

Eyes: Pupils equal reactive, sclera anicteric, no redness or inflammation noted.

Ears: No tenderness or discharge.

Nose: No tenderness or discharge.

Throat: Tongue midline, tonsils noted, Mallampati II airway; no exudate, lesions, or erythema noted.

Neck: Full range of motion. Soft and supple, no tenderness, jugular venous distention (JVD), nodes, or carotid bruits noted.

Chest: Clear to auscultation, no rhonchi, rales, or wheezes noted without labored breathing or use of accessory muscles.

Heart: S1 and S1 audible, regular rhythm, no murmurs, clicks, or rubs.

Breast: Deferred.

Abdomen: Soft, no tenderness, positive bowel sounds.

Musculoskeletal: Full range of motion, ambulates without difficulty.

Peripheral vascular: No edema, clubbing, or cyanosis.

Neurologic: Awake, alert, and oriented. Cranial nerves II–XII are grossly intact.

Database

Preoperative labs at preadmission testing approximately 3 days prior to surgery.

Laboratory Measurement	Result	Reference Range/Units
WBC	4.4	4–11 K/mcL
RBC	4.21	4.0–5.2 M/mcL
HGB	13.4	11.5–16 g/dl
HCT	40.0	34–46 %
MCV	88	82–98 fl
MCH	29	27–33 pg
MCHC	32.1	32–35%
Platelet	245	160–400 K/mcL
RDW	13.6	11.4–14.5%
Neutrophils	50	38–80%
Eosinophils	2	0–7%
Basophils	0.4	0–1.5%
Lymphocytes	27.1	12–48%
Monocytes	4.1	0–12%
Leukocytes	2.2	0–5%
Abs neutrophils	2.7	1.5–8.8 K/mcL

(continued)

Laboratory Measurement	Result	Reference Range/Units
Abs eosinophils	0.1	0–0.8 K/mcL
Abs basophils	0.01	0–0.16 K/mcL
Abs lymphocytes	1.1	0.5–5.3 K/mcL
Abs monocytes	0.2	0–1.3 K/mcL
Abs leukocytes	0.1	0–0.6 K/mcL
Pro time	11.2	9.8–13.7 seconds
Activated PTT	33.8	24.4–35.4 seconds
INR	0.98	.85–1.17 INR
Sodium	144	136–144 mEq/L
Potassium	4.1	3.5–5.1 mEq/L
Chloride	110	98–109 mEq/L
CO_2	26	24–30 mEq/L
Glucose	139	70–99 mg/dl
BUN	12	6–20 mg/dl
Creatinine	0.9	0.6–1.3 mg/dl
Total bilirubin	0.7	0–1.0 mg/dl
Total protein	6.8	6.3–8.1 g/dl
Albumin	4.5	4.0–5.2 g/dl
Calcium	8.6	8.5–10.5 mg/dl
AST	24	10–37 U/L
Alk phosphatase	67	0–115 U/L
ALT	21	5–37 U/L
Type and cross specimen	Blood type done	Received in lab and valid

Electrocardiogram (EKG): Normal sinus rhythm.
Chest radiograph: No active cardiopulmonary disease seen. Cardiac silhouette is normal.

Anesthesia Risk Classification

American Society of Anesthesiologists/Physical Status (ASA/PS) — Level II.

The ASA/PS classification system attempts to categorize patients based on the presence of co-morbid conditions. Although this system was not intended to be used as a predictor of outcomes, the ASA physical status generally correlates with perioperative mortality rate. This classification system has been shown in one prospective study to be a predictor of postoperative outcomes (Wolters, Wolf, Stutzer, & Schroder, 1996).

CEBM, level 1b.

Critical Appraisal

> Blood typing was done as a precaution. If the patient's blood contained an unusual antibody, it might take several hours to get blood products. It was our plan to not transfuse blood even in an emergency. However, if there was a major intraoperative problem, we would need to discuss with the family the possibility of imminent death if the patient was not transfused. Without previous blood typing we would essentially have no viable choice to offer the family (**D3, C1, PO B; D3, C3, PO A**).

Education

I discuss with patient the anesthesia plan, risks and benefits, and potential complications associated with general anesthesia. I explain that all forms of anesthesia involve some risks and that no guarantees or promises can be made concerning the results of the procedure. Although rare, unexpected severe complications with anesthesia can occur and include the possibilities of infection, bleeding, drug reactions, blood clots, loss of sensation, loss of limb function, paralysis, stroke, brain damage, heart attack, or death.

In addition to the general discussion regarding the risks of general anesthesia, it is important to discuss this patient's wishes in the peri- and postoperative period with regard to blood transfusions. This patient would not accept blood, platelets, fresh-frozen plasma, cryoprecipitate, or albumin. He would accept hetastarch (Hespan) and the use of cellsaver as long as it was a closed system (**D 3, C1, PO B**).

The patient has previously been started on epoetin alfa (Epogen) and ferrous sulfate (Feosol) supplements. The patient is also instructed at this time what to expect in the postoperative period in terms of pain management, probable postoperative intubation, and intensive care unit (ICU) management.

> *"Bloodless surgery" or surgery with the exclusive avoidance of the transfusions of blood products has been successfully implemented at many surgical centers and with many different types of high risk surgeries. The adoption of this idea is for many reasons; including patient's request for no blood products and emerging evidence of the detrimental effects of allogeneic blood transfusions such as increased rates of infection, longer hospital stays, increased rates of cancer reoccurrence, disease transmission and transfusion related lung injury. Bloodless surgery involves proper and comprehensive patient management across all specialties. The four basic tenets include preoperative patient optimization, maximizing hemopoiesis, minimizing intra-op blood loss and maximizing patient oxygenation (Martyn et al., 2002).*
>
> CEBM, level 5.

> *The use of cell salvage in oncologic surgery remains controversial. The recycling of blood cells that have been exposed and in close proximity to malignant tumor cells, in theory could contribute to the reoccurrence of primary*

tumors. There has been one retrospective study of patients undergoing radical cystectomies for bladder cancer. A review of three year survival rates showed no difference in groups that received cell salvage blood versus those who did not receive cell savage blood (Nieder, Manoharan, Yang, & Soloway, 2007).

CEBM, level 4.

The use of a leukocyte reduction filter along with cell salvage in one small study showed that when comparing samples of cell salvaged blood before and after the use a leukocyte reduction filter there were no remaining viable nucleated malignant cells in the samples (Catling et al., 2008).

CEBM, level 2b.

Plan of Anesthesia Care

Estimated length of procedure: 500 minutes (8.3 hours).
Estimated blood loss: 2,000 cc or greater.
Intraoperative: General anesthesia with a central line and arterial blood pressure monitoring. Cell salvage device for intraoperative blood collection and bloodless surgery with a closed circuit system **(D3, C1, PO B)**.

Critical Appraisal

This was an ethically challenging case for me because I had to evaluate my own personal biases. It is challenging when the patient's right to autonomy is pitted directly against the tenet of non-maleficence. The surgeon explained that this had the potential to be a very difficult and bloody surgery. It would be personally difficult for me to actively care for a patient while watching him exsanguinate with no possibility of "solving" the problem with a transfusion. This was a young, relatively healthy man with a family. It required frank discussion of the real chance of death from a probably preventable cause—blood loss. There has been debate in the health care community about conscientious objection in providing care for patients. Although I was specifically asked by my clinical chairman to participate in this case, I did have the option to say no. I chose to participate because I felt the patient's autonomy outweighed my personal biases. Based on this decision, I constructed the best plan I could that respected his wishes but provided for a high level of care that would help conserve blood loss. As discussed before, cell salvage in oncologic surgery is controversial, but with the use of a leukocyte reduction filter, the benefits of its use outweighed the risks. We agreed to the use of a closed system for cell salvage, which is not our usual procedure (D3, C3, PO A, B).

This patient required a special consent form because the anesthesia and surgical consent form is bundled into one document and has consent for use of blood products as part of the standard consent. The patient required separate surgical and anesthesia consents that were obtained in conjunction with the anesthesia attending post discussion with the patient (D3, C3, PO D).

Postoperative: Hydromorphone (Dilaudid) patient-controlled analgesia pump, propofol (Diprivan) drip for sedation as patient will likely remain intubated.

> *Epidural hematoma formations in the spinal canal due to epidural anesthesia are a rare but potentially devastating complication. The definitive treatment of such occurrences is surgical decompression within several hours to avoid long term neurologic sequelae. Since the incidence is rare there are no prospective studies available. However, a review of case studies in 1996 revealed that coagulopathies or the use of anticoagulant therapy are the predominant risk factors for the development of hematomas (Wulf, 1996). Further, the American Society of Regional Anesthesia and Pain Medicine came up with a consensus statement report in 2002 that was based on a collective experience of recognized experts in the field of neuraxial anesthesia and anticoagulation. These guidelines are based on case reports, clinical series, pharmacology, hematology, and risk factors for surgical bleeding. Essentially, they concluded to use good clinical judgment and gave some general guidelines for at risk patients (Horlocker et al., 2004).*
>
> CEBM, level 4 (Wulf, 1996), 5 (Horlocker et al., 2004).

Critical Appraisal

Estimated length and blood loss are based both on surgical textbooks and a discussion with the operating surgeon. Because the surgeon had the imaging of the tumor available and knew the clinical history, the surgeon played an integral part in planning the perioperative management. Due to the anticipated surgical length and large blood loss, this plan was the only viable option. The tumor was very vascular and not well circumscribed. The patient required general anesthesia with large-bore access for rapid fluid resuscitation. Additionally, postoperatively we anticipated that the patient would remain intubated due to large fluid shifts and a large blood loss. This surgery is associated with a large amount of postoperative pain because muscle and bone resections are part of the procedure. Postoperative pain control might include the placement of an epidural catheter prior to the induction of general anesthesia. However, this technique was not an option because this patient was at high risk for dilutional coagulopathies and anemia, which have been related to adverse neurologic sequelae in the presence of epidural catheters.

Anesthesia Care

Induction: Minute 30

Patient is transported to operating room. Five-lead EKG with automatic ST segment monitoring in leads II and V, pulse oximeter, and blood pressure cuff are applied.

Vital signs: Blood pressure 166/79, pulse 74, respirations 20.

A 20-gauge intravenous catheter is inserted and the patient is given 2 mg of midazolam (Versed) for anxiolysis and 2.5 mg intravenous metoprolol (Lopressor). The patient did not take his morning dose of metoprolol (Toprol).

Critical Appraisal

I administered a beta-blockade to this patient. I chose to start with a lower intravenous dose, recognizing that the patient was underhydrated due to NPO status and was about to receive several induction drugs that might cause profound hypotension.

Vital signs (five minutes from previous vital signs): Blood pressure 134/79, pulse 72, respirations 15.

The 2007 ACC/AHA guidelines for this particular patient state that beta blockers should be continued perioperatively in patients undergoing surgery who are receiving beta blockers to treat angina, symptomatic arrhythmias, hypertension (Fleisher et al., 2007).

CEBM, level 1a.

The patient is preoxygenated for three minutes. Induction of anesthesia is with 100 mg lidocaine (Xylocaine), 150 mcg of fentanyl (Sublimaze), 200 mg of propofol (Diprivan), and 60 mg of rocuronium (Zemuron). Subsequent laryngoscopy is atraumatic, and a size 8.0 endotracheal tube is placed and confirmed. Patient has a grade II airway; under direct laryngoscopy some but not all parts of the vocal cords are visualized.

Post-Induction: Minutes 40–70

Vital signs: Blood pressure 127/67, monitor heart rate 72 normal sinus rhythm. The patient is placed on the anesthesia ventilator on volume-controlled ventilation, tidal volume = 700, rate = 8, positive end-expiratory pressure = 5, fraction of inspired oxygen = 50%. Isoflurane (Forane) is turned to 0.8%. Clindamycin (Cleocin HCL) 900 mg is also administered.

Critical Appraisal

Standard induction of anesthesia includes preoxygenation and the administration of a sequence of drug classes. I administered lidocaine to attenuate airway reflexes during laryngoscopy and to decrease the burning sensation felt with the administration of propofol. Fentanyl was given for pain control during intubation. Propofol was given to induce amnesia and sedation, and finally rocuronium was given to produce muscle relaxation to facilitate intubation.

> *Surgical site infections complicate an estimated 780,000 operations in the United States each year. Despite solid evidence regarding the avoidance of potentially preventable surgical infections through appropriate use of anti-microbial agents and other means these practices are underutilized in hos-pitals across the country. In a 2005 study forty-four hospitals reported data on 35,543 surgical cases. Hospitals improved in several specific measures to prevent surgical site infections. The infection rate decreased 27%, [from 2.3% to 1.7%] in the first versus last three months. It is prudent that anesthesia pro-viders in conjunction with the entire surgical team apply these measures into their own practice. These measures include correct selection of antimicrobial agent based on surgery and allergy status, timing and duration of antibiotic administration, maintaining normothermia, oxygenation, euglycemia and appropriate hair removal (Dellinger et al., 2005).*
>
> CEBM, level 1b.

The right internal jugular vein is cannulated using sterile technique with a 12Fr gauge introducer. A left arterial catheter is placed for continuous moni-toring of blood pressure, and a 14-gauge left antecubital peripheral intrave-nous is placed. An 18Fr nasal gastric tube and an esophageal temperature probe are inserted atraumatically.

The patient is placed in a supine position, and the right hip is slightly elevated so the surgeon has access to the entire upper thigh area. The left arm is secured on an arm board, and the right arm is placed across the patient's body, padded, and secured.

Critical Appraisal

The types of intravenous lines were chosen based on Poiseuille's law as described by the following equation. Simply, the flow of a liquid (Q) passing per unit time through a tube is directly proportional to the pressure difference (delta p) between its ends and to the fourth power of its internal radius (r^4), and inversely proportional to its length (L) and to the viscosity (n) of the fluid. One important application of this principle is that the larger the diameter of the intravenous line and the shorter the length of the catheter, the quicker the flow of fluids, which is essential in rapid fluid resuscitation. A 12Fr double-lumen introducer central line and a 14-gauge peripheral intravenous are the largest available at this institu-tion. Also, a 12Fr introducer is much shorter than a triple-lumen catheter—hence quicker flow.

$$Q = \frac{\pi r^4 \Delta p}{8 \eta L}$$

Maintenance of Anesthesia: Minutes 75–450

Vital signs are stable throughout the procedure, with fluid boluses and phenylephrine (Neosynephrine) 40–80 mcg boluses given for systolic blood pressure < 80 mmHg. The patient is maintained on 0.7% isoflurane (Forane) that is titrated to preserve stable hemodynamic parameters.

Blood is drawn three times during the case, and the results at 430 minutes are shown below.

Laboratory Measurement	Value	Reference Range
Ph	7.41	7.35–7.45
PCO$_2$	38	35–45
PaO$_2$	231	85–199 mmHg
HCo$_3$	19	22–26 mEq/L
HGB	5.1	11.5–16.0 g/dl
HCT	15.4	34–46%
Ionized calcium	4.0	5.0–8.0 mg/dl
Glucose	156	70–99 mg/dl
Lactic acid	3.9	0.7–1.9 mEq/L

Estimated blood loss is 4,200 cc. The patient was given 8,200 cc of Normosol, 3 units of Hetastarch (Hespan), and 900 cc of cellsaver blood. One gram of calcium chloride was given for hypocalcemia.

Critical Appraisal

Abnormal lab results were anticipated because the patient had a large intraoperative blood loss (approximately 60 percent of total blood volume). The patient was anemic but hemodynamically stable with the use of liberal fluid replacement and pharmacologic interventions. Lactic acid can be used intraoperatively as one measure to determine the adequacy of fluid resuscitation. This patient's lactic acid level was high, which could indicate hypovolemia; however, the value can be influenced by multiple factors. The patient also had an increase in glucose as part of the stress response to surgery and blood loss, which I chose not to treat.

Emergence from Anesthesia: Minutes 350–450

Patient is transported to the ICU intubated and sedated. The patient is given 2 mg of midazolam (Versed) prior to transport and requires a low-dose phenylephrine (Neosynephrine) drip to maintain blood pressure. An additional 500 cc of Normosol is given during transport.

Categorical fluid replacement calculation:	Calculated replacement	Actual Given
NPO deficit (1.5 cc × kg × NPO hours)	~ 1,200 cc	1,200
Hourly maintenance fluids (kg + 40 cc)	~ 140 cc/hr	1,050
Insensible surgical loss (5 cc/kg) per hour	After 1st hour (6.5 hours total)	3,200
Estimated blood loss (EBL) (1 cc colloid per 1 cc blood loss) OR (3 cc crystalloid per 1 cc blood loss)	2,400 cc colloid 5,400 cc crystalloid	5,400

[a]The total by this calculation is approximately 10.8 L of crystalloid.

Perioperative fluid therapy is the subject of much controversy, the results of clinical trials investigating the effect of fluid therapy on surgical outcomes are contradictory and original studies on which fluids calculations were based are inadequate. A recent systematic review reached the following conclusions: current standard fluid therapy is not evidence-based; the evaporative loss from the abdominal cavity is highly overestimated; the non-anatomical third space loss is based on inconsistent methodology and may not even exist; and lastly the major rule that should be followed is that fluid lost should be replaced and fluid overload should be avoided (Brandstrup, 2006).

CEBM, level 3a.

Follow-up Care: Arrival in ICU, Minutes 450–515

The ICU is a closed unit with its own team of attending physicians, fellows, and nurse practitioners. I give a full report to the nurse practitioner and ICU attending physician, and they then assume care of the patient. Vital signs are stable, and the patient remains on a low-dose phenylephrine (Neosynephrine) drip at time of transfer.

Assessment

54-year-old African American male presented for general anesthesia (GA) for wide excision of a sarcoma on his right thigh. Past medical history was significant for HTN and type 2 DM. Anesthesia risk was as assessed as ASA

II. This patient was adequately prepared for surgery from both a medical and anesthesia perspective. Special preparation included epoetin alfa (Epogen) and ferrous sulfate (Feosol) supplementation prior to surgery. On the day of surgery the patient's wishes for no blood products were clarified and discussed among team members. Anesthesia and surgical concerns as well as sequelae related to the avoidance of blood and blood products were discussed with the patient and family members. The patient and family agreed with the plan of care to avoid blood, blood products, and albumin along with the use of a closed circuit cell salvage system and hetastarch. The patient had a 445-minute, wide excision of a right thigh mass. Intraoperative frozen section was reported as a high-grade sarcoma. The patient had an estimated blood loss (EBL) of 4,200 cc. The patient was given 8.2 L of crystalloid, 1,500 cc of hetastarch, and 900 cc of cell savaged blood. The patient's urine output was 950 cc. The patient was transferred to the ICU with four large Jackson-Pratt drainage devices. No hardware was placed during the procedure. Although blood loss was larger than expected, the surgery proceeded uneventfully and the patient was managed intraoperatively with crystalloids, hetastarch, and cell salvage techniques. The patient was stable when transferred to the ICU **(D3, C1, PO C)**.

ICD-9 Codes

171.9
401.9
250.0

Encounter Two (postoperative day 1; 16 hours after transfer to ICU)

Anesthesia Follow-up Visit in ICU

Subjective (S)—Patient intubated and family at bedside.

Objective (O)—Afebrile, blood pressure 85/50 (mean arterial pressure [MAP] = 61 mmHg), pulse 90. Phenylephrine (Neosynephrine) drip titrated to maintain a MAP of > 60 mmHg.

Neurologic: Intubated and sedated.

Respiratory: Lungs bilaterally clear to auscultation. No. 8.0 endotracheal tube at 22 cm at teeth secured with harness. Pressure-controlled ventilation, inspiratory pressure = 12, respiratory rate = 10, pressure support = 5, positive end-expiratory pressure = 5, fraction of inspired oxygen = 40%.

Heart: S1, S2 regular rhythm, no murmurs.

Abdomen: Soft, nondistended.

Skin: Large dressing on right thigh, multiple drains with serosanginous fluid.

Medications: Propofol (Diprivan) infusion for sedation, phenylephrine (Neosynephrine) for hemodynamic control.

Invasive lines: All intact and without evidence of infection—right internal jugular 12F introducer, left radial arterial line, 14-gauge right antecubital.

Database

Laboratory Measurement	Result	Reference Range/Units
WBC	7.1	4–11 K/mcL
RBC	?	4.0–5.2 M/mcL
HGB	6.1	11.5–16.0 g/dl
HCT	19.1	34–46%
Platelet	89	160–400 K/mcL
Pro time	14.4	9.8–13.7 seconds
Activated PTT	37	24.4–35.4 seconds
INR	1.6	0.85–1.17 INR
Sodium	144	136–144 mEq/L
Potassium	3.2	3.5–5.1 mEq/L
Chloride	110	98–109 mEq/L
CO_2	26	24–30 mEq/L
Glucose	158	70–99 mg/dl
BUN	14	6–20 mg/dl
Creatinine	1.1	0.6–1.3 mg/dl
Ph	7.41	7.35–7.45
PCO_2	38	35–45
PaO_2	231	85–199 mmHg
HCo_3	19	22–26 mEq/L
HGB	6.5	11.5–16.0 g/dl
HCT	19.3	34–46%
Ionized calcium	4.4	5.0–8.0 mg/dl
Glucose	151	70–99 mg/dl
Lactic acid	2.1	0.7–1.9 mEq/L

Assessment

54-year-old AA male POD1 after wide excision of right thigh sarcoma. Large EBL and no blood products given in observance of patient's religious beliefs. No adverse events as related to anesthetic management. Patient still requires vasoactive support for hemodynamic stability and remains intubated and sedated.

Plan

Defer to ICU team for day-to-day patient management.

CASE SUMMATION

This patient was managed in the ICU with five additional days of epoetin alfa (Epogen) (300 unit/kg/day) and restarted on ferrous sulfate (Feosol) via a nasogastric feeding tube until oral intake was tolerated. The team treated this patient based on supportive therapy and symptom management. Blood pressure was managed by fluid therapy and vasoactive drips, as needed. Electrolytes were replaced as needed, and nutritional support was given via a nasogastric tube. Pharmacologic support was given, and laboratory values were corrected until he could support his own airway. When this occurred, the patient was weaned from the ventilator.

Patient was extubated on POD6 and transferred to the surgical step-down unit on POD14. As per his orthopedic surgeon, the patient is currently several months post surgery, alive and well with limited functioning of right leg. He remains in intensive physical and occupational therapy **(D3, C1, PO C)**.

COMPETENCY DEFENSE

Domain 3, Competency 1. Construct and evaluate outcomes of a culturally sensitive, individualized intervention that addresses the specific needs of a patient in the context of family and community.

Defense. This competency was met by evaluation and assessment of the patient's needs in light of his religious beliefs. An immediate perioperative plan was discussed and implemented with the patient. This included the avoidance of blood products and the use of alternate methods of fluid resuscitation that included hetastarch and an intraoperative cell savage device with use of a leukocyte reduction filter. The plan was evaluated postoperatively, and the patient was found to be stable. Long-term follow-up shows the patient alive and in rehabilitation therapy.

Domain 3, Competency 1. Synthesize the principles of legal and ethical decision-making, and analyze dilemmas that arise in patient care, interprofessional relationships, research, or practice management to improve outcomes.

Defense. The competency was met by examination of my personal biases and consideration of the patient's autonomy versus my duty as a health care provider. I did, however, draw a blood sample for blood typing in case there was an intraoperative emergency. I felt that this action was within the principle of non-maleficence. Additionally, since the hospital's standard legal consent form could not be utilized, I helped to create a special informed consent for nonuse of blood products.

Medications

Drug: Cetirizine Hydrochloride (Zyrtec)

Dose range: 5–10 mg daily.

Method of administration in this case: By mouth.

Mechanism of action: Antihistamine that selectively inhibits the effect of peripheral H1-receptors.

Clinical uses: Allergic rhinitis.

Side effects (common): *Gastrointestinal:* Xerostomia. *Neurologic:* Headache, somnolence. *Other:* Fatigue.

Drug: Calcium Chloride

Dose range: Adults: 0.5–1.0 g/dose over 2–5 minutes (1g = 13.6 mEq [270 mg] of elemental Ca++).

Method of administration in this case: Intravenous.

Mechanism of action: Calcium salt; electrolyte supplement.

Clinical uses: Hypocalcaemia (serum calcium level < 8.5 mg/dL or an ionized calcium level < 4.2 mg/dL).

Side effects
Common: *Gastrointestinal:* Constipation, metallic taste, nausea, vomiting. *Endocrine metabolic:* Hypercalcemia, hypomagnesemia. *Musculoskeletal:* Muscle weakness. *Renal:* Hypercalciuria.
Serious: *Cardiovascular:* Bradyarrhythmia, cardiac arrest (with rapid IV injection), cardiac dysrhythmia (injection), hypertension (injection), hypotension, vasodilatation.

Drug: Clindamycin (Cleocin)

Dose range: 600 or 900 mg every 8 hours.

Method of administration in this case: Intravenous.

Mechanism of action: Binds to 50S ribosomal subunit, interfering with protein synthesis.

Clinical uses: Treatment of susceptible bacterial infections, mainly those caused by anaerobes, streptococci, pneumococci, and staphylococci; bacterial vaginosis (vaginal cream, vaginal suppository); pelvic inflammatory disease (IV); topically in treatment of severe acne; vaginally for *Gardnerella vaginalis*.

Side effects
Common: *Dermatologic:* Rash. *Gastrointestinal:* Diarrhea, nausea.
Serious: *Gastrointestinal:* Pseudomembranous enterocolitis (rare—black box warning). *Hepatic:* Increased liver function test, jaundice.

(continued)

Drug: Epoetin Alfa (Epogen)

Dose range: *Prophylaxis:* Hemoglobin level greater than 10 g/dL and up to 13 g/dL, 300 U/kg/day subcutaneously for 10 days before surgery, on the day of surgery, and for 4 days after OR 600 U/kg subcutaneously once weekly at 21, 14, and 7 days prior to surgery plus a fourth dose on the day of surgery; all patients should receive iron supplements, and deep vein prophylaxis should be strongly considered. *Anemia:* 10,000 U 3 times a week to 40,000–60,000 units once weekly.

Method of administration in this case: Subcutaneous.

Mechanism of action: Glycoprotein that exerts the same biological effects as endogenous erythropoietin, which is produced in the kidney. It stimulates the division and differentiation of committed erythroid progenitors in the bone marrow, increasing red blood cell production.

Clinical uses: Treatment of anemia.

Side effects
Common: *Dermatologic:* Pain of skin at injection site, pruritus, rash. *Gastrointestinal:* Constipation, diarrhea, indigestion, nausea, vomiting. *Musculoskeletal:* Arthralgia. *Neurologic:* Dizziness, headache, insomnia, paresthesias. *Respiratory:* Cough, dyspnea, pulmonary congestion, upper respiratory infection. *Other:* Fever.
Serious: *Cardiovascular:* Edema, hypertension.

Drug: Fentanyl (Sublimaze)

Dose range: 2–50 mcg/kg.

Method of administration in this case: Intravenous.

Mechanism of action: Opioid analgesic.

Clinical uses: Pain control.

Side effects
Common: *Cardiovascular:* Peripheral edema, tachyarrythmias. *Endocrine metabolic:* Dehydration, weight loss. *Gastrointestinal:* Abdominal pain, constipation, diarrhea, loss of appetite, nausea, vomiting. *Musculoskeletal:* Backache. *Neurologic:* Asthenia, confusion, dizziness, headache, sedation. *Renal:* Urinary retention. *Respiratory:* Cough.
Serious: *Respiratory:* Apnea.

Drug: Ferrous Sulfate (Feosol)

Dose range: *Prophylaxis:* Oral: 1–2 mg Fe/kg/day up to a maximum of 15 mg/day. *Treatment of mild to moderate iron-deficiency anemia:* Oral: 3 mg Fe/kg/day in 1–2 divided doses. *Treatment of severe iron-deficiency anemia:* Oral: 4–6 mg Fe/kg/day in 3 divided doses.

Method of administration in this case: By mouth.

(continued)

Mechanism of action: Iron is absorbed in the duodenum and upper jejunum; in persons with normal serum iron stores, 10 percent of an oral dose is absorbed; this is increased to 20 to 30 percent in persons with inadequate iron stores. Food and achlorhydria will decrease absorption.

Clinical uses: Exogenous iron supplement for the treatment of anemia.

Side effects (common): *Gastrointestinal:* Constipation, dark stools, epigastric pain, GI irritation, nausea, stomach cramping, vomiting, diarrhea, heartburn. *Genitourinary:* Discoloration of urine. *Other:* Contact irritation.

Drug: Hetastarch (Hespan)

Dose range: 500–1,000 mL IV per day; maximum 1,500 mL/day (approximately 20 mL/kg).

Method of administration in this case: Intravenous.

Mechanism of action: Volume expander—synthetic polymer derived from a waxy starch composed of amylopectin.

Clinical uses: Hypovolemia.

Side effects (serious): *Hematologic:* Blood coagulation disorder. *Hepatic:* Hepatotoxicity. *Neurologic:* Intracranial hemorrhage.

Drug: Hydromorphone (Dilaudid)

Dose range: Initial (opiate-naive patients), 0.75–1.00 mg IV every 2 hours as needed; usual, 1–2 mg IV (slow) every 4 to 6 hours as needed. Patient-controlled analgesia (PCA) = concentration 0.2 mg/mL; basal IV infusion up to 0.2 mg/hr; usual bolus dose is 0.1–0.2 mg (range 0.05–0.50 mg) with lockout period 5 to 15 minutes.

Method of administration in this case: Intravenous.

Mechanism of action: Pure opioid agonist.

Clinical uses: Acute or chronic pain.

Side effects
Common: *Gastrointestinal:* Loss of appetite, nausea, vomiting. *Neurologic:* Asthenia, dizziness, sedation somnolence. *Cardiovascular:* Hypotension (frequent). *Neurologic:* Confusion, myoclonus, seizure.
Serious: *Respiratory:* Apnea, respiratory depression.

Drug: Isoflurane (Forane)

Dose range: Minimum alveolar concentration (MAC) is 1.1%. (The MAC of an inhaled anesthetic is the alveolar concentration that prevents movement in 50 percent of patients in response to a standardized stimulus, such as a surgical incision. MAC mirrors brain partial pressure and allows comparisons of potency between agents.)

Method of administration in this case: Inhalation.

(continued)

Mechanism of action: Nonflammable volatile anesthetic.

Clinical uses: Main component of general anesthesia delivered via endotracheal tube.

Side effects
Common: *Cardiovascular:* Hypotension. *Respiratory:* Respiratory depression.
Serious: *Other:* Dysrhythmias. *Neurologic:* Seizures. *Other:* malignant hyperthermia, hepatotoxicity.

Drug: Lidocaine (Xylocaine)

Dose range: 0.7–1.4 mcg/kg, usually followed by a drip 1–4 mcg/min.

Method of administration in this case: Intravenous.

Mechanism of action: Amide local anesthetic that blocks voltage-gated sodium channels from inside the cell, preventing subsequent channel activation and interfering with the large transient sodium influx associated with membrane depolarization.

Clinical uses: Anti-arrhythmic, adjunct for local anesthesia or Blunts airway reflexes in response to instrumentation.

Side effects
Common: *Dermatologic:* Edema, erythema at injection site, injection site pain, pruritis. *Gastrointestinal:* Nausea, vomiting. *Musculoskeletal:* Backache. *Neurologic:* loss of consciousness (LOC), seizure, dizziness, headache, light-headedness, numbness, paresthesias, shivering, somnolence. *Ophthalmic:* Blurred vision, burning sensation in eye, diplopia. *Psychiatric:* Apprehension, confusion, euphoria, feeling nervous.
Serious: *Cardiovascular:* Bradyarrhythmia, hypotension, arrest, heart block.

Drug: Metformin (Glucophage)

Dose range: Initial: 500 mg orally twice daily or 850 mg orally once daily. Maintenance: 1,000–2,550 mg orally daily in 2 to 3 divided doses (maximum 2,550 mg/day).

Method of administration in this case: By mouth.

Mechanism of action: Lowers basal and postprandial glucose levels in type 2 diabetes patients through several mechanisms: decreases hepatic glucose production, decreases intestinal absorption, and increases peripheral glucose uptake and utilization by improving insulin sensitivity.

Clinical uses: Oral antihyperglycemic agent.

Side effects
Common: *Endocrine* metabolic: Cobalamin deficiency. *Gastrointestinal:* Diarrhea, flatulence, indigestion, nausea, vomiting. *Neurologic:* Asthenia.
Serious: *Endocrine metabolic:* Lactic acidosis (rare).

(continued)

Drug: Midazolam (Versed)

Dose range: 0.30–0.35 mg/kg over 20 to 30 seconds (allowing 2 minutes for effect). Dose adjusted for comorbidities.

Method of administration in this case: Intravenous.

Mechanism of action: Short-acting benzodiazepine central nervous system (CNS) depressant, reversibly interacts with gamma-amino butyric acid (GABA) receptors in the central nervous system.

Clinical uses: Sedative or adjunct to anesthesia.

Side effects
Common: *Gastrointexstinal:* Nausea and vomiting. *Neurologic:* Involuntary movement. *Psychiatric:* Agitation.
Serious: *Cardiovascular:* Cardiac arrest, usually in combinations with CNS depressant drug (rare), hypotensive episode (rare). *Respiratory:* Apnea, respiratory arrest with CNS depressant drugs (rare), respiratory depression.

Drug: Metoprolol (Toprol, Metoprolol)

Dose range: *Immediate release:* Initial: 50 mg twice daily (usual dosage range 50–200 mg twice daily; maximum 400 mg/day). Increase dose at weekly intervals to desired effect.
    Extended release: Initial: 100 mg/day (maximum: 400 mg/day).

Method of administration in this case: By mouth, intravenous.

Mechanism of action: Beta-adrenergic blocker with selective activity on beta 1-adrenoreceptors located mainly in cardiac muscles. At higher doses, it also inhibits beta 2-adrenoreceptors of bronchial and vascular smooth muscles.

Clinical uses: Control of hypertension, angina, congestive heart failure, arrhythmias, and myocardial infarctions.

Side effects
Common: *Cardiovascular:* Bradyarrhythmia, cold extremities, hypotension. *Dermatologic:* Pruritus, rash. *Gastrointestinal:* Constipation, diarrhea, indigestion, nausea. *Neurologic:* Dizziness, fatigue, headache. *Psychiatric:* Depression. *Respiratory:* Dyspnea, wheezing.
Serious: Heart failure.

Drug: Phenylephrine (Neosynephrine)

Dose range: Initial: 100–180 mcg/min. Continuous maintenance: 40–80 mcg/min or 0.5 mcg/kg/min; titrate to desired response. Dosing ranges between 0.4 and 9.1 mcg/kg/min have been reported.

Method of administration in this case: Intravenous.

(continued)

Mechanism of action: Sympathomimetic agent, differing from epinephrine only in lacking a hydroxyl (OH) group in the 4 position on the benzene ring. Powerful postsynaptic alpha-receptor stimulant with little effect on beta-receptors in the heart. Peripheral resistance increases considerably due to constriction of most vascular beds and both systolic and diastolic blood pressure increases. Marked reflex bradycardia can occur.

Clinical uses: Multiple uses, but when used for hypotension or shock, the drug is used in higher doses.

Side effects
Common: *CNS:* Anxiety, dizziness, excitability, giddiness, headache, insomnia, nervousness, restlessness. *Neuromuscular and skeletal:* Paresthesias, pilomotor response, tremor, weakness. *Renal:* Decreased renal perfusion, reduced urine output.
Serious: *Cardiovascular:* Arrhythmia (rare), decreased cardiac output, hypertension, pallor, precordial pain or discomfort, reflex bradycardia, severe peripheral and visceral vasoconstriction. *Endocrine and metabolic:* Metabolic acidosis. *Gastrointestinal:* Gastric irritation, nausea. *Local:* IV: Extravasation that may lead to necrosis and sloughing of surrounding tissue, blanching of skin. *Respiratory:* Respiratory distress. *Other:* Hypersensitivity reactions (including rash, urticaria, leukopenia, agranulocytosis, thrombocytopenia).

Drug: Propofol (Diprivan)

Dose range: 2.0–2.5 mcg/kg.

Method of administration in this case: Intravenous.

Mechanism of action: Short-acting sedative or hypnotic. Its mechanism of action has not been well defined.

Clinical uses: Induction agent, general anesthetic or sedation (dose dependent).

Side effects (serious): *Cardiovascular:* Bradyarrhythmia, heart failure, hypotension. *Immunologic:* Anaphylaxis (rare). *Neurologic:* Seizure, myoclonus. *Renal:* Acute renal failure.
    Reproductive: Priapism. *Respiratory:* Apnea, respiratory acidosis. *Other:* Bacterial septicemia, pain on injection.

Drug: Rocuronium (Zemuron)

Dose range: 0.6–1.2 mg/kg IV (intubation, higher dose range for rapid sequence intubation), 0.1–0.2 mg/kg IV push (maintenance).

Method of administration in this case: Intravenous.

Mechanism of action: Non-depolarizing neuromuscular agent with intermediate duration of action. It competes with acetylcholine for receptors at the motor endplate and results in neuromuscular blockade.

(continued)

Clinical uses: Muscle relaxation or to facilitate endotracheal intubation.

Side effects

Common: *Dermatologic:* Injection site pain.

Serious: *Cardiovascular:* Cardiac dysrhythmia (rare), hypertension, hypotension, tachyarrhythmia (rare). *Immunologic:* Anaphylaxis (rare).

Source: All drug information from Micromedex Healthcare Series—available through institutional or personal license at www.micromedex.com.

References

Barakat, O., Cooper, J.R., Jr., Riggs, S.A., Hoef, J.W., Ozaki, C.F., & Wood, R.P. (2007). Complex liver resection for a large intrahepatic cholangiocarcinoma in a Jehovah's witness: A strategy to avoid transfusion. *Journal of Surgical Oncology, 96*(3), 249–253.

Brandstrup, B. (2006). Fluid therapy for the surgical patient. *Best Practice and Research Clinical Anaesthesiology, 20*(2), 265–283.

Catling, S., Williams, S., Freites, O., Rees, M., Davies, C., & Hopkins, L. (2008). Use of a leucocyte filter to remove tumour cells from intra-operative cell salvage blood. *Anaesthesia, 63*(12), 1332–1338.

Clark, M.A., Fisher, C., Judson, I., & Thomas, J.M. (2005). Soft-tissue sarcomas in adults. *New England Journal of Medicine, 353*(7), 701–711.

Dellinger, E.P., Hausmann, S.M., Bratzler, D.W., Johnson, R.M., Daniel, D.M., Bunt, K.M., et al. (2005). Hospitals collaborate to decrease surgical site infections. *American Journal of Surgery, 190*(1), 9–15.

Dixon, J.L., & Smalley, M.G. (1981). Jehovah's Witnesses. The surgical/ethical challenge. *Journal of the American Medical Association, 246*(21), 2471–2472.

Faris, P.M., Ritter, M.A., & Abels, R.I. (1996). The effects of recombinant human erythropoietin on perioperative transfusion requirements in patients having a major orthopaedic operation. The American Erythropoietin Study Group. *Journal of Bone Joint Surgery of America, 78*(1), 62–72.

FDA. (2009). *Postmarket drug safety information for patients and providers—ESA.* Retrieved June 1, 2009 from http://www.fda.gov/Drugs/DrugSafety/PostmarketDrugSafetyInformation forPatientsandProviders/UCM109375

Fleisher, L.A. (2002). Preoperative evaluation of the patient with hypertension. *Journal of the American Medical Association, 287*(16), 2043–2046.

Fleisher, L.A., Beckman, J.A., Brown, K.A., Calkins, H., Chaikof, E.L., Fleischmann, K.E., et al. (2007). ACC/AHA 2007 guidelines on perioperative cardiovascular evaluation and care for noncardiac surgery: Executive summary: A report of the American College of Cardiology/American Heart Association Task Force on Practice Guidelines (Writing Committee to Revise the 2002 Guidelines on Perioperative Cardiovascular Evaluation for Noncardiac Surgery) developed in collaboration with the American Society of Echocardiography, American Society of Nuclear Cardiology, Heart Rhythm Society, Society of Cardiovascular Anesthesiologists, Society for Cardiovascular Angiography and Interventions, Society for Vascular Medicine and Biology, and Society for Vascular Surgery. *Journal of the American College of Cardiology, 50*(17), 1707–1732.

Gyamfi, C., & Yasin, S.Y. (2000). Preparation for an elective surgical procedure in a Jehovah's Witness: A review of the treatments and alternatives for anemia. *Primary Care Update for OB/GYNS, 7*(6), 266–268.

Horlocker, T.T., Wedel, D.J., Benzon, H., Brown, D.L., Enneking, K.F., Heit, J.A., et al. (2004). Regional anesthesia in the anticoagulated patient: Defining the risks. *Regional Anesthesia and Pain Medicine, 29*(Suppl 1), 1–11.

Magner, D., Ouellette, J.R., Lee, J.R., Colquhoun, S., Lo, S., & Nissen, N.N. (2006). Pancreaticoduodenectomy after neoadjuvant therapy in a Jehovah's witness with locally advanced pancreatic cancer: Case report and approach to avoid transfusion. *American Surgical Journal, 72*(5), 435–437.

Martyn, V., Farmer, S.L., Wren, M.N., Towler, S.C.B., Betta, J., Shander, A., et al. (2002). The theory and practice of bloodless surgery. *Transfusion and Apheresis Science, 27*(1), 29–43.

McAnulty, G.R., Robertshaw, H.J., & Hall, G.M. (2000). Anaesthetic management of patients with diabetes mellitus. *British Journal of Anaesthesia, 85*(1), 80–90.

Misra, A., Mistry, N., Grimer, R., & Peart, F. (2009). The management of soft tissue sarcoma. *Journal of Plastic Reconstructive Aesthetic Surgery, 62*(2), 161–174.

Nieder, A.M., Manoharan, M., Yang, Y., & Soloway, M.S. (2007). Intraoperative cell salvage during radical cystectomy does not affect long-term survival. *Urology, 69*(5), 881–884.

Singelenberg, R. (1990). The blood transfusion taboo of Jehovah's Witnesses: Origin, development and function of a controversial doctrine. *Social Science Medicine, 31*(4), 515–523.

Wolters, U., Wolf, T., Stutzer, H., & Schroder, T. (1996). ASA classification and perioperative variables as predictors of postoperative outcome. *British Journal of Anaesthesia, 77*(2), 217–222.

Wulf, H. (1996). Epidural anaesthesia and spinal haematoma. *Canadian Journal of Anaesthesia, 43*(12), 1260–1271.

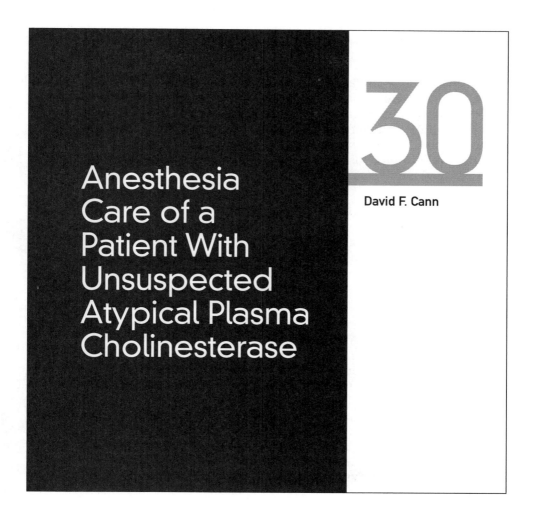

30

Anesthesia Care of a Patient With Unsuspected Atypical Plasma Cholinesterase

David F. Cann

This case narrative describes the care I provided for a 16-year-old female with commercial insurance who presented for extraction of impacted wisdom teeth. The case narrative focuses on one encounter that lasted approximately 420 minutes. After an uneventful surgical course, the patient failed to initiate spontaneous ventilations during the emergence from general anesthesia. Care was provided in the Ambulatory Surgery Center. This case narrative demonstrates my ability to meet the following Columbia University School of Nursing (CUSN) doctoral competencies for comprehensive direct patient care.

DOMAIN 1, COMPETENCY 1

Evaluate patient needs based on age, developmental stage, family history, ethnicity, and individual risk, including genetic profile, to formulate plans for health promotion, anticipatory guidance, counseling, and disease prevention services for healthy or sick patients and their families in any clinical setting.

PO A. Identify a potential genetic risk.

PO C. Evaluate individual patient needs based on age, developmental stage, family history, ethnicity, and individual risk.

PO D. Formulate a plan that addresses health promotion, anticipatory guidance, and/or disease prevention for the individual.

PO E. Develop a plan that addresses health promotion, anticipatory guidance, and/or disease prevention for the family.

DOMAIN 1, COMPETENCY 3

Formulate differential diagnoses and diagnostic strategies and therapeutic interventions with attention to scientific evidence, safety, cost, invasiveness, simplicity, acceptability, adherence, and efficacy for patients who present with new conditions and those with ambiguous or incomplete data, complex illnesses, comorbid conditions, and multiple diagnoses in all clinical settings.

PO A. Formulate a differential diagnosis for a patient who presents with new, undifferentiated signs and symptoms.

PO C. Discuss the rationale for the differential diagnosis.

PO D. Discuss the rationale for the diagnostic evaluation with attention to scientific evidence, safety, cost, invasiveness, simplicity, acceptability, adherence, and efficacy.

PO E. Discuss the rationale for the therapeutic intervention with attention to scientific evidence, safety, cost, invasiveness, simplicity, acceptability, adherence, and efficacy.

DOMAIN 1, COMPETENCY 5

Evaluate and direct care during hospitalization, and design a comprehensive discharge plan for patients from an acute care setting.

PO A. Assess the acuity of the patient's condition and determine the most appropriate inpatient treatment setting based on level of acuity.

PO B. Actively participate in the admission process to the appropriate inpatient treatment setting.

PO C. Actively co-manage patient care during hospitalization.

PO D. Formulate plan for ongoing care to be provided in a subacute setting, such as a long-term care facility, rehabilitation facility, or home or community setting.

PO E. Coordinate ongoing comprehensive care to be provided in a subacute setting, such as a long-term care facility, rehabilitation facility, or home or community setting.

ENCOUNTER CONTEXT

Encounter One (day of scheduled elective surgery)

DNP role: I am a certified registered nurse anesthetist (CRNA) and DNP resident assuming the responsibility of providing anesthesia and perioperative care for this patient.

Identifying Information

Site: Rural, 10-bed critical access hospital.

Setting: Outpatient surgery center.

Reason for encounter: Patient admission for extraction of wisdom teeth under general anesthesia.

Informant: Information is obtained from the patient and her mother. The patient's mother is present throughout the history and physical examination. Parental consent is obtained because the patient is a minor.

Initial encounter (zero minutes)

Chief complaint: "I need to have my wisdom teeth pulled. I have never had surgery before."

History of present illness: 16-year-old Caucasian female presents to the outpatient surgery center for extraction of four impacted wisdom teeth under general anesthesia. The patient has no prior history of having general anesthesia. Patient has had nothing by mouth for more than 10 hours. She denies history of adverse reaction to anesthetic agents.

> *Having had prior general anesthesia without a significant adverse outcome tells the CRNA that there is a high likelihood that the patient is not at risk for developing malignant hyperthermia, a genetically linked, potentially fatal reaction to anesthetic agents. Having had no significant adverse outcomes in the past will also lead the anesthetist to believe that airway management has been successful in the past and therefore will likely be a non-issue for an impending intubation (Merah, Wong, Foulkes-Crabbe, Kushimo, & Bode, 2005).*
> Oxford Centre for Evidence-Based Medicine (CEBM), level 2a.

She denies a history of cardiac, pulmonary, endocrine, hematologic, or neurologic disease.

Current medications: None.

Allergies: No known food, drug, or environmental allergies.

Hospitalizations: None.

Past medical history: Denies any medical illness including history of neurologic, cardiac, pulmonary, gastrointestinal, renal, metabolic, hematologic, or musculoskeletal disease.

Surgical history: Denies previous surgery and anesthesia experience.

Social history: The patient lives with her biological mother, stepfather, and two half-brothers. She is finishing her junior year of high school. She denies tobacco, alcohol, or drug abuse. She claims to not be sexually active. Her mother is supportive of her care.

Family history: Denies a family history of anesthetic complications.

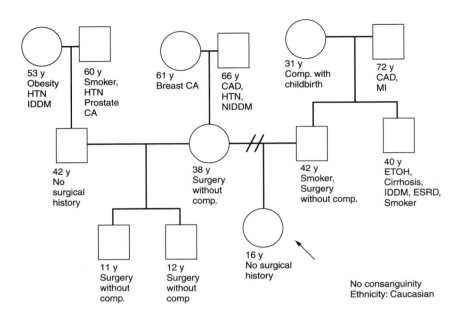

Review of Systems

Constitutional: Denies weakness, fatigue, fever, chills, or recent weight change.

Neurologic: Denies history of somnolence, loss of consciousness, convulsive states, alteration in gait, tremors, paresis, paralysis, headache.

HEENT: Denies history of head injury. Denies itching, redness, edema, laceration of eyes, or vision changes. Denies ear discharge, hearing loss, tinnitus, or vertigo. Denies history of sinusitis, rhinitis, nasal congestion, or epistaxis. No difficulty swallowing.

Respiratory: Denies current pulmonary problems, including pneumonia or bronchitis, pain, dyspnea, cough, abnormal sputum production, hemoptysis, wheezing.

Cardiac: Denies chest pain, dyspnea, syncope, hypertension, or heart murmur.

Vascular: Denies history or symptoms of claudication, varicose veins, phlebitis, edema, or cyanosis.

Gastrointestinal: Denies food intolerance, dysphasia, abdominal pain, vomiting, constipation, diarrhea, blood in stool, liver disease.

Gynecologic/Genitourinary: Denies urinary pain, oliguria, polyuria, hematuria, pyuria, or incontinence. Last menstrual period (LMP) one week ago.

Musculoskeletal: Ambulates without any difficulty. Denies pain, tenderness or weakness in extremities. No history of fractures.

Endocrine: Denies changes in growth or weight, polyuria, or excessive sweating.

Skin: Denies rashes, sores, itching, dryness, or changes in hair or nails.

Hematologic: Denies easy bruising or bleeding. Denies history of blood transfusion.

Physical Examination

Vital signs: Blood pressure 101/64 (patient is seated, small adult cuff), HR 80, temp 98.4°F, resp 20, SpO_2 on room air 100%, weight 59.1 kg, height 170.2 cm, BMI 21.3.

Appearance: Thin, healthy-appearing female.

Neurologic: Alert, oriented × 3, cooperative, and coherent. Cranial nerves II-XII intact. Pin prick and light touch intact. Motor 5/5 all extremities and equal bilaterally. Tone without rigidity. Coordination is intact.

Airway: Mucosa and gingivae are pink and intact. No bleeding observed. Teeth are intact without damage or decay. Full mandibular range of motion with a thyromental distance of 3 fingerbreadths (> 6 cm). Mallampatti classification of I reveals full view of uvula. She is thin stature, has full range of motion of her neck, and denies a history of neck, jaw or back injuries.

> *A Mallampatti classification of III or IV coupled with a thyromental distance of less than 6cm and decreased cervical range of motion indicates a potential for difficult intubating conditions (Merahet al., 2005).*
>
> CEBM, level 1.

Skin: Warm and dry. Nail without clubbing, brisk capillary refill. Appropriate hair distribution, no edema.

Head: Normocephalic, symmetric, no weakness noted. No trauma apparent.

Eyes: Pupils equal round, react to light, brisk responses. No redness or discharge present.

Ears: Tympanic membranes pearl-gray without redness, discharge, or inflammation. Hearing grossly intact.

Nose: No deformities, obstruction, or discharge.

Neck: Supple, no masses, tender in right mandibular region. Trachea midline, thyroid palpable. No jugular venous distention (JVD).

Chest: Respiratory rate regular and unlabored. Symmetric chest expansion. All lung fields without adventitious sounds.

Heart: S1, S2 present. Heart rate slow and regular, no murmurs.

Abdomen: Symmetric, non-obese, non-rigid, bowel sounds present in four quadrants, non-tender.

Musculoskeletal: No prostheses or scars. No open fractures or deformities. She ambulates without difficulty.

Laboratory Data Review
None ordered or reviewed.

Impression
16-year-old female with no significant medical history to undergo general anesthesia for removal of wisdom teeth.

Education:15 Minutes

I explain the anesthetic procedure, including risks and benefits to the patient and her mother. I answer all questions and obtain informed consent **(D1, C5, PO A, B).**

Time Line of Patient Care

20 Minutes

- A 20-gauge intravenous line is started by the registered nurse into the dorsal surface of the right hand.

30 Minutes

- I accompany the patient to the operating room, where I apply the standard monitors.
- Initial vital signs: Blood pressure 111/67, heart rate 88, respirations 24, 100% room air. Lead II = normal sinus rhythm (NSR).
- I administer midazolam (Versed) 2 mg and fentanyl (Sublimaze)100 mcg intravenously. I pre-oxygenate and induce with 120 mg of propofol (Diprivan) and 60 mg of succinylcholine (Anectine). I perform an atraumatic laryngoscopy, and tracheal intubation is achieved. I then administer desflurane (Suprane) 6.0% with 50/50 nitrous oxide/oxygen at a 2-liter/minute flow.

30–110 Minutes

- I maintain a level of general anesthesia for the patient while continuously monitoring for changes in condition.
- I document vital statistics, depth of anesthesia, blood loss, and fluid balance at a minimum of every five minutes. Blood pressures ranges from 80/52 to

121/69, heart rate ranges from 74 to 89, blood loss is minimal, and 900 mL of intravenous lactated Ringer's solution is administered.

110 Minutes

- Surgical wound is closed.
- I initiate the emergence from anesthesia. 100% FiO_2 is administered with desflurane (Suprane) off. I hypoventilate the patient to accumulate $PaCO_2$. No spontaneous ventilation by the patient is evident.
- I perform a peripheral nerve assessment with a train-of-four monitor, which reveals 0/4 twitches.

A train of four is a peripheral nerve monitoring technique that involves administration of four electrical stimuli, each 0.5 seconds apart, that are applied to the body surface over a predetermined nerve. Commonly used nerves are the facial and ulnar nerves. If there is a muscular response to 0/4 impulses then there is minimal neuromuscular activity present. If the response is 4/4, then there is maximum return of neuromuscular functioning. 1, 2 or 3 twitch responses indicate 25%, 50% or 75% return of neuromuscular functioning respectively (Rowlee, 1999).

CEBM, level 2a.

- A second peripheral monitor is used to rule out equipment problems. The result continues to be 0/4 twitches.
- I notify the surgeon.
- I reassure the patient verbally that I am helping her breathe right now and she will soon be able to do so herself.
- I started a propofol (Diprivan) infusion at 50 mcg/kg/min to maintain an adequate depth of anesthesia while she remains paralyzed, and I continue to monitor her vital signs, which are essentially unchanged from her baseline **(D1, C5, PO A, C).**

Assessment

An unanticipated prolonged neuromuscular blockade is observed in this patient, who had been given an intubating dose of 60 mg succinylcholine (Anectine) 80 minutes prior. During emergence from general anesthesia, the patient was to be weaned from the ventilator. When spontaneous ventilation was not initiated, a train-of-four test was performed. The findings demonstrated evidence of minimal return of neuromuscular functioning.

Succinylcholine (Anectine) is a commonly used depolarizing neuromuscular blocking agent that is used to facilitate endotracheal intubation. The unique benefit of this medication is its fast onset of 30–60 seconds and relatively short duration of action of four to six minutes. The short duration of action is due to its metabolism by plasma cholinesterase at the neuromuscular junction. A prolongation of action ranging from 10 minutes to 10 hours is seen when there is an impairment or deficiency in the plasma cholinesterase.

Prolonged neuromuscular blockade can be caused by factors other than atypical pseudocholinesterase, therefore, other factors must be ruled out prior to concluding that the paralysis is due to an inherited condition.

Hypokalemia, hypocalcemia, and hypermagnesaemia can produce prolonged neuromuscular blockade. Hypothermia and impaired ability to metabolize medications via renal or hepatic biotransformation must also be considered when there is an unanticipated prolongation of paralysis from neuromuscular blocking agents (Leadingham, 2007).

CEBM. level 1.

A deficiency or abnormality of plasma cholinesterase levels will prolong neuromuscular blockade when succinylcholine (Anectine) is used. Atypical pseudocholinesterase activity can be inherited or acquired as in the case of advanced renal disease, liver disease, malnutrition, burns or malignancy (Leadingham, 2007).

CEBM, level 1.

The incidence of inherited, homozygous atypical plasma cholinesterase function is estimated to be 1:3,200 (Morneault et al., 2007).

CEBM, level 1.

This 16-year-old woman has no underlying disease process that leads me to believe that the prolongation of paralysis is due to an acquired condition. She does not have evidence of hypothermia because her core temperature is 98.0. I will obtain a basic metabolic panel to evaluate serum potassium, calcium, and magnesium **(D1, C3, PO A, C, D, E)**.

120 Minutes

- I perform a peripheral venous blood draw for complete blood count (CBC) and basic metabolic profile (BMP).

140 Minutes

- I review the laboratory data. The CBC and BMP are within normal range, including calcium, potassium, magnesium, and total protein. There is no evidence of renal or liver disease.

145 Minutes

- I suspect the patient has a plasma cholinesterase dysfunction.
- Further diagnostic testing is indicated.
- I contact the laboratory regarding plasma cholinesterase level assessment and dibucaine number.
- I am informed that the laboratory will need to send this sample to an exterior location and the results will take a minimum of three days to be returned.

- I draw the blood samples and send them for analysis.
- The surgeon and I speak with the family about the suspected plasma cholinesterase dysfunction and explain her need for temporary ventilatory support **(D1, C1, PO A, C, D)**.

165 Minutes

- I transport the patient to the post-anesthesia unit with full monitoring.
- I continue the propofol (Diprivan) infusion and ventilator support.
- Train of four reveals 0/4 twitches.
- I continue to monitor vital signs, which remain stable. I am evaluating depth of anesthesia and degree of neuromuscular blockade on a continuum **(D1, C5, PO C)**.

220 Minutes

- Train of four reveals 1/4 twitches. Her vital signs remain stable.

245 Minutes

- Train of four reveals 2/4 twitches. Her vital signs are at baseline.

270 Minutes

- Train of four reveals 3/4 twitches. She maintains stable blood pressures and heart rate.

300 Minutes

- Train of four reveals 4/4 twitches with greater than 4/10 seconds of sustained tetany present. I discontinue the propofol (Diprivan) infusion. Sustained tetany combined with train-of-four results of 4/4 indicate that > 90 percent of neuromuscular functioning has returned. Because of this return, she will be able to resume spontaneous ventilations and will no longer require propofol (Diprivan) sedation **(D1, C5, PO C)**.

315 Minutes

- Patient spontaneously breathing with tidal volumes greater than 300 cc, demonstrating adequate return of neuromuscular functioning. I determine that she is able to follow commands and demonstrate a sustained head lift for greater than five seconds. I remove the endotracheal tube and she maintains spontaneous ventilations. SaO_2 100% on room air **(D1, C5, PO C)**.

330 Minutes

- Patient awake, alert, oriented, denies pain, denies nausea, and denies recollection of events during initial emergence.

420 Minutes

- I speak with the patient and her mother and give them a detailed letter explaining the events of her anesthesia course.
- I explain that the plasma cholinesterase levels and dibucaine number results will be sent directly to her surgeon and her primary care provider.
- I instruct the patient and her family to follow up with her primary care provider in the immediate future to discuss the likelihood of plasma cholinesterase dysfunction and how this will affect her and her family members in the future.
- I discharge the patient to home from the post-anesthesia care unit.
- I give a copy of the letter to the surgeon.
- I place a copy of the letter in her medical record.

(D1, C5, PO D, E.)

Case Summation

I administered general anesthesia to this 16-year-old female to facilitate comfort for removal of four wisdom teeth. During emergence from anesthesia following an uneventful surgical course, the patient was unable to initiate spontaneous ventilations. This finding led me to perform an assessment of neuromuscular functioning with a train-of-four monitor. Based on the 0/4 reading of the train of four, I determined that the patient was likely still paralyzed from the succinylcholine (Anectine) that was administered during induction of anesthesia.

Prolongation of the effects of succinylcholine (Anectine) is attributed to either a "phase two" block or atypical plasma cholinesterase. Since a phase two block was not possible due to the limited dosing of the medication, it was determined that the patient was likely experiencing the effects of atypical plasma cholinesterase.

ICD-9 Codes

Dental impaction (528.3)
Atypical plasma cholinesterase (289.89)

Addendum

Although I had no direct contact with this patient following this procedure, the surgeon informed me that the patient was stable with no reported surgical complications at both of her postoperative appointments. The surgeon also told me that the laboratory results indicated atypical plasma cholinesterase levels of 2,671 U/L (normal range = 5,200–12,800). The dibucaine number was 33 percent (normal is greater than 80 percent). Both indicated atypical plasma cholinesterase functioning. He assured me that the primary provider would follow up with the patient regarding referral for genetic counseling for both her and her family members.

Critical Appraisal

Much research has been focused on the detection and treatment of atypical plasma cholinesterase. In the situation in the operating room, it was of greatest importance to treat the immediate condition and then focus investigations on finding an underlying cause and possible treatment. The priority for this patient was to provide adequate ventilatory support, reassure the patient since the anesthetics had presumably worn off leaving the patient potentially coherent but paralyzed, and finally, provide adequate sedation until the patient was fully able to maintain her own respiratory efforts. When these conditions were met, it was then a priority to further investigate and draw laboratory diagnostics to establish possible causes for the condition.

> *Treatment goals include providing immediate reassurance, sedation, and venti-lation. Electrolyte values must be obtained and blood for plasma cholinesterase values should be obtained. Other causes should be considered and family history needs to be scrutinized for past problems with anesthesia. Sedation and venti-lation must be maintained until there is clear evidence of full neuromuscular functioning. After extubation, the patient and family, when applicable, must be counseled and referred for genetic testing (Ramirez et al., 2005).*
>
> CEBM, level 2c.

Screening all patients for this condition prior to administration of anesthesia is not feasible. Although advances have been made in identifying specific genotypes that might indicate the presence of abnormal plasma cholinesterase function, it is not practical to subject every patient to such screening. In addition to the added time and blood work required, it would also create a financial burden on both the patient and the health care providers.

> *The molecular genetic methods of genotyping must be both efficient and cost effective to be considered a viable pre-screening option. Although screening for a single genetic abnormality or sequencing an entire gene may be practical for someone with a suspected plasma cholinesterase abnormality, it would not be practical to fully screen all patients (Levano et al., 2005).*
>
> CEBM, level 3a.

Since genetic screening is not a viable option, the best screening method is based on patient history. Since the condition is primarily inherited, it can often be learned from parents or siblings that there is a possibility of the disorder being present. A surgical history might also reveal signs of the disorder. Careful atten-tion must be paid to any abnormal surgical history findings.

It is, however, practical to screen a patient and family members if there is a suspicion of the presence of deficient or atypical plasma cholinesterase function-ing. The patient in this scenario was referred to her primary care physician for further testing and genetic counseling.

(continued)

Conducting a routine evaluation by biochemical analysis of plasma cholinesterase activity as well as obtaining a dibucaine number is usually sufficient to confirm the presence of an abnormality of genetic origin. The benefit of screening family members and providing genetic counseling is evident (Cerf et al., 2002).

CEBM, level 2b.

A 2003 study of 32 patients showed that when a known or suspected case of atypical plasma cholinesterase comes to the operating room and requires a medication such as succinylcholine, careful titration and decreased intubating doses may be enough to offset the increased duration, increased potency, and decreased clearance of the drug (Ostergaard et al., 2003).

COMPETENCY DEFENSE

Domain 1, Competency 1. Evaluate patient needs based on age, developmental stage, family history, ethnicity, and individual risk, including genetic profile, to formulate plans for health promotion, anticipatory guidance, counseling, and disease prevention services for healthy or sick patients and their families in any clinical setting.

Defense. I evaluated the patient's specific needs as they related to her family history, individual risk, and genetic profile. I identified the potential genetic risk of atypical plasma cholinesterase as it coincided with her abnormal clinical presentation of prolonged paralysis following the administration of succinylcholine (Anectine).

Domain 1, Competency 3. Formulate differential diagnoses and diagnostic strategies and therapeutic interventions with attention to scientific evidence, safety, cost, invasiveness, simplicity, acceptability, adherence, and efficacy for patients who present with new conditions and those with ambiguous or incomplete data, complex illnesses, comorbid conditions, and multiple diagnoses in all clinical settings.

Defense. I identified the relationship of the patient's symptoms to the probable diagnosis of atypical plasma cholinesterase and implemented appropriate treatment to ensure appropriate patient care.

Domain 1, Competency 5. Evaluate and direct care during hospitalization, and design a comprehensive discharge plan for patients from an acute care setting.

Defense. I directed her care to prolong sedation while return of normal neuromuscular functioning was achieved. I actively participated in her co-management during hospitalization by monitoring her vital signs, maintaining ventilatory support, and ordering appropriate laboratory tests. My interventions for risk reduction for the individual were to counsel the patient and her family members about the risks of atypical plasma cholinesterase and to refer her for further testing. I also typed a detailed letter explaining the circumstances of her anesthetic course, gave a copy to the patient and to the surgeon, and added one to her medical record.

Medications

Drug: Midazolam (Versed)

Dose range: 0.30–0.35 mg/kg over 20 to 30 seconds (allowing 2 minutes for effect); dose adjusted for comorbidities.

Method of administration in this case: Intravenous.

Mechanism of action: Short-acting benzodiazepine central nervous system (CNS) depressant, reversibly interacts with gamma-amino butyric acid (GABA) receptors in the central nervous system.

Clinical uses: Sedative or adjunct to anesthesia.

Side effects
Common: Hypotensive episode, nausea and vomiting, involuntary movement, agitation, apnea, respiratory depression.
Serious: Cardiac arrest, respiratory arrest.

Drug: Fentanyl (Sublimaze)

Dose range: 2–50 mcg/kg.

Method of administration in this case: Intravenous.

Mechanism of action: Opioid analgesic.

Clinical uses: Pain control.

Side effects
Common: Dizziness, headache, sedation, cough, abdominal pain, constipation, diarrhea, loss of appetite, nausea and vomiting, backache, asthenia, confusion, urinary retention.
Serious: Peripheral edema, tachyarrhythmia, cough.

Drug: Propofol (Diprivan)

Dose range: *Induction:* 2.0–2.5 mcg/kg. *Maintenance:* 100–200 mcg/kg/min IV infusion (dose varies for age and surgery type).

Method of administration in this case: Intravenous.

Mechanism of action: Short-acting sedative/hypnotic. Mechanism of action has not been well defined.

Clinical uses: Induction agent, general anesthetic or sedation (dose dependent).

Side effects
Common: Apnea, bradyarrhythmia, hypotension, myoclonus, pain on injection.
Serious: Anaphylaxis (rare), seizure, acute renal failure, respiratory acidosis, bacterial septicemia, heart failure.

(continued)

Drug: Succinylcholine (Anectine)

Dose range: *Facilitate endotracheal intubation or provide skeletal muscle relaxation during surgery or mechanical ventilation:* 0.6 mg/kg IV (range 0.3–1.1 mg/kg). *Rapid-sequence intubation:* 1.0–1.5 mg/kg IV push.

Method of administration in this case: Intravenous.

Mechanism of action: Ultra-short-acting depolarizing skeletal muscle relaxant, mimics acetylcholine as it binds with the cholinergic receptors on the motor endplate.

Clinical uses: Surgical paralysis, depolarizing muscle relaxant.

Side effects
Common: Muscle rigidity, myalgia, prolonged raised intraocular pressure.
Serious: Bradyarrhythmia (especially in children), cardiac arrest, cardiac dysrhythmia, tachyarrhythmia, hyperkalemia, malignant hyperthermia, immune hypersensitivity reaction, rhabdomyolysis, apnea, respiratory depression.

Drug: Desflurane (Suprane)

Dose range: Minimum alveolar concentration (MAC) is 6 percent. (The MAC of an inhaled anesthetic is the alveolar concentration that prevents movement in 50 percent of patients in response to a standardized stimulus, such as a surgical incision. MAC mirrors brain partial pressure and allows comparisons of potency between agents.)

Method of administration in this case: Inhalation.

Mechanism of action: Nonflammable volatile anesthetic.

Clinical uses: Main component of general anesthesia delivered via endotracheal tube, laryngeal mask airway, or mask.

Side effects
Common: Alteration in heart rate, hypotension, excessive salivation, nausea, vomiting, headache, cough.
Serious: Bradyarrhythmia, cardiac arrest, cardiac dysrhythmia, heart failure, hypertension, malignant hypertension, shock, sinus arrhythmia, tachycardia, Torsades de pointes, hyperkalemia, malignant hyperthermia, acute pancreatitis, hepatic necrosis, hepatitis, liver failure, rhabdomyolysis, seizure, nephrotoxicity, apnea, laryngeal spasm, pharyngitis.

References

Cerf, C., Mesguish, M., Gabriel, I., Amselem, S., & Duvaldestin, P. (2002). Screening patients with prolonged neuromuscular blockade after Succinylcholine and mivacurium. *Anesthesia and Analgesia, 94,* 461–466.

Leadingham, C.L. (2007). A case of pseudocholinesterase deficiency in the PACU. *Journal of PeriAnesthesia Nursing, 22(4),* 265–274.

Levano, S., Ginz, H., Siegmund, M., Fillipovic, M., Voronkov, E., & Urwyler, A. (2005). Geno-
typing the butyrylcholinesterase in patients with prolonged neuromuscular block after
Succinylcholine. *Anesthesiology, 102*(3), 531–535.

Merah, N.A., Wong, D.T., Foulkes-Crabbe, D.J., Kushimo, O.T., & Bode, C.O. (2005). Modified
Mallampati test, thyromental distance and inter-incisor gap are the best predictors of difficult laryngoscopy in West Africans. *Cardiothoracic Anesthesia, Respiration and Airway,
52*(3), 291–296.

Morneault, K., Lacy, T.L., Connelly, N.R., & Dupont F. (2007). Prolonged neuromuscular block in
two patients undergoing abdominal surgery. *Internet Journal of Anesthesiology, 12*(1).

Ostergaard, D., Viby-Mogensen, J., Rasmussen, S.N., Gatke, M.R., Pedersen, N.A., & Skovgaard,
L.T. (2003). Pharmocokinetics and pharmacodynamics of mivacurium in patients phe-
notypically heterozygous for the usual and atypical plasma cholinesterase variants. *Acta
Anaesthesiologica Scandinavia, 47,* 1219–1225.

Ramirez, J.G., Sprung, J., Keegan, M., Hall, B.A., & Bourke, D.L. (2005). Neostigime-induced
prolonged neuromuscular blockade in a patient with atypical pseudocholinesterase.
Journal of Clinical Anesthesia, 17, 221–224.

Rowlee, S.C. (1999). Monitoring neuromuscular blockade in the intensive care unit: The
peripheral nerve stimulator. *Heart and Lung, 9*(10), 352–364

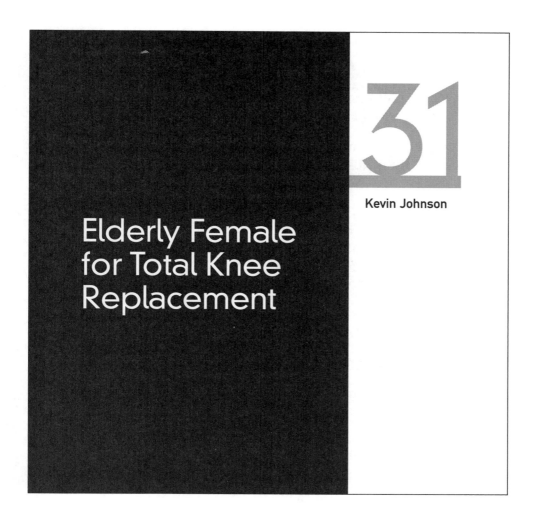

31

Kevin Johnson

Elderly Female for Total Knee Replacement

I chose this case narrative because it demonstrates the multidimensional care required in the management of anesthesia for a Medicare-insured 70-year-old woman who required a total knee replacement. This case addresses the following Columbia University School of Nursing (CUSN) doctoral competencies for comprehensive direct patient care.

DOMAIN 1, COMPETENCY 5

Evaluate and direct care during hospitalization, and design a comprehensive discharge plan for patients from an acute care setting.

PO A. Assess the acuity of the patient's condition and determine the most appropriate inpatient treatment setting based on level of acuity.
PO B. Actively participate in the admission process to the appropriate inpatient treatment setting.

PO C. Actively co-manage patient care during hospitalization.

PO D. Formulate plan for ongoing care to be provided in a subacute setting, such as a long-term care facility, rehabilitation facility, or home or community setting.

PO E. Coordinate ongoing comprehensive care to be provided in a subacute setting, such as a long-term care facility, rehabilitation facility, or home or community setting.

DOMAIN 2, COMPETENCY 1

Assemble a collaborative interdisciplinary network, and refer and consult appropriately while maintaining primary responsibility for comprehensive patient care.

PO A. Initiate referral to other health care professionals while maintaining primary responsibility for patient care.

PO B. Accept referrals from other health care professions and communicate consultation findings and recommendations to the referring provider and collaborative network.

PO C. Utilize consultation recommendations for decision-making while maintaining primary responsibility for care.

PO D. Evaluate outcomes of interventions.

PO E. Provide ongoing patient follow-up, and monitor outcomes of collaborative network interventions.

DOMAIN 2, COMPETENCY 2

Coordinate and manage the care of patients with chronic illness utilizing specialists, other disciplines, community resources, and family, while maintaining primary responsibility for direction of patient care and ensuring the seamless flow of information among providers as the focus of care transitions across ambulatory to acute, subacute, and community settings.

PO A. Coordinate care for a patient with chronic illness as the focus of care transitions across ambulatory, acute, subacute, and/or community settings.

PO B. Co-manage care for a patient with chronic illness as the focus of care transitions across ambulatory, acute, subacute, and/or community settings.

PO C. Coordinate care for a patient with chronic illness utilizing specialists, other disciplines, community resources, and family.

PO D. Direct care for a patient with chronic illness and ensure the seamless flow of information among providers as the focus of care transitions across settings.

PO E. Co-manage care for a patient with chronic illness, utilizing shared decision-making and teaching.

PO F. Co-manage care for a patient with chronic pain as the focus of care transitions across ambulatory, acute, subacute, and/or community settings.

DOMAIN 3, COMPETENCY 2

Evaluate gaps in health care access that compromise optimal patient outcomes, and apply current knowledge of the organization and financing of health care systems to ameliorate negative impact.

PO A. Identify gaps in access that compromise the patient's optimum care.

PO B. Identify gaps in reimbursement that compromise the patient's optimum care.

PO C. Demonstrate patient advocacy in the provision of continuous and comprehensive care.

PO D. Apply current knowledge of the organization to ameliorate negative impact.

PO E. Apply current knowledge of health care systems to ameliorate negative impact.

ENCOUNTER CONTEXT

Encounter One: Pre-Anesthesia Evaluation (day prior to admission to hospital)

DNP role: I am a certified registered nurse anesthetist (CRNA) and DNP resident.

Identifying Information

Site: A large teaching hospital.

Setting: Inpatient and admission to rehabilitation.

Reason for encounter: Initial pre-anesthesia evaluation and workup.

Informant: Patient.

Principle diagnosis: Degenerative joint disease.

Principal procedure planned: Total knee replacement with insertion of an inferior vena cava filter in the radiology department prior to going to the operating room.

Chief complaint: "I have constant pain in my knees and I am going to have a total knee replacement."

History of Present Illness

MJ is a 70-year-old white female who presents for a left total knee replacement. She has a long history of hypertension (HTN), hyperlipidemia, chronic obstructive pulmonary disease (COPD), and newly diagnosed type 2 diabetes mellitus (DM) that is currently diet controlled. Her history is complicated by a fall during an ice storm in 2004 that resulted in a deep vein thrombosis (DVT) in her left lower extremity. She denies any signs or symptoms of a pulmonary embolus (PE) at that time and was treated with anticoagulant therapy for six months.

MJ now presents with chronic discomfort and left leg pain that radiates from her thigh down to her calf. She has daily pain upon walking, difficulty with weight bearing, and pain with bending her left knee. Her exercise activity is limited due to the pain in her left leg. She states that the doctor told her that she has "bone on bone in her left knee." She is admitted to the hospital to undergo surgery for a left total knee replacement. She is hopeful that this surgery will take away the pain so she is able to enjoy a better quality of life.

Current Medications (see medications list at the end of the chapter)

Furosemide (Lasix) 40 mg by mouth once per day
Levothyroxine (Synthroid) 100 mcg by mouth once per day
Atenolol (Tenormin) 25 mg by mouth once per day
Acetylsalicylic acid (Aspirin) 81 mg by mouth once per day
Verapamil (Calan) 80 mg by mouth once per day
Losartan (Cozaar) 50 mg by mouth once per day
Simvastatin (Zocor) 20 mg by mouth once per day
Celecoxib (Celebrex) 200 mg by mouth once per day
Multiple vitamins by mouth once per day
Coenzyme Q10 50 mcq by mouth once per day
Albuterol (Ventolin) inhaler as needed

Allergies

She denies any drug or contrast allergies.

Hospitalizations

- 1970—Full mouth dental extraction and tonsillectomy
- 1974—Abdominal hysterectomy
- 1975—Umbilical hernia repair
- 1977—Open cholecystectomy and appendectomy
- 2002—Anemia requiring blood transfusions
- 2004—Deep vein thrombosis in left lower extremity

Medical History

- Hypertension (HTN)—10 years, controlled on medication
- Hyperlipidemia—treated with medication for two years
- Chronic obstructive pulmonary disease (COPD)—despite the fact that she has no history of smoking
- Type 2 diabetes mellitus (DM)—newly diagnosed. Diet controlled. She has been monitoring her blood sugar at home once in the morning and once in the evening before bed. She states that the doctor told her she was "border

line" diabetic and that she needed to watch her diet. Denies polydypsia, polyphagia, polyuria, visual changes

- Arthritis/degenerative joint disease (DJD)—treated with celecoxib (Celebrex)

Surgical History

- Bilateral cataract extraction—2006
- Cholecystectomy/appendectomy—1977
- Umbilical hernia repair—1975
- Hysterectomy—1974

Review of Systems

General health: Denies any fever, chills, weight loss, or weight gain. States she has no change in appetite and denies excessive fatigue or insomnia.

Skin: States that she has dry skin and develops skin sores from scratching.

Eyes: Denies any visual disturbances, redness, pain, or discharge or excessive tearing.

Ears: Denies hearing loss or tinnitus.

Nose: Denies nose bleeds or congestion.

Mouth and throat: Denies any hoarseness, changes in voice, trouble chewing, or swallowing.

Neck: Denies swollen lymph nodes or stiffness.

Neurologic: Denies any weakness, dizziness, seizures, loss of memory or balance, or history of stroke. She states that her lower leg and toes feel numb at times on her left side.

Respiratory: Denies any cough, asthma, and wheezing or frequent upper respiratory infections. No tuberculosis exposure, hemoptysis, or pleurisy. States she occasionally experiences shortness of breath on exertion, especially in cold weather. She denies using her inhaler for the past year.

Cardiovascular: Limited exercise tolerance related to shortness of breath on exertion and pain in legs. MJ denies any chest pain, angina, irregular heart rate or rhythm. No palpitations, dizziness, fainting spells, or myocardial infarction.

Gastrointestinal: Denies nausea, vomiting, heartburn, dysphagia, jaundice, or hemorrhoids.

Genitourinary: Denies itching, burning, dysuria, or inability to void.

Endocrine: See Medical History. Denies change in hair, constipation, cold or heat intolerance.

Musculoskeletal: Denies back pain, neck pain, or stiffness. See HPI.

Peripheral vascular: She has had a significant amount of varicose veins in both legs for about 40 years, and her ankles become "puffy" after being on her feet throughout the day.

Hematologic: Denies bruising or bleeding.

Psychiatric: MJ states that she has been sad and tearful on a daily basis since her son died six months ago. She was taking medication for depression but decided to take herself off the medication because she did not want to take it anymore. She feels she was on "too much medication" and she can deal with her loss without medicine.

Social History

MJ is a 70-year-old female who is a homemaker. She was married for 25 years and is widowed. She has never remarried. She has five male children that range from 43 to 52 years in age. Her youngest son died six months ago of heart failure, and she has been struggling with that loss. Her immediate support systems are her four surviving children, who live out of state, and the church that she attends on a weekly basis.

Education

MJ has a 12th-grade education level. She has appropriate understanding of her health condition and the pending surgical procedure.

Family History

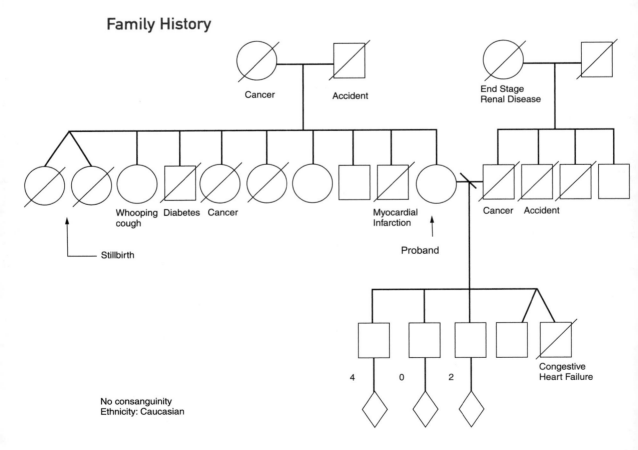

Physical Examination

General: MJ is a well-developed, obese white female with a depressed affect.

Vital signs: Blood pressure 160/84 in right arm, pulse 62; 156/90 in left arm. Temp 98.8°F. Weight 250 lb, height 5'6", calculated BMI 41.6 kg/m².

Airway: Full range of motion (FROM), three fingersbreaths mandibular to thyroid distance, Mallampatti class II.

Skin: Some skin excoriations noted in abdominal region from scratching, but no appearance of rash or ulcers. Warm and dry, with appropriate skin turgor. Extensive varicose veins are present in lower extremities bilaterally. Feet are warm and dry without ulcers.

Lymph: No lymphadenopathy bilaterally to neck, axilla, or groin.

HEENT: Hearing intact, oral mucosa clear, she is edentulous.

Neck: Carotid brachial and radial pulses are all 3+ in amplitude bilaterally, cervical bruits are not heard.

Lungs: Chest is without adventious sounds to auscultation in all fields.

Cardiac: Regular rhythm without murmurs or gallops.

Abdomen: Soft, no palpable masses, tenderness, or organomegaly.

Musculoskeletal: Pain on passive and active flexion to bilateral lower extremities.

Vascular: Lower extremity examination reveals the pulses to be 3+ in the femoral and the popliteals bilaterally. On the right, the posterior tibial and dorsalis pedis are absent. On the left, the posterior tibial and dorsalis pedis are 3+. Both feet are without atrophy or wasting. Extensive varicose vein formation on both lower extremities is present.

Genitalia: Deferred.

Neurologic: Cranial nerves II through XII grossly intact. Extraocular movements are intact. Deep tendon reflexes present 2+ equal bilaterally. Toes are down-going. Sensation is slightly decreased in lower extremities bilaterally, but intact to pressure, pain, and temperature.

Psychiatric: Alert and oriented to person, place, and time. Cooperative and has appropriate understanding of pending surgery.

Database

Diagnostic tests and consultations within past three months.

MRI of Lumbar Region of Spine

There is a significant multilevel facet arthropathy at L3-L4 through L5-S1 levels. There is a suggestion of mild spondylolisthesis at the L4-L5 level. Evidence of central and foraminal stenosis is present at this level, as well as a broad-base disc bulge. This is considered to be mild discogenic disease.

Venous Duplex Scan

This study is positive on the right, suggesting that she continues to have partial occlusive thrombosis to the left common femoral vein, superficial femoral, and popliteal vessels that appears to be chronic.

Recommendation (by vascular surgeon consulted by orthopedic surgeon in preparation procedure)

Recommendation by a vascular surgeon, given prior history of deep vein thrombosis (DVT), is to place a prophylactic inferior vena cava filter prior to reconstructive surgery. Anticoagulation therapy for at least four weeks post-operatively is recommended.

Cardiac Catheterization

Cardiac catheterization revealed an ejection fraction of 60 percent with no valvular abnormalities. Coronary arteries have mild diffuse lesions of 10 percent in the left main coronary artery (LMCA), left anterior descending artery (LAD), circumflex artery (CX), and right coronary artery (RCA). No evidence of increased pulmonary vasculature or ventricular dysfunction.

Cardiac Consultation

MJ is determined to have acceptable surgical risk for the planned procedure. She has minor clinical predictors of cardiovascular risk and describes functional capacity of greater than four (4) metabolic equivalent units (METS). The scheduled procedure is an intermediate-risk surgery according to American College of Cardiology/American Heart Association (ACC/AHA) criteria.

Patient Education (as part of preadmission evaluation)

I see MJ during her pre-admission evaluation for surgery and provide instructions for anesthesia for the date of her surgery. I inform her to not eat or drink after midnight the night before her procedure and instruct her on the appropriate medication to take the morning of her surgery. I educate her about her options for anesthesia: general anesthesia or regional anesthesia. We discuss the risk and benefits of both types of anesthesia, and she consents to general and/or regional anesthesia. MJ lives alone; therefore, she asks me to help locate a rehabilitation facility that could be utilized for recovery after hospital discharge.

Encounter Two: Admission for Surgery (24 hours after initial encounter)

Before assuming care for the patient, I review the chart.

Summary of morning events prior to my assuming care:

MJ presented to the hospital on the morning of her scheduled procedure for day surgery admission. An IVC filter was placed by a vascular surgeon in the radiology department. A radiology nurse administered intravenous (IV) sedation for comfort, and the procedure was performed under local anesthesia. MJ's electrocardiogram (ECG) rhythm on admission to the radiology department was sinus bradycardia (SB). During the procedure, MJ's heart rhythm became irregular and converted into an atrial fibrillation rhythm, with a ventricular rate of 70s–80s. She was otherwise asymptomatic. Upon completion of the procedure, she was taken to a short stay recovery room for monitoring and further cardiac evaluation because of the new arrhythmia.

A cardiology consult was requested to evaluate the etiology of the new-onset atrial fibrillation and exclude an acute myocardial infarction (MI). This consult was also obtained to determine if the scheduled surgery should proceed. A 12-lead ECG confirmed the rhythm of atrial fibrillation. Emergent laboratory studies were drawn for troponin, magnesium, electrolytes, and thyroid function. An echocardiogram was ordered by the cardiologist to rule out possible clot formation in the atria of the heart and to evaluate MJ's ventricular function.

Results from the echocardiogram revealed an ejection fraction of 60 percent with no evidence of emboli, which is consistent with a prior cardiac catheterization report. The ventricular rate continued to remain in the 70s and 80s, and the patient remained asymptomatic. Results of the laboratory studies revealed a troponin level that was negative with all other results within normal range, and a therapeutic thyroid stimulating hormone (TSH) level.

Assumption of Care

I initiate a discussion with the cardiologist regarding her condition, and he confirms that the procedure may proceed and that she is at moderate cardiac risk **(D2, C1, PO C)**.

Deep venous thrombosis is a common problem in orthopedics, and pulmonary embolism is a major cause of postoperative mortality. In the presence of surgical injury, emboli form because of venous stasis. During total-knee replacement, there is absolute stasis with the tourniquet inflated (Miller, 2005).
Oxford Centre for Evidence-Based Medicine (CEBM), level 5.

Atrial fibrillation is an excessively rapid and irregular atrial focus with no P waves appearing on the ECG. This is the most irregular rhythm; it is called irregularly irregular and may be associated with a pulse deficit. This rhythm is often associated with significant cardiac disease; however, idiopathic lone paroxysmal atrial fibrillation has become increasingly recognized (Miller, 2005).
CEBM, level 5.

Successful peri-operative evaluation and evaluation and treatment of cardiac patients undergoing non-cardiac surgery requires teamwork and communication between the patient, primary care physician, anesthesiologist, consultant, and surgeon (Berger et al., 2002).
CEBM, level 5.

The presence of an arrhythmia or cardiac conduction disturbance should provoke a careful evaluation for underlying cardiopulmonary disease, drug toxicity, or metabolic abnormality. Therapy should be initiated for symptomatic or hemodynamically significant arrhythmias, first to reverse the underlying cause and second to treat the arrhythmia (Picard, 2001).

CEBM, level 2c.

The addition of cardiac imaging such as echocardiography is of particular value for women and for patients whose EKG is difficult to interpret. Thromboemboli can be detected in the right side of the heart on echocardiography (Picard, 2001).

CEBM, level 2c.

Female patients with diabetes or with peripheral vascular disease fall into a category for which the risk of underlying CAD is intermediate or higher and are candidates for stress testing (Shaw et al., 2005).

CEBM, level 5.

Preoperative Discussion of Risks/Benefits of Anesthesia

- Zero minutes—I discuss with MJ an anesthetic plan of spinal anesthesia (SAB) with general anesthesia backup if the block is inadequate. I again discuss the risks of SAB, such as headache, backache, convulsions, persistent weakness, numbness, residual pain, chronic pain, and total spinal anesthesia. Risks of general endotracheal anesthesia (GETA) are mouth or throat pain, hoarseness, injury to mouth or teeth, vocal cords, eyes, and/or awareness of anesthesia.
- I explain to MJ, considering the events of the morning (a new onset of atrial fibrillation without clear reason), that a SAB will be a safer anesthetic for her cardiac status. I explain that I will provide enough sedation to keep her comfortable during her surgery and that she will be unaware of intraoperative events. I invite any questions and answer them to MJ and her family's satisfaction **(D1, C5, PO B, C).**

All anesthetic techniques and drugs have known cardiac effects that should be considered in the peri-operative plan. There appears to be no one best myocardium-protective anesthetic technique. Therefore, the choice of anesthesia and intraoperative monitors is best left to the discretion of the anesthesia care team, which will consider the need for postoperative ventilation, cardiovascular effects, sympathetic blockade, and dermatomal level of the procedure (Berger et al., 2002).

CEBM, level 5.

Plan: SAB with IV sedation, with GETA backup.

Spinal anesthesia reduces DVT rates after total-knee replacement by 20% (Miller, 2005).

CEBM, level 5.

Procedure Notes and Intraoperative Summary

- 10 minutes—After appropriate intravenous (IV) access is obtained, I give MJ 3 mg of midazolam (Versed) upon entrance into the operating room suite and apply all standard noninvasive monitors: electrocardiogram (ECG), noninvasive blood pressure cuff (NIBP), pulse-oximetry monitoring, and supplemental oxygen via nasal cannula are administered.
- 20 minutes—MJ is placed in the sitting position for the SAB. I perform a sterile betadine prep to the lumbar region and place a local skin wheal of 1% lidocaine (Xylocaine) at the L3-L4 interspace. A 25-gauge Pencan needle is passed to the subarachnoid space, and a free flow of cerebral spinal fluid (CSF) is obtained. No parathesia or blood is encountered. 1.8 cc of 0.75% bupivacaine (Marcaine) mixed with 10 mcq of morphine is injected into the subarachnoid space after a positive CSF aspirate. The needle is withdrawn and MJ is placed in the supine position. A sensory blockade is achieved to a dermatome level of T7. The circulating nurse then preps the surgical site per standard protocol of the operating room.

For knee surgery, analgesia is required in the dermatomes innervated by L2 and S2 nerve roots. Most knee procedures require a tourniquet around the thigh, which requires anesthesia up to the L1 nerve root (Raj, 2002).

CEBM, level 5.

The local anesthetic drug and dosage must be selected on the basis of expected duration of surgery and degree of motor blockade required. Local anesthetics are a class of drugs that are widely used in the diagnosis and/or treatment of acute as well as chronic pain. Bupivacaine is a long-lasting local anesthetic with highly desirable properties. Local anesthetics block the conduction of action potentials in peripheral nerves by preventing a rush of Na+ into axons (Raj, 2002).

CEBM, level 5.

Administration of a single dose of opioid may be efficacious as a sole or adjuvant analgesic agent when administered intrathecally or epidurally. One of the most important factors in determining the clinical pharmacology for a particular opioid is its degree of lipophilicity vs. hydrophylicity. Hydrophilic opioids (i.e., morphine and hydromorphone) tend to remain within the CSF and produce a delayed but longer duration of analgesia along with a generally higher incidence of side effects due to the cephalad spread of the hydrophilic opioid (Miller, 2005).

CEBM, level 5.

- 35 minutes—I initiate a propofol (Diprivan) infusion and titrate the dosage to achieve a level of sedation that will allow MJ to sleep during the surgery but to open her eyes when verbally stimulated. MJ continues to remain in atrial fibrillation with a ventricular rate in the mid to lower 60s. Vital signs remain stable and within 20 percent of her baseline. The procedure is completed without incident with an estimated blood loss (EBL) calculated to be 250 cc. IV fluid intake during the procedure is 2,200 cc with a urine output of 110 cc. No blood transfusion is required **(D2, C1, PO D, E)**.

Propofol is the most frequently used intravenous anesthetic today. It is a hypnotic used for induction and maintenance of anesthesia, as well as for sedation in and outside the operating room. When used as a continuous infusion the rate is titrated to individual requirements and the surgical stimulus (Miller, 2005).

CEBM, level 5.

Emergence from Anesthesia

- 125 minutes—I discontinue the propofol (Diprivan) infusion during closure of the subcuticular layer of the incision site; MJ awakens from the light sedation and is responsive to command. After dressings are placed over the surgical site, she is transferred to her bed and taken to the post-anesthesia care unit (PACU) in stable condition **(D1, C5, PO A, C).**

Propofol by continuous infusion provides a readily titratable level of sedation and rapid recovery once the infusion is terminated, irrespective of the duration of the infusion (Miller, 2005).

CEBM, level 5.

Post-Anesthesia Care Unit

- MJ remains in the post-anesthesia care unit for two hours with stable vital signs and without incident. Motor blockade from the SAB descends to a dermatome level below T–10 while her sensory blockade remains at T–7 **(D1, C5, PO A, C).**

Discharge from the Post-Anesthesia Care Unit

- 195 minutes—I discharge MJ in stable condition from the PACU to an orthopedic post-surgical floor with telemetry monitoring. I order oxygen at 2 L via nasal cannula for 24 hours with continuous pulse-oximetry monitoring. I order diphenhydramine (Benadryl) on an as-needed basis (PRN) for pruritus, but no other pain medications are ordered. I leave instructions to consult anesthesia if pain medicine is required **(D1, C5, PO A, B, C; D2, C1, PO B).**

Single-dose hydrophilic opioid administration provides effective post-operative analgesia. Delayed respiratory depression is primarily associated with hydrophilic opioids because of the cephalad spread of opioid, which typically occurs within 12 hours after the injection (Miller, 2005).

CEBM, level 5.

Pruritus is one of the most common side effects of intrathecal injection; it is relatively easy to treat and is not considered an important clinical outcome to avoid (Miller, 2005).

CEBM, level 5.

ICD-9 codes

715.96 Osteoarthrosis unspecified whether generalized or localized involving the lower leg

Postoperative Day 1, Hospitalization Day 2

I consult physical therapy (PT) to discuss with MJ the need for rehabilitation and the subsequent goals to achieve during her therapy. I visit MJ on the orthopedic floor where she is admitted with telemetry monitoring. I assist her with ambulation down the hallway with a walker. She is able to walk 100 feet.

I consult with cardiology regarding her history of deep vein thrombosis (DVT), and anticoagulation therapy with warfarin (Coumadin) is recommended by the cardiologist. I discuss with MJ the goals of anticoagulation therapy and the need to evaluate clotting times until therapeutic levels are obtained **(D1, C5, PO A, B, C; D2, C1, PO A).**

After 24 hours, atrial fibrillation may be associated with the development of atrial thrombi, with resultant pulmonary and systemic embolization. In the older individual or in the setting of specific risk factors, anticoagulation with warfarin should be strongly considered (Miller, 2005).

CEBM, level 5.

I request a pharmacy consultation to educate MJ on the importance of dietary choices while receiving warfarin (Coumadin) therapy **(D2, C1, PO A; D2, C2, PO C, D).**

MJ lives alone and has limited resources for help in her home. I consult with the orthopedic nurse manager to assist with arrangements for transfer to a rehabilitation center at the time of hospital discharge. Her vital signs remain stable. The opioid that I place in her spinal anesthesia begins to wear off, and subsequently pain is controlled with oxycodone (OxyContin) every 12 hours as needed and acetaminophen/hydrocodone (Lortab) every 6 hours for breakthrough pain. I order celecoxib (Celebrex) to be given for her chronic joint pain and to augment her current pain therapy regime **(D1, C5, PO D; D2, C1, PO E; D2, C2, PO C, D, E, F).**

MJ's urine output is marginal, and I order an IV fluid bolus to treat potential dehydration, then a continuous IV fluid infusion for the next 24 hours at 125 cc/hr. Her blood sugar is monitored every eight hours and treated with a sliding scale of regular insulin (Novalin R). She receives supplemental regular insulin (Novalin R) for a blood glucose result of 163 in the previous eight hours **(D1, C5, PO C).**

Postoperative Day 2, Hospitalization Day 3

I visit MJ in her hospital room. She appears tearful and depressed. She states she is depressed because of her new heart condition and the need to be on warfarin (Coumadin) therapy. She feels that her life is out of control since the death of her youngest son a few months prior to this admission. She proceeds to talk about how he had died.

I listen to her, encourage her to talk about her feelings, and provide emotional support while she cries. I explain she is recuperating as expected and it is not uncommon to feel "down" after surgery and anesthesia. I explain it is important that she talk about her son and that a support group may be beneficial. I obtain a psychiatric consult to evaluate the need to initiate antidepressant therapy and provide information about support groups available in the community for grieving parents **(D1, C5, PO D, E; D2, C1, PO A; D2, C2, PO A, C)**.

Research has shown that the experience of losing a child is by far the most painful grief experience. Bereaved parents have more intense symptomatology than adults grieving other types of family loss such as death of a parent or spouse (Jacobs, 1994).

CEBM, level 4.

Allow a bereaved mother to talk and cry openly for as long as she wants without stifling her release of emotions. Nurse practitioners must assist mothers in finding meaning in their child's death and help them identify appropriate ways to memorialize their child. Referring mothers to appropriate support groups and counselors can put grieving mothers in touch with others who are grieving so they can offer mutual support (Jacobs, 1994).

CEBM, level 4.

Her urine output increases with the continuous IV fluid infusion at 125 cc/hr. I encourage her to increase her oral intake of fluids so that the IV can be discontinued.

Treatment of pre-renal azotemia is directed at correcting intravascular volume deficits, improving cardiac function, restoring normal blood pressure, and reversing increases in renal vascular resistance (Morgan & Murray, 2006).

CEBM, level 5.

The physical therapist arrives in MJ's room to discuss with MJ, her oldest son, and her daughter–in–law the need to evaluate her home and remove any objects that may increase any risk of falls after returning home from rehabilitation. I provide teaching regarding the importance of removing any rugs or loose electrical cords that may be present to minimize the risk of unexpected falls **(D2, C2, PO A, C, E)**.

I contact a local community organization to arrange for home delivery of an elevated toilet seat, walker, three-prong cane, and shower chair as recommended by the PT consultant. This is to aid her in her activities of daily living once she is discharged from the rehabilitation center to her home **(D1, C5, PO D, E; D2, C1, PO E)**.

MJ's blood glucose remains elevated in the 150 to 160 ranges. They are treated per the regular insulin (Novalin R) sliding scale that is ordered. A diabetes consult is requested to assist in educating her about diabetes and proper nutrition once she is discharged from the hospital. I continue to monitor her blood glucose closely throughout her hospital stay **(D2, C1, PO C)**.

Achieving dietary change requires giving up long established patterns of eating habits and behavior and acquiring new tastes and habits. To be effective, diet self-management training must be individualized to suit the individual's lifestyle, likes and dislikes and must be reinforced to achieve agreed goals (Kapur et al., 2008).

CEBM, level 2c.

I contact MJ's insurance company at her request to inquire about the number of days covered by her insurance company in the rehabilitation facility. Approval is given for 20 days and will be covered at 100 percent. After 20 days in the rehabilitation facility, if further therapy is needed, MJ will have a $125.00/day co-payment.

MJ lives on a fixed income with limited resources. I contact her long-term care provider, at her request, to evaluate if assistance could be provided to lower her hospital co-payment. The plan administrator examines her policy and states that at 20 days the long-term care plan will pay MJ directly $100.00/day, therefore making her co-payment $25.00/day. I inform MJ of this, which relieves some of her anxieties.

I also inquire with her insurance company about the ability to have in-home physical therapy once she is discharged from the rehabilitation facility. Her insurance administrator explains that if physical therapy is medically necessary, they will pay 100 percent of the cost. This also relieves MJ's anxiety because of her limited resources (**D2, C2, PO A; D3, C2, PO A, B, C, D, E**).

Postoperative Day 3, Hospitalization Day 4 (discharge from hospital to rehabilitation facility)

MJ is discharged from the hospital and transported to a nearby rehabilitation facility. The surgeon initiates her transfer orders, and she is admitted to the facility for physical therapy two times per day. Acetaminophen/hydrocodone (Lortab) is ordered every six hours as needed for pain and is augmented with celecoxib (Celebrex) once daily. Anti-coagulation therapy with warfarin (Coumadin) is continued because of her persistent atrial fibrillation and the presence of the IVC filter. She resumes her daily regimen of blood pressure medications that she was taking before her hospital admission.

Postoperative Day 15, Rehabilitation Facility

I visit the rehabilitation facility to see MJ and inquire about her recovery. She states that her recovery is slow but that she feels she is "getting better." She continues to have a considerable amount of pain, especially after her physical therapy sessions are completed. I reinforce the importance of taking pain medicine on a consistent basis in order to keep her pain under control. I educate her about taking the pain medicine prior to her physical therapy for preemptive analgesia. MJ requests that I inquire with staff about the ability to have a physical therapist come to her home once she is discharged from the rehabilitation facility. I talk with the nursing staff and relay her request. The nursing staff state they will consult the social worker to make these arrangements and obtain approval from her insurance company.

MJ is discharged home from the rehabilitation facility on postoperative day 22.

Home Addendum

I contact MJ at her home to inquire about her transition to the home environment. She states that her pain is adequately controlled with the current medication regimen prescribed. She continues to take her celecoxib (Celebrex) as an adjunct to her arthritis and surgical pain. She states, "I am happy to be home."

She is satisfied with the results of her surgery at this point and feels she will be able to increase her activity with time. She continues to experience some emotional days regarding the loss of her son, and she now talks with a grief therapist in her home once a week. A home health nurse visits on a weekly basis to draw her blood to evaluate her coagulation studies. She monitors her diet and checks her blood sugar on a daily basis at home.

COMPETENCY DEFENSE

Domain 1, Competency 5. Evaluate and direct care during hospitalization, and design a comprehensive discharge plan for patients from an acute care setting.

Defense. I actively participated in multiple aspects of this patient's care from admission, through intraoperative and postoperative recovery, and formulated a comprehensive discharge plan.

Domain 2, Competency 1. Assemble a collaborative interdisciplinary network, and refer and consult appropriately while maintaining primary responsibility for comprehensive patient care.

Defense. I advocated for this patient in all settings and utilized the interdisciplinary team recommendations. I initiated consults when needed to address this patient's medical, emotional, and environmental needs.

Domain 2, Competency 2. Coordinate and manage the care of patients with chronic illness, utilizing specialists, other disciplines, community resources, and family, while maintaining primary responsibility for direction of patient care and ensuring the seamless flow of information among providers as the focus of care transitions across ambulatory to acute, subacute, and community settings.

Defense. This patient had multiple comorbid, chronic conditions. I provided comprehensive care that addressed her needs as she transitioned from pre-anesthesia evaluation through her hospital course to a subacute setting. I provided education and communicated with the health care team as well as family to ensure optimal outcomes. As a CRNA, I addressed her acute and chronic pain needs.

Domain 3, Competency 2. Evaluate gaps in health care access that compromise optimal patient outcomes, and apply current knowledge of the organization and financing of health care systems to ameliorate negative impact.

Defense. To ensure the best possible outcome, I communicated with this patient's health insurance and supplemental insurer so she could have adequate rehabilitation services at a facility and in her home.

Medications

Medication: Albuterol (Ventolin)

Dose: Two puffs every 4 hours.

Method of administration in this case: By mouth (inhaled) as needed.

Mechanism of action: Causes bronchodilation by action on B2 (pulmonary) receptors by increasing level of cyclic amp, which relaxes smooth muscle.

Clinical use: Adrenergic B2 agonist, sympathomimetic, bronchodilator.

Adverse effects: Tremors, anxiety, insomnia, headache, dizziness, palpitations.

Medication: Acetylsalicylic Acid (Aspirin)

Dose: 350–625 mg.

Method of administration in this case: By mouth daily.

Mechanism of action: Inhibits prostaglandin synthesis: Blocks prostaglandin synthetase action that prevents platelet aggregating substance thromboxane A2.

Clinical use: Inhibit platelet aggregation.

Adverse effects: GI bleeding, prolonged bleeding time, thrombocytopenia, hepatitis, and angioedema.

Medication: Atenolol (Tenormin)

Dose: 50–100 mg.

Method of administration in this case: By mouth daily.

Mechanism of action: Competitively blocks stimulation of B-adrenergic receptor within vascular smooth muscle; produces chronotropic activity, negative inotropic activity.

Clinical use: Non-specific beta-blocker, B1 and B2 blocker.

Adverse effects: Increased hypotension, bradycardia.

(continued)

Medication: Bupivacaine (Marcaine)

Dose: Up to 15 mg intrathecally or up to 5 mg/kg in epidural space.

Method of administration in this case: Intrathecal injection.

Mechanism of action: Inhibits Na+ ion channels, stabilizing neuronal cell membranes and inhibiting nerve impulse initiation and conduction.

Clinical use: Local anesthetic to temporally block sensory and motor sensation.

Adverse effects: Cardiac arrest with difficult resuscitation or death during epidural anesthesia in obstetric patients, seizures, underventilation with development of acidosis.

Medication: Celecoxib (Celebrex)

Dose: 100 mg two times per day; 200 mg.

Method of administration in this case: By mouth daily.

Mechanism of action: Inhibits prostaglandin synthesis by decreasing enzyme needed for biosynthesis; analgesic, anti-inflammatory, antipyretic properties. It is nonsteroidal anti-inflammatory, COX-2 inhibitor.

Clinical use: Anti-inflammatory.

Adverse effects: Fatigue, tachycardia, angina, MI, hypertension, fluid retention, GI bleeding, oliguria, azotemia.

Medication: Warfarin (Coumadin)

Dose: 2.5–10 mg/day. Adjust dosage to prothrombin time (PT) or international normalized ratio (INR).

Method of administration in this case: By mouth daily.

Mechanism of action: Interferes with blood clotting by indirect means; depresses hepatic synthesis of vitamin K-dependent coagulation factors (II, VII, IX, X).

Clinical use: Anti-coagulant.

Adverse effects: Diarrhea, hepatitis, hematuria, hemorrhage, agranulocytosis, leucopenia.

Medication: Losartan (Cozaar)

Dose: 25–50 mg.

Method of administration in this case: By mouth daily.

(continued)

Mechanism of action: Blocks the vasoconstrictor and aldosterone-secreting effects of angiotensin II; selectively blocks the binding of angiotensin II to the angiotensin I receptor found in tissues.

Clinical use: Anti-hypertensive.

Adverse effects: Angina pectoris, second-degree AV block; cerebral vascular accident, hypotension, myocardial infarction, dysrhythmias.

Medication: Morphine (Duramorph)

Dose: 0.2–1.0 mg.

Method of administration in this case: Intrathecal injection.

Mechanism of action: Binds to opiate receptors in the central nervous system, causing inhibition of ascending pain pathways, altering the perception of and response to pain; produces generalized CNS depression.

Clinical use: Analgesic, narcotic.

Adverse effects: Increased intracranial pressure, severe respiratory depression, and purititis.

Medication: Furosemide (Lasix)

Dose: 20–80 mg. Second dose in 6–8 hours: adjust up to 600 mg if needed.

Method of administration in this case: By mouth daily.

Mechanism of action: Furosemide blocks the absorption of sodium and chloride in the proximal and distal tubules, also in the loop of Henle, causing an increase in urine output.

Clinical use: Diuretic.

Adverse effects: Fever, vertigo, headache, volume depletion and dehydration, orthostatic hypotension, transient deafness, muscle spasm, and photosensitivity.

Drug: Regular Insulin (Novalin R)

Dose: Adjust to blood glucose level.

Method of administration in this case: Subcutaneous injection.

Mechanism of action: Insulin is the principal hormone required for proper glucose utilization in normal metabolic processes; stimulates peripheral glucose uptake, inhibits hepatic glucose production, inhibits lipolysis and proteolysis, regulating glucose metabolism.

Clinical use: Blood glucose control.

(continued)

Adverse effects: Palpitation, tachycardia, pallor, confusion, fatigue, loss of consciousness, and hypoglycemia.

Medication: Acetaminophen/Hydrocodone (Lortab)

Dose: 5–10 mg.

Method of administration in this case: By mouth every 4 hours as needed.

Mechanism of action: Lortab acts directly on the cough center in the medulla to suppress cough; binds to opiate receptors in CNS to reduce pain.

Clinical use: Opioid analgesic, non-opioid analgesic.

Adverse effects: Drowsiness, dizziness, convulsions, circulatory depression, and respiratory depression.

Medication: Midazolam (Versed)

Dose: 2–5 mg.

Method of administration in this case: Intravenous.

Mechanism of action: Depresses CNS at limbic and subcortical levels of brain, potentiating effects of GABA.

Clinical use: Sedation.

Adverse effects: Oversedation, hypotension, decrease respiratory rate.

Medication: Propofol (Diprivan)

Dose: 2.0–2.5 mg/kg for induction of anesthesia. 25 mcq/kg/min titrated to desired effect.

Method of administration in this case: Intravenous.

Mechanism of action: Produces dose-dependent CNS depression; action is unknown.

Clinical use: Sedation.

Adverse effects: Hypotension, apnea, flushing, phlebitis, hives, burning/stinging at injection site.

Medication: Simvastatin (Zocor)

Dose: 5–40 mg/day at night; not to exceed 80 mg/day.

Method of administration in this case: By mouth daily.

(continued)

Mechanism of action: Inhibits HMG-CoA reductase enzyme, which reduces cholesterol synthesis.

Clinical use: Anti-lipidemic.

Side effects: Liver dysfunction, myositis, rhabdomyolysis, muscle cramps, myalgia.

Medication: Levothyroxine (Synthroid)

Dose: 50–100 mg desired response, and then 75–125 mg daily as a maintenance dose.

Method of administration in this case: By mouth daily.

Mechanism of action: Increases metabolic rate, controls protein synthesis, cardiac output, renal blood flow, and O_2 consumption; exact mechanism unknown.

Clinical use: Thyroid hormone replacement.

Adverse effects: Thyroid storm, cardiac arrest, tachycardia, palpitations, hypertension, sweating, heat intolerance.

Medication: Verapamil (Calan)

Dose: 80–120 mg.

Method of administration in this case: By mouth up to three times daily.

Mechanism of action: Inhibits calcium ion influx across cell membrane during cardiac depolarization; produces relaxation of coronary vascular smooth muscle; dilates coronary arteries; decreases SA/AV node conduction.

Clinical use: Anti-hypertensive, anti-anginal.

Adverse effects: Congestive heart failure, bradycardia, hypotension, Stevens-Johnson syndrome.

References

Berger, P.B., Eagle, K.A., Calkins, H., et al. (2002). ACC/AHA guideline update for perioperative cardiovascular evaluation for non-cardiac surgery—executive summary. *Journal of the American College of Cardiology, 39*(3), 549–553.

Jacob, S.R, & Scandrett-Hibon, S. (1994). Mothers grieving the death of a child. *Nurse Practitioner, 19*(7), 60–65.

Kapur, K., Kapur, A., Ramachandran, S., et al. (2008). Barriers to changing dietary behavior. *Journal of the Association of Physicians of India, 56*, 27–32.

Mallampati, S.R., Gatt, S.P., Gugino, L.D., Desai, S.P., & Waraksa, B. (1985). A clinical sign to predict difficult tracheal intubation: A prospective study. *The Canadian Anaesthetists' Society Journal, 32*(4), 429–434.

Miller, R. (2005). *Miller's anesthesia* (6th ed., Vol. 1). New York: Elsevier Churchill Livingstone.

Morgan, G., Mikhail, M., & Murray, M. (2006). *Clinical anesthesiology* (4th ed.). New York: McGraw-Hill.

Picard, M.H., & Dennis, C.A. (2001). Assessing cardiac risk—How low (risk) should you go? *American Journal of Medicine, 111*, 73–74.

Raj, P. (2002). *Textbook of regional anesthesia*. New York: Churchill Livingstone.

Mieres, J.H., Shaw, L.J., Arai, A., et al. (2005). Role of noninvasive testing in the clinical evaluation of women with suspected coronary artery disease. *Circulation, 111*, 682–696.

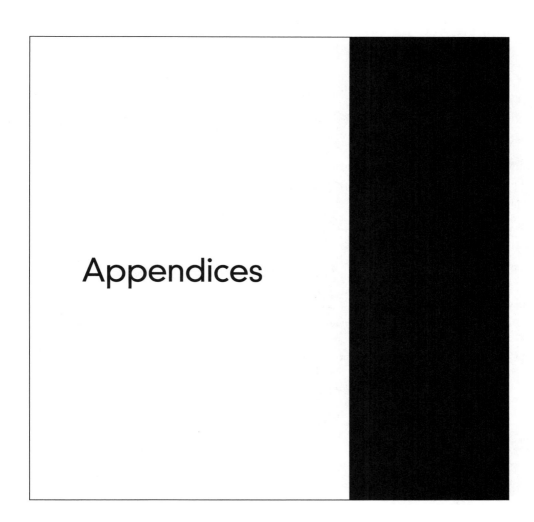

Appendices

DNP Resident Admission Order Documentation Guideline

Encounter number (day and time as related to case narrative time line)

Example: Encounter Two (day 0, 30 minutes since initial presentation to Emergency Department)

Admit to:
- Service
- Type of unit or setting
- DNP role

Diagnosis at time of admission

Condition
- Stable
- Guarded
- Serious
- Critical

Vital signs (As per floor protocol or per routine is not acceptable for portfolio documentation.)
- Frequency
  - Temperature
  - Pulse
  - Blood pressure
  - Respiratory rate
  - Weight
  - Central venous pressure

Allergies
- Medication
- Food
- Environmental (example: latex, adhesive tape)

Activity
- Include all therapeutically indicated activities
  - Bathroom privileges
  - Out of bed to chair
  - Walk with assistance, number of times a day

Nursing procedures, commonly including:
- Bed position
- Daily weights
- Dressing changes
- Parameters that require notifying DNP or team of change in patient's status, such as:
  - Temperature above 101°F
  - Heart rate > 100 beats per minute or < 60 beats per minute
  - Systolic blood pressure > 160 mmHg or < 100 mmHg
  - Diastolic blood pressure > 100 mmHg or < 60 mmHg
  - Respiratory rate > 30 respirations per minute or < 10 respirations per minute
- Respiratory care
- Urinary catheter
  - Straight catheterization with parameters
  - Foley catheter with parameters
- Wound care

Diet
- NPO
- Clear liquid
- Regular
- XXX-calorie ADA diet with no concentrated sweets for patients with diabetes mellitus
- Two-gram reduced sodium for hypertensive patients
- Reduced protein for renal patients
- Low cholesterol

Intake and output (includes all tubes)
- Arterial lines
- Drains
- Endotracheal tube
- Foley catheter
- Intravenous fluid type and rate
- Nasogastric tube

Medications
- Generic (Brand)
- Route
- Dosage
- Frequency

Laboratory tests
- Admission
- Daily orders
- Serial or repeating orders

Special (includes orders that do not fit into previous categories)
- Electrocardiogram
- Diagnostic imaging tests
- Consultation requests, including:
  - Physical therapy
  - Occupational therapy
  - Nutrition
  - Social services

DNP Resident On-Service Documentation Guideline

The on-service note is written when the DNP resident assumes care for a patient. The DNP resident reviews the hospital record and other patient records and briefly summarizes the hospital course to date. When writing the on-service note, the DNP resident forms an impression of the care provided and current patient needs and then integrates this information to work collaboratively as a member of the inpatient team to provide a seamless, ongoing plan of care and to address any newly identified problems. The on-service note contains the following sections.

Date of admission: *Example:* Admitted 23 days ago

Admitting diagnosis:

Procedures: List of procedures performed to date with results

Hospital course to date: Summary of hospitalization to date

Physical examination: Physical examination findings that are pertinent to the patient's identified problems

Pertinent laboratory data: Review of laboratory test results that inform the working diagnosis and treatment regimen

Impression: Description of the patient's general condition, description of changes in clinical status during the hospitalization, and assessment of each active clinical or psychosocial issue currently being addressed

Problem list

Plan
- Indicated diagnostic tests
- Therapeutic interventions
- Consultation requests
- Discharge planning

An off-service note is written when the DNP resident is no longer involved in providing care for the hospitalized patient before the patient is discharged. The off-service note briefly summarizes the hospital course to date to provide a mechanism for coordinating seamless delivery of ongoing care. The following sections are included:

Date of admission: *Example:* Admitted to medical unit from emergency department 4 days ago

Admitting diagnosis:

Procedures: A chronologic list of procedures and results

Hospital course to date: A summary of the important points of the hospitalization

Brief physical exam: Physical examination findings that are relevant to the identified patient problems

Pertinent laboratory data: Laboratory test results that inform the diagnosis and therapeutic plan

Impression
- A description of the patient's general status
- A general description of the patient's progress since admission
- An assessment of each active medical, surgical, or psychosocial issue currently being addressed

Problem list: Updated problem list

Plan
- Recommendations for further diagnostic testing
- Test results pending
- Therapeutic interventions currently planned
- Consults pending
- Discharge plan

DNP Resident Procedure Documentation Guideline

Procedure: Name of procedure

Indications: Specific reason procedure is required for this patient

Permission
- Explanation of risks and benefits
- Documentation that signed consent is in the medical record

Provider
- Describes the DNP role and responsibilities during the procedure
- Describes the team members present and their responsibilities during the procedure

Descriptions of procedure in paragraph form, including:
- Time out
- Preparation
- Positioning
- Anesthesia
- Vital signs
- Patient's status during procedure
- Instrumentation
- Time required for total procedure

Complications
- Presence or absence
- Description of any unanticipated complications or events

Estimated blood loss (EBL): Minimal or estimated amount lost

Specimens sent to laboratory

Findings if obtained during procedure

Disposition
- Patient's condition post procedure
- Patient location post procedure
- Professional designation of provider or team assuming post-procedure care

DNP Resident Intensive Care Unit Progress Note Documentation Guideline

The ICU progress note summarizes the events of the past 24 hours or the period of time being discussed in the case narrative.

Problem list
- Active problems
- Major inactive problems
- Allergies
- Past medical or surgical history relevant to the present illness

Events and procedures during the past 24 hours or period of time being discussed in the case narrative

Current medications

System-specific physical examination and pertinent flow sheet data, usually including:
- Central nervous system function
  - Neurologic assessment rating scores
  - Sedation level
- Cardiovascular function
  - Indicators of systemic perfusion
  - Blood pressure
  - Heart rate
  - Pressure monitoring data
- Pulmonary function
  - Ventilator settings
  - Arterial blood gas values
- Gastrointestinal function and nutritional status
- Fluids, electrolytes, and renal function
- Hematologic function
  - Complete blood count
  - Coagulation values
- Infectious disease status
  - Culture data
  - Antibiotic regimen and treatment duration
- Prophylaxis determined by patient risk assessment
  - Alcohol withdrawal
  - Deep venous thrombosis
  - Stress ulcers

- – Skin care
- Relevant laboratory and radiographic data

Additional systems and data are reported as appropriate to patient's presenting complaint, current status, and relevant health history.

Impression: As per general guideline; see Chapter 4.

Problem list
- Each problem on the list is assigned a number during the initial patient evaluation
- The problems are numbered in order of severity in the initial list
- During the course of the hospitalization problems are added chronologically to the list as they are identified
- The status of each problem is described as active or inactive throughout the hospitalization

ICD-9 codes

Plan: For each active problem address the following, as appropriate:
- Diagnostic tests
- Therapeutic interventions
- Counseling or education
- Consultations
- Goals for day
- Specialty hospital services

DNP Resident Discharge Summary Documentation Guideline

A formal discharge note is usually required when the patient is admitted for more than 24 hours. The discharge summary is written in the past tense, as documented in the medical record. The DNP resident gives special attention to HIPAA guidelines when transcribing the discharge summary into the case narrative. The discharge summary includes the following sections:

Date of admission: If the case narrative begins with admission to the hospital, this is day 0.

Date of discharge: The last day of hospitalization, such as day 24.

Admitting diagnosis:

Discharge diagnosis:

Attending service caring for patient

DNP role in the provision of care

Referring provider

Procedures
- Surgery
- Invasive diagnostic procedures

Summary of admission
- Important points from the admission history
- Important points from the admission physical examination
- Important points from the admission laboratory data

Hospital course
- Summary presented in chronologic order
- Includes evaluations, therapeutic interventions, and patient response
- Each identified problem addressed separately
- Events for each identified problem described in chronologic order

Condition at discharge
- Improved
- Unchanged
- Deteriorated

Disposition
- The location to which the patient is discharged, such as home, another acute care facility, rehabilitation center, or skilled nursing facility
- If patient is being transferred to another institution, the professional designation of the health care provider assuming responsibility for the patient's care

Discharge medications
- Medications list
- Generic (Brand)
- Dosage
- Route of administration
- Frequency
- Number of refills
- Medications reconciled at discharge

Discharge instructions and follow-up
- Diagnostic tests
- Referrals
  - Physical therapy
  - Occupation therapy
  - Social work
  - Visiting nurse
- Medications
- Therapeutic interventions
  - Nutrition instructions
  - Activity
  - Bathing
  - Wound care
- Counseling and education
- Return to work status
- Follow-up

Problem list
- Active problems
- Inactive problems

DNP Resident Pediatric Comprehensive Evaluation Documentation Guideline

Informant

Chief complaint: Reason for visit

History of present illness

Past medical history
- Prenatal history
  - Overall health of the mother
  - Prenatal care
  - Significant complication or infections
    - Tests for chlamydia, Group B strep, VDRL, HIV, hepatitis B, rubella titers
    - History of herpes
  - Medication use during pregnancy
  - Ultrasounds
  - Quadruple or triple screen results
- Perinatal history
  - Weeks of gestation
  - Type of delivery
  - Birth history: Birth weight, health of infant, Apgar scores (include medication used, problems at time of delivery, Apgar if available)
- Neonatal period
  - Congenital problems
  - Jaundice, infections
  - Admissions, parental or health care providers' concerns, extended hospitalization that required separation of mother and child
  - Early feeding history
- Common childhood illness
- Serious illness and operations
- Hospitalizations
- Accidents

Current medications
- Prescribed medications
- Alternative medications
- Over-the-counter medications

Allergies
- Medication (specify nature of allergic reaction)
- Food (specify nature of allergic reaction)
- Airborne (specify nature of allergic reaction)

Immunizations

Family history: Genogram

Social profile
- Household composition, type of dwelling, neighborhood
- Support systems
- Family relationships
- Culture
- Socioeconomic
- Employment, parental work schedule, career
- After-school activities, day care
- Religion, religious affiliation
- Family stresses (current, recent, and/or chronic)

Activities of daily living: NEEEDS
- **N**utrition
  - 24-hour recall
    - Infant: Type of feeding, amount (time for breast feeding), age of solid introduction, appetite
    - Child: Overall appetite, personal eating habits, mealtime pattern, and family interactions
  - Fluids consumed, including formula, juice, milk, or water
  - Vitamins
  - Any special diet
- **E**limination
  - Toilet training
  - Urinary characteristics
  - Enuresis or encopresis
    - Day and night
  - Bowel pattern
- **E**ducation
  - Grade
  - School performance
  - IEP
- **E**nvironmental health history
  - Parental occupation exposure
  - Smoke exposure
  - Carbon monoxide and smoke detectors
  - Pets
  - Heating, air conditioning, and ventilation
  - Drinking water and fluoridation
  - Sun exposure
  - Toxic chemicals

- – Radon
- – Extended travel
- **D**evelopment
  - – Fine and gross motor
  - – Language
  - – Cognitive
  - – Social
  - – Milestones
  - – Behavioral concerns
    - ▪ Parental, teacher, and day care provider's concerns
    - ▪ Relationship with sibling and peers
    - ▪ Approaches to discipline
- **S**leep
  - – Hours
  - – Night bottle usage
  - – Sleep environment
  - – Naps
  - – Snoring
  - – Enuresis
- **S**exual: Confidential communications
  - – 5 P's 2006 STD guidelines from the CDC: Partners, prevention of pregnancy, protection from STDs, practices, past history of STDs
  - – Menses: Age of menarche, dysmenorrhea, PMS, LMP, any concerns

If teen, consider HEADS I'M Very Good or GAPS assessment, as follows:

HEADS: I'M Very **G**ood
- **H**ome
  - – Household relationships
  - – Family dynamics and relationships
  - – Living arrangement
- **E**ducation and employment
  - – School attendance
  - – Grades
  - – Attitude about school relationships
  - – Best and worse subjects
  - – Homework goals
  - – Type of job, hours
- **A**ctivities
  - – Spare time
  - – Physical activity
  - – Screen time
  - – Friends
- **D**isabilities and drugs
  - – Tobacco
  - – Alcohol
  - – Recreational substance use by peers and self; frequency and quantity
  - – Disabilities in carrying out activities of daily living

- **S**leep, safety, self-image, sexuality, suicide, self-mutilation
  - History of harm to animals
  - History of harm to others
  - Suicide ideation
- **I**nternet and **M**edia
  - Time on Internet
  - Chat rooms
  - E-mail
  - Face-to-face meetings
  - Communication with strangers
  - Game time
  - Exposure to television violence
- **V**iolence
  - How conflicts are managed at home, school, work
  - Presence of guns in house as well as weapon carried
  - Nonconsensual sex, physical contact
- **G**ang
  - Member of gang, friends or family members in gangs, gang markings

Or

GAPS: Using appropriate history from **G**uidelines for **A**dolescent **P**reventive **S**ervices
  - Eating, weight
  - School
  - Friends and family
  - Weapons, violence, safety
  - Tobacco
  - Alcohol
  - Drug use
  - Self-esteem

Review of Systems

Physical examination

Impression: As discussed in general case narrative format; see Chapter 4

ICD-9 codes

Plan: For all active problems address the following, as appropriate:
- Diagnostic tests
- Therapeutic interventions
- Counseling and education
- Health care maintenance
- Referrals
- Follow-up

References

Levenberg, P.B., & Elster, A.B. (1995). *Guidelines for adolescent preventive services (GAPS): Implementation and resource manual.* Chicago: American Medical Association.

Cohen, E., Mackenzie, R.G., & Yates, G.L. (1991). HEADSS, a psychosocial risk assessment instrument: Implications for designing effective intervention programs for runaway youth. *Journal of Adolescent Health, 12,* 539–544.

DNP Pediatric Resident Interval Episodic Documentation Guideline

Informant

Chief complaint: Reason for visit

History of present illness

Interval pediatric assessment

Past medical history
- Pertinent medical history to presenting problem
- Any medical problems, emergency room visits, hospital admissions since last visit

Current medications
- Prescribed medications
- Alternative medications
- Over-the-counter medications

Allergies
- Medication (specify nature of allergic reaction)
- Food (specify nature of allergic reaction)
- Airborne (specify nature of allergic reaction)

Immunizations

Social profile: Include change in social profile

Activities of daily living: NEEEDS
- Nutrition
  - 24-hour recall, including fluids consumed
    - Infant: Feeding changes
    - Child: Appetite changes
- Elimination
  - Toilet training
  - Urinary characteristics
  - Enuresis or encopresis
  - Day and night
  - Bowel pattern

- **E**ducation
  - Grade
  - Concerns regarding school performances
- **E**nvironmental health history
  - Parental occupation exposure
  - Smoke exposure
  - Travel history
  - Environmental hazard exposure
- **D**evelopment
  - Pertinent to presenting problem
- **S**leep
  - Hours
  - Changes related to presenting problems
- If adolescent and pertinent to presenting problem, sexual: confidential communications
  - 5 P's 2006 STD guidelines from the CDC: Partners, prevention of pregnancy, protection from STDs, practices, past history of STDs
  - Menses: Age of menarche, dysmenorrhea, PMS, LMP, any concerns

Review of systems: Includes only those systems not addressed previously that are pertinent to presenting problem

Physical examination: Includes only those systems pertinent to reason for visit, presenting problem, or health maintenance needs

Impression: As discussed in general case narrative format; see Chapter 4

ICD-9 codes

Plan: For all active problems address the following, as appropriate:
  - Diagnostic tests
  - Therapeutic interventions
  - Counseling and education
  - Health care maintenance
  - Referrals

Initial encounter (zero minutes)

Chief complaint: "In patient's own words"

History of present illness
- Reason for anesthesia care
  - Preoperative diagnosis
  - Type of anesthesia
- Anesthesia history
- NPO status
- Relevant history of the following systems to assess anesthesia risk
  - Cardiac
  - Pulmonary
  - Endocrine
  - Hematologic
  - Neurologic disease
- Family history of adverse anesthetic outcome and risk factors

Current medications

Allergies

Hospitalizations

Past medical history

Surgical history

Social history

Family history: Genogram

Review of systems

Physical examination: Includes all sections of the comprehensive medical examination; for anesthesia, includes a detailed assessment of the airway:
- Condition of mucosa and gingiva
- Dentition status with chips or loose teeth noted and status of dentures
- Mouth opening with thyromental distance
- Mallampati classification
- Neck range of motion

Database
- Diagnostic laboratory tests with patient value and reference range in table format
- Imaging
- Other information

Education
- Specific to case
- Discussion of risk/benefits
- Informed consent

Anesthesia plan and rationale
- Estimated length of the procedure
- Estimated blood loss
- Anesthesia type
- Invasive monitoring
- Postoperative plan

Anesthesia care
- **Induction,** x minutes
  - Vital signs
  - Sequence of induction
  - Procedure notes
- **Anesthesia maintenance,** x minutes
  - Vital signs
  - Intraoperative notes, summary—include updated vital signs, laboratory values
  - Event notes
- **Emergence,** x minutes
  - Extubation or reason for remaining intubated
  - Total fluids—crystalloids, colloids, blood products
  - Total blood loss
  - Urine output
  - Patient condition—vital signs
- **Follow-up care,** x minutes
  - Transfer care to post-anesthesia care unit or intensive care unit
  - Orders
- **Discharge,** x minutes
  - Discharged from the post-anesthesia care unit
  - Condition—vital signs, including pain measurement, laboratory values, pertinent information
  - Discharge teaching as appropriate

Assessment: Clinician discussion of anesthetic considerations

ICD-9 codes

Continuum of care
- Follow-up care, inpatient or outpatient
- Focused note that describes follow-up and includes subjective and objective data as well as impression and plan

DNP Resident Comprehensive Psychiatric Evaluation Documentation Guideline

Chief complaint: Current problem in patient's own words

History of present illness (HPI)
Description of symptoms the patient is currently experiencing guides the HPI with attention to onset, duration, patient's perception of contributing external stressors, and effect of illness on daily life.

The information is presented in chronological order and includes prior diagnostic tests, related history, previous treatment for the problem, risk factors, pertinent family history, current medications, and relevant questions based on the *Diagnostic and Statistical Manual of Mental Disorders* (DSM-IV-R) signs and symptoms for the differential diagnoses being considered.

Detailed discussion of other significant ongoing problems directly related to the chief complaint may be included in separate paragraphs of the HPI section.

Past psychiatric history
- Age of onset
- Symptoms
- Suicidal behavior
- Violence
- Hospitalizations
- Medication trials
- Medication adherence
- Adverse events
- Outpatient treatment

Substance use history
- Tobacco
  - Age of first use
  - Route
  - Frequency
  - Pack years
  - Smoking cessation history
- Alcohol
  - Age of first use
  - Frequency and amount
  - Withdrawal symptoms
  - Tolerance

- Ambulatory treatment
- Detoxifications
- Inpatient rehabilitation
- Length of sobriety
- Prescription drugs and recreational substance abuse
  - Age of first use
  - Route
  - Frequency
  - Withdrawal symptoms
  - Tolerance
  - Treatment
  - Detoxification
  - Rehabilitation
  - Length of sobriety

Medical history
- Current medications
  - Prescribed medications
  - Over-the-counter medications
  - Vitamins
  - Herbals
  - Supplements
- Allergies to drugs and environment, including manifestations
- Surgeries
- Hospitalizations
- Transfusions
  - Type of blood product
  - Number of units
  - Adverse reactions if known
- Trauma
- Stable current problems
- Past problems unrelated to the HPI that have resolved
- Specific illnesses, documentation of presence or absence of common adult illnesses
  - Asthma
  - Bleeding disorders
  - Cancer
  - Diabetes (DM)
  - Emphysema
  - Hepatitis
  - Hypertension (HTN)
  - Kidney disease
  - Liver disease
  - Myocardial infarction (MI)
  - Sexually transmitted infections (STIs)
  - Stroke (CVA)
  - Peptic ulcer disorder (PUD)
  - Sexually transmitted infection (STIs)

- Thyroid disease
- Tuberculosis (TB)
- Health maintenance according to U.S. Preventive Services Task Force guidelines or other expert panel
- Immunizations according to CDC guidelines
- Nutrition
  - Recent weight loss or gain
  - Typical diet
  - Extensive focus on body weight or specific region of body
  - Unusual eating patterns, such as binging, purging, or extensive restriction
- Exercise
  - Frequency
  - Intensity
  - Duration
  - Type of physical activity
- Sleep pattern
  - Number of hours each night
  - Difficulty falling asleep
  - Frequent awakening
  - Nightmares
  - Sleepwalking
  - Sleep attacks
  - Hallucinations when falling asleep or when awakening

Childhood history
- Birth and delivery
  - History of intrauterine exposure to toxins, chemicals, or medications
  - Birth or delivery complications
- Development
  - Common childhood illness
  - Serious illness
  - Accidents
  - Delay in developmental milestones
  - Place of birth and upbringing
  - History of abuse
  - Relationship with siblings or only child
  - History of parental divorce or separation
  - Relationships with primary caretakers
  - Educational achievement as child

Travel history
- To regions where there is possible exposure to infectious agents
- To regions where there could be exposure to agents or chemicals that can affect the brain

Family history: Includes psychiatric, medical, and substance abuse history

Social history
- Education
- Military service
- Work history
- Relationship history
- Stressors and support (financial, family, work, clergy)
- Lifestyle risk factors
- Current marital status
- Children
- Sexual orientation
- Insurance and financial support
- Religion
- Hobbies
- Beliefs
- Living conditions

Review of systems: Identify possible physiologic etiologies that may contribute to the patient's presenting symptoms or current psychiatric illness, with special attention to neurologic, endocrine, and psychosomatic symptoms. The following sections may be included as appropriate to the situation:
- General health
- Skin
- Head, eyes, ears, nose, mouth, and throat
- Neck
- Breast
- Respiratory
- Cardiovascular
- Gastrointestinal
- Gynecologic
- Urinary
- Male genitourinary
- Endocrine
- Musculoskeletal
- Peripheral vascular
- Hematologic
- Neurologic
- Psychiatric: Included in HPI and past psychiatric history

Mental status examination
- General appearance
- Attitude and engagement
- Psychomotor activity
- Speech
- Thought process
- Thought content
- Perception
- Mood
- Affect

- Sensorium
- Insight and judgment

Physical examination: If the mental health nurse practitioner performs a physical examination, the following sections are included as appropriate. If a physical examination is performed by another health care provider, the time of examination and professional designation of the provider are documented, and the relevant sections and pertinent positive and negative findings are summarized by the mental health nurse practitioner in this section.
- Vital signs
- Skin
- Lymph nodes
- HEENT
- Neck
- Chest
- Heart
- Abdomen
- Male genital
- Pelvic
- Rectal
- Musculoskeletal
- Peripheral vascular
- Neurologic
  - CN exam
  - Motor exam
  - Cerebellum
  - Sensory
  - Reflexes

Diagnostic tests
- Laboratory test
- Imagining and other information

Impression
- For each new or undifferentiated problem or symptom, create a comprehensive list of possible diagnoses *in paragraph form* from most to least likely diagnosis. Based on the patient's medical, psychiatric, and family history, risk factors, presence and absence of examination findings, and diagnostic tests, determine the probability of each diagnosis according to DSM-IV-R criteria. State the most likely diagnosis and provide a rationale. This diagnosis will form the basis for the plan.
- For each ongoing problem, separately discuss the status of the condition. This diagnosis will form the basis for the ongoing plan for that condition.
- If appropriate, usually in the setting of ongoing care, for each previously identified acute or self-limiting diagnosis, state the resolution and note whether problem is inactive and you need not consider ongoing care.
- Health maintenance and immunizations should be addressed according to established guidelines, if appropriate. Address the patient's health

maintenance needs at appropriate intervals and include in the plan of care under health maintenance.

Diagnostic impression
- Axis I
- Axis II
- Axis III
- Axis IV

Risk assessment
- Suicidal ideation
- Homicidal ideation
- Impulse control
- Overall risk of harm rate

ICD-9 codes

Plan: For all active problems, address the following, as appropriate:
- Diagnostic tests
- Therapeutic interventions
- Counseling and education
- Health care maintenance
- Referrals
- Follow-up

DNP Resident Adult Comprehensive Documentation Guideline

Chief complaint: Current problem in patient's own words

History of present illness (HPI)
Description of symptoms the patient is currently experiencing guide the HPI, with attention to onset, frequency, duration, progression, quality, quantity, anatomic location, radiation, aggravating, alleviating, and associated factors, patient's perception of contributing external stressors, and effect of illness on daily life.

The information is presented in chronological order and includes prior diagnostic tests, related history, previous treatment for the problem, risk factors, family history, medications, and pertinent review of systems relevant to differential diagnoses being considered.

Other significant ongoing problems should be included in the HPI in a separate paragraph in detail if they relate to the chief complaint.

Health history
- Current medications
  - Prescribed medications
  - Herbal supplements
  - Over-the-counter medications
  - Supplements
  - Vitamins
- Allergies
  - Drugs and environment, including manifestations
- Operations
- Hospitalizations
- Transfusions
  - Type of blood product
  - Number of units
  - Adverse reactions
- Trauma
- Stable current problems
- Past problems unrelated to the HPI that have resolved
- Documentation that adult patients have been questioned about the following illnesses
  - Usual childhood illness or immunizations
  - Anemia
  - Asthma
  - Anxiety

- – Bleeding disorders
- – Cancer
- – Depression
- – Diabetes (DM)
- – Elevated lipids
- – Emphysema
- – Hepatitis
- – HIV
- – Hypertension (HTN)
- – Kidney disease
- – Liver
- – Myocardial infarction (MI)
- – Peptic ulcer disorder (PUD)
- – Stroke (CVA)
- – Sexually transmitted infection (STIs)
- – Thyroid
- – Tuberculosis (TB)
- Health maintenance, according to U.S. Preventive Services Task Force guidelines or other expert guidelines
- Immunizations, according to CDC guidelines

Family history: Genogram

Psychosocial history
- Patient profile
  - – Beliefs as related to health
  - – Children
  - – Marital status
  - – Past or present employment
  - – Sexual orientation
  - – Insurance
  - – Financial support
  - – Education
  - – Religion
  - – Hobbies
  - – Household composition
  - – Sleep
  - – Leisure
  - – Stressors and support
- Lifestyle risk factors
  - – Tobacco
  - – Alcohol
  - – Substance use
  - – Caffeine use
  - – Diet and exercise

Review of systems
- General health
- Skin

- Head
- Eyes
- Ears
- Nose
- Mouth and throat
- Neck
- Breast
- Respiratory
- Cardiovascular
- Gastrointestinal
- Female genitourinary
- Male genitourinary
- Endocrine
- Musculoskeletal
- Peripheral vascular
- Hematologic
- Neurologic
- Psychiatric

Physical examination
- General
- Vital signs
- Skin
- Lymph nodes
- HEENT
- Neck
- Chest
- Heart
- Breast
- Abdomen
- Male genital
- Pelvic
- Rectal
- Musculoskeletal
- Peripheral vascular
- Neurologic
    - Mental status exam
    - CN exam
    - Motor exam
    - Cerebellum
    - Sensory
    - Reflexes

Diagnostic tests
- Laboratory test
- Imagining and other information

Impression

- For each new or undifferentiated problem or symptom, create a comprehensive list of possible diagnoses *in paragraph form* from most to least likely diagnosis. Based on the patient's history, which includes presence and absence of pertinent findings, physical examination, diagnostic tests, and risk factors, determine the probability of each diagnosis. State the most likely diagnosis and provide a rationale. This diagnosis will form the basis for the plan.
- For each ongoing problem, separately discuss the status of the condition. This diagnosis will form the basis for the ongoing plan for that condition.
- If appropriate, usually in the setting of ongoing care, for each previously identified acute or self-limiting diagnosis, state the resolution and note that problem is inactive and you need not consider ongoing care.
- Health maintenance and immunizations should be addressed according to established guidelines, if appropriate. Address the patient's health maintenance needs at appropriate intervals and include in the plan of care under health maintenance.

ICD-9 codes

Plan: For all active problems address the following, as appropriate:
- Diagnostic tests
- Therapeutic interventions
- Counseling and education
- Health care maintenance
- Referrals
- Follow-up

DNP CRNA Resident Pre-Surgical Documentation Guideline

History of present illness (HPI)
- Concise and chronological discussion of presenting condition that requires surgical intervention
- Significant ongoing problems included in separate paragraphs

Allergies

Past medical history
- Stable current problems
- Past problems unrelated to the HPI that have resolved
- Documentation that adult patients have been questioned about the following illnesses:
  - Asthma
  - Bleeding disorders
  - Cancer
  - Diabetes (DM)
  - Emphysema
  - Hepatitis
  - Hypertension (HTN)
  - Kidney disease
  - Liver
  - Myocardial infarction (MI)
  - Peptic ulcer disorder (PUD)
  - Stroke (CVA)
  - Sexually transmitted infection (STIs)
  - Thyroid
  - Tuberculosis (TB)
- Hospitalizations
- Transfusions
  - Type of blood product
  - Number of units
  - Adverse reactions
- Trauma
- Health maintenance, according to U.S. Preventive Services Task Force guidelines
- Immunizations, according to CDC guidelines

Past surgical history

Medications
- Prescriptions, over-the-counters, and herbals
- Frequency that "as needed (PRN) medications" are used
- Milligrams of acetaminophen taken per day

Family history
- Genogram
- Anesthetic family history

Social history
- Stressors and support (financial, family, work, clergy)
- Lifestyle risk factors
- Tobacco
- Alcohol
- Substance use
- Caffeine use
- Diet and exercise
- Patient profile, including marital status, children, past or present employment, sexual orientation, insurance and financial support, education, religion, hobbies, beliefs, living conditions

Review of systems

Physical examination

Diagnostic tests
- Laboratory tests
- Imaging and other information
- Review of other health care providers' consults, if present

Impression: Discuss the status of each identified ongoing health problem. It is imperative to optimize patient health status so that the patient is an appropriate candidate for anesthesia. The diagnostic impression will form the basis for the anesthetic plan.

ICD-9 codes

Plan: Ensures that the patient is an appropriate candidate for anesthesia
- Diagnostic tests
  - Electrocardiogram (EKG)
  - Echocardiogram
  - Pulmonary function tests
  - Laboratory tests
- Therapeutic interventions
- Counseling and education
- Referrals (specialty consults)
- Follow-up

History of present illness
- Reason for anesthesia care
  - Type
  - Preoperative diagnosis
- Anesthesia history
- NPO status
- Relevant history for anesthesia risk
  - Cardiac
  - Pulmonary
  - Endocrine
  - Hematologic
  - Neurologic disease
- Family history of adverse anesthetic outcome or risk factors

Current medications

Allergies

Hospitalizations

Past medical history

Surgical history

Social history

Family history

Review of systems: Most likely a focused history for a healthy patient who requires anesthesia services for an office procedure

Focused physical examination

Database
- Laboratory test with patient values and reference range in table format
- Imaging and other information

Impression: Clinician discussion of anesthetic considerations

Education
- Specific to case
- Discussion of risk/benefits

Informed consent: Documentation that signed informed consent is in the medical record

Anesthesia plan and rationale
- Estimated length of the procedure
- Estimated blood loss
- Anesthesia type
- Postoperative plan

Anesthesia care induction, x minutes
- Vital signs
- Sequence of induction
- Procedure notes

Anesthesia maintenance, x minutes
- Vital signs
- Intraoperative notes, summary
- Event notes

Emergence, x minutes
- Total fluids
- Total blood loss
- Urine output
- Patient condition
- Vital signs

Follow-up care, x minutes
- Transfer care to post-anesthesia care unit or home
- Orders

ICD-9 codes

Discharge summary note, x minutes
- Time of admission
- Time of discharge
- Admitting diagnosis
- Discharge diagnosis
- Procedure
- Brief history and pertinent physical findings
- Condition at discharge
  - Improved
  - Unchanged
  - Worse

- Disposition
- Discharge medications
  - Generic (Brand)
  - Strength
  - Route of administration
  - Frequency
  - Refills or number dispensed
- Discharge instructions and follow-up
  - Clinic return date
  - Diet instructions
  - Activity restrictions
  - Wound care
  - Referrals
    - Physical therapy
    - Occupational therapy
    - Social work
    - Visiting nurse services
  - Return to work status

Initial encounter (zero minutes)

Consultation: Reason CRNA is called to emergency department (ED)

Allergies

Current medications

Past medical history

Hospitalizations

Surgical history

Social history

Patient evaluation
- *Subjective:* Patient's current condition using patient's words or perspective as appropriate to patient clinical status and level of acuity
- *Objective:* Focused physical examination. The following systems are always included in this section. Additional systems are assessed according to patient presenting complaint.
  - General
  - Vital signs
    - Temperature
    - Blood pressure
    - Heart rate
    - Respiratory rate
    - Pulse oximetry
    - Pain assessment using standardized scale
  - Airway
    - Dentition
    - Mallampati score
    - Mouth opening
    - Thyromental distance
  - Chest: Breath sounds
  - Heart

- Neurologic
    - Mental status exam
    - Cranial nerve exam

Impression: Assessment of patient's condition as related to the reason the CRNA has been asked to participate in care

Plan
- Interventions
- Therapeutics
- Medications
- Orders
- Special tests

DNP CRNA Resident Labor and Delivery Anesthesia Documentation Guideline

Initial encounter (zero minutes)

Allergies

Current medications

Pregnancy history

Past medical history

Hospitalizations

Surgical history

Social history

Patient current status
- Subjective: Brief statement of how patient feels and her perceived needs at the time of evaluation
- Focused physical examination
  - General: Description of patient physically and emotionally as well as significant others present
  - Vital signs: Temperature, blood pressure, heart rate, respiratory rate, pain measurement, and status of fetus
  - Airway: Mallampati class, mouth opening, thyromental distance
  - Chest: Breath sounds
  - Heart: Rate, description of S1, S2, murmurs, rubs
  - Skin: Rash, tattoos
  - Neurologic: Mental status exam, cranial nerve exam, sensory examination
  - Musculoskeletal: Range of motion and power in extremities
- Database: Labor stage and dilation as reported by obstetric service or midwife
- Laboratory tests with patient value and reference range in table format
- Impression: Clinician assessment of maternal fetal status
- Plan
  - Candidate for labor epidural
  - Orders

- Education and counseling
  - Risk/benefits explained
  - Alternatives

ICD-9 codes

Anesthesia procedure, x minutes
- Procedure: Name of procedure, such as labor epidural or combined spinal epidural
- Indications: Specific reason procedure is required for this patient
- Permission: Risk and benefits explained, consent signed and placed in the chart
- Provider: Professional designations of the team members present and their responsibilities during the procedure

Descriptions of procedure in paragraph form, including:
- Preparation
- Positioning
- Level placed and catheter measurement
- Medications utilized
- Description, vital signs, maternal fetal tolerance of procedure
- Post-procedure pain relief

Complications: Presence or absence of complications, including description of events if any occurred

Interval assessment, x minutes
- Vital signs: Maternal blood pressure, heart rate, respiratory rate, pain measurement, and update of fetal status
- Follow-up of the patient's condition following the procedure, written in paragraph format and including:
  - Assessment of intervention
  - Labor progression
  - Additional type and volume of medication given for uncontrolled pain
  - Sensation and patient movement
  - Anesthesia related complications—presence or absence

Interval assessment, x minutes
- Additional patient assessments
- Additional medication administration
- Catheter manipulation
- Intubation
- Surgical cesarean section

The anesthesia perioperative encounter template is used if the patient requires operating room care.

Post-vaginal delivery note, x minutes (paragraph form)
- Vital signs
- Documentation of safe epidural catheter removal and site inspection
- Extremity movement
- Presence or absence of paresthesias
- Anesthesia-related complications
- Newborn assessment
  - Delivery time
  - Appearance
  - Pulse
  - Grimace
  - Activity
  - Respiration
  - Apgar scores

DNP CRNA Resident Postoperative Care Unit (PACU) Documentation Guideline

Initial encounter (zero minutes)

Allergies

Current medications

Past medical history

Hospitalizations

Surgical history

Social history

Current admission and assessment of present status
- Subjective: Brief statement describing patient current status.
- History of present illness
- Preoperative diagnosis
- Surgery type
- Type of anesthesia
- Fluids used
  - Crystalloids
  - Colloids
  - Blood products
- Estimated blood loss
- Urine output
- Medications used during anesthesia care
- Intraoperative events (if any)
- Objective: Focused physical examination, which includes the following systems.
  - General
  - Vital signs
    - Temperature
    - Blood pressure
    - Heart rate
    - Respiratory rate
    - Pain measurement
  - Airway status

- Intubated
- Natural airway
- Nasal cannula, face mask, nasal airway, or oral airway in place
- Chest: Breath sounds
- Heart: Rate, description of S1, S2, murmurs, rubs
- Abdomen: Shape, bowel sounds, bruits, masses, rebound, tenderness
- Vascular: Palpation of peripheral pulses, edema
- Skin: Surgical site inspection
- Neurologic
  - Mental status exam
  - Cranial nerve exam
- Database
  - Laboratory tests with patient value and reference range in table format
  - Imaging and other information
- Impression: Assessment of patient status in the postoperative period
- PACU admission orders
  - Vital sign frequency
  - Fluids—type and rate
  - Pain medications and delivery route (intravenous, epidural, or by mouth)
  - Other medications
  - Ventilator orders and weaning orders as needed
  - Laboratory tests ordered: special tests (EKG, CXR, Troponin, etc.)
  - Consults needed
  - Discharge planning from PACU

ICD-9 codes

Indexes

DOMAIN AND COMPETENCY INDEX

HEALTH CARE SETTING INDEX

SUBJECT INDEX

Note: Page numbers followed by a t indicate that the reference is to a table on the designated page.